MW00514600

LANCASTER GENERAL HOSPITAL
Pacemaker Services
555 North Duke Street
Lancaster, PA 17604
(717)290-5511 Ext. 7894

IMPLANTABLE CARDIOVERTER DEFIBRILLATOR THERAPY: THE ENGINEERING - CLINICAL INTERFACE

Developments in Cardiovascular Medicine

C.A. Nienaber and U.Sechtem (eds.): Imaging and Intervention in Cardiology.
1996   ISBN 0-7923-3649-6
G. Assmann (ed.): HDL Deficiency and Atherosclerosis. 1995
                                                 ISBN 0-7923-8888-7
N.M. van Hemel, F.H.M. Wittkampf and H. Ector (eds.): The Pacemaker Clinic of
the 90's. Essentials in Brady-Pacing. 1995
                                                 ISBN 0-7923-3688-7
N. Wilke (ed.): Advanced Cardiovascular MRI of the Heart and Great Vessels.
1995   ISBN 0-7923-3702-4
M.LeWinter. H. Suga and M.W. Watkins (eds.): Cardiac Energetics: From Emax to
Pressure-volume Area. 1995   ISBN 0-7923-3721-2
R.J. Siegel (ed.): Ultrasound Angioplasty. 1995
                                                 ISBN 0-7923-3722-0
D.M. Yellon and G.J. Gross (eds.): Myocardial Protection and the Katp
Channel.   ISBN 0-7923-3791-3
A.V.G. Bruschke. J.H.C. Reiber. K.I. Lie and H.J.J. Wellens (eds.): Lipid Lowering
Therapy and Progression of Coronary Atherosclerosis. 1996
                                                 ISBN 0-7923-3807-3
A.S.A. Abd-Elfattah and A.S. Wechsler (eds.): Purines and Myocardial Protection.
      1995   ISBN 0-7923-3831-6
M. Morad, S. Ebashi, W. Trautwein and Y. Kurachi (eds.): Molecular Physiology
and Pharmacology of Cardiac Ion Channels and Transporters. 1996
                                                 ISBN 0-7923-3913-4
A.M. Oto (ed.): Practice and Progress in Cardiac Pacing and Electrophysiology.
1996   ISBN 0-7923-3950-9
W.H. Birkenhager (ed.): Practical Management of Hypertension. Second Edition.
1996   ISBN 0-7923-3952-5
J.C. Chatham, J.R. Forder and J.H. McNeill(eds.):*The Heart In Diabetes*.
1996   ISBN 0-7923-4052-3
M. Kroll, M. Lehmann (eds.): Implantable Cardioverter Defibrillator Therapy: The
Engineering-Clinical Interface   ISBN 0-7923-

IMPLANTABLE CARDIOVERTER DEFIBRILLATOR THERAPY: THE ENGINEERING - CLINICAL INTERFACE

Edited by:

Mark W. Kroll, PhD
Vice President, Tachycardia Business Unit
Pacesetter Inc., A St. Jude Medical Company
Sylmar, California, USA

and

Michael H. Lehmann, MD
Clinical Associate Professor of Medicine
Wayne State University School of Medicine
Director, Arrhythmia Center
Sinai Hospital
Detroit, Michigan, USA

Distributors for North America:
Kluwer Academic Publishers
101 Philip Drive
Assinippi Park
Norwell, Massachusetts 02061 USA

Distributors for all other countries:
Kluwer Academic Publishers Group
Distribution Centre
Post Office Box 322
3300 AH Dordrecht, THE NETHERLANDS

Library of Congress Cataloging-in-Publication Data

A C.I.P. Catalogue record for this book is available
from the Library of Congress.

Copyright © 1996 by Kluwer Academic Publishers

All rights reserved. No part of this publication may be reproduced, stored in a
retrieval system or transmitted in any form or by any means, mechanical, photo-
copying, recording, or otherwise, without the prior written permission of the
publisher, Kluwer Academic Publishers, 101 Philip Drive, Assinippi Park, Norwell,
Massachusetts 02061

Printed on acid-free paper.

Printed in the United States of America

To our parents,

Irene, Bill, Betty, and Bert;

our wives,

Lori and Annie;

and our children,

Braden, Mollie, Ryan, Chase, Jonah, David, and Ruth.

This book is based on information and facts believed to be accurate at the time of publication. The views of the authors do not necessarily reflect those of their employers and institutions.

TRADEMARKS:
The following are trademarks and registered trademarks:
AICD, Ventak, Endotak, Mini, Mini AV, and PRx (Guidant Corp. - CPI);
PCD, Active Can, Jewel, Jewel Plus, Marker Channel, T-Shock, AMD, and Transvene (Medtronic);
Guardian, EnGuard, Sentry (Telectronics);
Res-Q (Intermedics);
Cadence, Cadet, TVL, and Contour (Ventritex);
Defender (ELA Medical);
Aegis, and Autocapture (Pacesetter);
Angeflex and Hot Can (Angeion).

NOTICE:
The medications described in this book do not necessarily have specific approval by the US Food and Drug Administration for the situations and dosages described. The package insert for each drug should be consulted as it contains the usage as approved by the Food and Drug Administration.

Table of Contents

Contributing Authors

Ted P. Adams, MSEE
Chairman & CEO
St. Croix Medical
Minneapolis, MN
612-574-0570

Masood Akhtar, MD
Professor of Medicine
Chief, Cardiovascular Disease Sec.
Univ. of Wisconsin Medical School
Milwaukee Clinical Campus
Director, Arrhythmia Services
Sinai Samaritan Medical Center
Director, Clinical Electrophysiology
Laboratory
St. Luke's Medical Center
Milwaukee, WI
414-219-7686

J. Todd Alderfer, MD
Pennsylvania State University
Hershey Medical Center
Hershey, PA
717-531-8521

Kathi Axtell, RN
Sinai-Samaritan
Milwaukee, WI
414-283-7686

Stanley M. Bach, BSEE, MD
Arden Hills, MN
612-635-9514

John J. Baga, MD
Clinical Assistant Prof. of Medicine
Wayne State University
Arrhythmia Center
Sinai Hospital
Detroit, MI
313-493-6395

Susan M. Blanchard, PhD
North Carolina State Univ.
Raleigh, NC
919-515-6726

Zalmen Blanck, MD
University of Wisconsin
Milwaukee Clinical Campus
St. Luke's Medical Center
Wisconsin Electrophysiology Gp.
Milwaukee, WI
414-649-3390

Dennis A. Brumwell
Bloomington, MN
612-893-0503
cmoswizard@AOL.COM

Randolph A.S. Cooper, MD
Duke University
Durham, NC
919-660-5100

Sanjay Deshpande, MD
Assistant Professor of Medicine
Univ. of Wisconsin Medical School
Milwaukee Clinical Campus
Sinai-Samaritan
Milwaukee, WI
414-219-7686

Anwer Dhala, MD
Assistant Professor of Medicine
Univ. of Wisconsin Medical School
Milwaukee Clinical Campus
Staff Electrophysiologist
St. Luke's Medical Center
414-649-3378

Stephen M. Dillon, PhD
Philadelphia Heart Institute
Presbyterian Medical Center
Philadelphia, PA
215-662-9582
SDillon@IX.Netcom.com

Joel B. Ennis
Director of Engineering
Maxwell Labs.
San Diego, CA
619-576-7685

Richard N. Fogoros, MD
Professor of Medicine
Allegheny University of the Health
Sciences
Director, Clinical Electrophysiology
Allegheny General Hospital
Pittsburgh, PA
412-359-6444

Byron L. Gilman
Chairman & CEO
SurVivaLink
Mpls, MN
612-939-4181

Wolfram Grimm, MD
ZIM-Kardiologie
Philipps Univ.
Marburg, Germany
49-6421282772

Michael L. Hardage, MSEE
Ventritex Inc.
Sunnyvale, CA
713-361-5677
73763.402@Compuserve.com

Curtis F. Holmes, PhD
Vice President, Technology
Wilson Greatbatch, Ltd.
Clarence, NY
716-759-6901

Raymond Ideker, MD, PhD
Professor of Medicine
Professor of Physiology
Professor of Biomedical Engineering
U Alabama at Birmingham
Cardiology,
Birmingham, AL
205-975-4710
REI@CRML.UAB.edu

Veronica Ivan, BSEE
Medtronic Inc.
Mpls, MN
612-574-4067

Mohammad R Jazayeri, MD
Associate Professor of Medicine
Univ. of Wisconsin Medical School
Milwaukee Clinical Campus
Sinai-Samaritan
Milwaukee, WI
414-219-7686

Douglas J. Lang, PhD
Director of Therapy Research
Cardiac Pacemakers Inc.
St. Paul, MN
612-638-4000

Michael J. Kallok, PhD
Angeion Corp.
Plymouth, MN
612-550-9388

Kai Kroll
St. Croix Medical
Minneapolis, MN
612-574-0570
Krol0009@Gold.TC.UMN.edu

Francis E. Marchlinski, MD
System Director and Section Chief
Cardiac Electrophysiology
Allegheny University
Philadelphia, PA
215-842-6408

Paul Monroe, PE
Janesville, WI
608-752-2574

Morton M. Mower, MD
Cardiac Pacemakers, Inc.
St. Paul, MN
410-243-1127

Randall Nelson
Engineering Project Manager
Angeion Corp.
Plymouth, MN
612-550-9388

Walter Olson, PhD
Tachycardia Arrhythmia Research
Sr. Research Fellow
Medtronic Inc.
Mpls, MN
612-574-6170

Luis A. Pires, MD
Clinical Assistant Prof. of Medicine
Wayne State University
Arrhythmia Center
Sinai Hospital
Detroit, MI
313-493-6395

Mark E. Rosenthal, MD
Dir. of Cardiac Electrophysiology
Abington Memorial Hospital
Abington, PA
215-517-1000

Claudio D. Schuger, MD
Clinical Assistant Prof. of Medicine
Wayne State University
Arrhythmia Center
Sinai Hospital
Detroit, MI
313-493-6395

Edward Shapland, PhD
President
Cortrak Medical Inc.
Minneapolis, MN
612-362-0597

Richard B. Shepard, MD
Professor of Surgery
Division of Cardio Thoracic Surgery
U Alabama at Birmingham
Birmingham, AL
205-934-4672
RShepard@UAB.edu

William S. Staewen, CCE
Medical Engineering Consultant
Selbyville, DE
302-436-5461

Jasbir S Sra, MD
Associate Professor of Medicine
Univ. of Wisconsin Medical School
Milwaukee Clinical Campus
Staff Electrophysiologist
St. Luke's Medical Center
Wisconsin Electrophysiology Gp.
Milwaukee, WI
414-649-3390

Russell T. Steinman, MD
Clinical Assistant Prof. of Medicine
Wayne State University
Arrhythmia Center
Sinai Hospital
Detroit, MI
313-493-6395

Jerry Supino
Pharmatarget
Maple Grove, MN
612-420-5344

Michael L. Sweeney
Ventritex Inc.
Sunnyvale, CA
408-738-4883

Patrick Tchou, MD
Cleveland Clinic
Cleveland, OH
216-444-6792

J. Marcus Wharton, MD
Associate Professor of Medicine
Director Clinical Cardiac
Electrophysiology
Duke University Medical Center
Durham, NC
919-681-6478
Whart002@MC.Duke.edu

Preface

THE IMPLANTABLE CARDIOVERTER DEFIBRILLATOR, or "ICD," is arguably the most technologically challenging type of therapy that physicians utilize today. At the same time, engineers who design ICDs are being called upon by clinicians to extend even further the technological envelope in quest of building the "ideal" device. To the extent, however, that physicians who utilize ICDs are not sufficiently comfortable with or familiar with the engineering principles that guide ICD function, the full clinical potential of even an ideal device will not be realized. In complementary fashion, engineers require as full an appreciation as possible of the real world "boundary conditions" and clinical impact of various ICD features, if the latter are truly to be perfected. This book is intended to serve as an educational tool to foster mutual understanding and communication among physicians, engineers, and other professionals involved in ICD therapy, with the ultimate purpose of enhancing patient care.

The highly varied backgrounds of such a diverse audience posed obvious challenges in the preparation of this volume. Given the overwhelmingly greater involvement of clinicians in the day-to-day management and follow-up of ICD recipients, we gave high priority to the presentation of oftentimes complex yet relevant engineering concepts in a manner that could be understandable to most clinicians. The majority of the topics covered herein relate to principles of operation of the ICD and its various subsystems with the aim of facilitating an in-depth understanding of ICD function and malfunction, independent of the specific manufactured device a patient receives. At the same time, features of specific ICD models are frequently introduced to provide practical clinical examples that are intended to complement the theoretical treatment. Topics for the mainly clinically oriented chapters are not intended to be all-inclusive but rather are focused on areas that we felt deserve emphasis for the larger purpose of optimizing care of the ICD patient.

The twin challenges of striking a proper balance of content and seeking clarity of technical language were compounded by the rapid pace of technologic evolution (spanning the first four generations of ICD devices) over the time period that this book was prepared. In order to arrive at text that would meet our objectives while maintaining technologic relevance, most chapters had to undergo multiple (and, at times, substantial) revisions. We cannot thank our author colleagues enough for the patience, understanding and close collaborative support they provided, without which this book would not have been possible.

In addition to the listed authors, we would like to especially thank Nabil Kanaan, PhD for proofreading; Sabine Jaensch and Sandra Crumlish for reference checking; Kathy Davis, Karen Beal, and Diane Szubeczak for superb secretarial support; and Karl Kroll for many drawings.

Finally, we are deeply grateful to our families who lovingly tolerated the countless hours of our unavailability during the course of this project.

MARK W. KROLL, PHD
MICHAEL H. LEHMANN, MD

1

Sudden Cardiac Death
Prevalence, Causes,
Underlying Substrates,
and Triggers

Masood Akhtar, MD, Mohammad R Jazayeri, MD, Jasbir S Sra, MD, Zalmen Blanck, MD, Sanjay Deshpande, MD, Anwer Dhala, MD, and Kathi Axtell, RN

S UDDEN DEATH is defined by the World Health Organization as death occurring from natural causes within 24 hours of the onset of acute illness.[1,2] Sudden death remains one of the major unresolved public health problems in the United States accounting for approximately 15-20% of all fatalities.[3,4] Even though a variety of cardiovascular and noncardiovascular ailments can culminate in sudden death, cardiac etiology is overwhelmingly the most common underlying pathology in these individuals.[3,5,6]

Sudden cardiac death (SCD) accounts for more that 50% of cardiovascular mortality.[5] The incidence of SCD has progressively decreased over the last three decades and this decline parallels the reduction in the overall deaths from cardiovascular causes. Several factors may have contributed toward this trend, including the changes in dietary habits and life style, cessation of smoking, and possibly improvement in health care. Although difficult to estimate, contemporary cardiovascular interventions such as anti-ischemic drug therapy, thrombolysis, myocardial revascularization, etc., probably have made some impact in this regard. Nonetheless, it is safe to state that even now, more than 300,000 lives are lost annually in the United States due to SCD.[5,6] It is estimated that more than 100,000 of these individuals are less than 65 years old.

Some aspects of terminology and definitions need clarification at the outset. Individuals classified as SCD victims in many series include patients who survive the episode because of timely intervention. In such circumstances the terminology of cardiovascular collapse and cardiac arrest may be more appropriate.

Depending upon the nature of trigger, the death may be instantaneous or take several hours. Duration of acute illness before the actual demise is helpful in speculating about the nature of the underlying process. For example, most arrhythmic deaths are instantaneous or occur in less than one hour. On the other hand, deaths from pump failure are likely to take somewhat longer.

Clinical Circumstances of SCD

Contrary to the lay perception, SCD is not due to "heart attack." The latter term should be reserved for patients who suffer acute myocardial infarction. Data from autopsy series and resuscitation cases suggest that approximately 80% of the victims do not have evidence of transmural myocardial infarction (MI).[7,8] On the other hand, a critical degree of coronary artery narrowing is present in more than 75% of the cases.[9-12] Occlusive coronary lesions, however, are present in less than 30% of the cases.[13] Resuscitation cases, when followed with serial ECG and cardiac enzymes, do not reveal a pattern of recent MI in most cases. A typical victim is a male with known cardiac pathology, generally coronary artery disease, and a healed MI.[14] With this relatively stable substrate, lethal arrhythmic events such as ventricular tachycardia and ventricular fibrillation can be initiated with a variety of triggers, leading to SCD (Fig. 1). It should be pointed out that although coronary artery disease is the most common associated structural abnormality; other forms of heart disease i.e., dilated or hypertrophic cardiomyopathy may be the sole pathology.[15,16] In some cases no obvious structural abnormality can be identified.[17]

Although several vascular and nonarrhythmic cardiac diseases can cause SCD, such events are *not* common. Table 1 lists some of the more frequent nonarrhythmic etiologies of SCD encountered in clinical practice.[18] Rarely will these patients survive, even in a monitored setting. Fortunately, such mechanisms of SCD collectively account for a minority of cases. *Cardiac arrest, secondary to arrhythmic causes, is the most common form of SCD (Fig. 1) and certainly the main mechanism of preventable SCD.* In this communication, henceforth, the description of SCD will imply arrhythmic forms, ventricular tachycardia (VF) or fibrillation (VF) in most cases, unless stated otherwise. Since SCD is the end result of an interplay

Table 1. Nonarrhythmic causes of sudden death.

Cardiac rupture
Acute pericardial tamponade
Acute extensive myocardial infarction
Massive pulmonary embolism
Aortic dissection
Acute cerebral hemorrhage

between underlying chronic substrates and acute triggers (Fig. 2), the role played by these factors is separately detailed below.

Myocardial Substrates

It is uncommon to witness the occurrence of SCD in individuals with normal myocardium; although a massive sudden metabolic change in the myocardium can create lethal circumstances. On the other hand, there is a strong association between myocardial scarring and SCD.[8,14] The replacement of the myocardium by scar tissue either as a result of prior MI, or a nonspecific process may lead to (1) overall poor cardiac systolic function and (2) creation of reentrant pathways which can provide a suitable milieu for VT/VF. Although acute MI can also produce an unstable, arrhythmogenic environment, in most cases there is no evidence of a recent myocardial infarction and at times even the role of ischemia is difficult to prove.[19]

The relationship between poor systolic function as measured by left ventricular ejection fraction (EF) and cardiovascular mortality is well known.[20] There is an inverse relation between the value of EF and SCD. Although the exact mechanism by which the low EF influences SCD is not clear and may be quite complex, it may be in part due to the extent of myocardial fibrosis. Acute and chronic myocardial damage, mainly produced by coronary lesions, has been extensively studied both in the experimental model and the clinical pathological cases.[8,14,21] However, myocardial fibrosis from other cardiac structural abnormalities may have similar sequelae. For example, in patients with idiopathic dilated cardiomyopathy, monomorphic VT may be indistinguishable from those seen with chronic fibrosis due to coronary artery disease.[22]

Aside from fibrosis, other organic myocardial changes such as hypertrophy and inflammation, can also increase the prevalence of SCD in the afflicted population.[5,15,16] A significant proportion of patients with hypertrophy; die suddenly, and arrhythmic mortality in this population may account for up to 60% of cardiovascular deaths. As indicated earlier, SCD can occasionally occur in individuals with no gross evidence of structural cardiac abnormality.

Regardless of the precise mechanism, the presence of myocardial structural changes somehow make such hearts vulnerable to SCD from VT/VF. The latter has been documented as the initiating event, when electrocardiographic monitoring is available at the time of collapse. In a series of 157 such cases reported by Bayes de Luna et al, VT/VF was noted in 83%.[23] However, by the time a rescue team arrives (typically 5-10 minutes later) one-fourth of the victims have bradycardia or asystole Fig. 1.[24] Bradycardia and/or asystole rarely causes SCD, unless the resultant heart rate slowing leads to pause-dependent torsade de pointes (see below). The best documented examples of SCD where bradycardia alone precedes the onset of SCD, are in patients with end stage heart disease.[25] SCD, in these patients is most likely due to hemodynamic collapse and cardiac pacing, therefore, is not followed by detectable improvement in survival.[25] When bradycardia follows VT/VF (due to a lapse of time [Fig. 1]), the recovery and survival statistics are also dismal despite resuscitation efforts including cardiac pacing, suggesting irreversible myocardial damage by that time.[26]

Unique substrates for SCD may be present in the absence of myocardial pathology i.e. in patients with Wolff-Parkinson-White and long QT syndromes. In a small percentage of patients with WPW syndrome, the accessory pathway is able to conduct rather rapidly during atrial flutter-fibrillation. The latter, when initiated, could lead to VT in some patients with a short refractory period of the accessory pathway.[27] This is a preventable form of SCD if the condition is recognized in time.

Prolongation of myocardial electrical recovery (long QT) can either be acquired or exist on a congenital basis.[28] The associated polymorphic VT (torsade de pointes), is presumed to be due to the emergence of early after-depolarizations and can degenerate into VF.[28] The acquired form of torsade de pointes is often initiated or aggravated by bradycardia, hypokalemia, hypomagnesemia, and drugs which prolong the QT interval.

Congenital long QT syndrome is also associated with torsade de pointes which is often triggered or aggravated by autonomic nervous system arousal and release of adrenalin (e.g. from exercise, or startle reaction). Although underlying structural heart disease is often present in the acquired form of long QT syndrome, the occurrence of torsade de pointes in either the congenital or ac-

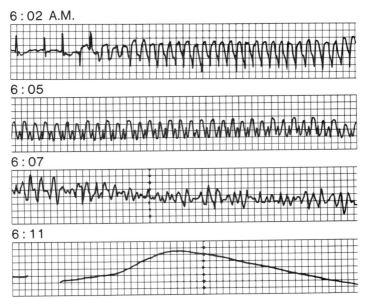

Figure 1. Monitored onset of sudden cardiac death. The sudden onset of mono-morphic VT occurs at 6:02 AM. There is QRS widening followed by ventricular fibrillation and finally asystole. The odds of successful resuscitation progressively decreases with the passage of time. When the asystole ensues, the chances of successful resuscitation are less than 1%.

quired QT interval syndrome is not dependent upon underlying structural myocardial pathology.

Triggers for SCD

Myocardial Ischemia

Since the majority of SCD victims do have a critical degree of coronary artery stenosis narrowing, it is natural to implicate myocardial ischemia as a triggering event. However, the actual part played by ischemia is not clear in many individuals since acute coronary occlusion of a critical degree is not demonstrable in the majority.[13,19] Whether added coronary artery spasm is responsible for production of critical narrowing at the time of collapse is conjectural. The fact that calcium channel blockers (vasodilators) do not prevent SCD argues against a significant role played by coronary artery spasm.[29] Patients who survive SCD with pre-existing MI generally have inducible VT, demonstrated by programmed electrical stimulation in the cardiac electrophysiology laboratory, indicating the presence of a chronic arrhythmogenic substrate.[30] Conversely, patients with VT/VF seldom develop these arrhythmias during graded exercise, a maneuver designed to create an ischemic environment.[19] One clinical setting where acute myocardial ischemia may be contributing to the onset of VT/VF is when polymorphic VT occurs in association with a normal QT interval.[31,32] Acute ischemia remains a major cause for such an arrhythmia, when concomitant critical coronary artery disease and/or spasm can be documented.[31,32] When LV function is preserved, these patients rarely have inducible VT in the electrophysiology laboratory.

Based upon some of the reasons provided above, it seems reasonable to state that the exact role of acute myocardial ischemia in SCD victims is not clear in many instances, particularly those with preexisting poor LV function related to healed MI. In some cases a combination of healed MI and acute ischemia may be responsible for the fatal arrhythmic event.[6,33] SCD, in the settings of noncoronary artery disease substrates, can obviously occur in the absence of acute ischemia.

Electrolyte Abnormalities

Many patients with high risk of SCD have a history of congestive heart failure or hypertension are on diuretic therapy to reduce or minimize fluid retention. Depletion of potassium through urinary losses is not uncommon in this population unless the are carefully monitored and abnormalities are corrected or prevented by potassium supplementation. Ventricular arrhythmias related to potassium or magnesium depletion are accompanied by prolongation of myocardial recovery and, consequently, the QT interval.[22] The resultant VT, (torsade de pointes), can often lead to VF or, per se, can cause hemodynamic collapse. In the series of patients with monitored SCD quoted earlier, torsade de pointes was observed in 13% of the cases,[23] making it a rather important concern since in the vast majority, long QT is iatrogenic and hence preventable.

Neurohumoral Factors

The influence of the autonomic nervous system on the sinus rate and atrioventricular nodal conduction is well known, but its effect on ventricular arrhythmogenesis is somewhat more controversial. However, in a variety of clinical settings this role may be more apparent. Some examples include:

1. Torsade de pointes, in association with congenital long QT, is frequently initiated or aggravated by catecholamine stimulation and controlled with beta blockers.[28]

2. Some forms of monomorphic VT are induced with exercise and can be more readily replicated with isoproterenol administration rather than programmed electrical stimulation alone in the electrophysiology laboratory.[22]

3. Sympathetic stimulation can produce a significant increase in oxygen consumption by increasing both the heart rate and myocardial contractility. In patients with critical degree of coronary stenosis, an increased oxygen demand could lead to myocardial ischemia culminating in VT/VF.

4. Severe bradycardia and asystole can be induced with vagal stimulation as seen frequently in association with neurocardiogenic/presyncope.[34] The resultant bradycardia, per se, may not be fatal but pause dependent torsade de pointes could emerge, leading to SCD.

Additional evidence for a possible role of the autonomic nervous system in the initiation of sustained VT or VF comes from documentation of a circadian pattern of appropriate ICD shock frequency (greatest in the morning hours)[35,36]—similar to that observed in relation to various other acute cardiac events.[37] The observation of reduced long term R-R interval variability in post-MI patients prone to sustained VT suggests altered autonomic dynamics in these cases.[38]

Pharmacologic Agents
A variety of pharmacologic agents have been implicated for facilitating or aggravating ventricular arrhythmogenesis. Some clinical circumstances and agents that may be responsible are outlined here:

1. Antiarrhythmic drugs that prolong the QT interval can produce torsade de pointes which represents a potentially fatal new arrhythmia in these patients.[22] The usual culprits include Class IA (quinidine, procainamide, and disopyramide), and Class III agents e.g., sotalol and at times even amiodarone. Women are at relatively increased risk of developing this proarrhythmic complication.[39] In the experimental model, it has been shown that quinidine induced early after-depolarizations with QT prolongation can be aggravated by both heart rate slowing and reduction in extracellular potassium concentration.[40] To what extent these aggravating factors play an additional role in clini-

cal situations is unclear, but such factors could create the arrhythmic milieu in patients who have been chronically stable on a given dose of an antiarrhythmic agent.

2. Several groups of drugs, Class IC antiarrhythmic drugs in particular, prolong His Purkinje system and intramyocardial conduction and aggravate existing arrhythmias, i.e., causing increased frequency or conversion to incessant forms.[41] The most likely underlying electrophysiologic basis for this is a critical degree of conduction slowing without comparable or greater prolongation of refractoriness in existing reentrant circuits.   At times, this type of effect is more subtle, manifesting as inducible monomorphic VT, not present at baseline state.[42] The magnitude of this problem is unknown and is hopefully smaller since the results of CAST (Cardiac Arrhythmia Suppression Trial) have been known.[43]

3. The mechanism of SCD in CAST is still unclear but the available data suggest that (a) proarrhythmic drug effect may occur months after the initiation of therapy and (b) interaction between flecainide/encainide and other factors such as rate acceleration, sympathetic stimulation, and/or myocardial ischemia may create a lethal environment.[44] It is conceivable that such interactions may occur with other drugs as well.

4. On occasion, other agents including antidepressants, digitalis, bronchodilators, and sympathomimetics may cause or aggravate ventricular arrhythmias. The scale of this problem among the SCD population is also not clear at this time.

Electrical Triggers
Electrical (i.e., arrhythmic) triggers per se may be responsible for initiation of the sustained VT or VF, either arising de novo or brought about by other factors already discussed. The contribution of these electrical triggers to SCD could take several forms:

1. Intramyocardial reentry. The presumed mechanism of VT/VF related to myocardial scarring is reentry.[22] In this model, areas of fibrosis interspersed by viable myocardial cells provide the optimal conditions of anatomic obstacle, anisotropic conduction, and pathways for re-excitation. Potential reentrant circuits can be triggered into sustained VT or VF by introduction of ventricular premature beats. This can be accomplished in the

laboratory by the technique of programmed ventricular stimulation and has been most convincingly demonstrated in patients with spontaneous sustained monomorphic VT in the setting of an old myocardial infarction.[30] Less frequently, a similar type of VT can also be induced in patients with primary myocardial disease. Since these tachycardias can be replicated in the laboratory with introduction of extrastimili, it is sometimes assumed that a clinical episode of monomorphic VT is also initiated by spontaneous ventricular premature beats. This assumption is further reinforced by the well known relationship between ventricular premature beats and SCD.[20]

There is, however, ample evidence to the contrary - that the spontaneous ventricular premature beats seldom initiate the episodes of VT/VF. In fact, the ventricular premature beats may be, and in all likelihood are, just another expression of the same underlying process (reentry in this case). Some of the reasons which support this hypothesis are outlined below:

a) Spontaneous ventricular beats seldom initiate VT/VF in patients with structurally normal hearts. It is the underlying myocardial abnormality rather than premature beats which create the necessary conditions for sustained VT/VF.

b) In post MI populations marked suppression of premature beats with certain drugs (such as flecainide, encainide, and moricizine) is associated with a higher incidence of SCD.[43,44]

c) The spontaneous onset of monomorphic VT is seldom triggered by ventricular premature complexes arising in sites remote from the location of the circuit (or scar). In this setting the morphology of the first and all subsequent beats is the same suggesting a similar origin. [45,46] The first beat interrupts the sinus rhythm, and hence, is premature by definition but is not necessarily the cause of subsequent beats or tachycardia.

We believe that the emergence of monomorphic VT is frequently a manifestation of continuous abortive reentry that occurs during penetration of reentrant circuits with each sinus beat.[45] This abortive reentrant impulse may be what is recorded as abnormal late potential on a signal averaged ECG. Its overt manifestation is prevented by refractoriness of the surrounding tissue created by the immediately preceding sinus beat. The emergence of the reentrant impulse into the surrounding myocardium can cause a premature beat, couplets, or nonsustained and sustained monomorphic VT, depending upon the number of completed revolutions by the reentrant wave form. Changes in the conduction characteristics of intramyocardial circuits or refractoriness of the boundary can be brought about by several factors including heart rate variability, changes in anatomic tone, electrolyte imbalance, ischemia, and hemodynamic factors. This hypothesis is strengthened by the observation that in patients with monomorphic VT, the QRS morphology of sustained VT is often similar to the isolated premature beats.[45,46]

2. In a small number of cases, spontaneous ventricular premature beats may trigger sustained VT/VF. This seems likely when the initiating ventricular premature beat (or beats) have a different QRS appearance as compared to the sustained ventricular tachycardia. It is quite conceivable that in many situations the mechanism triggering the occurrence of ventricular premature complexes may be unrelated to the underlying myocardial fibrosis. It is also possible that frequent, consecutive, and particularly early ventricular premature beats could trigger ventricular fibrillation in rare circumstances. It should be pointed out, however, that the true nature of initial and subsequent events in these situations has seldom been studied, particularly when the resultant VT is polymorphic in appearance. The role of premature beats for the initiation of supraventricular tachycardia and atrial fibrillation in patients with Wolff Parkinson White syndrome is well established. In these settings, a life threatening situation can be created by atrial and/or ventricular premature beats.

3. In patients with idiopathic as well as ischemic cardiomyopathy, another mechanism of VT is observed at times. The reentry pathway here, incorporates both of the bundle branches, the His bundle, and the interventricular septum.[47,48] The resultant bundle branch reentry tachycardia tends to be rapid and frequently presents with syncope and/or cardiac arrest. In our experience, this tachycardia constitutes a relatively common form of induced monomorphic VT in patients with idiopathic dilated cardiomyopathy accounting for approximately 40% of the cases. Degeneration into VF is likely because of the tachycardia's rapid rate and also poor underlying cardiovascular status. Most documented initiation of spontaneous bundle branch reentrant

tachycardia also do not seem to start with premature beats (unpublished observations).

4. VT can occur in the absence of obvious structural heart disease.[22] The underlying substrates and triggers are poorly understood as are the electrophysiologic mechanisms. In some of these patients, the induction techniques suggest reentry, but in others it may be triggered activity related to afterdepolarizations. Fortunately, these types of VT infrequently lead to VF. However, it should be pointed out that SCD with documented VF does occur in patients without detectable structural abnormality.[17]

Hemodynamic Decompensation

Hemodynamic decompensation with resultant pulmonary congestion, hypoxia, acidosis, etc., can acutely destabilize or create an arrhythmogenic environment leading to a variety of arrhythmias inducing VT/VF. This is an ever present possibility in patients with moderate to severe heart disease and can be triggered by several factors. Precipitating factors include supraventricular tachycardia, positive or negative inotropic pharmacologic agents, changes in peripheral resistance, blood volume, etc. These are the most likely mechanisms of SCD in patients with chronic congestive heart failure, but could also be operative in individuals with only periodic cardiac decompensation.[49]

Management and Prevention of SCD

From the foregoing discussion, it should be apparent that SCD is a major cause of death, and most SCD are arrhythmic in nature with VT/VF initiating the event in more than 80% of the cases. A large pool of patients have no warning and many who have known heart disease have nonspecific symptoms prior to SCD.[24] Nonetheless, a significant number of individuals are known to be at high risk of SCD, such as those who survive cardiac arrest and patients with VT related syncope, near syncope, or hypotension. The prevention and management of SCD, therefore, must incorporate consideration of patients with and without prior history of cardiac arrest.

In patients without prior warning the only realistic solution is out-of-hospital resuscitation with the help of rescue squads. Many communities have emergency care networks but the arrival of rescue teams in less than four minutes (critical for prevention of

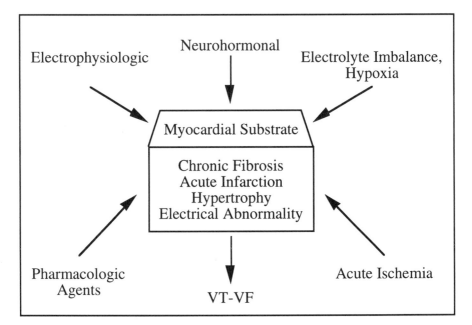

Figure 2. Substrate triggers of SCD. The schema shows a variety of myocardial substrates, which are usually chronic, interact with triggers that are often acute to precipitate VT/VF.

neurologic deficit), and hence a favorable final outcome is not common. Clearly this area needs further improvement which can only be achieved with significantly more funding that is presently inadequate in most communities.

For those who have known risk factors, the options of therapy include antiarrhythmic drugs, VT surgery, catheter ablation, and ICD.[6] Realizing all the substrates and triggers that can contribute to SCD in any given patient (Fig. 2), it is inconceivable that any pharmacologic intervention will prevent SCD to a measurable extent. Similarly VT surgery and catheter ablation are designed to correct the pre-existing VT. The native disease process i.e., myocardial ischemia, poor left ventricular function, etc., is likely to progress causing SCD from different mechanisms in the same patient. It is for this reason we believe that ICD, by virtue of its broad spectrum of effectiveness against VT/VF of any mechanism, is the best, currently available, interventional approach for individuals at high risk for SCD.

ACKNOWLEDGMENTS:

Fig. 1 is courtesy of Mark Josephson and has appeared in the Annals of Internal Medicine.[6]

1. World Health Organization. Manual of the international statistical classification of diseases, injuries, and causes of death. Based on the recommendations of the Ninth Revision of Congress, 1975, and adopted by the twenty-ninth World Health Assembly, 1975 revision. Geneva, World Health Organization, 1977 p 470.
2. Corday E. Symposium on identification and management of the candidate for sudden cardiac death - introduction. Am J Cardiol 1977;39:813-815.
3. Kuller L. Sudden and unexpected non-traumatic deaths in adults: A review of epidemiological and clinical studies. J Chronic Dis 1966;19:1165-1192.
4. Burch GE, DePasquale ND. Sudden unexpected natural death, Am J Med Sci 1965;249:86-97.
5. Myerburg RJ, Kessler KM, Castellanos A. Sudden cardiac death: structure, function and time-dependence of risk. Circulation 1992;85:I2-I10.
6. Akhtar M, Garan H, Lehmann MH, et al. Sudden cardiac death: Management of high risk patients. Ann Intern Med 1991;114:499-512.
7. Cobb LA, Baum RS, Alvarez H III, et al. Resuscitation from out of the hospital ventricular fibrillation: 4 years followup. Circulation 1975;52:223-228.
8. Reichenbach DD, Moss NS. Myocardial cell necrosis and sudden death in humans. Circulation 1975;52:60-69.
9. Baba N, Bashe WJ, Keller MD, et al. Pathology of atherosclerotic heart disease in sudden death. I. Organizing thrombosis and acute coronary vessel lesion. Circulation 1975;52:53-59.
10. Perper JA, Kuller L, Cooper M. Arteriosclerosis of coronary arteries in sudden, unexpected deaths. Circulation 1975;52:27-33.
11. Friedman M. The pathogenesis of coronary plaques, thromboses, and hemorrhages: an evaluative review. Circulation 1975;52:34-40.
12. Weaver WD, Lorch GS, Alvarez HA, et al. Angiographic findings and prognostic indicators in patients resuscitated from sudden cardiac death. Circulation 1976;54:895-900.
13. Davies, MJ. Anatomic features in victims of sudden coronary death: Coronary artery pathology. Circulation 1992;85:19-24.
14. Lie JT, Titus JL. Pathology of the myocardium and the conduction system in sudden coronary death. Circulation 1975;52:43-52.
15. Messerli FH, Ventura HO, Elizardi DJ, et al. Hypertension and sudden death: Increased ventricular ectopic activity in left ventricular hypertrophy. Am J Med 1984;77:18-22.
16. Anderson KP. Sudden death in hypertrophic cardiomyopathy. Cardiovasc Res 1984;5:363-377.
17. Wilber DJ, Garan H, Finkelstein D, et al. Out-of-hospital cardiac arrest Use of electrophysiologic testing in the prediction of long-term outcome. N Engl J Med 1988;318:19-24.
18. Akhtar M, Wolf F, Denker S. Sudden cardiac death, in Pollock ML, Schmidt DH (ed): Heart Disease and Rehabilitation, 2nd edition, New York, John Wiley & Sons, 1986 pp 115-130.
19. Meissner MD, Akhtar M, Lehmann MH. Nonischemic sudden tachyarrhythmic death in atherosclerotic heart disease. Circulation 1991;84:905-912.
20. Bigger JT, Fliess JS, Kleiger R, et al. Multicenter postinfarction research group: The relationship among ventricular arrhythmias, left ventricular dysfunction and mortality in the two years after myocardial infarction. Circulation 1984;69:250-258.
21. Wit AL, Allessie MA, Bonke FIM et al. Electrophysiologic mapping to determine the mechanism of experimental ventricular tachycardia initiated by prema-

ture impulses: experimental approach and initial results demonstrating reentrant excitation. Am J Cardiol 1982;49:166-185.

22. Akhtar M. Clinical spectrum of ventricular tachycardia. Circulation 1990;82:1561-1573.

23. Bayes deLuna A, Coumel P, Leclercq JF. Ambulatory sudden cardiac death: mechanisms of production of fatal arrhythmia on the basis of data from 157 cases. Am Heart J 1989;117:151-159.

24. Liberthson RR, Nagel EL, Hirschman JC, et al. Pathophysiologic observations in prehospital ventricular fibrillation and sudden cardiac death. Circulation 1974;49:790-798.

25. Luu M, Stevenson WG, Stevenson LW, et al. Diverse mechanisms of unexpected cardiac arrest in advanced heart failure. Circulation 1989;80:1675-1680.

26. Myerburg RJ, Conde CA, Sung RJ, et al. Clinical, electrophysiologic and hemodynamic profile of patients resuscitated from prehospital cardiac arrest. Am J Med 1980;68:568-576.

27. Wellens HJ, Durrer D. Wolff-Parkinson-White syndrome and atrial fibrillation: relation between refractory period of accessory pathway and ventricular rate during atrial fibrillation. Am J Cardiol 1974;34:777-782.

28. Jackman WM, Friday KJ, Anderson JL, et al. The long QT syndromes: A critical review, new clinical observations and a unifying hypothesis. Prog Cardiovasc Dis 1988;31:115-172.

29. Bigger JT, Coromilas J, Rolnitzky LM, et al. Multicenter diltiazem postinfarction trial investigators: Effect of diltiazem on cardiac rate and rhythm after myocardial infarction. Am J Cardiol 1990, 65:539-546.

30. de Bakker JMT, van Capelle FJL, Janse MJ, et al. Reentry as a cause of ventricular tachycardia in patients with chronic ischemic heart disease: Electrophysiologic and anatomic correlation. Circulation 1988;77:589-606.

31. Tchou P, Atassi K, Jazayeri M, et al. Etiology of long QT. J Am Coll Cardiol 1989;13:21A. (abstract)

32. Myerburg RJ, Kessler KM, Mallon SM, et al. Life-threatening ventricular arrhythmias in patients with silent myocardial ischemia due to coronary artery spasm. N Engl J Med 1992;362:1451-1455.

33. Garan H, McComb JM, Ruskin JN. Spontaneous and electrically induced ventricular arrhythmias during acute ischemia superimposed on 2-week-old canine myocardial infarction. J Am Coll Cardiol 1988;11:603-611.

34. Sra JS, Anderson AJ, Sheikh SH et al. Unexplained syncope evaluated by electrophysiologic studies and head-up tilt testing. Ann Intern Med 1991;114:1013-1019.

35. d'Avila A, Wellens F, Andries E, et al. At what time are implantable defibrillator shocks delivered? Evidence for individual circadian variance in sudden cardiac death. Eur Heart J 1995;16:1231-1233.

36. Behrens S, Galecka M, Brüggerman T, et al. Circadian variation of sustained ventricular tachyarrhythmias terminated by appropriate shocks in patients with an implantable cardioverter defibrillator. Am Heart J. 1995;130:79-84.

37. Muller JE, Tofler GH, Stone PH. Circadian variation and triggers of onset of acute cardiovascular disease. Circulation 1989;79:733-743.

38. Huikuri HV, Seppänen T, Koistinen MJ, et al. Abnormalities in beat-to-beat dynamics of heart rate before the spontaneous onset of life-threatening ventricular tachyarrhythmias in patients with prior myocardial infarction. Circulation 1996;93:1836-1844.

39. Makkar RR, Fromm BS, Steinman RT, et al. Female gender as a risk factor for torsade de pointes associated with cardiovascular drugs. JAMA 1993;270;2590-2597.

40. Davidenko J, Cohen L, Goodrow R, et al. Quinidine-induced action potential prolongation, early after-depolarizations and triggered activity in canine purkinje fibers: Effects of stimulation rate, potassium, and magnesium. Circulation

1989;79:674-686.
41. Winkle RA, Mason JW, Griffin JC, et al. Malignant ventricular tachyarrhythmias associated with use of encainide. Am Heart J 1981;102:857-864.
42. Ruskin JN, McGovern B, Garan H, et al. Antiarrhythmic drugs; a possible cause of out-of-hospital cardiac arrest. N Engl J Med 1983; 309:1302-1306.
43. The Cardiac Arrhythmia Suppression Trial (CAST) investigators. Preliminary report: effect of encainide and flecainide on mortality in a randomized trial of arrhythmia suppression after myocardial infarction. N Engl J Med 1989;321:406-412.
44. Akhtar M, Breithardt G, Camm AJ, et al. Task force of the working group on arrhythmias of the European Society of Cardiology: CAST and beyond: implication of the Cardial Arrhythmia Suppression Trial. Circulation 1990;81:1123-1127.
45. Niazi I, Jazayeri M, McKinnie J, et al. New insights into initiating mechanisms of clinical ventricular tachycardia. Circulation 1988;78:II-71. (abstract)
46. Berger MD, Waxman HL, Buxton AE, et al. Spontaneous compared with induced onset of sustained ventricular tachycardia. Circulation 1988;78:885-892.
47. Caceres J, Jazayeri M, McKinnie J et al. Sustained bundle branch reentry as a mechanism of clinical tachycardia. Circulation 1989;79:256-270.
48. Tchou P, Jazayeri M, Denker S, et al. Transcatheter electrical ablation of right bundle branch: a method of treating macroreentrant ventricular tachycardia attributed to bundle branch reentry. Circulation 1988;78:246-257.
49. Packer M. Sudden unexpected death in patients with congestive heart failure: A second frontier. Circulation 1985;72:681-685.

2

History of the ICD

William S. Staewen, CCE and Morton M. Mower, MD

TOWARDS the latter part of the 1960s, cardiac defibrillation, by external means, was considered an effective treatment for terminating ventricular fibrillation. Elective cardioversion, using the same external defibrillating devices, was also a commonly used therapy for the conversion of ventricular tachycardia, atrial fibrillation, and atrial flutter to more normal rhythms. These cardioversion devices utilized a synchronization of the defibrillator discharge with the patient's own R-wave so as to prevent induction of ventricular fibrillation from cardioversion shocks that otherwise may have been delivered during the vulnerable portion of the cardiac cycle (the early portion of the T-wave). The history of the ICD also began during this period, at the time when the idea was first conceptualized by Michel Mirowski.

While Mirowski was working in Israel in the late 1960s, his Chief of Medicine and close personal friend, Harry Heller died following a short history of repeated episodes of ventricular arrhythmias. Knowing that each episode was potentially life threatening, and frustrated by the lack of a means for therapeutic intervention, Mirowski conceived of a miniaturized defibrillator capable of being implanted and delivering a defibrillating shock to the heart via a transvenous catheter.

In 1969, Sinai Hospital of Baltimore was constructing a new Coronary Care Unit and Mirowski was recruited from Israel to be its first Director. He brought with him and presented to us his idea of an automatic implantable defibrillator. The need for such a device was founded on several observations. First, in the United States alone, approximately 450,000 people were thought to be dying of sudden cardiac death each year. It was suspected that most of these deaths were due to ventricular fibrillation. Secondly, it was adequately demonstrated in the then early coronary care units, that defibrillation shocks delivered promptly could successfully revert ventricular fibrillation and ventricular tachycardia to

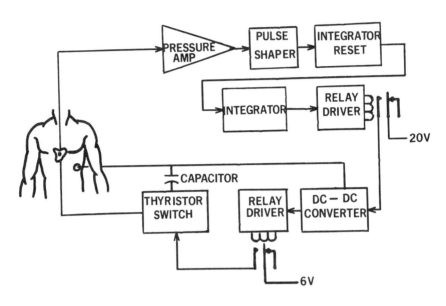

Figure 1. - The block circuit diagram of the original prototype of the automatic implantable defibrillator. Two separate relays initiate charging of the capacitor and discharge of the pulse to the subject respectively.

normal rhythms even in the presence of severe underlying cardiac disease. It was noted that ventricular fibrillation was frequently preceded by a brief period of ventricular tachycardia. Finally, it was acknowledged that most victims of sudden cardiac death outside of the hospital could not be reached in time to implement effective external defibrillation therapy.

Working in the hospital's clinical engineering and animal research facilities, we designed, constructed, and successfully tested a prototype automatic defibrillator in dogs in 1969.[1] This was achieved in less than three months work, and without any institutional or outside financial support. The prototype employed a right ventricular pressure sensor to detect ventricular fibrillation. Defibrillation was achieved through a modified pacing catheter electrode inserted in the right ventricle and a small circular electrode implanted in the anterior chest wall. The pacing catheter was modified by virtue of permanently soldering the stylet in it to reduce the resistance of the catheter electrode.

We utilized an exponential capacitor discharge defibrillation waveform in our prototype. Defibrillation was successfully achieved about 15 s after the onset of fibrillation, typically with 10 J of energy. In subsequent experiments we used damped sinusoidal waveforms by discharging the capacitor through a 100 mH inductor and were able to accomplish defibrillation with as little as 3 J delivered to the animal.

A block diagram of our prototype is shown in Fig. 1. The RAMP GENERATOR was set to develop a sawtooth waveform that would eventually rise to a voltage level sufficient to turn on the transistor in the RELAY DRIVER. Each time a pressure pulse was detected, the sawtooth (ramp) signal would however be reset to 0 V. In the absence of a pressure signal, the RELAY DRIVER would activate the DC-DC CONVERTER and begin charging the 16 μF capacitor. When the capacitor voltage reached the energy level we had pre-selected, the transistor in a second RELAY DRIVER was biased on, causing the THYRISTOR SWITCH to conduct and allow the capacitor to discharge through the patient electrodes. The device then automatically returned to the standby mode, awaiting the next episode of arrhythmia.

This prototype performed quite reliably in the animal experiments. It was larger than what we would have considered desirable for implantation and the current drain was higher than wanted for long battery life. However, we made no special effort to enhance these features in our original prototype. The goal was to simply demonstrate that such a device could be reasonably designed and constructed to perform the task of automatic defibrillation. The experimental model clearly demonstrated the practicality of the concept.

Because the sensing circuit of the prototype could detect any cardiac malfunction that largely resulted in the abolition of the phasic nature of the right ventricular pressure curve, the device could be used to deliver shocks for the treatment of ventricular tachycardia as well as fibrillation.

Later experimental models included significant changes in the sensing method.[2] The pressure transducer used in the original prototypes was considered to be too fragile and expensive for practical widespread use, and it was replaced with a catheter based system that monitored a combination of cardiac contraction derived from resistive changes in the catheter when the lead body was flexed, and the endocardial electrogram signal. During ventricular fibrillation, the absence of both R-waves on the electrogram and phasic output from the contraction sensor would initiate a charging cycle. This schema was then again replaced in the first clinical units with the more advanced and sophisticated probability density function detection system which was exceptionally specific for ventricular fibrillation.

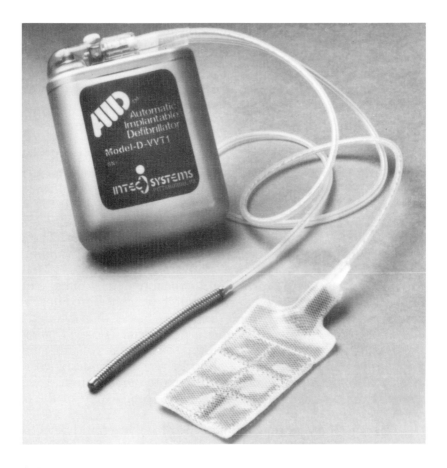

Figure 2. The initial clinical model of the Automatic Implantable Defibrillator (AID) with its superior vena cava and apical patch electrodes. This design was tested chronically in the animal laboratory for a number of years before the first human application.

The original prototype successfully achieved ventricular defibrillation between the right ventricular electrode catheter and a subcutaneous precordial electrode (metal plate) placed under the skin of the anterior chest wall. However, we also considered it preferable to have a totally intravascular electrode system because it could potentially lower the energy requirements for defibrillation.

Such an electrode system could also greatly simplify the implantation procedure and allow the use of the same catheter system for defibrillation, sensing, and cardiac pacing in future applications. Experiments were performed in healthy dogs using a dual electrode bearing catheter that was passed through the jugular vein, with the distal electrode placed in the right ventricular apex and the proximal electrode located in the venous system just outside of the heart.[3] These experiments demonstrated that ventricular defibrillation was attainable through a single intravascular catheter with energies as low as 10 J.

John Schuder was also able to demonstrate experimental success with this single intravascular catheter lead system.[4] His experiments were quite successful using low energy truncated pulses. He reported that truncated waveforms having an initial current of 7 A, a final current of 3 A, and time constants of 10 and 20 ms were 50% and 81% effective, respectively. Pulses with an initial current of 10 A, a final current of 5 A and time constants of 5 and 10 ms were 60% and 98% effective.

An investigation to determine human defibrillation requirements was then performed during bypass surgery using a catheter electrode in the right ventricular apex and a platinum electrode with saline soaked sponge clamped to the superior vena cava simulating a single transvenous catheter system.[5] Defibrillation was accomplished using energies of 5-15 J with truncated pulses through this system.[6] Although these experiments validated the effectiveness of low energy defibrillation shocks through a transvenous catheter system, there were some practical negative aspects of this approach that precluded it's use in the initial clinical models. These included the sensitive nature of the catheter's dependence on positioning within the right ventricle, and the possibility of dislodgement of the electrode from the apex. There was also the theoretical possibility of myocardial damage from the high current density through the small electrode surface area, and a significantly uneven electric field distribution of the defibrillation pulse. In 1972 the Mirowski group began it's collaboration with Medrad Inc. (Pittsburgh, Pa.) on the development of the clinical model (Fig. 2) of the Automatic Implantable Defibrillator (AID). One of the initial priorities of this phase of the work was to explore alternatives to the single intravascular catheter system.[7]

Their experiments clearly indicated that by far the most consistent and stable defibrillation energy thresholds were achieved with insulated conformal electrodes placed on both the base and the apex of the heart. This electrode configuration also resulted in the lowest energy requirements for successful defibrillation. Truncated exponential waveforms were adopted. They required low peak voltage and current for effective defibrillation and the circuits required to generate them were simple. Initial shocks were delivered at 25 J approximately 15 s after the detection of ventricular fibrillation.

As mentioned earlier, the first clinical units developed by Medrad (their later subsidiary was called Intec) employed a sensing system based on the analysis of the probability density function. The basic premise of the probability density function as a means of detecting ventricular fibrillation is that a significant portion of the normal electrogram is occupied by the isoelectric line (the quiescent electrical portions of the cardiac cycle), whereas the electrical signal representing ventricular fibrillation does not contain significant isoelectric periods. Therefore, the signal conditioning elements in the probability density function (PDF) circuits were designed to detect the absence of the isoelectric line in the electrogram. This was facilitated by differentiating the input signal and providing filtering cutoffs at 15 and 100 Hz to eliminate the influence of elevated ST segments and high-frequency interference, respectively. The concept of the PDF is illustrated in Fig. 3.

During the period from 1972 to 1976, a considerable effort was amassed by the Medrad/Intec group to design a defibrillator that would eventually be suitable for human implantation. Reliability and safety were paramount in their design objectives. This was an enormous responsibility that the designers accepted. The design had to be virtually unflawed. It had to reliably sense ventricular fibrillation and deliver a high energy electric shock to correct the arrhythmia in less than one minute. This had to be accomplished with a device placed remotely in the hostile environment of the body. It had to function as designed for years and must not, if it would fail for any reason, cause injury to the patient. There were some in the medical and engineering communities who doubted that it would be possible. Even the very concept and possible clinical usefulness were challenged editorially in prominent medical and engineering journals by eminently qualified experts in the fields of cardiology and medical instrumentation.[8, 9]

In addition to having established the critical design criteria for the optimal electrode system, defibrillating energy/waveform, and a fibrillation detection circuit, the design team had to address several other important features because of the uniqueness of this implanted device. They needed to incorporate design features that would not permit circuit failures to inhibit processing and detection of the patient's signals. Circuitry had to be designed to prevent accidental charging of the unit due to component failures. Similarly, a circuit was added to prevent accidental charging of the circuit during implantation because of 60 Hz interference being injected

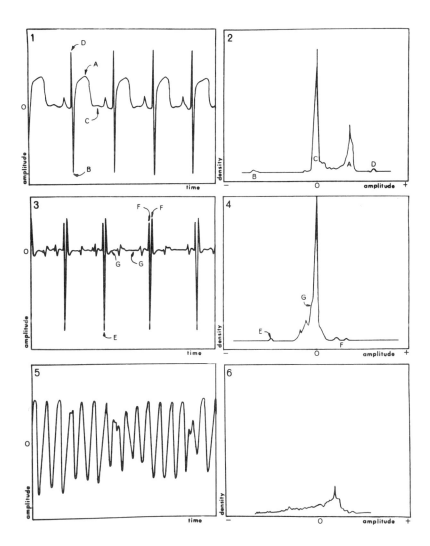

Figure 3. Normal (1), filtered (3), and fibrillation (5) electrograms with corresponding probability density functions (2, 4 and 6). The peak at zero amplitude (C) indicates that the signal spends considerable time near the baseline. Filtering augments this peak (G). The absence of such a peak (Frame 6) reflects the short time the signal is near baseline and indicates fibrillation.

through the electrode leads while being handled. This was necessary because a 60 Hz sine wave could be easily interpreted as a fibrillation signal by this method.

The energy storage capacitors used in an ICD needed to be as small as possible. Aluminum electrolytic capacitors were selected because they were able to provide high capacitance values (240 µF) with the capability of storing high voltage (680 V) in a small volume. These capacitors were chosen over other types in spite of their less than optimal leakage current characteristics. It was determined that the tradeoff of possibly greater leakage current than in other type capacitors, due to deformation of the oxide layer in the absence (for long periods) of applied voltage was manageable. Later models of the AID used special aluminum electrolytic capacitors of German origin that exhibited significantly lower leakage currents.

Two lithium vanadium pentoxide batteries were selected as the power source. Important selection criteria included a high energy density and low output impedance in addition to long life. A hermetically sealed titanium case was selected for encapsulation of the devices for human implantation.

A means of testing the implanted defibrillator was also incorporated into the design. Since there would likely be extended periods of time between normal operation (therapeutic) of the implanted defibrillator, a noninvasive means of testing and verifying that it functions was considered essential. The test mode that was added to the unit also allowed periodic charging of the capacitors. This helped to minimize capacitor leakage. After charging the capacitors in the test mode they were automatically discharged into an internal test load. The charge time was transmitted by radio telemetry to an external monitor that provided a digital display of the capacitor charging time. Progressive increases in charge time indicated depletion of battery energy or capacitor leakage problems.

The device was ready for the first chronic implants in animals in 1976. In order to demonstrate that the device could perform as intended, it was necessary to be able to repeatedly induce ventricular fibrillation on demand in active, conscious animals.

An implantable "fibrillator" was designed for this purpose. It consisted of a battery powered 60 Hz phase shift oscillator that was activated by a magnetic reed switch triggered by a magnet placed over the site of the implant. This unit delivered a fibrillating current of approximately 50 mA directly to the heart of the animal through a right ventricular catheter electrode. This provided a convenient and reliable experimental model of sudden arrhythmic death in active animals.[10] The action of the fibrillator and defibrillator were dramatically illustrated in movies that were filmed during several experimental demonstrations. An example is shown in Fig. 4. In the very near future these fibrillation-defibrillation sequences

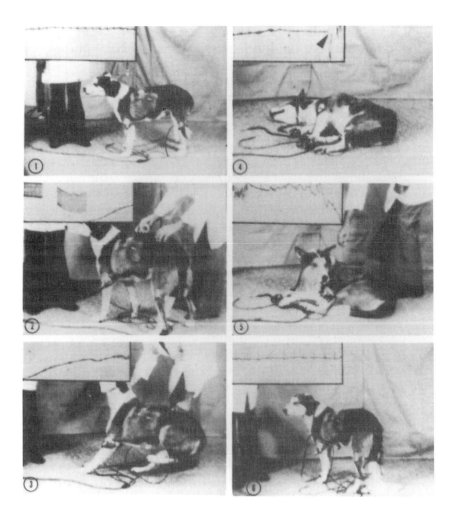

Figure 4. Scenes from a famous movie. (1) Normal Sinus Rhythm in a conscious dog, (2) induction of ventricular fibrillation with a magnet placed over the implanted fibrillator, (3) resultant syncope (4) automatic internal shock is delivered 15 s after induction, (5) the animal 3 s after defibrillation, and (6) 15 s after defibrillation.

were to become routine events during clinical electrophysiological studies.

The pre-clinical studies were conducted on a series of 25 animals that resulted in 60 defibrillator-implant months. Twenty-four fibrillation-defibrillation episodes were observed to have been successfully reverted. Lead damage, 1 caused by the animal and 3 caused by surgery, led to a total of 4 failures. Pre-clinical testing also included analysis of long term in vitro performance of the defibrillator and how it was affected by various physical and electrical stresses. Many of the tests exceeded the conditions required for validating implantable pacemakers. The anatomic effects of chronic electrode implantation and defibrillatory discharges were studied for up to 11 months following implant. Minimal effects were observed.

The Applied Physics Laboratory of the Johns Hopkins University made an independent evaluation of the AID under a special grant from the National Aeronautics and Space Administration (NASA). They reviewed the basic device design, analyzed the components, conducted provocative challenges to the sensing system, reviewed the pre-clinical test data, and evaluated the manufacturing and quality control procedures. They also employed NASA techniques in their evaluations, such as radiographic analysis of the laser weld zones and microcalorimetry analysis of the device batteries. Statistical analysis of device reliability was also performed at both the component and system level. The Johns Hopkins University School of Medicine also challenged the manufactured AID defibrillators with arrhythmias that they had recorded on FM magnetic tape. It was determined by the independent reviewers in July of 1979 that the AID Defibrillator was suitable for limited clinical trials in selected patients who presented with a high risk of encountering one or more attacks of ventricular fibrillation. In 1980 the Institutional Review Board (IRB) of the Johns Hopkins Hospital and the US Food and Drug Administration (FDA) approved the clinical investigation of the AID Defibrillator. Clinical validation was the next step in the saga of the implantable defibrillator.

The first implant of an AID device in a human took place on February 4, 1980 at the Johns Hopkins Hospital. This model was eventually implanted in 37 patients and was highly successful in detecting and terminating ventricular fibrillation. However, it soon became apparent that many survivors of sudden cardiac death who were referred for implantation also suffered from hemodynamically unstable ventricular tachycardias at the onset which degenerated to ventricular fibrillation only at a later stage. This underscored the need to incorporate significant modifications that would make the system responsive to the entire range of ventricular tachyarrhythmias. This necessitated adding rate determination and R-wave synchronization capability to the unit. The second generation defibrillator with cardioverting capability was renamed the automatic implantable cardioverter defibrillator (AICD) and was designated the AID-B. This unit was incorporated into the clinical study in April of 1982. A close bipolar right ventricular electrode catheter was added to convey the electrogram signals to the new rate analysis circuit. This provided independent input signals (separate from the defibrillating electrodes) for accurate rate determination and R-wave synchronization of the shocks. This bipolar electrode was also planned for use eventually as a pacing electrode.

The AID-B was physically akin to the early pacemakers, as can be appreciated from Fig. 6 although the unit is partially obscured by a donut shaped magnet. The pulse generator weighed 293 grams with a volume of 162 cc. It's dimensions were 11.2 X 7.1 X 2.5 cm. The electronic circuits consisted of over 300 discrete components and were housed in an inner can with the capacitors, lithium batteries, and a test-load resistor. The titanium outer can was hermetically sealed with a laser beam weld. Magnetically triggered coded audio signals were emitted from a piezoelectric crystal located near the center of the can. These signals could be used to check the sensing function and to determine whether the unit was active or inactive. If the device was active, the unit beeped synchronously with the R-waves allowing the clinician to verify that each QRS complex was being sensed and that there was no miscounting due to T-wave sensing.

The external monitoring device, also seen in Fig. 5, was designated AIDCHECK-B. It allowed testing the battery strength and determining the cumulative number of pulses that were delivered to the patient. The test devices magnet could also be used to activate or deactivate the device, as desired. The battery charger for the AIDCHECK-B was found useful during implantation as a source of low-level alternating current to induce malignant arrhythmias for testing the proper function of the unit.

The AID-BR was introduced in mid 1982 and employed ventricular rate as it's only detection criteria. It was used primarily in patients who exhibited "spikey" ventricular tachycardia morphologies. The probability density function criteria were not as suitable for reliable detection of these morphologies. The AID-BR was also a discrete component device. This facilitated design modifications by Medrad/Intec but production was labor intensive, with over 200 man-hours required to produce a single device. Problems with the original leads surfaced early in the clinical trials. The conductors were made from silver tinsel wire because it had excellent electrical conductivity characteristics. However, the silver tinsel wire was replaced with Teflon coated drawn brazed strand (DBS) wire after several cases of electrical discontinuity occurred. The DBS wire enhanced lead fatigue resistance and strength while still maintaining high electrical conductivity. DBS wire also had a successful history of use in implantable cardiac pacemaker leads.

The original clinical trials lasted from February of 1980 through October of 1985 . At that time the AID-B and AID-BR received approval from the FDA for market release. Intec was acquired by Cardiac Pacemakers Incorporated (CPI) and its parent company, Eli Lilly and Company in May of 1985.

CPI's Ventak-C unit (originally designated AICD or AID-C by Intec) was released in March of 1986. This third generation device was a hybrid electronic module utilizing integrated circuit technology in place of discrete components. The Ventak-C did not incorporate any new functions but it did include some design enhancements as well as a more efficient manufacturing process. It introduced some mild improvements in the probability density function and automatic gain control circuitry and the output energy storage capacitors were replaced with newer and smaller units having even higher energy density characteristics. These improvements resulted in a smaller, thinner, and lighter defibrillator. It weighed 250 grams, its volume was 148 cc, and had dimensions of 10.8 X 7.6 X 2.0 cm. The Ventak-C proved to be remarkably reliable and quickly accounted for the majority of patients who received units. However, it's parameters (as well as those of it's AID-B/BR predecessors) were set during assembly at the plant and could not subsequently be changed.

The Ventak-P is a multiprogrammable integrated circuit unit whose parameters could be changed at will by the physician. This unit was introduced into clinical studies in September of 1988. It permitted programmability of rate cutoff (110-200/min). Delivered energy could be set by the physician between 0.1 and 30 J. Delay after detection prior to initiation of charging the capacitors could be programmed between 2.5 and 10 s. The probability density function could also be programmed on or off, thus eliminating the need to produce separate models. The Ventak Model 1550 was approved for general use by FDA in early 1989. It was essentially identical to the Ventak-P with a somewhat more limited programming capability.

The first non-thoracotomy system was implanted in late 1986.[11] It consisted of a right ventricular catheter (cathode) and a subcutaneous platinum-iridium mesh patch electrode (anode). The transvenous defibrillating lead, called the Endotak, is designed to be implanted similar to conventional pacemaker leads. The subcutaneous patch controls the direction of the shock pulses given through this lead system.

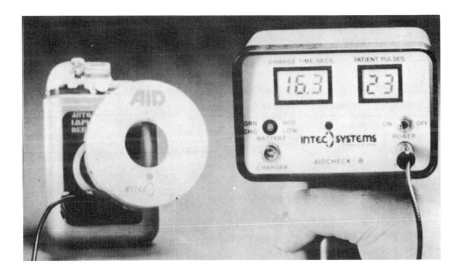

Figure 5. The ICD with its testing system, the AIDCHECK-B, and a magnet in place. The digital display on the left indicates the capacitor charging time, while that on the right shows the number of shocks delivered to the patient.

In 1989 other manufacturers introduced devices for clinical trial.[12] Ventritex began trials in the United States with the Cadence device. It was a software-driven, multifunction ICD offering programmable anti-tachycardia (and backup bradycardia) pacing, selection of cardioverting and defibrillating functions, and sophisticated arrhythmia detection algorithms to distinguish between arrhythmias of concern. The Cadence also features the first use of the biphasic waveform and electrogram storage. A smaller version, the Cadet, with 73 cm^3 volume was introduced in late 1995.

The primary direction in the 1990's has been towards smaller devices (Chap. 12) and the use of totally nonthoracotomy lead systems. The Medtronic Jewel, with a volume of 83 cm^3 and Active Can electrode, was commercially released in the US in 1994; its compact version, the Micro Jewel, was released in June of 1996. The CPI Mini, with a volume of 68 cm^3 was USA followed shortly at the end of 1995. The even smaller Mini II (59 cm^3) was introduced in the summer of 1996. The Ventritex Contour (57 cm^3) was first implanted in June 1996.

The Angeion Sentinel (also distributed as the Pacesetter Aegis), with a 60 cm^3 volume and dual battery technologies for greater longevity (Chap. 10, Appendix) began clinical trials in 1996. The devices also have a programmable Hot Can so only one model need be used for both pectoral and abdominal implants.

Dual chamber functionality is on the horizon. The ELA Defender has been implanted in Europe and features dual chamber arrhythmia detection algorithms and DDD pacing. The CPI Mini AV is slated for clinical introduction in late 1996 and will also feature dual chamber detection algorithms and DDD pacing. The Medtronic AMD 7250 will provide both atrial and ventricular defibrillation and is scheduled for late 1996 first implant. The InControl Metrix atrial ICD began clinicals in early 1996.

1. Mirowski M, Mower MM, Staewen WS, et al. Standby automatic defibrillator: An approach to prevention of sudden coronary death. Arch Intern Med, 1970;126:158-161.
2. Mirowski M, Mower MM, Staewen WS, et al, The development of the transvenous automatic defibrillator. Arch Intern Med 1972;129:773-779.
3. Mirowski M, Mower MM, Staewen WS, et al. Ventricular defibrillation through a single intravascular catheter electrode system. Clin Res 1971;19:328. (abstract)
4. Schuder JC, Stoeckle H, West JA, et al. Ventricular defibrillation in the dog with a bielectrode intravascular catheter. Arch Intern Med, 1973;132:286-290.
5. Mirowski M, Mower M, Gott VL, et al. Transvenous automatic defibrillator: Preliminary clinical tests of the defibrillating subsystem. Trans Amer Soc Artif Int Organs 1972;18:520-525.
6. Mirowski M, Mower MM, Gott VL, et al. Feasibility and effectiveness of low energy catheter defibrillation in man. Circulation 1973;47:79-85.
7. Langer A, Heilman MS, Mower MM, et al. Considerations in the development of the automatic implantable defibrillator. Medical Instrum 1976;10:163-167.
8. Lown B, Axelrod P. Implanted standby defibrillators. Circulation 1972;46:637-639.
9. Editorial. J Assoc Advanc Med Instr, 1971;5:310.
10. Mirowski M, Mower MM. The automatic implantable defibrillator: Some historical notes. Brugada P and Wellens H (eds), Cardiac Arrhythmias: Where To Go From Here? Mount Kisco NY, Futura Publishing Company, Inc., 1987
11. Moser S, Troup P, Saksena S, et al. Non-thoracotomy implantable defibrillator system. PACE 1988;11:887. (abstract)
12. Troup P. Early development of defibrillation devices. IEEE Eng Med Biol 1990;9:19-24.

3

The Electrophysiological Effects of Defibrillation Shocks

Stephen M. Dillon, PhD

THIS VOLUME describes the remarkable progress made in the technical development and the clinical application of the implantable cardioverter-defibrillator. Such progress is more remarkable for having been made in the absence of a complete understanding of how electrical shocks terminate arrhythmias. However, nearly a century after the start of scientific investigations into the mechanisms of defibrillation, we may only now be at the threshold of attaining such an understanding. This chapter will discuss what has been thought and what we have learned about the electrophysiological effects of shocks and how these effects relate to the overall defibrillation process.

Background

Scientific investigation of electrical defibrillation has been underway since the turn of the century beginning with the work of Prevost and Battelli.[1] It was much later after this work that the underpinnings of our understanding of the electrophysiological mechanisms of electrical defibrillation were developed by Gurvich and Yuniev[2] who recognized that defibrillation shocks were also stimulating agents. This is in contrast to then earlier hypotheses[3] which proposed that defibrillation shocks temporarily suppressed electrical activity, an opinion likely due to the observation of asystole after application of the relatively long duration shocks used at the time. Gurvich and Yuniev speculated that stimulation by an electrical shock caused defibrillation in the same way that stimulated extrasystoles terminated circus movement in rings of tissue - premature stimulation of excitable myocardium in advance of the reentrant wavefront.[2] This idea still persists in current theories of defibrillation[4,5] and is the main component of the familiar critical mass hypothesis.[6,7]

That shocks extinguished fibrillation wavefronts through stimulation was a powerful, elegant and readily understood concept which seemingly accounted for many experimental observations. Thus, from a conceptual and quantitative standpoint, defibrillation was regarded as large-scale tissue stimulation.[8] This notion of a defibrillation shock as a form of stimulus will be the starting point for the discussion of the electrophysiological mechanisms of defibrillation. As our later results will show, defibrillation shocks cannot be considered to be exactly analogous to ordinary stimulation since they can evoke responses from myocardium which is otherwise refractory to normal forms of stimulation.[9,10] This additional range of action for defibrillation shocks may be important for a complete understanding of the defibrillation process.

Before further discussion of defibrillation mechanisms, it is helpful to briefly review the basic electrical phenomena of the heart. The two main topics pertaining to this chapter are the electrophysiological processes underlying myocardial stimulation and those processes responsible for the propagation of the cardiac impulse. Though these topics are covered in greater depth in several books and reviews,[11-14] the following discussion will remind the reader of the basic concepts described in this chapter.

Among clinicians and bioengineers the most familiar expressions of the heart's electrical activity are the electrocardiogram and the contact electrogram. These signals arise from extracellular voltage gradients generated by the propagation of the cardiac impulse.[15,16] But, for scientific investigations of the electrophysiology of defibrillation shocks, one of the most important indications of cardiac electrical activity is the *action potential*, i.e. the time course of the transmembrane voltage seen during electrical activation of the myocardium. Fig. 1 illustrates the basic features of the cardiac action potential.

Cardiac muscle undergoes a stereotypical electrical response when stimulated; the membrane voltage rapidly *depolarizes* from its normal negative resting potential and remains depolarized for several hundred milliseconds before it spontaneously *repolarizes* back to resting potential. The initial rapid transition is called the upstroke phase and it is caused by the regenerative activation of the sodium current. The upstroke phase can be completed within 1 ms or so. The transient period of maintained depolarization following the upstroke is called the plateau phase and, although some depolar-

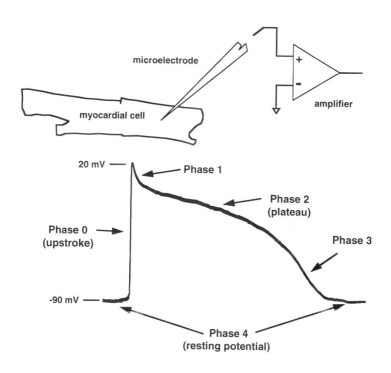

Figure 1. The cardiac action potential. The top of the figure shows impalement of a myocardial cell by a glass microelectrode. This permits measurement of the intracellular potential by a high impedance amplifier. The bottom of the figure shows a cardiac action potential recorded by microelectrode from canine epicardial muscle. The resting potential is -90 mV during the diastolic phase (*Phase 4*). Stimulation of the myocardium causes a rapid upstroke (*Phase 0*) in membrane potential to a level of 20 mV. The upstroke is followed by a phase of early rapid repolarization (*Phase 1*), a prolonged phase of slow repolarization (*plateau* or *Phase 2*) and a terminal phase of rapid repolarization (*Phase 3*).

izing current persists during the plateau, other currents activate at this time which return the membrane potential to resting levels. Ventricular myocardium will remain at the resting potential unless excited by some stimulus or by a cardiac impulse. Excitation occurs when the depolarizing current from an external electrical stimulus or from the leading edge of a propagating cardiac impulse brings the cellular membrane potential up to a threshold potential for excitation.

When the cell membrane is brought up to the threshold potential, the membrane will continue to depolarize on its own accord and in the process give rise to the depolarizing deflection characteristic of the upstroke phase. The upstroke phase is generated by the rapid and intense inrush of sodium ions across the cellular membrane through specialized protein pores called ion channels. The self-sustaining nature of the upstroke phase is due to the fact that these sodium channels sense membrane voltage and, though normally closed, will open when the membrane potential reaches or exceeds the threshold potential. Since the current flow through sodium channels further depolarizes the myocardial cell, a positive feedback cycle is initiated which leads to the rapid depolarization of the cell. This depolarization process comprises the phenomenon of myocardial stimulation.

Most if not all of the electrical determinants of cardiac stimulation, i.e. the intensity and duration of the electrical stimulus (Chap. 4), can be understood from the point of view of raising the cardiac membrane potential to the threshold potential.[17] Another characteristic of cardiac excitability cycle, that of myocardial refractoriness, is also due to the behavior of the sodium channel. The refractory period is that time when a pacing stimulus, if applied too soon after a previous stimulus, is unable to stimulate an action potential. This is because once the myocardial membrane is depolarized, the sodium channel spontaneously closes and enters an inactivated state. Inactivation is maintained throughout the action potential while the membrane is depolarized. Upon repolarization, the sodium channel leaves the inactivated state and is again available for activation by membrane depolarization. This behavior accounts for the fact that pacemaker stimuli are ineffective when applied to already depolarized and hence refractory myocardium. Myocardial cells residing at the resting potential are excitable because a large fraction of the sodium channels are available for activation by a depolarizing stimulus.

An understanding of fibrillation and of the consequences of defibrillation shocks is intimately related to how the cardiac impulse propagates. The leading edge of a cardiac impulse is formed by the upstroke phase of the action potential. The cardiac impulse propagates outward into the heart from the point of origination, whether from a natural cardiac pacemaker or a stimulating electrode, by exciting action potentials in adjacent cells. Fig. 2 illustrates the basic features of action potential propagation.

A portion of the depolarizing current developed during the action potential is spread from cell to cell. This is because myocardial cells are electrically connected to each other through specialized structures called gap junctions. Although cardiac cells are comprised of insulating lipid membranes, electrical continuity between adjacent cells is established by protein channels residing at

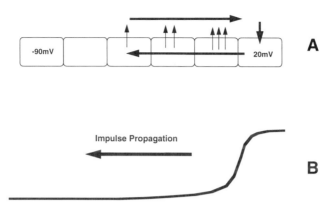

Figure 2. Propagation of the cardiac action potential (not drawn to scale). Panel A shows a linear "cable" of myocardial cells. The rightmost cell is depolarized to 20 mV by prior excitation. The leftmost cells reside at a resting potential of -90 mV. Depolarization of rightmost cell establishes a flow of current in a loop along the direction of the intercellular voltage gradient (*left arrow*), across the cellular membranes (*small up arrows*), into the extracellular fluid (*right arrow*), and back into the depolarized cell (*down arrow*). The number of small up arrows across the cellular membranes indicate the relative intensity of current flow. Panel B shows a plot of membrane potential versus distance (corresponding to voltage gradient scenario in Panel A) inducing leftwards propagation of an action potential. The leftward propagating action potential establishes a slight elevation (foot) in cellular membrane potential ahead of the upstroke phase which eventually brings cells to the excitation threshold.

the gap junctions. Thus, current can flow in a loop from cells which are depolarized (positive membrane potential) to cells which are resting (negative membrane potential) by taking a path through the electrolytes comprising the extracellular and intracellular media.

The spread of depolarizing current away from the edge of the cardiac impulse brings the membrane potential of adjacent cells up toward the threshold potential whereupon these cells are able to develop their own action potential upstroke phases in the manner described above. The combination of the passive spread of depolarization, called electrotonus, and the active generation of the upstroke is responsible for the spread of the cardiac action potential throughout the ventricles.

The Optical Recording Method

High voltage shocks required for defibrillation overwhelm and temporarily incapacitate the sensitive electrical recording instrumentation needed to study the heart's electrical activity. Recent years have seen the development of electrical recording methods which mitigate or reduce the effects of the "shock artifact".[18-21] Our laboratory introduced the optical recording technique to defibrillation research.[9,10]

The usual method for recording myocardial action potentials is by glass microelectrodes. Such recordings are obtained by impaling myocardial cells with sub-micron size tips of glass microelectrodes in order to establish electrical contact with the interior cellular potential. (Fig. 1) This method has been and continues to be applied to studies of defibrillation in order to understand the fundamental electrical processes underlying the effects of electrical shocks.[18,21] The microelectrode technique provides precise, accurate measurements of membrane potential. However, recordings are difficult to obtain, particularly in beating hearts; are rarely simultaneously obtained at more than one site; and, lastly, like all electrical methods, are subject to shock artifact. Optical recording makes it possible to obtain continuous, artifact-free action potential recordings,[9,10,22-24] to record action potentials at a hundred or more sites at once[25-30] and to record the voltage changes arising in portions of a single cell.[24]

The basis of the optical recording method is the ability of certain dyes to transduce the membrane potential of cells into an optical signal.[31-33] (Fig. 3) To use this method, the myocardium must first be stained with the voltage sensitive dye, typically by adding the dye to the solution perfusing the heart or by injection of dye into the coronary circulation. The dye molecules either reside in the extracellular compartment or adsorb onto the cellular membrane.

Those molecules on the cell membrane come under the influence of the electrical field established by the transmembrane potential, and under that influence, alter their optical properties. The dyes used in our laboratory respond to changes in membrane potential by linearly and rapidly changing the strength of their fluorescent emission. The mechanism of this sensitivity is not yet understood for all dyes but in general involves a membrane potential-dependent change in dye molecule orientation or membrane binding.[31,34,35] Optical recording is insensitive to shock-induced artifacts because the dye molecules sense only the transmembrane potentials and do not respond to voltage gradients developed inside or outside of the cell. Appropriate optical instrumentation is needed to stimulate and collect the optical signals generated by the voltage-sensitive dye.

This laboratory has used a laser to excite dye fluorescence and a photodiode-based detector to measure fluorescence. We have developed fiber optic methods for delivering the laser light and collecting the fluorescence so that optical recordings could be made

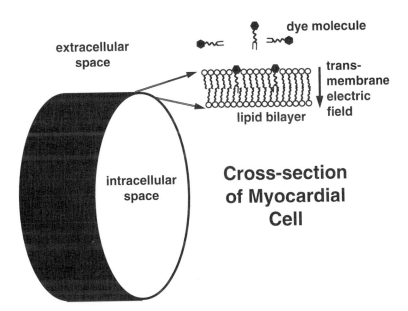

Figure 3. Voltage-sensitive dye mechanism. A cross-section of the a myocardial cell is shown along with a close-up of the lipid bilayer comprising a section of the cell membrane. Voltage-sensitive dye molecules reside in the extracellular space and adsorb onto the outer membrane leaflet of the myocardial cellular membrane. These dye molecules come under the influence of the transmembrane electric field established by the cellular membrane potential. The electric field is shown here directed inwards while the cell is at the resting potential.

from intact hearts.[36] We have also developed a technique called laser scanning in order to make multiple site optical recordings.[25] In laser scanning a single laser spot is repeatedly and rapidly scanned across a series of pre-determined sites on the surface of the heart while the resulting fluorescence emission is continuously recorded. An important example of the power of optical recording to study defibrillation is the report from another laboratory where a microscope-based method was used to record the responses of individual membrane segments within a single cell.[24]

Electrical Defibrillation

An understanding of defibrillation encompasses phenomena and mechanisms operating across a variety of levels. The summary flow chart in Fig. 4 begins with a cardiac fibrillatory process (*FIBRILLATION*). According to Moe, the rapid, disorganized elec-

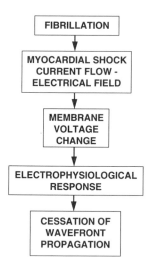

Figure 4. Flowchart of phenomena involved in defibrillation. See text for discussion.

trical activity characteristic of fibrillation is due to the simultaneous propagation of multiple cardiac impulses (wandering wavelet hypothesis).[37] These impulses undergo a continuous process of collision and splitting and so vary in number and size. This process is considered to be self-sustaining so that once it is initiated, it will not terminate on its own. (Fibrillation has been called perniciously stable.[13])

Moe developed his hypothesis using computer modeling, but Allessie demonstrated, during atrial fibrillation, the presence of multiple wavefronts which followed continuously shifting pathways in the course of spawning other wavefronts or dying out.[38] Whenever electrical propagation ceased in an atrium, it was always observed to restart following activation by an impulse arising from the other atrium. This led to the observation that atrial fibrillation required a minimum number of wavelets in both atria in order to sustain itself. Thus, even if a given wavefront spontaneously terminates, others survive and spawn new "daughter" wavelets which perpetuate fibrillation. Other investigators have mapped electrical activity during ventricular fibrillation and demonstrated similar multiple wavelets of activation.[39-41] Ventricular fibrillation has not been as completely mapped (as the atrium) because it supports propagation in a large, 3-dimensional mass.

Highly detailed mapping has been carried out on parts of the epicardial surface[42] but comparable electrode densities of intramural recording sites would render the ventricle a veritable pin cushion of needle electrodes. This task also represents a formidable engineering challenge since it is estimated to require 30,000 simultaneous electrogram recordings to adequately map fibrillation on the epicardium alone.[43] Near-term information about fibrillation will have to come from the use of smaller hearts or computer simulations. For example, the topological construct called a spiral wave describes a form of 3-dimensional reentry capable of reproducing the erratic activation characteristic of fibrillation.[44]

There will be a wide disparity in electrical activation states throughout the ventricle during fibrillation. Some areas of myocardium will be depolarized and so are refractory to ordinary stimulation, whereas other areas will be repolarized, although usually not completely to the resting potential,[45] and so are capable of excitation by electrical stimulation. Other areas of the ventricle will occupy intermediate levels of membrane potential at the moment of shock delivery. This characteristic non-uniformity of electrical state will exert a strong influence on the electrophysiological responses of the myocardium to a defibrillation shock.

The next step in the flow chart of Fig. 4 is the application of a high voltage defibrillation shock (*MYOCARDIAL SHOCK CURRENT FLOW - ELECTRICAL FIELD*). It is widely accepted that it is the flow of current through the heart which causes defibrillation. It has been established that defibrillation requires establishing a certain minimum electrical field throughout the heart.[46] Therefore, electrode systems which produce non-uniform electrical fields within the heart fail to minimize defibrillation thresholds because a shock strong enough to elevate all of the heart beyond a threshold field strength will raise some areas beyond the minimum value needed for defibrillation.

The third step in the flow chart considers the nature of the coupling between the shock electrical field and the myocardial membrane (*MEMBRANE VOLTAGE CHANGE*). The shock will give rise to changes in cellular potential wherever shock current traverses the myocardial membrane. Even though a shock is applied to the fluids bathing the heart, the flow of shock current is split between the intercellular and extracellular conductive compartments. Shock current is forced to cross cellular membranes wherever it leaves or enters the intercellular compartment. The flow of current across the cardiac membrane causes a voltage drop which will either elevate (depolarize) or lower (hyperpolarize) the membrane potential. When the shock current crosses into the cell from the extracellular space it hyperpolarizes the cell because the resulting membrane

voltage drop causes the inside of the cell to become more negative
with respect to the outside. When the shock current crosses from
the inside of the cell to the outside, a depolarization results.[a] Given
that a shock electrical field induces changes in membrane potential,
the electrical response of the myocardium to such voltage changes
can be expected to strongly depend on the magnitude, polarity and
distribution of these voltage changes.

The fourth step in the flow chart (*ELECTROPHYSIOLOGI-
CAL RESPONSE*) concerns the focus of this chapter. Action potential stimulation is an example of what is considered an electrophysiological response. Earlier it was described how depolarization
of cardiac membrane from the resting potential results in stimulation of an action potential. The same would be expected to occur
during defibrillation when those membranes which are sufficiently
repolarized, and hence excitable, are brought to the stimulation
threshold by shock-induced depolarization. Stimulation cannot be
the only electrophysiological response to a defibrillation shock.
First, the ventricle can be expected to reside at a variety of membrane potentials at the moment of shock delivery. Second, the shock
electrical field can be expected to vary in strength from place to
place. Third, the shock electrical field can be expected to develop
either depolarizing or hyperpolarizing voltage changes. Therefore, a
variety of electrophysiologic responses can be expected to arise as a
consequence of a shock. The major portion of this chapter will describe the type and nature of the responses observed.

The last step in the flow chart is *CESSATION OF
WAVEFRONT PROPAGATION*. The most commonly accepted hypothesis for defibrillation is that stimulation of excitable myocardium causes termination of the fibrillation wavefronts which support fibrillation. There are two assumptions embodied in this
concept. The first is that fibrillation relies upon the ability of the
"wandering wavelets" to continuously encounter myocardium which
is able to generate an action potential upstroke, i.e. excitable tissue.
If a wavefront invades an area of myocardium still refractory from
earlier activation, or if it cannot generate a sufficient amount of depolarizing current, this wavefront is expected to die out for lack of
ability to stimulate. The second part of this hypothesis is the belief
that if a shock stimulates the excitable myocardium in a portion of

---

a.   These patterns of membrane voltage changes should not be confused with those
     arising from the inward and outward movements of ionic channel currents. In
     the case of defibrillation the electromotive force (the defibrillator) lies outside
     of the membrane while in the case of ionic channel currents the electromotive
     force is generated across the membrane.

the ventricle, then the resulting depolarization prevents continued propagation of the wavelets needed to support fibrillation. Two contending theories of defibrillation, the *critical mass hypothesis*[5-7] and the *upper limit of vulnerability hypothesis*,[4] both feature fibrillation wavefront termination by this means. The critical mass hypothesis maintains that eliminating most or all fibrillation wavefronts in this manner will cause defibrillation. The upper limit of vulnerability hypothesis maintains that elimination of fibrillation wavefronts in this manner is a necessary but not sufficient condition for defibrillation.

This chapter will discuss how the electrophysiological effects of shock lead to defibrillation from the point of view of wavefront termination according to the above mechanisms. It will also discuss other possible pathways to defibrillation which exploit electrophysiological effects other than stimulation.

Electrophysiological Effects of Shocks

The question of whether defibrillation shocks actually stimulate myocardium—and, if so, how—was first addressed by Jones and co-workers.[18] They found that high electrical field strength shocks stimulated action potentials in myocardial cell cultures. The action potentials evoked by the shocks, except for the very high strength ones, were normal in appearance. The cell culture preparation permitted the investigators to cancel the artifacts caused by the shocks. However, use of cell cultures left open the possibility that actual defibrillation in whole hearts would reveal significantly different stimulating processes.

Our laboratory was able to verify that defibrillation shocks stimulated normal appearing action potentials by using the technique of optical recording to study the response to defibrillation threshold strength shocks applied during either pacing[9,22,47] or fibrillation.[48,49] Fig. 5 shows action potential stimulation in an isolated rabbit heart caused by shocks applied during steady pacing. A paced heart rather than a heart in fibrillation was used in order to investigate the effects of shocks under controlled conditions. The optical traces in Fig. 5 show pairs of action potentials elicited by a pacing stimulus (left) and a shock applied through defibrillation electrodes (right). The shock timings were adjusted so that they fell after full repolarization of the previous action potential and were delivered while the myocardium was fully excitable. The strength of the shock was adjusted to produce shock strengths in the range of

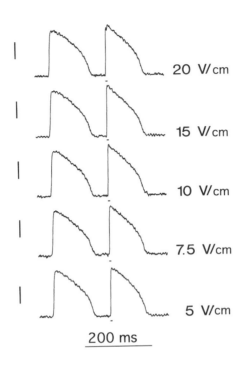

Figure 5. Shock applied during diastole. This figure shows optical action potentials recorded on the surface of a rabbit ventricle. The leftmost action potentials were stimulated by ventricular pacing. The rightmost action potentials were stimulated by the shock. The time and duration of the shock is indicated by the short black bar underlying the rightmost optical action potentials. The local shock electrical field strength in V/cm is indicated on the right. The vertical bars indicate the height of a 1% change in fluorescence intensity.

5-20 V/cm at the recording site. It can be seen that strong shocks elicited normal appearing action potentials which differed little from those produced by the pacing stimulus. Thus, for shocks applied during diastole, defibrillation shocks appear to behave as ordinary stimuli.

The fibrillating heart will have areas of myocardium in all states of refractoriness and excitability and thus the model was used to investigate the dependence of the response on the action potential phase. Fig. 6 shows optical recordings in cases where the shock fell at the earliest portion of the relatively refractory phase.

Pacing stimuli applied this soon before full repolarization cannot always be expected to elicit propagated responses.[50] This is because the inward sodium current responsible for the propagation of the cardiac impulse is largely inactivated by membrane depolarization. Rather, strong pacing stimuli evoke graded responses which

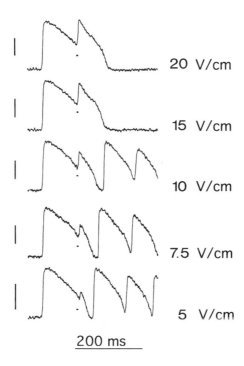

Figure 6. Shock applied during late repolarization. This figure is similar to Fig. 5 except that the shock was applied during late repolarization. The action potentials were stimulated by ventricular pacing. Graded responses were stimulated by the 5 and 7.5 V/cm shocks. The Additional Depolarization Time (ADT) response (delaying final repolarization of the myocardium) was elicited by the 10, 15, and 20 V/cm shocks. Extrasystolic action potentials arose after the 5, 7.5 and 10 V/cm shocks. The time and duration of the shock is indicated by the very short horizontal black bar underlying the optical action potentials.

indicate local depolarization of the membrane. Graded responses are diminished, slowly developing, sub-threshold responses which sometimes give rise to a delayed propagated response if the myocardium surrounding the electrode has repolarized sufficiently to become excitable again.[50]

The bottom two traces of Fig. 6 show that shocks of low to moderate field strengths (5-7.5 V/cm) were able to evoke a graded response like those elicited by strong pacing stimuli. These optical records are similar to microelectrode recordings taken from an in situ canine heart by Zhou and co-workers.[21]

In contrast, the response of the rabbit myocardium to shocks of higher field strength, ≥ 10 V/cm, departs from that predicted for shocks acting as ordinary stimuli. Here we see that the shocks evoked larger and more sustained depolarizations. Shocks of 15-20

V/cm gave rise to responses which are best characterized as new, extrasystolic action potentials. This result could not be obtained using ordinary local stimulation. Therefore, the analogy between defibrillation shocks and stimuli breaks down for shocks producing a high field strength at times when the myocardium is still halfway repolarized from the preceding action potential.

The result of strong shocks applied before full repolarization of the action potential is to produce additional membrane depolarization which, in effect, prolongs the time until full repolarization. The additional depolarization time induced by the shock increases with the shock strength. The effect of high strength shocks, many times the diastolic pacing threshold strength of 0.6-1.8 V/cm, applied to partially depolarized myocardium produced rapidly developed, long lasting depolarizing responses far different from the usual sort of graded response produced by ordinary stimulation.[51]

The traces in Fig. 6 also illustrate a phenomenon emphasized as a possible component of the defibrillation process, namely the upper limit of vulnerability.[4] It is known that a stimulus can cause fibrillation if delivered at a critical time during the T-wave of the ECG (the vulnerable period), i.e. a range of shock strengths and timings were found to induce extrasystoles and fibrillation.[52-54] The extrasystolic action potentials seen arising after repolarization of the first action potential in the bottom 3 traces of Fig. 6 result from just such arrhythmic activity (elsewhere in the preparation) induced by the shock (top 2 traces of Fig. 6). As has been found in the canine,[54] these arrhythmias in the rabbit decrease in likelihood with increasing shock strength.

The effects of a shock applied to myocardium recently depolarized by a preceding wavefront must also be considered when developing an understanding of defibrillation mechanisms. Fig. 7 shows the effects of shocks applied early during the plateau phase of the action potential (when the myocardium should be absolutely refractory). The lowest shock strength, 5 V/cm, had no effect on the action potential, as would be predicted for ordinary stimuli. (The extrasystole following the paced action potential is due to the vulnerability phenomenon, i.e. the higher intensity shocks caused an activation elsewhere which spread throughout the preparation.)

In the remaining traces, the increased shock strengths caused depolarizing deflections which increased in amplitude and duration with the increases in shock strength. Because the time course of the shock response traces out the phases of action potential repolarization, we have hypothesized that the shock evoked a new action po-

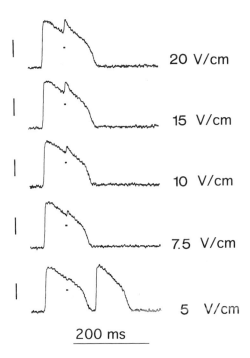

20 V/cm

15 V/cm

10 V/cm

7.5 V/cm

5 V/cm

200 ms

Figure 7. Shock applied during the plateau phase. This figure is similar to Fig. 6 except that the shock was applied during the plateau phase. There was no local response to the 5 V/cm shock. The 7.5 V/cm shock caused a small depolarizing deflection. The Additional Depolarization Time (ADT) response was elicited by the 10, 15 and 20 V/cm shocks. The ADT response delayed final repolarization of the myocardium. The action potentials were stimulated by ventricular pacing. The time and duration of the shock is indicated by the very short horizontal black bar underlying the optical action potentials.

tential, the upstroke of which arose from a depolarized level. The fact that shocks were able to elicit active responses from myocardium already depolarized (and, hence, expected by classical theory to be absolutely refractory to stimulation) lends strong credence to the notion that defibrillation shocks cannot be considered to act as ordinary electrical stimuli.

The literature had no prior reports of an additional phase of depolarization in response to a strong shock. Shocks were expected to cause stimulation in excitable myocardium but to have no effect on refractory myocardium.[55] Instead we found that defibrillation threshold strength shocks evoked active responses from supposedly refractory myocardium. We described this phenomenon as the *Additional Depolarization Time response*.[22] It was found that this additional depolarization time was accompanied by an equal prolonga-

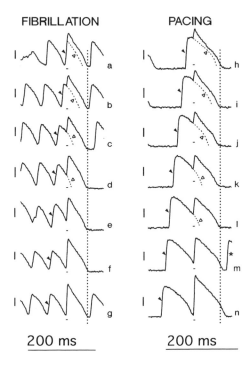

Figure 8. Shocks applied during fibrillation and pacing. Optical recordings compare shock responses obtained at the same site during fibrillation and pacing at a 300 ms cycle length. Traces *a-g* (*FIBRILLATION*) were obtained from the same site as traces *h-n(PACING)*. Shock times and durations are indicated by the very short horizontal black bars under each trace. Shocks were applied just at end of (*a*) or following (*b-g*) action potential upstroke. Filled arrowheads indicate the upstroke phase immediately preceding each shock. Open arrowheads in traces *a-d* mark dashed curves showing likely time course of repolarization (based on contour of immediately preceding action potential) had the shock not been applied. In traces *h-l*, dashed curves, indicated by open arrowheads, show the repolarization phase of a control action potential. Vertical dashed line shows Constant Repolarization Time response following defibrillation shock delivery during fibrillation but not during pacing. Asterisk indicates induced extrasystole. All shocks were 1.25 J.

tion of the effective refractory period. This result introduced a new component into hypotheses for defibrillation since, in addition to the proposed ability to extinguish wavefronts through stimulation, shocks could extend the refractoriness of myocardium already depolarized by prior impulses.[47,56]

The initial data for the action potential prolonging effects of shocks on depolarized myocardium was obtained during steady pacing. The question of whether the same phenomenon would be observed during fibrillation was resolved by another study.[49] Fig. 8 shows an illustration taken from this work in which the effects of a shock applied during fibrillation and pacing are compared. The traces were obtained from separate defibrillation episodes in which the shock was delivered 30 s after the start of fibrillation. Some defibrillation traces show repolarization to a steady level after the shock (traces *d-f*) while the rest show extrasystoles occurring before quiescence.

The shocks caused action potential stimulation when they arrived late in the repolarization phase (traces *e-g*) and caused the production of additional depolarization time when they arrived while the myocardium was depolarized (traces *a-d*). Thus, defibrillation shocks have been found to prolong the action potential just as seen for shocks applied during pacing.

The most remarkable difference between the effects of defibrillation threshold strength shocks applied during pacing and fibrillation was that, during the latter, the shock caused the myocardium to repolarize at a constant time after the shock. This constancy is indicated by the dashed vertical line running through the fibrillation/defibrillation traces of Fig. 8 at the moment of full repolarization We called this striking behavior the *Constant Repolarization Time* (CRT) response.[49] This constancy in post-shock repolarization time was not seen for shocks applied during pacing (e.g. right side of Fig. 8).

We have found that shocks which are not strong enough to reliably defibrillate do not typically evoke the CRT response. Such shocks are able to prolong depolarization time through the additional depolarization time mechanism. This suggests that there is a "threshold" for the CRT response.

Acute Deleterious Electrophysiologic Effects of Shocks

The preceding discussion focused upon what might be considered to be the "normal" effects of shocks and not the ability of very high shock fields to transiently or permanently damage the cells. Jones and co-workers found that shocks of strength in excess of 50 V/cm caused tachyarrhythmia, relaxed arrest followed by transient tachyarrhythmia and arrest with contracture and cellular fibrillation in studies of cultured cells.[18] These arrhythmias were accompanied by cellular depolarization thought to be due to electro-mechanical disruption of the sarcolemma leading to either transient or permanent membrane damage. Moore and Spear also showed that a single shock could cause prolonged membrane depolarization and myocardial inexcitability in Purkinje fibers.[19] Microelectrode studies of superfused papillary muscles also showed that shocks in excess of 50 V/cm caused prolonged depolarization and pacing failure although the inability to pace was not entirely explained by membrane depolarization.[57]

Studies of conduction disturbances in the in situ canine heart confirmed the predictions of the in vitro studies by finding persistent impulse slowing and block in the area experiencing high shock field strengths.[58] These indications of shock damage may account for the decrease in defibrillation success rate for shock strengths beyond the defibrillation threshold.[59] Also, the observation that biphasic waveforms produce less damage and fewer arrhythmias than monophasic waveforms is hypothesized to explain, in part, the greater efficacy of the biphasic shock waveform over that of the monophasic shock.[58,60] While these deleterious effects of shocks no doubt influence the overall process of electrical defibrillation, it remains to be proven that these processes significantly affect ordinary defibrillation (i.e., at energies not in excess of 100% probability of defibrillation).

Effects of Shocks on Cardiac Membrane Voltage

It was surprising to find that shocks evoked active responses while the myocardium was in a state of "absolute" refractoriness. This is because the sodium current responsible for the generation of the action potential should have been inactivated by membrane depolarization and because the prior literature spoke of the "depolarizing" effects of shocks.[8,55] It was not clear whether "depolarization" was meant to be synonymous with action potential stimulation or whether it was meant that shocks explicitly depolarized cardiac membranes. If the latter were true, then shocks could not evoke active responses because such a short depolarizing current pulse could not give rise to the prolonged depolarization seen on the optical recordings. The view that shocks only depolarized cardiac membranes was eventually refuted in a seminal paper by Plonsey and Barr[61] which modeled the effects of shock fields (currents) on a one-dimensional cable of cells. These authors demonstrated that shocks could give rise to both depolarizing and hyperpolarizing membrane voltage changes. We have adopted the general idea of bipolar shock-induced membrane voltage changes and used it to explain how strong shocks cause an additional period of depolarization in activated cells.

Our laboratory has conducted preliminary experiments to examine whether membrane depolarization by the shock is responsible for producing the Additional Depolarization Time using an

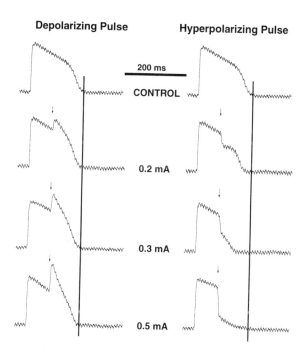

Figure 9. Effects of uniform myocardial membrane voltage changes. Optical action potentials recorded from the tip of a perfused rabbit papillary muscle. Brief current pulses (5 ms duration; indicated by arrows) were applied along the length of the papillary muscle. The leftmost traces show the effects of depolarizing voltage changes; the rightmost the effects of hyperpolarizing voltage changes. The vertical lines indicate the expected moment of full repolarization following the control action potentials. The strength of the current applied to the bundle is given in mA.

isolated, coronary-perfused papillary muscle from a rabbit heart.[62] This biologically simulated a one-dimensional cable of cells and allowed us to experimentally impose either hyperpolarizing or depolarizing changes in membrane potential at the tip of the papillary muscle. Fig. 9 shows optical action potentials recorded in response to purely depolarizing or purely hyperpolarizing membrane voltage changes imposed by the application of current along the length of the papillary muscle. The left column of optical action potentials shows the effect of depolarizing membrane potential changes. As expected, increasing amounts of depolarizing current caused larger depolarizing changes in membrane potential. However, these current-induced depolarizations did not prolong the duration of the action potential. This is because, even though the membrane was depolarized by the current pulse, the cardiac cell responded passively.

This is in contrast with the results in Fig. 7 which show an active depolarizing response which delayed final repolarization. Electrophysiological studies of myocardium using the intracellular current injection have also shown that a depolarizing pulse will not prolong the action potential.[63] The right column of optical recordings shows the effects of hyperpolarizing current pulses applied midway through the action potential. Increasing the strength of the hyperpolarizing current increased the amplitude of the downward deflection on the optically recorded membrane potential. A hyperpolarizing voltage change alone caused a shortening of the action potential rather than a prolongation of the depolarized state.

One consequence of the membrane hyperpolarization illustrated on the right of Fig. 9 was that the myocardium regained its excitability because the membrane potential was quickly reduced to its resting level. This suggested a possible hypothesis, as yet unproven, of how defibrillation shocks produce the Additional Depolarization Time response.

Fig. 10 shows a cylindrical cross-section of a myocardial fiber as a simplified representation of the unit bundle structure of the myocardium. The myocardial fiber is immersed in a left-to-right flow of shock current, some of which, as indicated by the arrows, enters and exits the cell by crossing the myocardial membrane. The portion of shock current which enters the left half hyperpolarizes (H) that patch of the membrane while the right side is depolarized (D). The hypothetical responses of the left and right sides of the cell are shown in the corners. A shock is applied during the plateau phase. The shock causes the right side of the cell to undergo further membrane depolarization. Since the sodium channels in this membrane patch are already inactivated, the shock does not give rise to an active response (as shown by the example in Fig. 9). The membrane potential of the right side of the cell is shown decaying back to plateau potential after the end of the shock. The left side of the cell is shown undergoing prompt hyperpolarization down to the vicinity of the resting potential.

The sodium channels in this abruptly hyperpolarized membrane patch are now able to undergo restoration of excitability since the negative membrane potential shifts the sodium channels out of their inactivated states. At the end of the shock, or perhaps during it, these channels undergo prompt excitation under the depolarizing influence of the right side of the cell.

This left patch of the membrane has had its ongoing action potential prematurely terminated by the shock through hyperpolarization and, through reactivation of the sodium channel, experi-

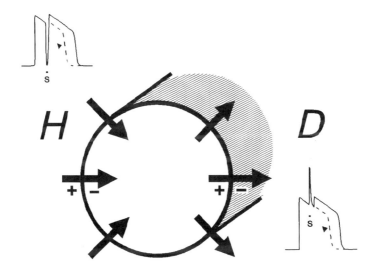

Figure 10. Hypothetical mechanism for Additional Depolarization Time. A cross-section of an idealized myocardial cell is shown. Shock current (*bold arrows*) is shown flowing into and out of the cell, from left to right, by crossing the cellular membrane. The halves of the cell that undergo membrane hyperpolarization and depolarization as a result of this current are indicated by *H* and *D*, respectively. Two hypothetical, shocked action potentials from each side of the cell are shown on the upper left and lower right side of the figure. The small black bar labeled *S* indicates the time and duration of the shock current. The repolarization phase of a hypothetical, control action potential is shown by the dashed tracing indicated by the filled arrowhead. Shock induced premature hyperpolarization, by shifting sodium channels out of their inactivated state, could permit their prompt reactivation from nearby depolarized membrane — resulting in a secondary action potential.

ences a new action potential. It is the depolarizing influence of this newly excited action potential which maintains the entire cell at a depolarized potential for a prolonged period outlasting the duration of the depolarization expected for the original action potential.

The optical recording method used here did not demonstrate these separate processes because it registered the integrated voltage responses of the entire cell. The optical signal showed the intrinsic depolarizing response of the reactivated sodium channels and the subsequent action potential which gives rise to the apparent additional depolarization time. According to this scheme the additional depolarization evoked by the shock is actually the duration of the reexcited action potential. The Constant Repolarization Time response seen in defibrillation (Fig. 8) is a manifestation of a constant duration of the reexcited action potential evoked by the shock from a fibrillating ventricle (see Dillon[49] for an explanation for the Constant Repolarization Time response).

The above mechanism explains the time and shock strength dependence of the shock responses and has the advantage of not requiring any novel electrophysiology: the larger the shock strength, the deeper the membrane is hyperpolarized and with it the greater the degree of sodium channel reactivation and the larger and longer the subsequent depolarizing response.[47] Weak shocks applied late in the action potential would excite responses based on their ability to bring sodium channels up to their excitation threshold level. Such shocks applied at earlier times would find sodium channels in less excitable states and so refractory to stimulation through depolarization. As shock field strength is increased, the shock is capable of restoring the sodium channels to greater levels of excitability and thus provoking active responses. Thus shocks would be capable of eliciting any of a continuum of shock responses depending upon the level of membrane potential and the local shock field strength. Ultimately the shock field strength could attain a level capable of eliciting a new action potential at any point during the action potential save during the upstroke phase itself.

Although the hypothetical mechanism illustrated in Fig. 10 remains unproven, there are experimental results which support its feasibility. For example, Knisely and co-workers used optical recording to demonstrate that externally applied shocks could develop bipolar changes of membrane potential.[24] These recordings were obtained from a single cell and so may not exactly mirror the response of myocardial fibers to electric fields. However, these results clearly show that it is possible to develop large differences in membrane potential across very short distances—in this case, the length of a single cell. Thus it is reasonable to expect that shocks could produce bipolar voltage changes across the width of a single myocardial unit bundle.

A computer model of the interaction between the shock's electrical field and the membrane potential has been developed by Krassowska and co-workers.[64] This model indicates that bipolar changes in membrane potential may arise at the ends of myocardial cells within a column of connected cells. These voltage changes arise because of discontinuities in intercellular conductivity due to the electrical resistance of the gap junctions connecting the cells.

Another crucial component of the hypothetical mechanism illustrated in Fig. 10 is the ability to rapidly bring the sodium channel out of the inactivated state. Swartz and Jones have shown that it was possible to accelerate the recovery of excitability in cells during the late phase of repolarization.[65]

Electrophysiological Responses and Fibrillation

Recent information makes it clear that there is no one electrophysiological phenomenon which can be said to characterize electrical defibrillation; rather, a variety of membrane responses can be found during defibrillation. This is because electrode systems presently in use create a non-uniform distribution of effective shock strength throughout the ventricle. (Chaps. 5 and 8) Also, fibrillation disrupts the electrical organization of the ventricle such that a shock will find the myocardium in a variety of excitability states. Thus, the electrophysiological response to a shock in any given area of the ventricle will be a function of state of electrical activation and the local effective shock strength.

Fig. 11 shows a schematic diagram of the ventricle and how the electrophysiological effects of a shock could be distributed throughout this myocardial mass. The schema is based upon measurements of shock voltage gradient found for shocks applied between electrodes placed on the ventricular apex and the right atrium.[66] (Be cautioned that this schematic representation is based on experimental data employing only one kind of electrode placement scheme. Other, possibly more complicated, patterns will result from different electrode placement schemes.)

The result, after some simplification, shows that the shock voltage gradient increases from base to apex and that, for the purposes of illustration, the shock strength ranges from values which have no discernible effect to those which cause membrane damage. It is assumed that a shock is applied during fibrillation.

At the base of the ventricle (A) there will be a zone where the shock will be so weak that it will have no effect on the action potential time course or on impulse propagation so that arrhythmic excitation there will continue unabated. In the next segment down towards the apex (B) the shock strength is strong enough to cause action potential stimulation in the most excitable myocardium.

This stimulation process also causes the affected myocardium to undergo a period of refractoriness which temporarily prevents it from participating in the fibrillation process. The fibrillating ventricle seldom attains the full resting potential so that the shock will most often be stimulating an action potential in partially refractory myocardium.[45] Further, the differing abilities of monophasic

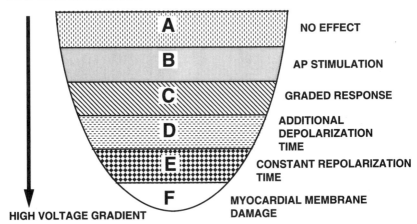

Figure 11. Schematic model of electrophysiological responses in the whole heart. The shock voltage gradient (*VG*) increases from the top towards the bottom of the heart. It is assumed that there is a distribution in membrane potentials representing all action potential phases at each of 6 different layers (*A-F*) in the heart. These layers are expected to yield a variety of electrophysiological responses to a shock as listed on the right side.

and biphasic waveforms to stimulate partially depolarized myocardium has been proposed to explain the ability of some biphasic shocks to defibrillate more readily than monophasic shocks.[67,68]

In the adjoining segment of ventricle (*C*) the shock has a sufficiently high intensity to evoke depolarizing responses from partially recovered myocardium, i.e. producing a graded response (e.g. bottom trace of Fig. 2) in addition to stimulating recovered myocardium. The brief period of depolarization elicited by the graded response could transiently block activation through the myocardium undergoing a graded response.[68] This transient block serves to set the stage for refibrillation according to the upper limit of vulnerability hypothesis.[12]

Further down (*D*) the shock field is strong enough to produce an Additional Depolarization Time response from relatively and absolutely refractory myocardium. The shock would delay the repolarization of the already depolarized myocardium and so make it refractory to immediate activation by cardiac impulses which may persist after the shock.

In addition to extending refractoriness within level *D*, the shock also exerts a homogenizing effect on the spatial disparity in repolarization times. As illustrated in Figs. 5-7, prolongation of the depolarized phase by a shock depends not only upon its strength but also on the timing of the shock relative to the membrane potential at the time of the shock. In the regime of shock strengths within myocardium represented by level D, the greatest prolongation of the depolarization will result from stimulation of the most repolarized myocardium while the least prolongation will be produced by the Additional Depolarization Time response elicited from the most depolarized (least repolarized) myocardium. Thus, after the shock, a complete action potential will ensue in the most repolarized myocardium while repolarization already underway in the most depolarized myocardium will continue, albeit slightly delayed. But, however small the amount of action potential prolongation produced in this most depolarized myocardium, it would still cause it to repolarize closer in time to that of the most repolarized myocardium stimulated by the shock.

A still stronger shock would cause even more of a prolongation of repolarization time in the most depolarized myocardium, while stimulating nearly the same action potential in the most repolarized myocardium, thus causing repolarization in these disparate areas of myocardium to occur even closer in time. In fact, we have found that graded increases in shock strength cause a progressive homogenization of the post-shock repolarization time during fibrillation.[69] This is because as the shock strength increases, the shock becomes capable of eliciting more of a complete, new action potential arising from a given level of membrane potential. The ultimate expression of the progressive homogenization of repolarization with increasing shock strength would occur when the shock becomes capable of stimulating an action potential of constant duration when applied at any level of membrane voltage during the action potential.

This phenomenon, the Constant Repolarization Time response, would occur within the higher regime of shock strengths encountered in the next myocardial level (E) in our hypothetical model of shock effects. The shock would thus eliminate the dispersion in refractoriness present in that part of the fibrillating ventricle and thus could make it resistant to prompt reentry induction. Thus, a cardiac impulse would be either uniformly conducted or blocked in this region but would not likely undergo immediate reentrant excitation.

Lastly, in the area of the apical shock electrode (F), the shock field strength causes temporary or permanent membrane damage such that impulse conduction is impaired and tachyarrhythmias possibly arise after the shock.

Present defibrillation hypotheses posit that any cardiac impulses present after the shock either result from failure to terminate all pre-shock wavefronts[5-7] or arise from reentrant activity induced by the shock itself.[4] As described above, the presence or absence of post-shock activity is determined by the ability of the shock to stimulate action potentials or graded responses. Our work suggests that stimulation may not be the only electrophysiological response underlying defibrillation.[11,22,49]

The crux of understanding the defibrillation process lies in being able to integrate the spatial and temporal interactions of shock-evoked electrophysiological responses. That is, how do these responses affect the fibrillation wavefronts existing at the time of the shock and how does ventricular activation proceed after the shock? We used laser scanning [22,30] to follow the time course of the action potential before, during and after the shock at 100 sites on the surface of a perfused rabbit heart. These data show that *sub-threshold* shocks can stimulate the myocardium in front of the fibrillation wavefront. The resulting depolarization, however, itself propagated and so arrhythmic activity in this area continued.

This suggests that an electrophysiological response other than simple premature stimulation of the most excitable myocardium is needed to terminate propagating activity during fibrillation. Figs. 6 and 7 show that strong shocks are able to evoke an active depolarizing response out of already depolarized myocardium (Additional Depolarization Time). Fig. 8 shows that the combined effects of stimulation and Additional Depolarization Time causes a Constant Repolarization Time in the rabbit heart during defibrillation.

We have shown that a shock which defibrillates, resynchronizes repolarization observed on the ventricular surface.[49] In general, the disparity in post-shock repolarization times was dependent on shock strength.[70] This is because a local effective shock field strength strong enough only to stimulate an action potential from excitable myocardium will cause the excitable areas to repolarize much later than those areas of the heart which were refractory. These refractory areas will continue to repolarize with the asynchrony imposed on them by their disparity in activation times.

By contrast, a shock strong enough to produce the Additional Depolarization Time response will not only cause delayed repolarization in the myocardium which is stimulated by the shock, it will also delay repolarization in the areas already depolarized. The power of this resynchronizing ability is that it conditions the ventricle to resist continued fibrillation by any impulses which persist after the shock. If a shock is strong enough to cleanly and promptly defibrillate (Pattern 1[6] or Type A[4] defibrillation), then the synchrony of post-shock repolarization times could be irrelevant.

The synchrony of repolarization would be important when electrical activation persists in some area of the ventricle after the shock since it would have the potential to undergo reentrant excitation if it encounters asynchronously repolarizing tissue. In these cases the shock may only transiently organize ventricular activation before full fibrillation resumes.[6] In other cases, defibrillation may ultimately occur after a run of one or more post-shock extrasystolic activations (Pattern 2[6] or Type B[4] defibrillation) The degree of repolarization resynchronization and the fraction of myocardium undergoing resynchronization may determine the outcome of a shock.

Conclusion

This chapter has described the range of electrophysiological responses shocks are capable of evoking in a fibrillating ventricle. We have also attempted to relate these responses to the overall defibrillation process. Other discussions of how these responses arise and interact to cause defibrillation can be found elsewhere (see reviews[11-13,69] and discussion of Dillon[49]). It is clear from Fig. 11 however that any complete description of defibrillation, whether successful or failed, must account for the variety of interactions which arise as a result of the non-uniform distribution of both shock strength and myocardial action potential phases.

The experimental electrophysiologic data from our laboratory presented in this review were obtained from isolated perfused rabbit hearts. Sweeney and co-workers[56] have demonstrated a prolongation of refractoriness due to moderate shocks which they attributed to stimulation of a graded response. We have similarly investigated the effects of shocks on effective refractory period using strong shocks. We found the same dependence of refractory period prolongation on the shock strength and timing in the in situ canine as found for the prolongation of the optically recorded action potential in the in vitro rabbit heart.[47] Furthermore, our preliminary optical investigations of defibrillation in the intact canine model have demonstrated the Additional Depolarization Time response (Fig. 12), an important finding since it had only previously been demonstrated in vitro.

Lastly, Franz and co-workers have made monophasic action potential recordings in humans during defibrillator implantation

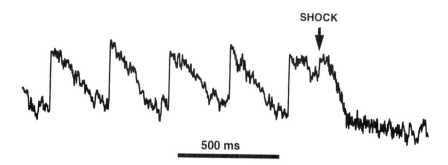

Figure 12. In situ optical recording of defibrillation from the canine. This in situ optical recording shows the last 2 s of arrhythmia before termination by a shock delivered at the time indicated by the arrow. This shock evoked an Additional Depolarization Time response and so demonstrates that this phenomenon is not peculiar to the isolated, perfused rabbit heart where it was first observed.

testing. (In this method, the injury potential produced by the catheter traces out the time course of the action potential.) They found that recordings from two widely separated locales not only showed an increase in post-shock repolarization time with increasing shock strength, but also an increasing synchrony in post-shock repolarization time which was associated with successful defibrillation.[71]

ACKNOWLEDGMENTS:

We would like to acknowledge the support of the Sidney Kimmel Cardiovascular Research Center and Program Project Grant HL 30557 and Grant HL 49246 from the Heart Blood and Lung Institute of the National Institutes of Health. Fig. 3 is adapted with permission.[22] Fig. 8 is adapted with permission from Circulation.[49] Fig. 10 is adapted with permission from Circulation Research.[23]

1. Prevost JL, Battelli F. Sur quelques effets de decharges electriques sur le coeur des mammiferes. Comptes Rendus Acad Sci 1899;129:1267-1268.
2. Gurvich NL, Yuniev GS. Restoration of regular rhythm in the mammalian fibrillating heart. Am Rev Sov Med 1946;3:236-239.
3. Hooker DR, Kouwenhoven WB, Langworthy OR. The effects of alternating electrical currents on the heart. Am J Physiol 1933;103:444-454.
4. Chen PS, Shibata N, Dixon EG, et al. Activation during ventricular defibrillation in open-chest dogs. Evidence of complete cessation and regeneration of ventricular fibrillation after unsuccessful shocks. J Clin Invest 1986;77:810-823.
5. Witkowski FX, Penkoske PA, Plonsey R. Mechanism of cardiac defibrillation in open-chest dogs with unipolar DC-coupled simultaneous activation and shock potential recordings. Circulation 1990;82:244-260.
6. Mower MM, Mirowski M, Spear JF, et al. Patterns of ventricular activity during catheter defibrillation. Circulation 1974;69:858-861.

7. Zipes DP, Fischer J, King RM, et al. Termination of ventricular fibrillation in dogs by depolarizing a critical amount of myocardium. Am J Cardiol 1975;36:37-44.
8. Geddes LA, Niebauer MJ, Babbs CF, et al. Fundamental criteria underlying the efficacy and safety of defibrillating waveforms. Med & Biol Eng & Comput 1985;23:122-130.
9. Dillon S, Wit AL. Transmembrane voltage changes recorded during counter-shock in normal rhythm. Circulation 1987;76:IV-242.(abstract)
10. Dillon SM, Wit AL. Use of voltage sensitive dyes to investigate electrical defibrillation. Proc IEEE Eng in Med and Biol 1988;10:215-216.
11. Dillon SM: The electrophysiological effects of defibrillation shocks, In: Josephson ME, Wellens HJJ (eds) Tachycardias: Mechanisms and Management. Mount Kisco, NY, Futura Press, 1993 pp 457-477.
12. Chen PS, Wolf PD, Ideker RE. Mechanism of cardiac defibrillation. A different point of view. Circulation 1991;84:913-919.
13. Witkowski FX, Kerber RE. Currently known mechanisms underlying direct current external and internal cardiac defibrillation. J Cardiovasc Electrophysiol 1991;2:562-572.
14. Ideker RE, Wolf PD, Tang ASL: Mechanisms of defibrillation, In: Tacker WA (ed) Defibrillation of the heart. ICDs, AEDs, and Manual. St. Louis, Mosby, 1994 pp 15-45.
15. Spach MS, Barr RC, Serwer GA, et al. Extracellular potentials related to intercellular action potentials in the dog purkinje system. Circ Res 1972;30:505-519.
16. Biermann M, Shenasa M, Borgreffe M, et al. The interpretation of cardiac electrograms, In: Shenasa M, Borgreffe M, Breithardt G, et al (eds) Cardiac Mapping. Mount Kisco, NY, Futura, 1993 pp 11-34.
17. Pearce JA, Bourland JD, Neilsen W, et al. Myocardial stimulation with ultrashort duration current pulses. PACE 1982;5:52-58.
18. Jones JL, Lepeschkin E, Jones RE, et al. Response of cultured myocardial cells to countershock-type electrical field stimulation. Am J Physiol 1978;235:H214-H222.
19. Moore EN, Spear JF: Electrophysiologic studies on the initiation, prevention, and termination of ventricular fibrillation, In: Zipes DP, Jalife J (eds) Cardiac Electrophysiology and Arrhythmias. Orlando, Grune & Stratton Inc., 1985, pp 315-322.
20. Witkowski FX, Penkoske PA. A new fabrication technique for directly coupled transmural cardiac electrodes. Am J Physiol 1988;254:H804-H810.
21. Zhou X, Knisley SB, Wolf PD, et al. Prolongation of repolarization time by electric field stimulation with monophasic and biphasic shocks in open-chest dogs. Circ Res 1991;68:1761-1767.
22. Dillon SM: Use of optical recording for investigating electrical defibrillation, In: Clinical Application of Modern Image Technologies II. Proceedings SPIE Progress in Biomedical Optics. Bellingham, WA, SPIE, 1994, pp 387-396.
23. Dillon SM. Optical recordings in the rabbit heart show that defibrillation strength shocks prolong the duration of depolarization and the refractory period. Circ Res 1991;69:842-856.
24. Knisley SB, Blitchington TF, Hill BC, et al. Optical measurements of transmembrane potential changes during electrical field stimulation of ventricular cells. Circ Res 1993;72:255-270.
25. Dillon S, Morad M. A new laser scanning system for measuring action potential propagation in the heart. Science 1981;214:453-456.
26. Hill BC, Courtney KR. Design of a multi-point laser scanned optical monitor of cardiac action potential propagation. Ann Biomed Eng 1987;15:567-577.
27. Fujii S, Hirota A, Kamino K. Optical recording of the development of electrical activity in embryonic chick heart during early phases of cardiogenesis. J Physiol (Lond) 1981;311:147-160.

28. Davidenko JM, Pertsov AV, Salomonz R, et al. Stationary and drifting spiral waves of excitation in isolated cardiac muscle. Nature 1992;355:349-351.
29. Hirano K, Sawanobori T, Hiraoka M. Circus movement tachycardia examined by the optical recording and by the computer simulation. Jap Heart J 1982;23:109-111.
30. Dillon SM: Optical mapping, In: Shenasa M, Borgreffe M, Breithardt G, Haverkamp W, Hindricks G (eds) Cardiac Mapping. Mount Kisco, NY, Futura, 1993, pp 587-606.
31. Waggoner AS, Grinvald A. Mechanisms of rapid changes of potential sensitive dyes. Ann NY Acad Sci 1977;303:217-241.
32. Cohen LB, Salzberg BM. Optical measurement of membrane potential. Rev Physiol Biochem Pharmacol 1978;83:35-88.
33. Waggoner AS. Dye indicators of membrane potential. Ann Rev Biophys Bioeng 1979;8:47-68.
34. George EB, Nyirjesy P, Basson M, et al. Impermeant potential-sensitive oxonol dyes. I. Evidence for an "On-Off" mechanism. J Memb Biol 1988;103:245-253.
35. Fluhler E, Burnham VG, Loew LM. Spectra, membrane binding, and potentiometric responses of new charge shift probes. Biochem 1985;24:5749-5755.
36. Dillon SM, Wit AL. Voltage sensitive dye recordings from intact hearts using optical fibers. Biophys J 1988;53:641a. (abstract)
37. Moe GK. Computer simulation of atrial fibrillation. Comp Biomed Res 1965;2:217-238.
38. Allessie MA, Lammers WJEP, Bonke FIM, et al. Experimental evaluation of Moe's multiple wavelet hypothesis of atrial fibrillation, In: Zipes DP, Jalife J (eds) Cardiac Electrophysiology and Arrhythmias. Orlando, Grune & Stratton Inc., 1985, pp 265-275.
39. Janse MJ, van Cappelle FJ, Morsink H, et al. Flow of "injury" current and patterns of excitation during early ventricular arrhythmias in acute regional myocardial ischemia in isolated porcine and canine hearts: evidence for two different arrhythmogenic mechanisms. Circ Res 1980;47:151-165.
40. Pogwizd SM, Corr PB. Electrophysiologic mechanisms underlying arrhythmias due to reperfusion of ischemic myocardium. Circulation 1987;76:404-426.
41. Harumi K, Smith CR, Abildskov JA, et al. Detailed activation sequence in the region of electrically induced ventricular fibrillation in dogs. Jap Heart J 1980;21:533-544.
42. Bayly PV, Johnson EE, Wolf PD, et al. A quantitative measurement of spatial order in ventricular fibrillation. J Cardiovasc Electrophysiol 1993;4:533-546.
43. Ideker RE, Wolf PD, Simpson E, et al. The ideal cardiac mapping system, In: Shenasa M, Borgreffe M, Breithardt G, Haverkamp W, Hindricks G (eds) Cardiac Mapping. Mount Kisco, NY, Futura, 1993, pp 649-653.
44. Winfree A: Theory of spirals, In: Zipes DP, Jalife J (eds) Cardiac Electrophysiology. From Cell to Bedside. 2nd ed. Philadelphia, W.B. Saunders, 1994, pp 379-389.
45. Zhou X, Guse P, Wolf PD, et al. Existence of both fast and slow channel activity during the early stages of ventricular fibrillation. Circ Res 1992;70:773-786.
46. Wharton JM, Wolf PD, Smith WM, et al. Cardiac potential and potential gradient fields generated by single, combined, and sequential shocks during ventricular defibrillation. Circulation 1992;85:1510-1523.
47. Dillon SM, Mehra R. Prolongation of ventricular refractoriness by defibrillation shocks may be due to additional depolarization of the action potential. J Cardiovasc Electrophysiol 1992;3:442-456.
48. Dillon SM. Constant repolarization time after a defibrillation shock. FASEB J 1990;4:A682.(abstract)
49. Dillon SM. Synchronized repolarization after defibrillation shocks. A possible component of the defibrillation process demonstrated by optical recordings in rabbit heart. Circulation 1992;85:1865-1878.

50. Kao CY, Hoffman BF. Graded and decremental response in heart muscle fibers. Am J Physiol 1958;194:187-196.
51. Frazier DW, Krassowska W, Chen PS, et al. Extracellular field required for excitation in three-dimensional anisotropic canine myocardium. Circ Res 1988;63:147-164.
52. Wiggers CJ, Wegria R. Ventricular fibrillation due to single, localized induction and condenser shocks applied during the vulnerable phase of ventricular systole. Am J Physiol 1940;128:500-505.
53. Chen PS, Shibata N, Dixon EG, et al. Comparison of the defibrillation threshold and the upper limit of ventricular vulnerability. Circulation 1986;73:1022-1028.
54. Shibata N, Chen PS, Dixon EG, et al. Influence of shock strength and timing on induction of ventricular arrhythmias in dogs. Am J Physiol 1988;255:H891-H901.
55. Zipes DP. Electrophysiological mechanisms involved in ventricular fibrillation. Circulation 1975;52:120-130.
56. Sweeney RJ, Gill RM, Steinberg MI, et al. Ventricular refractory period extension caused by defibrillation shocks. Circulation 1990;82:965-972.
57. Li HG, Jones DL, Yee R, et al. Defibrillation shocks increase myocardial pacing threshold: An intracellular microelectrode study. Am J Physiol 1991;260:H1973-H1979.
58. Yabe S, Smith WM, Daubert JP, et al. Conduction disturbances caused by high current density electric fields. Circ Res 1990;66:1190-1203.
59. Jones JL, Jones RE. Postshock arrhythmias - a possible cause of unsuccessful defibrillation. Crit Care Med 1980;8:167-171.
60. Jones JL, Jones RE. Improved defibrillator waveform safety factor with biphasic waveforms. Am J Physiol 1983;245:H60-H65.
61. Plonsey R, Barr RC. Effect of microscopic and macroscopic discontinuities on the response of cardiac tissue to defibrillating (stimulating) currents. Med & Biol Eng & Comput 1986;24:130-136.
62. Dillon SM. Action potential prolongation by defibrillation shocks may be due to reactivation of the rapid sodium current. Biophys J 1994;66:A82. (abstract)
63. Goto M, Brooks CM. Membrane excitability of the frog ventricle examined by long pulses. Am J Physiol 1969;217:1236-1245.
64. Krassowska W, Pilkington TC, Ideker RE. Periodic conductivity as a mechanism for cardiac stimulation and defibrillation. IEEE Trans Biomed Eng 1987;34:555-560.
65. Swartz JF, Jones JL, Jones RE, et al. Conditioning prepulse of biphasic defibrillator waveforms enhances refractoriness to fibrillation wavefronts. Circ Res 1991;68:438-449.
66. Chen PS, Wolf PD, Claydon FJ, et al. The potential gradient field created by epicardial defibrillation electrodes in dogs. Circulation 1986;74:626-636.
67. Swartz JF, Jones JL, Fletcher RD. Symmetrical biphasic defibrillator waveforms enhance refractory period stimulation in the human heart. J Am Coll Cardiol 1991;17:335.(abstract)
68. Jones JL: Waveforms for implantable cardioverter defibrillators (ICDs) and transchest defibrillation, In: Tacker WA (ed) Defibrillation of the Heart. ICDs, AEDs, and Manual. St. Louis, Mosby, 1994, pp 46-81.
69. Witkowski FX, Penkoske PA. Refractoriness prolongation by defibrillation shocks. Circulation 1990;82:1064-1066.
70. Wang T, Kwaku KF, Dillon SM. Repolarization resynchronization may underlie the efficacy of biphasic shocks. Circulation 1994;90:I-446.(abstract)
71. Fabritz CL, Kirchhoff PF, Fletcher RD, et al. Post-shock repolarization time dispersion measured by two monophasic action potential recordings predicts defibrillation success in humans. Circulation 1994;90:I-446.(abstract)

4

Defining the Defibrillation Dosage

Mark W. Kroll, PhD, Michael H. Lehmann, MD, and Patrick J. Tchou, MD

THE DOSAGE is an essential part of any therapy prescription. This is true whether the therapy is a pharmacological agent or an electrical intervention. Unfortunately, there has been no standardization for the dosage of the electrical shock of an ICD.

It is important to accurately quantify defibrillation dosage for the following reasons:

1. Implanted devices must be programmed to provide a sufficient safety margin with a device output above the patient's defibrillation threshold. (Chap. 5)

2. A physician should be able to equate threshold readings from an external cardioverter defibrillator (analyzer) device with a prospective ICD. At present, readings from external devices are not always accurately transferable to an implantable device even if both are from the *same* manufacturer.

3. When a patient receives a replacement device, it is desirable to be able to compare outputs of the explanted device and the replacement device.

4. A comparison of electrode and ICD system efficacy between device manufacturers can only be accomplished with standardized dosage measurements.

The easiest ICD electrical output parameter to measure is *energy*. However, two decades of animal research has clearly demonstrated that the *average current* is a better measure of the heart's defibrillation requirements. The best measure of the heart's requirements is the *rheobase current* which is the average current required for an infinite duration pulse. (The analog for device output is the *effec-*

tive current defined in Equation [Eq.] 4, below) The discrepancy between the device parameter energy and the heart's actual defibrillation requirement continues to inhibit dosage standardization and understanding.

Units of Electricity

To find appropriate units for the dosage for electrical defibrillation, we must begin by reviewing the six basic units of electricity that are directly relevant to the ICD. These are: the coulomb, ampere, volt, ohm, farad, and joule. Electricity is rarely visualized and thus the electrical units are typically taught by means of fluid or hemodynamic analogies.

The *coulomb* is a unit of charge equal to 6×10^{18} electrons. This number is analogous to the mole in chemistry which is 6×10^{23} molecules. A mole of electrons would thus be about 100,000 coulombs and there is an unfortunate difference between the fundamental units of electricity and chemistry.

The *ampere* is the unit of current and is equal to the flow rate of 1 coulomb per second. A fluid analogy is a flow rate of 1 liter per minute.

The *volt* is the unit of voltage. Voltage is electrical pressure and represents the force driving the current through its path. The volt is usually defined empirically as 98.2% of the voltage of a certain (cadmium mercury) electrochemical cell. The fluid analogy of voltage is pressure, for example, mmHg.

The *ohm*, usually written Ω, is the unit of electrical resistance. It is defined by "Ohm's law" as the ratio of the voltage to the current. For example, a typical defibrillation pulse has an average voltage of 400 V and an average current of 8 A. The inter-electrode resistance is thus $50 \Omega = 400 \text{ V}/8 \text{ A}$. This definition makes intuitive sense in that one would expect that a path of greater resistance would require more voltage (i.e., higher pressure) to force a given current (i.e. flow) through it. The hemodynamic analogy is peripheral resistance which is typically expressed as mmHg/liter·min. While the terms "impedance" and "resistance" are often used interchangeably, a purist would reserve the term resistance to describe the impedance of an electrical circuit that had no energy storage capability. Since the ICD load (electrodes plus heart) has a small capacitive component,[1,2] impedance is the more accurate term.

The *farad* is the unit of capacitance. The capacitance simply measures the ability of a capacitor to store charge. Here the fluid

Table 1. Basic electrical units.

Parameter	Unit	Symbol	Definition	Analogy
charge	coulomb	C	6×10^{18} electrons	liter or mole
current	ampere	A	coulomb/second	liter/minute
voltage	volt	V	98.2% of CdHg cell voltage	mmHg pressure
resistance	ohm	Ω	volts/ampere	mmHg/liter/minute
capacitance	farad	F	coulombs /volt	ml/mmHg compliance
energy	joule	J	volt·ampere·second	calorie

analogy of compliance is very helpful. Imagine an elastic bladder of a certain compliance which is being used to store a fluid. The compliance is the ratio of volume to pressure and a typical unit is ml/mmHg. Thus the formula for volume may be written algebraically as:

volume = compliance · pressure

Analogously:

charge = capacitance · voltage

Capacitance is defined as the ratio of the charge to the voltage. A capacitor is essentially two conducting plates separated by an insulator. For a given technology (and fixed insulator thickness) the capacitance is proportional to the surface area of these plates. The charge formula means: "To increase the charge in a capacitor, one can either increase the surface area (to produce more capacitance) or increase the voltage (which is analogous to storing under a higher pressure). See Chap. 11 for a more complete discussion.

The final basic unit is the *joule* of energy. Energy can be expressed in various units depending on what type of energy one is dealing with (e.g. electrical, heat, etc.). The joule is about 1/4 of a calorie, for example. The joule is (electrically) the energy of a pulse of one volt and one ampere lasting one second. Algebraically:

energy = voltage · current · time

This formula is exact for steady voltages and currents but is only an approximation when they are changing throughout the pulse. It is precise for rectangular waveforms but not for capacitive discharge waveforms, whose energy is calculated from Eqs. 12 and 13 below.

A rectangular defibrillation pulse of 400 V, 8 A, and 8 ms would have 25.6 J (= 400 V · 8 A · 0.008 s) of energy.

Space Normalized Units of Electricity
Anyone who has jump-started a car trusts that 12 V between the limbs has no stimulating effect. However, a 9 V transistor radio battery across the tongue provides an obvious neural stimulation. The primary difference is the significantly higher *electric field* in the second case. (Another difference is the reduced impedance from the saliva.) The electric field, or potential gradient, is defined as the voltage difference per distance. A typical unit is volts per centimeter. In the case of the 9 V battery, the inter-electrode spacing is about 0.6 cm and the electric field is 15 V/cm = 9 V/0.6 cm which is well within the range required to stimulate tissue.

The analogous unit for current is the *current density* with typical units of milliamperes per cm^2 or mA/cm^2. A typical ICD epicardial patch electrode may have a surface area of 40 cm^2. With an average current of 8 A the current density (near the electrode) is given by 200 mA/cm^2 = 8 $A/40 \ cm^2$.

The space normalized unit of resistance is the *volume resistivity* whose unit is the Ω·cm. It is defined as the ratio of the electric field to the current density. The volume resistivity of blood is about 200 Ω·cm. This means that a cube, 1 cm on edge, of blood will have a resistance of 200 Ω between opposite faces. The volume resistivity of lungs, for example, is about 2000 Ω·cm.

Defibrillation Parameters

Defibrillation at the Tissue Level
Present theories suggest various mechanisms for electrical defibrillation which are not necessarily exclusive and may be overlapping. They require the current to be strong enough to extinguish wavefronts in either a large portion[3,4,5] or in all of the myocardium.[6] In addition, the ability of shocks to extend the refractoriness of depolarized myocardium[7,8] may also play a role in defibrillation, perhaps by resynchronizing repolarization.[9] See Chaps. 3 and 7 for further discussion. Whatever the merits and relative contributions of the various mechanisms are, the cell membrane must be stimulated electrically. At the cellular level, this is regarded as being caused by the local electrical field.

Theoretical modeling[10] and animal myocyte studies[11] have shown that the field required for stimulation with the field perpendicular to the cell's long axis, is approximately 2-6 times that required for a field parallel to the cell. However, the electrical volume resistivity of the myocardium is also highest for perpendicular current flows in approximately the same ratio. Since the current density equals the electric field divided by the volume resistivity, the current density required for stimulation is fairly constant regardless of orientation.

Indeed, in a canine myocardium model, it has been demonstrated that the current density for far-field stimulation varies insignificantly with cell fiber orientation.[12] Thus while the electric field is probably responsible for electrical defibrillation on the cellular membrane level, the current density may be the best descriptor on a tissue level.

The Rheobase and Chronaxie

In the late 19th century Weiss found a linear relationship between the charge (Q) required for tissue stimulation and the duration (d) of the pulse.[13] His pulse generator, the ballistic rheotome, comprised a battery source and a rifle shot of known velocity to first cut a shunting wire and then to cut a series wire located a known distance away.[14] He reported that the charge required for stimulation was given by:

$$Q = K_1 d + K_2$$

Lapicque[15] divided the Weiss equation by d giving the required (average) current as:

Eq. 1 $$I_{ave} = K_1 + \frac{K_2}{d}$$

Lapicque also defined two useful terms. The first is the "rheobase" for the value K_1 which is the current required for an infinite duration pulse. Lapicque defined the "chronaxie" as that duration which required a doubling of the rheobase current.

The chronaxie time d_c is thus given by:

$$d_c = \frac{K_2}{K_1}$$

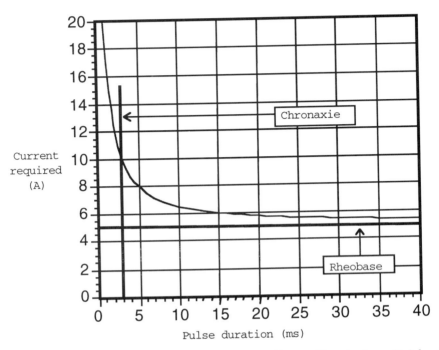

Figure 1. Sample strength-duration curve for defibrillation. The rheobase (5 A here) represents the asymptote of the average current required for an infinitely long pulse. The chronaxie (3 ms here) is that duration at which the required current is doubled from the rheobase level.

Defining I_r as the rheobase current (K_1) and rearranging Eq. 1 gives:

Eq. 2 $$I_{ave} = I_r\left[1 + \frac{d_c}{d}\right]$$ (for pulses of a given duration d)

In 1978, Bourland showed that defibrillation shocks followed an *average current law*. That is, *the average current of a pulse is the best measure of its effectiveness when compared to other pulses of the same width regardless of shape*.[16] This held true for pulses of 2-20 ms in width regardless of the droop or "tilt" (see Eq. 7 below). Other studies demonstrated that the average current law extended to pulse durations of 40 ms.[17] More importantly, Bourland implicitly showed that defibrillation nicely followed a Weiss-Lapicque strength-duration curve as in Fig. 1.

What this all means is that *the rheobase current is essentially the defibrillation threshold (DFT) expressed as a current.* Importantly, it is expressed as a current from a standardized (infinite) pulse width and is thus independent of the pulse width used for DFT testing.

Experimental studies using the calf,[18] pony,[19,20] dog,[21-24] and cultured chick cells[25] have shown that *the defibrillation chronaxie duration is in the range of 2-4 ms with a representative value of 3 ms.* This value will be used throughout this chapter. Typical pulse durations used clinically are at least double this value. The defibrillation chronaxie time for humans has recently been shown to be 3.2 ms.[26]

Typical rheobase currents in man are 2.3-5.6 A. This can be easily calculated from Eq. 11 (below) assuming a 140 µF capacitor, 50 Ω impedance, 65% tilt waveforms, a 3.2 ms chronaxie, and DFTs of 5-30 J. While Eq. 11 is for effective current, this is equal to the rheobase for shocks exactly at the DFT.

The following paradigm may be helpful for understanding the relevance of the chronaxie time. Consider the defibrillation pulses as shown in Fig. 2. Both are rectangular pulses, i.e., they have a constant voltage and current throughout the active portion of the pulse. These pulses are being applied to a patient assumed to have a 5 A rheobase threshold for defibrillation. The pulse on the left, which is "very wide" (essentially of infinite duration), has a 5 A amplitude and, hence, would be sufficient for defibrillation. This is, after all, the definition of the rheobase current. The pulse on the right has a duration equal to the chronaxie time. Therefore, it must supply an average current equal to twice that of the rheobase—i.e., 10 A. These two simple waveforms capture the gist of the strength-duration relationship for defibrillation and should be well understood before proceeding.

A pulse of 40 ms duration qualifies as "very wide" with acceptable accuracy. Using Ohm's law, and assuming a typical resistance of 50 Ω, we see that a voltage of 250 V $= 50\,\Omega \cdot 5$ A is required for defibrillation by the "very wide" pulse. The corresponding energy is then 50 J $= 250$ V $\cdot 5$ A $\cdot 0.04$ s. In turn, the energy corresponding to the pulse on the right (Fig. 2) will be 15 J $= 500$ V $\cdot 10$ A $\cdot 0.003$ s. Note that the pulse delivered with a duration equal to the chronaxie time has a significantly lower threshold energy. Indeed it has been shown that, for rectangular pulses, the lowest energy requirement, for any electrical stimulation, does occur when the duration equals the chronaxie time.[27] This is analogous to the reduced energy during cardiac pacing with the use of shorter duration higher current pulses.

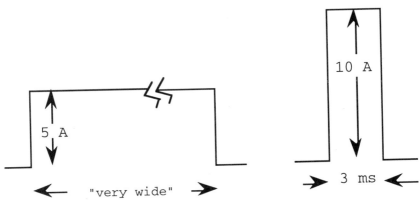

Figure 2. Two equivalent pulses for a patient with a 5 A rheobase defibrillation threshold and a 3 ms chronaxie time.

While allowing for easier calculations, the rectangular pulse is not practical for an implantable device, as it would require an enormous power supply. The *capacitive discharge waveform* is used exclusively in the ICD (Chaps. 7 and 13). With this waveform, the relationship between pulse efficiency and the chronaxie duration is slightly more complex but the basic ideas remain applicable. For example, the strength-duration curve still applies in the sense that wider pulses require a lower average current for defibrillation. However, the average current produced by the capacitive discharge pulse falls off rapidly as the capacitor voltage decreases. Therefore extending the pulse duration to "deliver more energy" is usually of limited benefit with capacitive discharge shocks.

Effective Current
Imagine that a given pulse is exactly at the defibrillation threshold for a given patient. This pulse will have a known average current and duration. The rheobase may now be calculated for this patient from a simple rearrangement of Eq. 2:

Eq. 3 $$I_r = \frac{I_{ave}}{1 + \dfrac{d_c}{d}}$$

Note that the average current is merely divided by the "duration correction" factor, i.e. $\left[1 + \frac{d_c}{d}\right]$, to obtain the rheobase.

An important dosage measurement is *the maximum rheobase current which a given pulse can satisfy.* This parameter has been referred to as the Effective Current (I_{eff}) of the pulse.[28] Whereas the rheobase, as specified in Eq. 3, is a physiological parameter (quantifying the heart's requirements), I_{eff} is primarily an electronic parameter which quantifies the output of a defibrillator. The formulas, however, are identical:

$$\text{Eq. 4} \qquad I_{eff} = \frac{\text{average current}}{\text{duration correction}} = \frac{I_{ave}}{1 + \dfrac{d_c}{d}}$$

The effective current of a pulse simply measures its average current corrected for the duration. For example, a pulse with an average current of 5 A that was "very wide" (so that d_c/d is close to zero) would have an effective current of 5 A as well. However, a pulse with an average current of 10 A and a pulse duration of 3 ms would also have an effective current of 5 A (assuming a chronaxie time of 3 ms). Similarly, an output pulse of 20 A with a pulse duration of 3 ms would have an effective current of 10 A. *What makes effective current useful is that it is a measure of the ICD output that directly relates to the defibrillation requirements of the heart, i.e. the rheobase.*

The power of the effective current calculation lies in its ability to easily consider the effects of changing durations, capacitance values, and resistances. It should be emphasized that the effective current calculation applies to any strength pulse—not just to one exactly at the DFT.

Imagine a capacitive discharge pulse from a capacitance C charged to a voltage V, termed "leading edge voltage," "initial voltage," "peak voltage," or "charge voltage"—all synonymous with respect to present monophasic or biphasic ICD waveforms (Fig. 3). If the capacitor is discharged over pulse duration d to a "final " (or "trailing") voltage V_f thereby truncating the terminal portion of the exponential voltage decay, then the average current is:

$$\text{Eq. 5} \qquad I_{ave} = \frac{C\,(V - V_f)}{d}$$

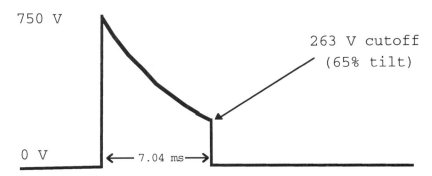

Figure 3. Typical monophasic capacitive discharge (truncated exponential) waveform with a leading edge voltage of 750 V and a trailing edge voltage of 263 V. Time course of voltage decay follows an exponential curve that is truncated upon completion of prespecified pulse width or achievement of voltage that yields a prespecified tilt.

This formula is correct for a monophasic waveform and also for the first phase of a biphasic waveform. It may be rewritten in terms of *tilt* [where tilt = $\dfrac{V - V_f}{V}$]:

Eq. 6 $I_{ave} = \dfrac{CV \cdot tilt}{d}$ (for tilt given as a fraction—not %)

      The equation may seem to imply that increasing the tilt increases the average current. However, since the duration increases faster as a function of the tilt (Eq. 8 below), the average current actually *decreases* with increasing tilt. If the tilt is not specified a priori, it may be calculated (expressed here again as a fraction—not as a percentage) from d, R, and C using a standard formula from electrical circuit theory:

Eq. 7 $tilt = 1 - e^{-d/RC}$ implying:

Eq. 8 $d = -R C \cdot \log_e(1\text{-tilt})$

      Eq. 8 describes how, for fixed R and C, the duration of the capacitive discharge pulse prolongs as the tilt is increased. Some manufacturers, who believe that the achievement of a certain tilt (typically 65%) is very important for defibrillation efficacy, provide Eq. 8 in the form of a table so that the physician can set the pulse duration to arrive at this desired tilt.

The product of R and C is in units of time (seconds) and is referred to as the *time constant*. For example 7 ms = 0.007 s = 50 Ω · 140 μF. This gives the time needed for the resistor to drain the capacitor down to 37% of its initial voltage. This parameter is the same as the "turnover time" used in biochemistry and is analogous to, but slightly larger than, the "half-time" of washout or clearance used in pharmacology.

Combining Eqs. 4 and 6, and multiplying through by d, gives:

Eq. 9
$$I_{eff} = \frac{C\,V \cdot tilt}{d + d_c}$$

Substituting Eq. 7 for tilt yields (for a fixed pulse duration d):

Eq. 10
$$I_{eff} = \frac{C\,V\,[1 - e^{-d/RC}]}{d + d_c}$$

while using Eq. 8 for a tilt based pulse gives (again, where tilt is expressed as a fraction):

Eq. 11
$$I_{eff} = \frac{CV \cdot tilt}{-RC \cdot \log_e(1\text{-tilt}) + d_c}$$

A typical capacitive discharge waveform is shown in Fig. 3. This represents the discharge of a 140 μF capacitor into a 50 Ω impedance. Note that the pulse has an initial voltage of 750 V and is truncated after the voltage drops to 263 V. This truncation represents a tilt specification of .65 (65%). The average current (Eq. 6) is 9.75 A and the effective current may be calculated (Eq. 11) as 7.0 A, which means that this pulse will defibrillate any patient with a rheobase threshold of under 7.0 A.

The capacitive discharge pulse provides us with another way of looking at the chronaxie duration. By calculating the effective current at each duration (using Eq. 10), one can determine the defibrillation ability of a capacitive discharge pulse at increasing durations. The results are shown in Fig. 4 for a typical scenario of a 140 μF capacitor, initially charged to 750 V, discharging into a load of 50 Ω. This curve is correct only for the assumed time constant of 7 ms = 50 Ω · 140 μF and will be shifted to the right

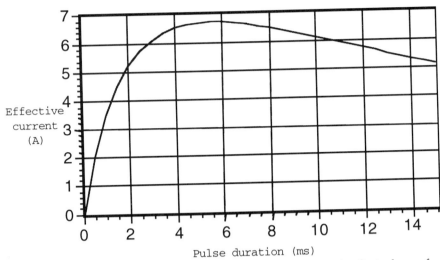

Figure 4. Effective current vs. pulse duration of a monophasic (or first phase of a biphasic) shock generated by a 140 µF capacitor charged to 750 V. Assumes a chronaxie time of 3 ms and an electrode resistance of 50 Ω. This curve will be qualitatively similar but shifted for other RC time constants. Note that the optimal duration is about 6 ms.

(towards longer durations) for increasing resistances. The stored energy is a constant 39.4 J.

There are two items of note in the graph of Fig. 4. First, the effective current rises rapidly for the first 3 ms of pulse duration. The vast majority (>90%) of the effective current is attained in this first 3 ms of the pulse. Equivalently, there is minimal additional benefit from energy delivered after the chronaxie duration. Second, the effective current declines after a duration of 6 ms. Thus, current delivered after the first 6 ms is utilized less efficiently. This is why the truncation of the capacitive discharge pulse has been found to be so beneficial.

All points on the curve in Fig. 4 represent shocks of the same stored energy. In spite of this there is a significant range of defibrillation capability as measured by the effective current—because of the varying durations. *Thus, the DFT, as measured by energy, will be minimized with the shock duration corresponding to the apex of the curve in Fig. 4.*

In a later section we will see that not all joules are created equally. However, if one ICD can deliver an effective current of 12 A and another ICD delivers an effective current of 16 A (both at maximum output), one can say with confidence that the second device has a higher defibrillation capability than the first (assuming both waveforms are monophasic or both are biphasic) regardless of the voltage, capacitance value, and pulse duration. The same cannot be said for a simplistic parameter such as energy.

While the effective current is directly comparable to the rheobase it cannot be specified exactly *a priori* for an ICD. This is because the current calculation requires knowledge of the defibrillation electrode resistance. Nevertheless, one could assume a standard resistance of 50 Ω and rate an ICD for the effective current on that basis. A more minor problem is the chronaxie value which can vary from 2-4 ms for various animal models. There is no harm in using a chronaxie value of 3 ms for all calculations as the differences in results from using this value versus the extremes of 2-4 ms are relatively minor.

Parameters for the Biphasic Waveform
The first phase of a practical biphasic appears to act as does a monophasic shock.[29] The first phase duration (for a fixed typical second phase duration) also follows the same hyperbolic strength-duration relationship that the monophasic shock does.[30] Theoretical models, with retrospective validation, suggest that the first phase does indeed behave as a monophasic shock.[31]

Thus, for biphasic waveforms one should use the duration, average current, and effective current of the first phase for dosage measurements. Of course, this does not mean that the second phase is irrelevant; the latter clearly acts as a powerful catalyst to significantly reduce the electrical requirements of the first phase.[31] However, as seen in Fig. 5, the second phase is much smaller in amplitude and has a much more complex strength-duration relationship. Thus there is no obvious benefit in including its electrical parameters with the first phase measurements.

For biphasic waveforms the conclusions of increased efficiency through optimal pulse durations are still true—at least qualitatively. Recent clinical studies have shown significant lowering of DFTs from the use of biphasic waveforms with each phase duration nearer the chronaxie.[32,33] A shock with a first phase of about 3.5 ms (42% tilt) had delivered energy thresholds that were *half* that of the biphasics with a conventional width first phase of 7 ms (65% tilt).[32]

To quantitate the *energy* associated with biphasic waveforms, the portion (first phase or overall shock) chosen for measurement is not critical. For ease of calculations, one may wish to use the energy of the whole waveform, as the delivered energy (Eq. 13, below—using V_f of second phase) is then typically equal to the stored energy (E_{del} = 90-99% of E_{std}). For calculations of average or

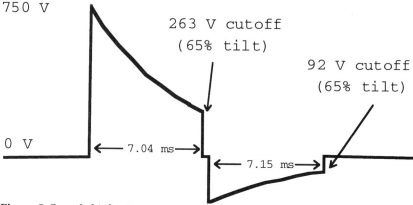

Figure 5. Sample biphasic capacitive discharge (truncated exponential) waveform with a 65% tilt for both the positive and negative phases (Medtronic Jewel). Note that the leading edge voltage of the second phase is equal in absolute value to the trailing edge voltage of the first phase. (This is not the case with the Ventritex Contour and its predecessors—see Chap. 13, "Other Biphasic Waveform Circuitry.") The second phase is slightly longer than the first due to the increased resistance seen with the lower voltages of the second phase.[1,2] The slight gap (<1 ms) between the phases is to allow for delays in the semiconductor switches (see Chap. 13) and has no physiological relevance (for gaps significantly less than the myocyte membrane time constant of about 3 ms).

effective currents, the first phase must be used. See Chap. 7 for more details on the biphasic waveform.

Energy as a Parameter

Stored vs. Delivered Energy

The energy of a capacitive discharge ICD pulse is easy to calculate. The *stored energy* (E_{std}) is given by :

Eq. 12. $E_{std} = 0.5 \, C \, V_i^2$

where C is the capacitance in farads and V_i is the initial (or leading edge) voltage.

The *delivered energy* (E_{del}) from the capacitor (i.e., actually taken from the capacitor and giving the highest value of all of the definitions for delivered energy) can be derived by calculating the energy stored in the capacitor before and after the pulse and then taking the difference (V_f is the final or trailing edge voltage):

Eq. 13. $E_{del} = 0.5 \, C \, (\, V_i^2 - V_f^2 \,)$

A simpler calculation, which is a good estimate for the typical monophasic waveform, is merely to take 90% of the stored energy as an approximation for E_{del}. (Note that as V_f gets closer to zero, i.e., high tilt, Eqs. 12 and 1 become more nearly identical.) For example, assuming a capacitance of 140 μF, the waveform of Fig. 3 has a stored energy of 39.4 J and a delivered energy of 34.7 J. The delivered energy is 88% of the stored energy in this case. This rule of thumb will overestimate the delivered energy if the tilt is significantly below 65%. For typical biphasic shocks, the delivered energy is about 95% of the stored energy (because of the low V_f of the second phase and the high overall tilt); thus, there is no reason to distinguish between the two measurements for this waveform.

There is no consistent definition of delivered energy. One manufacturer, Guidant/CPI, merely discounts the stored energy by 11% and labels the result as the "delivered energy." The actual energy delivered (as a fraction of the stored) from the capacitor is about 95%; past the semiconductor switches about 90%; to the end of the leads (and varying with the leads added) about 80-90%; and past the interfacial layer[2] (electrode-tissue interface) about 70-90%. However, the energy actually delivered "into" the heart (i.e., more than 1 mm past the electrodes) can be calculated to be as low as 10% of the stored energy, using actual tissue measurements of voltage gradients found in animal studies![34] This further highlights the advantage of current-based description of defibrillation. Each manufacturer calculates the delivered energy as a different fraction of the stored energy which further adds to the confusion and detracts from its meaningfulness. Thus, "Delivered Energy," while very popular jargon among non-researcher clinicians, has no physiological relevance and has no consistent definition; the authors recommend against its usage.

There is no theoretical model which suggests that either of the energies (stored or delivered) has any relationship to the biological processes involved in defibrillation. However, the delivered energy (into the myocardial tissue) is a measure of the impact of the shock in terms of myocardial heating. By contrast, the stored energy (for a maximal shock) is a function of the physical size of the capacitor and is a measure of the battery drain per shock charging cycle. For the rectangular shocks produced by large laboratory amplifiers, there is not necessarily any relevant stored energy, although the delivered energy can always be calculated.

Limitations of the Energy Parameter

Although a popular defibrillation parameter clinically, energy is *not* directly related to the defibrillation requirements of the heart. A simple example readily demonstrates this. Imagine a 10 V pulse of 10 s duration and a 50 Ω impedance. This is a rectangular (not a capacitive discharge) waveform and thus Eqs. 12 and 13 are not applicable. However, since we know from Ohm's law that the (average) current is 0.2 A, we can calculate the energy of the pulse (see "Units of Electricity" section) as 20 J = 10 V · 0.2 A · 10 s. This energy is above the DFT of the typical patient yet will not defibrillate, since the average current is well below the typical rheobase current (1-10 A). Thus, the energy of a pulse does not necessarily predict its ability to defibrillate the heart.

There are three specific problems in the use of energy as a dosage: its dependence on resistance, pulse width, and capacitance. To simplify the calculations, the first two analyses (dependence on resistance and pulse width) will be done for the case of ideal rectangular waveforms. The results are similar, although harder to arrive at, for the practical capacitive discharge waveforms. For the case of the dependence on the capacitance value we will, of course, analyze the capacitive discharge waveform.

Dependence on Resistance

Let us return briefly to the rectangular pulse of Fig. 2 in order to simplify a calculation. Again it is assumed that the patient has a defibrillation rheobase of 5 A. Let us also assume that a pulse width of 3 ms (concordant with the chronaxie time) is being used, so that the current is twice the rheobase, or 10 A. During implantation the defibrillation electrode resistance is 50 Ω. The average current law (see discussion following Fig. 1) may be used to calculate the required delivered energy. The required voltage is 500 V = 10 A · 50 Ω and the pulse energy, therefore, is 15 J = 500 V · 10 A · 0.003 s. A year later, local tissue fibrosis increases the electrode resistance to 80 Ω. The required voltage thus increases to 800 V and the threshold energy is now 24 J = 800 V · 10 A · 0.003 s. Thus, the threshold energy increased by 9 J with the change in resistance.

In view of even greater uncertainties in transthoracic resistance, modern external defibrillators are moving away from the use of energy for the dosage measurement.[35,36] With external defibrillators, there is a strong trend towards the use of current as a measure of shock strength, although it is often euphemized as "resistance-corrected energy".[37]

Dependence on Pulse Duration
Let us now assume a patient with a 3 A defibrillation rheobase and a 50 Ω impedance. To simplify the calculations we again assume the use of a rectangular pulse with a duration equal to the chronaxie. Since at the chronaxie duration (i.e. 3 ms) the required current is twice the rheobase, the required voltage will be 300 V = 6 A · 50 Ω. Accordingly, the threshold energy required for the 3 ms pulse will be 5.4 J = 300 V · 6 A · 0.003 s. Suppose we now implant an ICD that happens to have a pulse duration of 9 ms. We wish to maintain the same defibrillation capability. The following calculations will allow us to predict the delivered energy that will be required for the new device. The new average current required is given by algebraically rewriting Eq. 4:

$$I_{ave} = 3\,A\left[1+\frac{3\,ms}{9\,ms}\right]$$

$$= 4\,A$$

$$V = 4\,A \cdot 50\,\Omega = 200\,V \quad \text{(Ohm's law)}$$

$$Energy = 7.2\,J = 200\,V \cdot 4\,A \cdot 0.009\,s$$

Thus the mere change of pulse duration from an ideal 3 ms value to one closer to clinical usage (9 ms) has increased the threshold energy by a significant 33% to 7.2 J from 5.4 J.

This discussion on the energy dependence on resistance and pulse duration used ideal rectangular pulses. The relationships for capacitive discharge pulses are actually very similar even though the calculations are more complex.

Dependence on Capacitance
Another disadvantage of the use of energy as a defibrillation dosage is that this form of measurement is dependent on the capacitor used to deliver that dose. This is because very large capacitors take much more time to deliver their charge than the optimal 3 ms. A smaller capacitor delivers its bolus of charge much more quickly and hence has higher efficiencies and lower energy thresholds associated with it.[38-40]

This phenomenon may be illustrated by comparing the DFTs for the same patient with the use of two different capacitance values. Two capacitance values that have been used in ICDs are

Table 2. Dependence of stored energy DFT on capacitor value, despite equal rheobases.

Capacitance Value	Shock Duration	Voltage	Stored Energy	Average Current	Effective Current
120 µF	6.3 ms	750 V	33.8 J	9.29 A	6.29 A
180 µF	9.4 ms	669 V	40.3 J	8.28 A	6.29 A

All waveforms are monophasic with 65% tilt. Resistance of 50 Ω and 3 ms chronaxie assumed.

120 µF and 180 µF. Imagine that the 120 µF capacitor is charged to 750 V and is used to deliver a 65% tilt shock. Assuming a resistance of 50 Ω and chronaxie of 3 ms, Eq. 11 may be used to calculate a resulting effective current of 6.29 A. The stored energy (Eq. 12) is 33.8 J.

What voltage and stored energy are required with the 180 µF capacitor to achieve the same effective current? Using Eq. 11 (again assuming a 50 Ω resistance) shows that the 180 µF capacitor must be charged to 669 V to deliver an effective current of 6.29 A. By Eq. 12, this results in a stored energy of 40.3 J. (See Table 2—which uses Eq. 8 to calculate the durations.) Thus, the larger capacitor will have (energy) thresholds about 20% larger and will require more physical volume for the same defibrillation capability. This larger stored energy requirement also reduces the number of shocks which the ICD can deliver.

This dependence of the DFT on the capacitor value can be a significant matter if one seeks to switch to a different manufacturer during generator replacement or use an external cardioverter defibrillator (ECD) system to set thresholds in advance of implanting an ICD. *Thus, if two devices have different capacitor values, the defibrillation energy thresholds are not necessarily transferable from one device to the other.*

This problem actually existed with the first ICD systems. The ECD had a capacitance of 145-150 µF while the ICD had a capacitance of about 125 µF.[41] Thus the thresholds from the external box did not accurately reflect the ICD thresholds. Fortuitously, the error was in the direction of providing extra safety margin for the ICD. Had the internal capacitor had a larger value, the safety margin would have been partly compromised. The recent trend toward "device based" DFT testing (i.e., directly via the ICD) during implantation obviates the potential capacitance mismatch problem.

This problem is again relevant now that many older high capacitance devices (130-150 µF) are being replaced with newer ICDs with capacitances down to 90 µF. Again, this direction of change will provide extra safety margin. Changing in the opposite direction will lower the safety margin.

For an excellent review of the effect of capacitance changes, as well as many other waveform topics, see Block et al.[42]

Specification of the Duration: Time , Tilt, or Both ?

The duration of the shock is typically specified as either a fixed time (e.g., 7 ms) or a fixed tilt (e.g., 65%). Each of these specifications has advantages and disadvantages. The primary difference is in the way each form of specification responds to changes in the electrode resistance. This is important as the resistance will frequently increase significantly after implantation.[43] Surprisingly, the fixed tilt devices do well for impedance decreases.[27] However, as discussed in the next section, the tilt specification is slightly inferior to the fixed time specification for dealing with impedance increases. For another approach to the question of optimal durations, which gives similar results, see Irnich.[44]

An approach which may be equal to or better than either approach, at all impedances, is the *composite duration specification* (e.g., 44% tilt followed by a fixed time extension of 1.6 ms). This is equivalent to a time duration equal to a weighted average of the RC time constant and the chronaxie duration (d_c):[27]

Eq. 14 $d = 0.58 \, (R \, C + d_c)$

Note that this is neither a pure fixed time specification nor a pure tilt specification, but rather a hybrid which is designed to capture the best features of both. This formula recites the necessary compromise between the electronics (sufficient duration to discharge the capacitor) and the heart's defibrillation requirement (shock duration near the chronaxie time).

The Tilt Specification and "Constant Energy"

The tilt specification guarantees a certain delivered energy because the capacitor is always drained down to a certain final voltage level, hence always releasing a fixed amount of energy (see Eq. 13). One marketed ICD accordingly guarantees its delivered energy since it uses a duration specification of a 65% tilt. This is guaranteed (hence "constant energy") for resistances up to a maximum of 178 Ω. Unfortunately, since duration is proportional to the resistance (for tilt based devices), the duration, given by Eq. 8, could be as high as 26 ms with the device's 140 μF capacitor. For an impedance of 178 Ω and a chronaxie duration of 3 ms, an initial voltage (maximum charge) of 750 V will result in a shock with an effective current of only 2.33 A (Eq. 10 or 11).

The theoretical optimum pulse duration for the corresponding RC time constant, in this example, is 16 ms (Eq. 14). This duration yields an effective current of 2.65 A (Eq. 10). This is still a very low effective current and may be insufficient to defibrillate. Nevertheless, shortening the pulse, to 16 ms, increased the effective current by 14%. For the tilt specified pulse (d = 26 ms) to achieve the same effective current as the 16 ms pulse, the voltage on the capacitor would have to be increased by the same 14% (Eq. 9). This translates (Eq. 12) into an increase of 23% in the capacitor stored energy requirement for defibrillation. Thus, the tilt specification has significantly increased the DFT (measured in units of energy).

Some comments are in order for this example. First, an impedance of 178 Ω is rare and the implanting physician would most likely seek a lower impedance electrode system. For a more moderately elevated impedance of 100 Ω, the tilt based devices still are inferior in performance to a device with the optimal duration but the differences are less than 10% in terms of energy. (For an impedance in the neighborhood of the common clinical value of 50 Ω, there is no clinically measurable difference.) Second, the theoretical optimum duration of 16 ms is significantly longer than the 3 ms chronaxie and even longer than the 6 ms optimum shown in Fig. 4. Is there a contradiction? No. Fig. 4 is based on a resistance of 50 Ω— not 178 Ω. The 16 ms duration represents the necessary "compromise" between the chronaxie time and the very large RC time constant in this example.

Thus, a large increase in the duration was warranted and the philosophy behind the tilt-based devices has some merit. The problem with the tilt approach, however, is that the increase in duration may be excessive and the safety margin for defibrillation might be partially compromised. If the device did not increase the pulse duration proportionally to the resistance (as done automatically with a tilt-based device)—but rather increased it judiciously to obtain the optimal pulse width—then the safety margin would be less compromised. The net effect with small resistance changes (<10 Ω) is insignificant clinically, but for a large (50Ω) change the lowered efficiency of the wide waveform could consume all of the original safety margin and result in ineffective therapy.

A similar approach to tilt has been referred to as "pseudo-tilt." Here, the implanting physician programs a fixed duration to effect a certain tilt based on the impedance found during implant. (See the discussion following Eq. 8.)

Table 3. Output analysis of a device with increasing durations, with demonstration of "negative safety margin" for defibrillation.

Delivered Energy	Initial Voltage	Shock Duration	Resulting Tilt	Average Current	Effective Current
20 J	581 V	6.0 ms	55%	8.00 A	5.33 A
25 J	649 V	6.0 ms	55%	8.93 A	5.96 A
33 J	680 V	11.5 ms	78%	6.96 A	5.52 A

A resistance of 50 Ω and chronaxie of 3 ms are assumed.

Variable Pulse Widths and the "Negative Safety Margin"

The Telectronics 4210 had a highest delivered energy shock of 33 J. Its unique feature was that its pulse durations changed automatically with the programmed *delivered* energy level. The physician was unable to set the durations independently of the energy setting. For example, the 20 J shock always had a pulse duration of 6 ms and an initial voltage of 650 V, while the 33 J shock always had a duration of 11.5 ms and an initial voltage of 680 V. Both were delivered from a 150 μF capacitor.

A straightforward use of Eq. 10 may be used to compare these two pulses for effective current, assuming an electrode resistance of 50 Ω and a chronaxie of 3 ms. (The average currents may be calculated with the use of Eqs. 6 and 7.) The results are shown in Table 3 along with the intermediate shock of 25 J. Note that the 33 J shock has less effective current than does the 25 J shock. If a patient had a threshold of 25 J then the use of the maximum output of 33 J would appear to give a safety margin of 8 J. (Chap. 5) However this shock actually has *less* defibrillation capability (5.52 A vs. 5.96 A). Note that the 20 J shock has essentially the same effective current as does the 33 J shock (5.33 A vs. 5.52 A.). Thus, the maximum output of this type of device offers minimal advantage over the 20 J setting.

Since the higher energy shock (33 J) has significantly less defibrillation ability than a lower energy one (25 J), it could be said that the device has a *negative safety margin*. Qualitatively, squeezing the last drops of charge out of the capacitor to "deliver more energy" results in extremely low final currents and voltages, and consequently lower average and effective currents.

It must be pointed out this problem exists only for devices which use *increasing* pulse widths to achieve higher delivered energies. This is not a concern with either fixed time duration or fixed tilt devices.

So Why Use Energy?

Energy remains a simple dosage parameter to calculate; hence it is favored by most manufacturers. It also has the advantage of being available on most programmers. In spite of some accuracy limitations it has the further advantage of correlating with decades of publications and over a decade of clinical experience.

The basic limitation of energy as a dosage parameter is that it has no direct relationship to the defibrillation requirements of the heart. *Energy is meaningful only when resistance, capacitance, and duration (either the time or the tilt) are all fixed.* This condition is satisfied in most clinical situations and with most devices.

Caution is warranted, however, when significant changes are anticipated in the capacitance, electrode resistance, or pulse duration. Electrode resistances can change with time.[36] Also, for ICD replacement—with the old electrodes remaining—one must be alert for changes in either the capacitance or pulse durations. These changes could arise from a generator model change or when switching from an external (perioperative) device to the implantable unit. Such considerations are particularly important in patients with high defibrillation thresholds.

It may be prudent to insist that a device manufacturer disclose the devices capacitance value, pulse durations, and voltage so that appropriate output comparisons can be made. This would allow the calculation of the device output in terms of the effective current. It would also allow *restatement of the DFT in terms of a rheobase current.*

Recall that exactly at the threshold for defibrillation, the device effective current is equal to the rheobase current. *The effective current formula may thus be used to calculate the rheobase* as follows: The DFT, as a leading edge voltage, is recorded. (If not available it is calculated from the DFT energy using Eq. 12. and solving for V_i.) The effective current corresponding to this voltage is then calculated with Eq. 9, and is equal to the rheobase.

Summary

The dosage for defibrillation is an important and subtle concept. Many dosage parameters have been proposed.

The defibrillation requirements of the heart, at the tissue level, are given as electric fields and current densities. At the whole heart level (i.e., between electrodes—see Table 4) the heart's defibrillation requirements follow an average current law for both monophasic

Table 4. Electrical measures of dosage relevant at the electrode level.

Parameter	Accurately Measures	Clinical Advantage	Clinical Disadvantage
average current	stimulation ability at electrode level for fixed pulse duration	accurately relates heart's defibrillation requirements regardless of resistance	cannot be guaranteed for ICD without knowing electrode resistance*
effective current	stimulation ability at electrode level for arbitrary pulse duration	directly related to rheobase; relates to heart's requirements regardless of resistance and pulse duration	cannot be guaranteed a priori for ICD without knowing electrode resistance*
initial voltage	capacitor charge	easy to measure and known a priori for all resistances	no direct relation to heart's requirements
stored energy	capacitor size, battery drain	can be guaranteed for all ICDs, widely used.	no direct relation to heart's requirements
delivered energy	myocardial heating	can be guaranteed a priori for tilt based pulses; widely used.	may give negative safety margins with changing durations; no direct relation to heart's requirements.

* But, for comparative purposes standard values of 50 Ω resistance and 3 ms chronaxie could be used.

defibrillation shocks and the first phase of biphasic shocks. These requirements also obey the Weiss-Lapicque strength-duration curve which is defined by the chronaxie duration and the rheobase current. The rheobase current is the defibrillation threshold expressed as a current of infinite duration. The chronaxie duration is that which requires a doubling of the rheobase current for defibrillation

The effective current expresses the ICD output in terms of its defibrillation capability as defined by the strength-duration curve. The effective current allows for the easy calculation of the effect of waveform parameter changes. Whereas the rheobase is a physiological parameter (quantifying the heart's requirements), the effective current is primarily an electronic parameter (quantifying the defibrillator output). The effective current is useful since it is a measure of the ICD output that directly relates to the defibrillation requirements of the heart, i.e., the rheobase.

The effective current can be calculated for the monophasic truncated exponential using only the leading edge voltage, capacitance, resistance, duration, and chronaxie. The first phase parameters are used for the biphasic waveform calculation.

Energy is easy to calculate but energy thresholds are affected by changes in resistance, capacitance, and pulse duration. The optimum pulse duration depends on the RC time constant (product of the ICD energy storage capacitance and the defibrillation electrode resistance). Deviations from this optimum value will result in increased defibrillation thresholds. Pulse durations which change with the energy level can result in negative safety margins. While very popular, the usage of delivered energy has no physiological basis, or consistent definition (as it depends on the point of measurement), and is not recommended by the authors.

The dependence of the defibrillation (energy) threshold on the capacitor value can be a significant matter if one seeks to switch to a different manufacturer during generator replacement or use an external cardioverter defibrillator system to set thresholds in advance of implanting an ICD. Thus, if two devices have different capacitor values, the defibrillation energy thresholds are not necessarily transferable from one device to the other.

It is hard to improve on the 1978 admonition of Charles Babbs:

> Since there is no agreement at present as to the essential property of the electrical stimulus that causes defibrillation the lack of exact descriptions of the voltage and current waveforms employed in experimental studies seriously compromises the future utility and comparability of much hard-won experimental data.[45]

There is indeed no ideal dosage unit for defibrillation. The energy is meaningful *only* when the resistance, capacitance, and duration (expressed either as time or tilt) are all fixed. Fortunately, this is true in most clinical situations and with most devices. The possible occurrence of exceptions, however, is important to bear in mind, especially in the settings of high DFT.

It is important for clinicians to be able to compare ICD outputs in a meaningful way. We propose the effective current as a standard for rating ICD output. This would be calculated with a standard resistance of 50 Ω and chronaxie time of 3 ms. The defibrillation threshold would be determined in a conventional fashion. The value in terms of either a voltage or energy would then be converted into the rheobase current, and the safety margin would be the difference between the effective current of the ICD shock and the rheobase current. (In keeping with the strict definition of safety margin used in the following chapter, the rheobase current used would be that current that succeeds 99% of the time.)

1. Brewer JE, Tvedt MA, Adams TP, et al. Low voltage shocks have a significantly higher tilt of the internal electric field than do high voltage shocks. PACE 1995;18:214-220.
2. Kim Y, Schimpf PH. Electrical behavior of defibrillation and pacing electrodes. Proc IEEE 1996;84:446-456.
3. Mower MM, Mirowski M, Spear JF, et al. Patterns of ventricular activity during catheter defibrillation. Circulation 1974;49:858-861.
4. Zipes DP, Fischer J, King RM, et al. Termination of ventricular fibrillation in

dogs by depolarizing a critical amount of myocardium. Am J Cardiol 1975;36:37-44.
5. Witkowski FX, Penkoske PA, Plonsey R. Mechanism of cardiac defibrillation in open chest dogs with unipolar DC-coupled simultaneous activation and shock potential recordings. Circulation 1990;82:244-260.
6. Chen PS, Shibata N, Dixon EG, et al. Comparison of the defibrillation threshold and the upper limit of ventricular vulnerability. Circulation 1986;73:1022-1028.
7. Dillon SM. Optical recordings in the rabbit heart show that defibrillation strength shocks prolong the duration of depolarization and the refractory period. Circ Res 1991;69:842-856.
8. Zhou X, Knisley SB, Wolf PD, et al. Prolongation of repolarization time by electric field stimulation with monophasic and biphasic shocks in open-chest dogs. Circ Res 1991;68:1761-176.
9. Dillon SM. Synchronized repolarization following defibrillation shocks. A possible component of the defibrillation process demonstrated by optical recordings in the rabbit heart. Circulation 1992;85:1865-1878.
10. Irnich W. The fundamental law of electrostimulation and its application to defibrillation. PACE 1990;13:1433-1447.
11. Tung L , Sliz N, Mulligan MR. Influence of electrical axis of stimulation on excitation of cardiac muscle cells. Circ Res 1991;69:722-730.
12. Frazier DW, Krassowska W, Chen PS, et al. Extracellular field required for excitation in three dimensional anisotropic myocardium. Circ Res 1988;63:147-164.
13. Weiss G. Sur la possibilite' de rendre comparable entre eux les appareils survant a l'excitation electrique. Arch Ital de Biol 1901;35:413-446.
14. Fredericq H. Chronaxie: Testing excitability by means of a time factor. Physiol Rev 1928;8:501-545.
15. Lapicque L. Definition expèrimentalle de l'excitabilitè. Proc Soc Biol 1909;77:280-285.
16. Bourland JD, Tacker WA, Geddes LA, et al. Comparative efficacy of damped sine wave and square wave current for transchest ventricular defibrillation in animals. Medical Instrum 1978;12:38-41.
17. Koning G, Schneider H, Hoelen AJ, et al. Amplitude-duration relation for direct ventricular defibrillation with rectangular current pulses. Med Biol Eng 1975;13:388-395.
18. Gold JH, Schuder JC, Stoeckle H, et al. Transthoracic ventricular defibrillation in the 100 Kg calf with unidirectional rectangular pulses. Circulation 1977; 56:745-750.
19. Bourland JD, Tacker WA, Geddes LA. Strength duration curves for trapezoidal waveforms of various tilts for transchest defibrillation in animals. Med Instr 1978;12: 38-41.
20. Geddes LA, Bourland JD, Tacker WA. Energy and current requirements for ventricular defibrillation using trapezoidal waves. Am J Physiol 1980; 238: H231-H236.
21. Wessale JL, Bourland JD, Tacker WA, et al. Bipolar catheter defibrillation in dogs using trapezoidal waveforms of various tilts. J Electrocardiol 1980;13:359-366.
22. Niebauer MJ, Babbs CF, Geddes LA, et al. Efficacy and safety of defibrillation with rectangular waves of 2 to 20-milliseconds duration. Crit Care Med 1983; 11:95-98.
23. Geddes LA, Niebauer MJ, Babbs CF, et al. Fundamental criteria underlying the efficacy and safety of defibrillating current waveforms. Med Biol Eng Comp 1985; 23:122-130.
24. Tang AS , Yabe S, Wharton M , et al. Ventricular defibrillation using biphasic waveforms: the importance of phasic duration. J Am Coll Cardiol 1989;13:207-

214.

25. Jones JL, Jones RE. Determination of safety factor for defibrillator waveforms in cultured heart cells. Am J Physiol 1982;242:H662-H670.

26. Gold MR, Foster AH, Shorofsky SR. The relationship between pulse width and defibrillation. Eur J.C.P.E. 1994;4:136.(abstract)

27. Pearce JA, Bourland JD, Neilsen W, et al. Myocardial stimulation with ultrashort duration current pulses. PACE 1982; 5: 52-58.

28. Kroll MW. A minimal model of the monophasic defibrillation pulse. PACE 1993;16:769-777.

29. Hillsley RE, Walker RG, Swanson DK, et al. Is the second phase of a biphasic defibrillation waveform the defibrillating phase? PACE 1993;16:1401-1411.

30. Feeser SA, Tang AS, Kavanagh KM, et al. Strength-duration and probability of success curves for defibrillation with biphasic waveforms. Circulation 1990;82:2128-2141.

31. Kroll MW. A minimal model of the single capacitor biphasic waveform. PACE 1994;17:1782-1792.

32. Swartz JF, Fletcher RD, Karasik PE. Optimization of biphasic waveforms for human nonthoracotomy defibrillation. Circulation 1993;88:2646-2654.

33. Natale A, Sra J, Krum D, et al. Relative efficacy of different tilts with biphasic defibrillation in humans. PACE 1996;19:197-206.

34. Daubert JP, Frazier DW, Wolf PD, et al. Response of relatively refractory canine myocardium to monophasic and biphasic shocks. Circulation 1991;84:2522-2538.

35. Lerman BB, Clark C, Deale OC. Current-based thresholds are independent of transthoracic resistance. Clin Res 1986;34:320A.(abstract)

36. Lerman BB, Halperin HR, et al. Relationship between canine transthoracic impedance and defibrillation threshold: evidence for current based defibrillation. J Clin Invest 1987;80:797-803.

37. Kerber RE, Martins JB, Kienzle MG, et al. Energy, current, and success in defibrillation and cardioversion: clinical studies using an automated impedance-based method of energy adjustment. Circulation 1988;77:1038-1046.

38. Leonelli FM, Kuo CS, Fujimura O, et al. Defibrillation thresholds are lower with small output capacitor values. PACE 1995;18:1661-1665.

39. Rist KE, Tchou PJ, Mowrey K, et al. Small capacitors improve the biphasic waveform. J Cardiovasc Electrophys 1994;5:771-776.

40. Swerdlow CD, Kass RM, Chen P-S, et al. Effect of capacitor size and pathway resistance on defibrillation threshold for implantable defibrillators. Circulation 1994;90:1840-1846.

41. Troup PJ. Implantable cardioverters and defibrillators. Curr Prob Card 1989;14:737-738.

42. Block M, Breithardt G. Optimizing defibrillation through improved waveforms. PACE 1995;18:526-538.

43. Schwartzman D, Hull ML, Callans DJ, et al. Serial defibrillation lead impedance in patients with epicardial and nonthoracotomy lead systems. J Cardiovasc Electrophysiol August 1996;7: (in press).

44. Irnich W. Optimal truncation of defibrillation pulses. PACE 1995;18:673-688.

45. Babbs CF, Whistler SJ. Evaluation of the operating internal resistance, inductance, and capacitance of intact damped sine wave defibrillators. Med Instrum 1978;12:34-37.

5

The Defibrillation Threshold

Igor Singer, MBBS and Douglas Lang, PhD

EFFICACY of implantable cardioverter defibrillator therapy is critically dependent on the ICD's ability to terminate ventricular tachycardia and ventricular fibrillation in a variety of clinical circumstances. To ensure that a device is reliable, adequate testing procedures are required at the time of the implant to determine effective defibrillation energies. This information is needed to determine whether the ICD can be programmed with adequate energy margins so that the shock of the implanted device is sufficient to defibrillate the heart given the lead system and waveform.

Defibrillation Success Curve and Energy Margins

Defibrillation requirements (expressed in terms of energy, voltage or current) are best described by a dose-response curve. (Fig. 1) The probabilistic character of defibrillation efficacy inherent in this curve may be due to random variation in the size of the myocardial mass,[1] conductive properties of myocardial cells[2] or systematic alteration of cellular or tissue electrophysiological characteristics involved in the initiation and perpetuation of VF.[3] The precise mechanisms are still unknown. Repeated defibrillation attempts at different energy levels are required to plot an exact energy dose-response curve. However, in practice this is impractical and may be potentially hazardous. The conceptual framework of a dose-response relationship, however, is important, since it has significant experimental and clinical implications.

ICD therapy has at its foundation the concept of the *defibrillation success curve*, since implant requirements dictate that the patient has an adequate safety margin between the curve and the output of the device. *Safety margin* may be defined as the difference between the ICD output (E_{ICD} in Fig. 1) and the minimum shock

strength required for consistent defibrillation (E_{99}, the energy yielding 99% defibrillation success. Since the relationship between successful defibrillation and shock energy is a sigmoidal probability
curve (Fig. 1), the lower boundary of the safety margin corresponds
to the curve's upper corner (E_{99}). Hence, the safety margin is a
measure of the width of the plateau between the ICD output and
the upper corner of the patient's defibrillation curve. The safety
margin should be large enough to accommodate shifts in this curve
to a less favorable (i.e., rightward) position at higher energies. Such
shifts in the defibrillation requirements may occur as a result of
shifts in position of endocardial lead systems, prolonged fibrillation
time, progression of the underlying disease, ischemia, altered antiarrhythmic drugs or other, as yet undefined, factors.

In scientific studies investigating the effects of various interventions on defibrillation energy requirements, the position of the
defibrillation success curve is often summarized by particular
points on the curve such as energy associated with 50% or 90%
likelihood of defibrillation (E_{50} and E_{90} respectively).

It must be stressed that in clinical practice the true safety
margin cannot be precisely determined, given practical constraints
that preclude an accurate delineation of the defibrillation success
curve. *Consequently, the measured defibrillation threshold (DFT) more
likely than not corresponds to an energy value less than* E_{99}. In other
words, the difference between E_{ICD} and measured DFT - constituting
the *measured energy margin* (confusingly termed "safety margin" in
common clinical parlance) - usually *overestimates the true safety margin.* The extent of this overestimation, termed the *efficacy margin,*
will depend on the accuracy with which a defibrillation test protocol locates the defibrillation success curve. For each of the various
DFT testing methods to be discussed below, we will also provide
an estimate of the minimum E_{ICD} that will yield an "adequate" energy margin—one that assures that E_{ICD} will be $\geq E_{99}$ (with a true
safety margin $\geq$ zero joules).

*The theoretical treatment of energy, safety, and efficacy margins
and the various protocols for their determinations provided herein is
based on experimental data using monophasic shocks. Although DFTs
(and their increases under adverse conditions) appear to be lower with
biphasic shocks, we expect that the margin calculations hold accurate and
that the protocols will give correct results.*

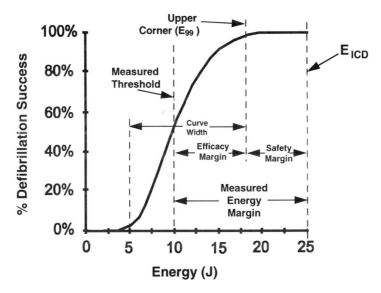

Figure 1. The defibrillation success curve: % probability for successful defibrillation versus shock energy. The *safety margin* for the device is defined as the difference between the ICD output (E_{ICD}, shown here programmed to 25 J) and the upper corner of the defibrillation success curve corresponding to (E_{99}) the energy having a 99% likelihood of achieving defibrillation. The *energy margin* measured during defibrillation threshold (DFT) testing (E_{ICD}-DFT) includes this true safety margin and an efficacy margin, which represents the increase in energy required to move from the measured DFT up the curve to energies that consistently defibrillate (E_{99}). The efficacy margin indicates the amount by which the measured energy margin overestimates the actual safety margin for the device due to the variability in the location of the DFT along the defibrillation success curve. Energy margin must be ≥ efficacy margin (i.e. E_{ICD} ≥ DFT + efficacy margin) to assure 99% defibrillation success and a nonnegative true safety margin. The energy difference (12 J) between the upper and lower "corners" (17 J and 5 J, respectively) is termed *curve width*.

Methods for Evaluating Energy Margins

Methods for assessing energy margins fall into two general categories: threshold techniques and verification techniques. *Threshold methods* are more rigorous, with a test sequence of repeated fibrillation-defibrillation episodes at various shock intensities that continues until one encounters energies that succeed at defibrillation and others, nearby, that fail. (Chap. 17) The DFT and enhanced DFT+ and DFT++ protocols (described later) belong to this category. These techniques determine the general location of the patient's defibrillation success curve so that an adequate energy margin can be provided.

In contrast, *verification techniques* are more clinically pragmatic, often requiring fewer fibrillation episodes. These techniques
are abbreviated because they do not require the patient to be tested
with energies that fail to defibrillate. While verification protocols
also verify energy margins for the patient, they do not locate the
defibrillation success curve as accurately as a threshold protocol.

In a verification procedure, intermediate energies that provide an adequate energy margin for the device are tested to verify
defibrillation success. If all test shocks defibrillate the patient, the
device is assumed to have an adequate energy margin for implant.
As will be outlined below, tests methods in this category are the
single-energy success protocols (3S, 2S or 1S = number of defibrillations at that energy) and the step-down success (SDS) protocol
(successful defibrillations at two neighboring energy levels).

As outlined in the following sections, energy margins required for ICD implant will depend on the specific protocol used
for evaluation the patient.[4,5] Based on our analysis of energy margins (see "Selecting the Best Protocol" below), we recommend the
step-down success protocol as the test procedure of choice. (Fig. 2)

According to the step-down success method, defibrillation
success is tested at two energies: if the initial defibrillation test is
successful, a second test is performed one step lower. While Fig. 2
depicts this protocol with a starting energy of 20 J, lower initial energies could be used as well. If the second test is also successful,
energy margins can be verified and the device implanted.

Failed defibrillations during these verification tests indicate
that the patient has moderate to high thresholds. To assure adequate energy margins for implant, threshold protocols must now be
used. (Fig. 2) If the initial shock fails, the patient can be evaluated
at higher energies to find the DFT energy that results in defibrillation. Enhanced (DFT+ and DFT++) procedures can be used to
validate the implant when the energy margin at the DFT is not adequate for a simple threshold protocol. When the initial shock in a
step-down success protocol succeeds, but the second shock fails,
the DFT is equal to the initial test energy. If this DFT does not have
adequate energy margin for implant, an enhanced DFT+ protocol
could be used. If these test methods indicate that the patient does
not have adequate energy margin for implant, the system should be
revised by repositioning the lead, adding additional defibrillation
electrodes, changing the waveform morphology or switching waveform polarity.

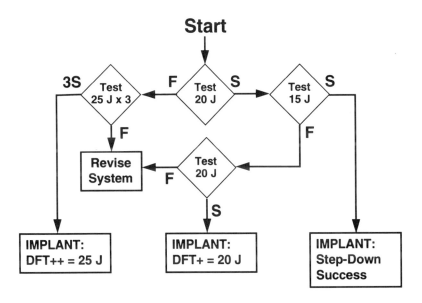

Figure 2. A defibrillation testing regimen incorporating both verification and threshold protocols for assessing implant margins. The figure illustrates the procedure for a device with a 30-34 J output, beginning at 20 J with a step-down success (SDS) protocol. If lower output ICDs are involved, the SDS protocol would begin at an energy one step higher than that equal to 50% of the maximum output. *(a)* If the initial SDS energy successfully defibrillates, the next lower energy (E_{SDS2}) is evaluated (e.g., 15 J in the figure). If both tests are successful, the minimum recommended ICD energy for implant equals 2.0 E_{SDS2}. *(b)* If the second test at E_{SDS2} fails to defibrillate, the starting energy then becomes equivalent to the standard decremental-step DFT measurement. Testing should return to the DFT to confirm defibrillation at the starting energy (i.e., DFT+), so that the minimum ICD energy can be 1.5 · DFT+. If this second test at the DFT starting energy DFT fails, the ICD lead system should be revised and testing repeated. *(c)* If the initial SDS energy fails at the beginning of this testing plan, testing should continue at the next higher energy to determine if adequate margins exist. Enhanced threshold protocols may be needed at this upper energy level, depending on the ICD output. In this figure, the upper energy level is 25 J, which requires a DFT++ (double confirmation) to provide the 1.2 · DFT++ energy margin for implant. If tests at this level encounter failure, the lead system should be revised. *F* and *S* are failed and successful defibrillations, respectively.

Energy Margins for Threshold Protocols

Threshold protocols are well established methods in the literature for assessing energy margins and are often used in clinical research. While clinical practice appears to favor verification protocols, we will first describe energy margins for the threshold methods to form a foundation for establishing energy margins for the more pragmatic verification techniques.

One threshold procedure commonly used in clinical research is the *standard DFT*. A DFT is determined by using a test sequence of repeated fibrillation-defibrillation trials with defibrillation attempts at successively increasing or decreasing energies using an external cardioverter-defibrillator or ICD. If the initial test energy is successful, subsequent defibrillation shock energies are decreased in succeeding trials until failure is encountered. If the initial energy fails to defibrillate, subsequent energies are incremented in later episodes until a successful defibrillation is obtained. By either testing sequence, the standard DFT is defined as the *minimum energy producing defibrillation success*. This measure is referred to, below, as simply DFT.

When assessing energy margins, the DFT is best viewed as a method for finding the general location of the defibrillation success curve. Due to the probabilistic nature of defibrillation, the bulk of the DFT measurements will be distributed along the sloping part of the curve.[6] The accuracy of the DFT as a method for estimating the energy margin will depend on the extent of this DFT distribution. Analysis of defibrillation probability indicates that DFTs obtained using a decreasing step protocol ($DFT_{decr\ steps}$) are distributed asymmetrically toward the upper end of the dose-response curve (Fig. 3),[a] with the average location at the energy that yields 71% defibrillation success (E_{71}, range E_{25} to E_{100}).[6] These results are very consistent with *in vivo* studies.[7-9] For example, the mean value for experimentally measured $DFT_{decr\ steps}$ was 10 ± 3.4 J, with energies that yielded defibrillation success probabilities ranging from 25% to 88% (mean $71 \pm 26\%$).[9] Thus, both probability analysis and animal studies agree that the DFT with decreasing steps is located along the upper three fourths of the defibrillation success curve, with the most probable location near 70% success and a distribution skewed to the upper part of the curve.

The variability in DFT each time it is repeated imposes certain restrictions on the selection of appropriate defibrillation energy

---

a.   The distribution of DFTs along the defibrillation success curve is influenced by the direction in which energies are changed during the DFT protocol.[6] DFT procedures that involve only decreasing energy steps have the distribution mentioned above in the text, with an average location at E_{71}. DFTs can also be measured with an increasing step protocol ($DFT_{incr\ steps}$), beginning first with energies *unlikely* to defibrillate. The $DFT_{incr\ steps}$ are distributed asymmetrically towards the *lower* end of the dose-response curve, with the average location near E_{35} (range E_1 to E_{75}, Fig. 3).[6] A DFT protocol starting near the midpoint of the curve ($DFT_{midpoint}$) could yield increasing or decreasing steps depending on the outcome of the first conversion attempt. The midpoint DFT protocol results in a DFT distribution centered at E_{56} with a range from E_{25} to E_{75} (Fig. 3).[13]

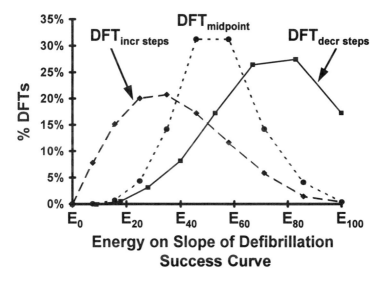

Energy on Slope of Defibrillation Success Curve

Figure 3. Distribution of DFT placements along the defibrillation success curve for three types of DFT protocols all using 20% energy steps. Threshold distributions along the curve were derived from an analysis of probabilities underlying the successful and failed defibrillation attempts involved in these protocols.[6] The DFT protocol using decreasing steps (DFT$_{decr steps}$) began with initial energies on the 100% success plateau beyond the success curve and stepped down in energy until an attempt failed. The decreasing step DFTs (*solid line*) are located along the upper 3/4 of the success curve, with a distribution skewed to the upper end. The midpoint DFT protocol (DFT$_{midpoint}$) began with initial energies near the midpoint of the success curve and stepped up or down to find the minimum energy yielding success. The distribution for the DFT$_{midpoint}$ (*dotted line*) is also located along the upper 3/4 of the defibrillation success curve, but the distribution is centered more to the middle of the curve. The increasing step DFT protocol (DFT$_{incr steps}$) began with initial energies near the bottom and increased in steps until a successful energy was found. The increasing step DFTs (*dashed line*) are located along the lower 3/4 of the defibrillation success curve, with the distribution skewed to the lower part.

margins for the patient's ICD.[4,5,7,10] If the DFT is located high on the defibrillation success curve (as in Fig. 4, curve *A*, with the DFT near E_{99}), the measured energy margin (E_{ICD} - DFT) closely approximates the actual safety margin, i.e., the width of the plateau between the curve and the output of the device (E_{ICD} - E_{99}). However, if the DFT is low on the curve (Fig. 4, curve *C*), the measured energy margin (E_{ICD} - DFT) will appear larger than the actual safety margin along the plateau (E_{ICD} - E_{99}). In this case, the measured energy margin includes both the safety margin between E_{99} and E_{ICD}, and an efficacy margin, which is the energy required to move up the curve from the measured DFT (E_{50} for curve C) to energies that consistently defibrillate, such as E_{99}. (Fig. 1)

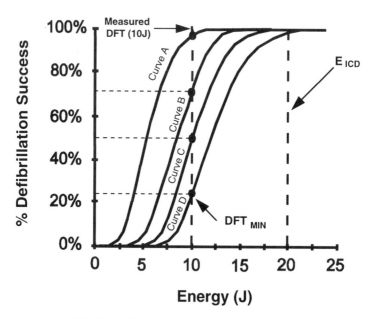

Figure 4. Four possible defibrillation success curves consistent with a DFT of 10 J.
Curve *A* represents a patient with low defibrillation energy requirements with the
DFT located near the top of the curve. Curves *B* and *C* represent patients with intermediate defibrillation energies with the DFT located at E_{75} and E_{50}, respectively.
Curve *D* represents the patient with the highest defibrillation energy curve possible
for a step-down DFT of 10 J. An energy margin of 2.0 DFT would place the minimum E_{ICD} at 20 J. For curve *D*, this places the ICD output at E_{99}. For the patient represented by curve *A*, this energy margin places the output of the device out on the
plateau with a safety margin of 10 J. Patients with intermediate defibrillation
curves (*B* and *C*) have somewhat smaller safety margins. For the patient depicted
by curve *B* (with a DFT = E_{75}), the minimum E_{ICD} is out on the plateau with a safety
margin of 8 J beyond E_{99} (see Appendix A, footnote *h*). For the patient in curve *C*
(DFT = E_{50}), the 2.0 · DFT energy provides a safety margin of only 5 J beyond the
defibrillation success curve (see Appendix A, footnote *g*). Note that curves *B-D*
could also represent various rightward (i.e., unfavorable) shifts in the defibrillation success curve due to ischemia or certain antiarrhythmic drugs, etc.

Since the standard DFT protocol does not indicate whether
the DFT is high or low on the curve, there is some uncertainty
whether the energy margin truly reflects the full safety margin for
the patient. *Thus, one should provide ICD shock energies with large
enough margins above the DFT to guarantee that even those patients
with DFTs that happen to end up low on the defibrillation success curve
will receive adequate therapy.* In determining the energy margin that
should be applied to all patients, one must consider the worst case
DFT: the patient for whom the defibrillation success curve is as far
to the right as the method allows (Fig. 4, curve *D*) with the DFT located at the lowest point on the curve (indicated by the term

DFT_{MIN} in Fig. 4). To properly assure patient safety, one must estimate how much of this energy margin is taken up by the efficacy margin along the curve and how much is left over for the margin of safety on the plateau.

For a DFT measured with decreasing steps, the lowest DFT position for the worst case patient is 25% success ($DFT_{MIN \, decr \, steps} = E_{25}$). To reach the top of the curve from this worst case DFT requires approximately $(2.0 \pm 0.3) \cdot DFT_{MIN}$ (see Appendix A), which corresponds to an increase in energy equal to approximately 75% of the defibrillation curve width.[6,9] This agrees with the reported energy increment required beyond the $DFT_{decr \, steps}$ for 100% defibrillation: energy to reach 100% success for all measured DFTs = 1.7 · DFT.[8]

Our theoretical analysis of DFT energy margins is also consistent with clinical work by Jones et al.,[11] who evaluated (during arrhythmia surgery) defibrillation success of test shocks above and below the DFT in patients with accessory pathways but otherwise normal hearts. Slightly larger energy margins were needed for 100% defibrillation of all patients ($2.6 \cdot DFT$),[11] since they used an increasing step DFT protocol in their study (see Appendix A). The $DFT_{incr \, step}$ protocol requires larger margins because the lowest DFT_{MIN} position is near the bottom of the defibrillation success curve.[6] The margin to reach the top of the curve corresponds to the full curve width, which equals $2.7 \cdot DFT$, according our analysis of defibrillation probability (see Appendix A). This agrees very closely with Jones' clinical results.

Thus, patients with decreasing step DFTs ≤ 15 J can be implanted with a 30-34 J device based on the standard DFT alone. The approximate $2.0 \cdot DFT$ energy margin required for these patients is within the energy output of the device. However, patients with higher defibrillation thresholds (≥ 20 J) may require more than a simple threshold measurement to satisfy implant energy margins. Lang et al.[7] have proposed an *enhanced DFT protocol* to help clarify energy margins in these situations. They recommended doing one or possibly two additional defibrillation trials at the measured DFT energy to allow implant with smaller energy margins.

For the enhanced protocol, if the first additional defibrillation test is successful, it is described as a DFT+. If two extra defibrillation tests are successful at the DFT, these are indicated as DFT++. If either DFT+ or DFT++ is encountered, there is a greater chance that the DFT is high on the defibrillation success curve. Thus, the energy margins for ICD implant can be smaller: $1.5 \cdot DFT+$ and $1.2 \cdot DFT++$ (see Appendix A). For a 30-34 J ICD, these smaller energy margins would allow ICD implant for patients with a DFT+ = 20 J or a DFT++ = 25 J. For ICDs with lower maximum output, the enhanced protocols could be used in a similar fashion to implant patients requiring smaller margins: e.g., for an ICD with a 20 J maximum output, implant could proceed with DFT+ = 12-13 J or DFT++ = 14-16 J.

Energy Margins for Verification Protocols
Verification protocols minimize the number of shocks delivered to the patient and are, therefore, more clinically pragmatic than the threshold protocols for assessing ICD energy margins. Of the two types of verification methods, the *step-down success* (SDS) protocol shares much in common with the DFT technique and will be discussed first.

Even though the SDS protocol does not necessarily end with a standard DFT measure, the initial stages of the SDS and DFT procedures are identical. (Fig. 2) Thus, if the SDS protocol ends with both the first and second tests successful, it defines an upper limit to the DFT. If one had continued the SDS protocol beyond the second SDS energy level (E_{SDS2}) and encountered a failed defibrillation, the E_{SDS2} energy would have equaled the DFT. If the energy one step below E_{SDS2} had been successful, then the DFT would have been lower than E_{SDS2}. Given that $DFT_{decr\,steps} \leq E_{SDS2}$, the worst case situation for the SDS protocol is that $E_{SDS2} = DFT_{decr\,steps}$. This link gives the E_{SDS2} all of the characteristics of the decreasing step DFT: its average location on the defibrillation curve is $\geq E_{71}$ with the worst case position for $E_{SDS2} = E_{25}$. Because of this, the energy margins for the step-down success protocol are similar to those for the decreasing step DFT: implant if $E_{ICD} \geq 2.0\,E_{SDS2}$ (where E_{SDS2} is the lower of 2 successful neighboring energy levels tested).

This implant margin provides some guidance for the initial starting energy for the step-down success protocol. To satisfy the "$E_{ICD} \geq 2.0\,E_{SDS2}$" criterion for a 30 J device, the highest energy for E_{SDS2} is 15 J, which places the initial SDS energy one step higher at 18-20 J. For a 20 J device, the maximum E_{SDS2} should be 10 J with the initial energy one step higher near 14-15 J.

Single-energy success protocols (3S, 2S or 1S) serve as alternatives to the SDS verification protocol.[10] These testing procedures differ from the SDS method in that the desired ICD energy margin is selected before testing and evaluated with a predetermined number of shocks. As for the SDS procedure, these single-energy success protocols do not locate the defibrillation success curve, but establish its upper (i.e., rightmost) boundary. Since the single-energy

Table 1. Adequate ICD energy margins for various threshold and verification protocols.

Test Method	Worst-case Location on Defibrillation Success Curve	Minimum Energy Recommended for 99% Defibrillation Success*
$DFT_{decr\ steps}$	E_{25}	$2.0 \cdot DFT$
DFT+	E_{50}	$1.5 \cdot DFT+$
DFT++	E_{75}	$1.2 \cdot DFT++$
Step-Down Success (SDS)	E_{25}	$2.0\ E_{SDS2}$
Single Energy 3S	E_{40}	$1.7\ E_{3S}$
Single Energy 2S	E_{25}	$2.0\ E_{2S}$

* Values derived from mathematical extrapolations of data reported by Davy et al[9] from defibrillation experiments in normal canines. (See Appendices) E = energy; S = success; E_{SDS2} = the lower of successful neighboring energy levels tested.

protocols have varying degrees of accuracy for defining the position of the defibrillation success curve, they each will have different energy margins for ICD implant (see Appendix *B* for derivation of 3S, 2S, and 1S energy margins). The more rigorous 3S protocol collects the greatest amount of information about the patient and requires the smallest implant margins, comparable to the DFT+: $E_{ICD} \geq 1.7\ E_{3S}$. The 2S protocol gains slightly less information and has energy margin requirements comparable to the $DFT_{decr\ steps}$: $E_{ICD} \geq 2.0\ E_{2S}$ for implant. The 1S protocol yields the least information about the patient and has the greatest energy margins among the verification techniques: $E_{ICD} \geq 2.7\ E_{1S}$ for implant.

Selecting the Best Protocol

Table 1 summarizes the energy margins for both threshold and verification protocols. (These parameters, as derived in Appendices A and B, should be taken only as approximate guidelines for patients with organic heart disease, since listed values for minimum ICD energies are based on experimental data from animals with normal hearts.) Note that for $DFT_{decr\ steps}$ and DFT+, there exist verification procedures with similar energy margin requirements. Since the verification methods often require fewer shocks and shorter defibrillation test durations, they are more attractive clinically than their threshold counterparts. Among the verification procedures, the step-down success (SDS) and 2S protocols have similar energy margins, but differences between these protocols indicate that the SDS method is preferred.

The step-down success protocol has several advantages over the single energy method. While the implant criterion with the SDS protocol ($E_{ICD} \geq 2.0\ E_{SDS2}$) is the same as the 2S protocol ($E_{ICD} \geq 2.0\ E_{2S}$), the SDS energy margin is based on the lower energy level

(E_{SDS2}). This allows the SDS protocol to start at a slightly higher energy than the 2S, improving the chances of VF defibrillation. Since neither protocol offers an energy margin advantage, the SDS is clinically more attractive as it subjects the patient to lower risk of experiencing failed defibrillation attempts.

In addition, the SDS protocol forms a seamless interface to the threshold techniques, should failed defibrillations be encountered in a high threshold patient. If the first SDS attempt fails, one can proceed to higher energies to find the DFT (or if margins are small, the DFT+ or DFT++). If the defibrillation attempt at the lower E_{SDS2} energy fails, the DFT is equal to the initial SDS energy. If this energy provides an adequate energy margin for a simple DFT, then the device can be implanted. If the energy margin is small, one can return to the initial energy to perform an enhanced DFT+ protocol. Since the SDS protocol starts at higher energies, a high threshold patient would be identified more quickly and with fewer failed defibrillations than with the 2S method.

Another favorable SDS aspect is its similarity with the DFT technique. Due to its decreasing step nature, the E_{SDS2} shares many of the characteristics of the decreasing step DFT: most importantly, its skewed distribution toward the top of the defibrillation success curve.[6] This skewed distribution has a significant impact on the range of energy margins provided by the $DFT_{decr\ steps}$ and SDS methods.

Since the $2.0 \cdot DFT$ energy margin for the decreasing step DFT protocol is based on a worst case patient (at the bottom of the 95% confidence interval), this margin will provide the fringe of the population with low positioned DFTs and ICD shock energy at the beginning of the plateau. (Fig. 5) Since almost all patients have DFTs located above this worst case DFT position, the $2.0 \cdot DFT$ margin will place the output of their ICDs to the right of the defibrillation curve out on the 100% success plateau. (Fig. 5, solid curve)

Almost all patients (90% = 100% - 10%) in Fig. 5 will have ICD energies $\geq 1.75\ E_{50}$, giving them safety margins $\geq$ one quarter curve width ($0.25\ E_{50}$) out beyond the defibrillation success curve. Proceeding slightly further out on the plateau, 75% of patients (i.e., those with $E_{ICD} \geq 2.0\ E_{50}$ in Fig. 5) have safety margins $\geq$ one half curve width; half the patients (i.e., those with $E_{ICD} \geq 2.25\ E_{50}$) have safety margins $\geq$ three-fourths curve width; and almost one third (i.e., those with $E_{ICD} \geq 2.5\ E_{50}$) have safety margins $\geq$ one full curve width beyond the edge of the defibrillation success curve. The E_{SDS2} shares this skewed distribution towards the high end of the defi-

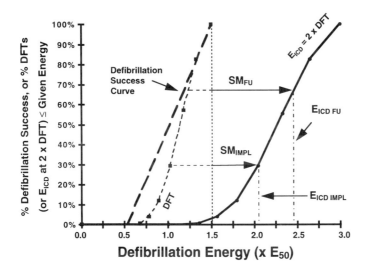

Figure 5. Cumulative distribution curves for the possible locations of $DFT_{decr\,steps}$ and $E_{ICD} = 2.0 \cdot DFT_{decr\,steps}$ plotted against defibrillation energy normalized to the midpoint of the defibrillation success curve. The straight *long-dashed line* represents the defibrillation success curve extending from $0.5\,E_{50}$ to $1.5\,E_{50}$ (i.e., curve width of $1.0\,E_{50}$). The *short-dashed curve* represents the cumulative distribution of $DFT_{decr\,steps}$ along the defibrillation success curve. The *solid curve* represents the cumulative distribution of ICD shock energies (E_{ICD}) providing a minimum energy margin of $2.0 \cdot DFT$. Each point on the E_{ICD} curve (exemplified by the dots) is generated by doubling, in the horizontal direction, the energy corresponding to a given point on the DFT cumulative distribution curve (exemplified by the solid squares). Note that all ICD energies $> 1.5\,E_{50}$ represent values along the plateau of the defibrillation success curve; the safety margin (*SM*), therefore, is defined by the horizontal segment extending from an energy of $1.5\,E_{50}$ to E_{ICD}. Due to the skewed distribution of the $DFT_{decr\,steps}$ towards the top of the defibrillation success curve, it is evident that the $2.0 \cdot DFT$ margin also provides safety margins to the majority of patients. (See text) This graph also demonstrates that if measured DFT is *artifactually* higher at follow up (FU) versus implantation (IMPL), i.e., solely from statistical variation of replicate measurements, increasing ICD output to twice the "new" DFT (i.e., to $E_{ICD\,FU}$) will widen the safety margin; however, the original safety margin would in no way be compromised if ICD output remained at $E_{ICD\,IMPL}$.

brillation success curve. Therefore, a worst case energy margin of $2.0\,E_{SDS2}$ will yield safety margins for the population that are equal to, if not greater than, the safety margins described above for the DFT. (Fig. 5)

By contrast, the 2S protocol does not have a testing bias influencing the 2S distribution along the defibrillation success curve, since it does not incorporate a decremental sampling of probabilities along the curve which yields this bias. The 2S distribution along the curve will be the same as the baseline E_{SDS2} distribution prior to the creation of its step-down sampling bias; it is primarily determined by the distribution of defibrillation thresholds within the population of ICD patient configurations near the E_{SDS2} energy. The heightened skewed distribution of the E_{SDS2} energies towards the top of the success curve yields a greater percentage of patients further out on the 100% success plateau with a 2.0 E_{SDS2} margin compared to the safety margin distribution with the 2.0 E_{2S} margin. This is another fundamental reason to use the step-down success protocols when verifying defibrillation energy margins for the patient.

On the surface, the 2S method is attractive since it is very straightforward with only one test energy. Due to this simplicity, some clinical centers have used a 2S protocol at 20 J for justifying ICD implant with 30-34 J devices. While a 2S protocol at 15 J would be sufficient to verify energy margins in this case, a 2S test at 20 J does not carry the same level of certainty. The 2.0 E_{2S} margin is based on a 95% confidence interval for the 2S method (see Appendix B). If one were to relax this level of confidence to 75%, then the 2S protocol would require only a 1.5 E_{2S} margin, which would support a 30 J device implant with 2S at 20 J. Use of this lower confidence level means that if the 2S test energy were somewhere on the slope of the defibrillation success curve, one has up to a 25% chance that the "1.5 E_{2S}" rule would not provide adequate energy margins to put the ICD energy on the plateau beyond the top of the defibrillation success curve. The actual therapeutic risk one experiences with the "2S at 20 J" implant criterion may be lower than this if the bulk of patients receiving this ICD/lead system have defibrillation thresholds far below the 2S energy. In this case, only those patients with thresholds within the vicinity of the 2S energy would be exposed to the increased risk of the 75% confidence interval: e.g., if only 25% of patients at a clinical center have thresholds near 15-20 J, approximately 6% of all patients evaluated at that center would be exposed to the risk of a substandard energy margin with the use of a "2S at 20 J" implant guideline [6% patients at risk = (25% of patients with high thresholds near 2S)·(25% chance of getting a low margin)].

Given that a 20 J step-down success protocol typically involves the same number of shocks as the "2S at 20 J" protocol, yet carries much less therapeutic risk, we recommend the use of the step-down success approach over the latter. This SDS recommendation still holds when considering the "2S at 15 J" protocol (which incurs none of the 20 J risks), due to the similarities between the SDS and DFT techniques and the seamless interface between the step-down method and the threshold protocols for high DFT patients.

Criteria for Adequate Energy Margins: Relation to "10 J Rule"
Historically, a minimum measured energy margin of 10-15 J has been used as an implant criterion. This "rule of thumb" has provided adequate energy margins for the CPI Ventak systems, judging by the low incidence of sudden death mortality seen with these devices. For E_{ICD} set at 30-34 J these 10 J energy margins are consistent with those specified in Table 1, assuming defibrillation threshold values ≤ 15 J or that an enhanced protocol (especially DFT++) is utilized when thresholds reach into the 18-25 J range.

Introduction of new leads and waveforms yielding lower measured DFTs or the deployment of smaller ICD devices with lower maximum energy output may change ICD guidelines from this absolute 10 J rule to one in which ICD energy margins are programmed based on some multiple of the measured DFT, as in Table 1. For example, assuming a 20 J maximum output device, a 15 J DFT violates the 10 J energy margin rule for implantation; yet, if the 15 J value is verified by a DFT++ protocol, the guidelines in Table 1 would justify implant, since defibrillation success is predicted for shock energies ≥ 18 J $= 1.2 \cdot 15$ J (i.e. within the device's capability.) Further study is needed to establish the role (and safety) of the energy margins (for ICD implant or high energy shock programming) as specified in Table 1 vs. the currently accepted empiric 10 J rule.

Time Dependent DFT Changes: Chronic and Acute
The key purpose for providing a patient with an adequate energy margin is to assure device function in the face of temporary or chronic increases in DFT. This may be due to chronic changes in threshold between implant and followup, possible temporary effects on threshold with prolonged VF duration or effects of an altered drug regimen. We will address the first 2 scenarios here and the last later in this chapter.

For *epicardial* lead systems, chronic changes in defibrillation threshold between implant and followup do not appear to be an issue. Animal and human studies with epicardial leads indicate that DFTs for patch leads do not shift substantially between generator replacements.[12-15] However, recent reports on the stability of defibrillation thresholds for *endocardial* lead systems are less consistent. Some studies indicate that DFTs do not change over time for monophasic and biphasic waveforms,[16-20] while others report a significant rise or fall in mean threshold[21-24] (three monophasic studies

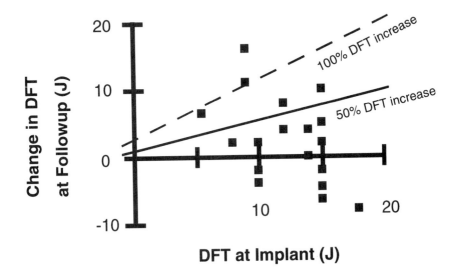

Figure 6. Change in defibrillation threshold for an endocardial defibrillation lead system between implant and followup (average 9.5 months) plotted as a function of the DFT at implant.[16] The mean defibrillation threshold at implant (12.4 + 0.7 J) was not significantly different from the mean threshold at followup (14.5 + 1 J). The majority of patients in this study (73% of 19 patients) evidenced DFT changes less than 50% above implant, since they fell below the line marked *50% DFT increase*. Two patients (11%) had DFTs that increased 50-100%, and they fell above this line, but below the dark solid line for *100% DFT increase*. Note that 3 patients (16%) had increases > 100%. These magnitudes of DFT changes are not seen with biphasic shocks in the *average* patient.[27]

show a 19%,[25] 32%[23] and 35%[26] increase; two biphasic studies show a 46%[24] increase and a 15%[27] decrease). When present, significant changes in mean thresholds were found to occur primarily between implant and predischarge several days later.[23-27]

Most of these studies follow similar patterns: a majority of patients evidenced only small DFT changes, with varying percentages having significantly higher or lower thresholds at followup, yielding the different outcomes of the various studies. The threshold trends for individual patients from one of the studies (which found no significant mean rise in DFT) is shown in Fig. 6.[16] The majority of patients in this study (73% of 19 patients) evidenced DFT changes less than 50%. Two patients (11%) had DFTs that increased 50-100% above implant, and three patients (16%) had threshold increases greater than 100%.

In a study of 146 patients with comparable numbers receiving monophasic and biphasic devices, the differences between the DFT changes was significant.[27] For the monophasic patients the mean DFT at implant, predischarge, and followup was 15.1 J, 18.3 J, and 17.0 J respectively. Both the predischarge and followup DFTs were significantly higher than the implant DFT. For biphasic patients the results were nearly reversed with DFTs of 13.3 J, 12.2 J, and 10.8 J for implant, predischarge, and followup. The followup mean was significantly *lower* than that of the implant. A clinically significant DFT rise ($\geq$ 2 energy steps—which was always $\geq$ 5 J) was seen in 11% of the monophasic patients but only in 1 (2%) of the biphasic patients. One could conclude that, while the probabilities of untoward therapy failure is lower, there is still a need for a true safety margin even with biphasic shock devices.

These changes in threshold could be due to the variation of repeated DFTs or a rightward shift in the defibrillation success curve. (E.g., Fig. 4) Changes in threshold due to replicate DFTs do *not* represent a true shift in the defibrillation success curve and, thus, will not affect the initial safety margin programmed for the device. Since the curve has not moved, the relative position between the top of the curve and the distribution of all possible E_{ICD} locations on the plateau for $2.0 \cdot DFT$ (Fig. 5) is unchanged. At implant, the $2.0 \cdot DFT$ guideline specifies an implant safety margin within this E_{ICD} distribution, $E_{ICD\ IMPL}$. (Fig. 5) If the DFT at followup were different due to replicate variability, reprogramming the device by reapplying the $2.0 \cdot DFT$ rule would specify a new location within this distribution of ICD energies, $E_{ICD\ FU}$. (Fig. 5) While the new safety margin at followup (SM_{FU}) is different from the implant safety margin (SM_{IMPL}), the original implant safety margin still remains valid because the curve has not shifted. If the device remained programmed to $E_{ICD\ IMPL}$, the patient would retain the original safety margin that justified the implant, even though the DFT has changed.

Our estimates of the threshold changes expected for repeated $DFT_{decr\ step}$ indicate that the replicate factor could contribute no more than $\pm$ 50% of the curve width and probably contributes half of this on average (see Appendix C). In the study depicted in Fig. 6, the majority of patients (73%) evidenced changes in DFT that were of this magnitude. Since these small changes are within the error of the evaluation technique, these threshold shifts are not clinically significant and might not even impact the safety margin obtained at implant.

Defibrillation threshold changes greater than 50% in Fig. 6 cannot be attributed to replicate DFT variation alone, and probably also reflect contributions of a rightward shift in the defibrillation success curve. For DFTs that increase 50% to 100%, the replicate DFT factor may have contributed from one quarter to one half of the increase, possibly more. For thresholds that have increased more than 100%, the majority of the threshold change is due to a shift in the position of the defibrillation success curve. Mechanisms for rightward shifts in this curve could include microdislodgement of the lead,[28] changes in myocardial substrate,[23] or altered pharmacologic exposure.

An acute factor that may influence defibrillation threshold is the *duration of VF*.[29-36] Animal studies indicate that prolonged fibrillation may be associated with moderately increased defibrillation thresholds.[29-32] Mean defibrillation energies in dogs and rabbits (DFT or E_{50}) increased 17-26% for VF durations of 30-40 s compared to arrhythmia durations of 10-15 s.[29-31] In swine, defibrillation thresholds out to 90 s did not influence the efficacy of test shocks with a 40% safety margin above the DFT.[32] While prolonged VF beyond 40 s may not have increased thresholds dramatically, it did increase the incidence of post-shock cardiac or respiratory dysfunction in most models.[29,31,32]

While these earlier studies involved primarily monophasic waveforms, preliminary data from canine experiments using biphasic shocks are consistent in showing (at each level of phase 1 tilt) progressive rises in DFT as VF duration increases from 3 s to 10 s to 40 s.[36]

In humans, defibrillation thresholds do not appear to change significantly for VF durations of 15-20 s compared to shorter arrhythmia durations of 5-10 s.[33,34] One clinical study found significantly increased defibrillation thresholds determined after failed sub-DFT shocks in 14 patients (21 ± 9 J after a mean VF duration of 28 ± 6 s) compared to standard threshold measurements (12 ± 7 J after a duration of 12 ± 4 s).[35] While it is conceivable that VF duration could have contributed to this increase, the authors proposed that the higher threshold measurements after failed sub-DFT shocks were associated with the effect of their multiple shock protocol.[35] After the failed sub-threshold shock, repeated defibrillation shocks were given to the patient in 100 V increments until defibrillation. While these multiple shocks delivered in rapid succession may have influenced defibrillation success, other evidence suggests that single sub-threshold defibrillation attempts do not influence the outcome of subsequent defibrillation attempts.[37]

Thus, clinical defibrillation thresholds are stable out to at least 20 s of fibrillation. Whether DFTs rise in humans for durations beyond 20 s is not clear; if they do rise with prolonged arrhythmias, animal studies suggest that the increase would be no greater than 26-40% for durations out to 40 s or more. According to AICD product experience,[38] 91% of arrhythmias receiving high energy therapy are converted by the first or second shock. Depending on the shock energy, these first two shocks would be delivered within the 20-30 s time frame. Since VF episodes treated by these early ICD shocks have stable defibrillation thresholds, the energy margins at implant are applicable, barring chronic changes in threshold from some other mechanism. By the third and fourth shock, 96% and 99% of arrhythmias have been converted by high energy shocks, respectively.[38] For the small percentage of episodes (1-4%) that continue out to this prolonged duration, defibrillation thresholds may have increased up to 26-40%. This does not appear to be a major therapeutic problem for ICDs, since most patients (75% or more) with a $2.0\ E_{SDS2}$ (or $2.0 \cdot DFT$) energy margin have defibrillation safety margins $\geq 50\%$ of the width of the defibrillation success curve. (Fig. 5) These safety margins are large enough to assure that the ICD operates in the face of extremely prolonged VF.

If clinical circumstances arise that lead one to suspect that the defibrillation success curve might shift rightward to higher energies, one should evaluate the efficacy of ICD high voltage therapy at followup to monitor the adequacy of ICD energy margins. If the curve has shifted rightward, the ICD may need to be programmed to higher energies, e.g., $E_{ICD} \geq 2.0 \cdot DFT$ for the new threshold. At implant, if one has adequate leeway for selecting larger energy margins, the device could be programmed to shock energies greater than the minimum requisite energy margin for that test protocol. If DFT changes occur chronically, selection of these slightly larger margins at implant may sustain proper energy margins for all patients.

Safety of Defibrillation Testing

Clinical experience indicates that intraoperative death as a result of DFT testing is rare although intractable VF has been reported.[39,40] Concern over this possibility has prompted the recommendation that physicians use the minimum number of VF inductions to verify adequate energy margins.[41] Unfortunately, it appears impossible to estimate the DFT a priori.[42] Little clinical data exist, however, regarding possible less extreme deleterious effects of DFT testing. There is anecdotal information about the effects of DFT testing on left ventricular function.[43,] One study reported that patients with ejection fractions < .30 can suffer prolonged reductions in their cardiac index even with endocardial systems;[44] another study found no such reduction.[45]

Another area of concern is the potential for adverse effects of transient episodes of hypotension during DFT testing on cerebral perfusion. Repeated episodes of fibrillation do lead to changes in the EEG.[46,47] We have studied this by plotting the changes in real time on a topographical color spectrum display, or in an analog fashion, to monitor continuous EEG during DFT testing.[43] The duration and the number of defibrillation episodes appear to be critical. More than six VF episodes lasting > 20 s have produced persistent EEG changes lasting up to several minutes. The significance of these changes is unknown at present, although similar changes during coronary artery bypass surgery have been shown to be associated with postoperative confusional states and, at times, local neurologic deficits.[46] Continuous EEG monitoring during DFT testing may enhance the safety of the testing procedures and help minimize the potential for transient cerebral dysfunction resulting from repeated fibrillation-defibrillation episodes during ICD testing. Similar techniques may also be used to help program the third-generation ICD devices and to optimize therapy with respect to the perfusion.

Upper Limit of Vulnerability Method

Assuming sufficient device energy, the dosage question also arises. It is tempting to simply program the device to its maximum output. This however, may not be the optimal tactic.[48] Higher energies increase battery drain, but additionally may have important electrophysiological consequences, including increased propensity for *de novo* arrhythmia development,[49-52] decreased myocardial contractility,[53] and myocardial damage.[54] Even though the biphasic waveforms have been shown to be less likely to cause electrophysiological abnormalities than monophasic waveforms[2] there may be some advantage to programming the first few shocks to a minimum appropriate energy margin over the DFT. This suggests the desirability of a simple method of determining the DFT (as opposed to merely verifying an adequate ICD output margin); ideally this would be done with a minimum number of fibrillation episodes.

One possible method for achieving this goal is to determine the upper limit of vulnerability (ULV) and to use it to assess DFTs.

With this approach, a high energy shock is delivered into the T-wave during a paced rhythm (typically at a basic rhythm of 500 ms). The lead with the latest peaking monophasic T-wave is selected and shocks are delivered after the eighth basic pace beat, at coupling intervals corresponding to 0 ms, 20 ms, 40 ms, and 60 ms before, and 20 ms after the peak of the T-wave.[55,56] Test shock energy is progressively reduced until fibrillation is induced. The highest level at which VF is induced is referred to as the ULV. Recent clinical and experimental studies have demonstrated a correlation between the DFT and the ULV.[55-59] Ideally, a DFT can be estimated with only 1 fibrillation episode.

If fibrillation is induced during this procedure, the defibrillation attempt (moderate energy "quasi-rescue" shock) could be used as a part of a standard testing protocol (DFT, 2S or 3S), or the patient could be rescued immediately to minimize exposure to VF. The energy of the quasi-rescue defibrillation shock could be chosen to be optimal by a certain formula based on the levels of the preceding ULV shock energies.[60] The result (success or failure) of the moderate energy quasi-rescue shock could then be used to increase the accuracy of the DFT estimate by a related formula.

The ULV process is also probabilistic.[58] Paralleling the defibrillation success curve, the ULV curve also exhibits a sigmoidal shape. The ULV value is sensitive to the exact placement of the shock in the T-wave.[61] Good correlations between ULV and DFT have been shown, in humans, as long as the T-wave shocks are delivered with the proper timing.[62,63] The ULV plus 3 J appears to be a good estimate for the E_{90} value;[55] and ULV plus 5 J for E_{99}.[56] It should be noted that these energy estimates for probability of defibrillation success were derived using pulses delivered from 133 μF capacitors[55] (nominal value of about 120 μF—see Chap. 11); the safety margin for ULV with other devices having capacitors of different (most likely smaller) values may be better defined by current or even voltage rather than by energy. (Chap. 4) For example, the first shock output could be set at about 0.7 A of average current or about 60 V of leading edge voltage above the ULV.

Effects of Antiarrhythmic Drugs on Defibrillation

Pharmacological therapy is often used in patients with ICDs to minimize the frequency of therapy delivery by the device. Since some antiarrhythmic drugs also affect DFT, the effects of antiarrhythmic therapy on DFT are important to consider when estab-

Table 2. Effects of various drugs on DFT.

Increase	No Change	Conflicting Reports	Decrease
Encainide[75]	MODE[75]	Quinidine[84,88]	Amiodarone[66,67] (acute)
ODE[75]	Procainamide[80,85]	Bretylium[84,88,89]	Clofilium[73,89]
Flecainide[76]		Isoproterenol[72,93]	Sotalol[74,92]
Recainam[77]		Mexiletine[71,79]	NAPA[92]
Amiodarone[65-71] (chronic)		Lidocaine[78,80,81]	
Atropine[72]			

lishing safety margins during the ICD implant and/or testing, and when the pharmacological therapy is modified. Relatively little data are available on this subject, and some data are conflicting. The discrepancies are at least in part related to the lack of the standardized testing procedures per se. A summary of the data is provided in Table 2.[64]

Drugs That Increase DFT
Class 1C drugs have been shown to increase DFT.[75,76] For example, this has been demonstrated for encainide, a Class 1C drug. Fain et al[75] examined the effects of intravenous encainide and its two major metabolites, o-dimethyl encainide (ODE) and 3-Methoxy-ODE (MODE), on the energy requirements for defibrillation in open-chest dogs. Following intravenous administration of encainide and ODE, the mean energy required to achieve 50% success of defibrillation (E_{50}) increased by $129 \pm 43\%$ and $76 \pm 34\%$ respectively, from control values. These values returned to the baseline after the washout of both drugs, demonstrating reversibility of the drug effect. No significant increase in E_{50} was observed after administration of MODE.

Another Class 1C drug, flecainide, has also been shown to increase DFT in a dose-dependent fashion.[76] The investigational Class 1C drug, recainam, has also been shown to elevate DFT.[77]

In general, Class 1B drugs cause a reversible concentration-dependent increase in energy requirements for successful defibrillation.[78,79] Lidocaine causes a reversible, concentration dependent increase in energy requirements for successful defibrillation.[80] This result may, however, be restricted to monophasic waveforms.[81] Another orally administered Type 1B antiarrhythmic drug, mexiletine, has been associated with increased DFTs in a single patient.[79] However, no controlled studies in either animals or in humans are available at present to corroborate this clinical observation. The possibility that the Class 1B action of phenytoin (Dilantin) may be associated with increased defibrillation energy requirements has not been investigated, to our knowledge.

Amiodarone, a Class 3 drug, has also been associated clinically with elevated DFTs. Amiodarone has multiple electrophysiologic properties, and the experimental and the clinical data are conflicting. The effect of amiodarone on DFT appears to be dependent on timing. Acute administration may lower the DFT.[66,67] On the other hand, a clinical case report and other studies suggest that chronic oral administration of amiodarone may result in elevation of DFT.[65,68-70] In experimental animals, Haberman et al[65] found two separate time-dependent manifestations; DFTs progressively increased the longer the animal had been exposed to the drug and the longer the VF was permitted to persist.

Fogoros described a patient in whom amiodarone appeared to elevate the DFT, with a return of DFT to an acceptable level following amiodarone discontinuation.[68] Guarnieri et al found striking increases in DFTs at the time of generator changes in ICD patients taking amiodarone.[69] The mean DFT increased from 10.9 ± 4.3 J at the time of the initial implant, to 20 ± 4.7 J at the time of the generator replacement. In contrast, DFTs decreased in patients taking either no antiarrhythmic drugs or only Class 1A antiarrhythmics.

Epstein et al in a multicenter retrospective study of 1,946 patients found that 90 patients (4.6%) had an elevated DFT ($\geq$ 25 J). [70] Fifty-two percent of these patients were receiving amiodarone, and 26% received other antiarrhythmic drugs. Elevated DFTs apparently related to amiodarone may reflect preselection bias of patients with less favorable prognosis (i.e., arrhythmias unresponsive to other antiarrhythmic drugs or other variables that may influence DFTs, e.g., myocardial mass) and may not necessarily reflect a deleterious effect of amiodarone on DFTs per se. Nevertheless, these data suggest possible adverse effect of amiodarone on DFT.

In summary it appears that amiodarone lowers the DFT when administered acutely, intravenously or orally, but chronically it may elevate DFT. The differences observed in the acute dog model and the chronic effects of amiodarone on DFTs clinically may be related to its metabolite, as well as the total body stores of the drug.[82] The drug metabolite, desethylamiodarone, and amiodarone accumulate in the myocardium, which may explain the delayed onset of the drug's antiarrhythmic action and the increase in DFTs in patients taking the drug chronically.[82,83]

Drugs With Minimal Effects or With Conflicting Reports
Class 1A drugs do not appear to alter DFT significantly. Dorian et al[84] found no significant effects on defibrillation energy requirements after quinidine infusion. Another Type 1A drug, Procainamide, was found to have no significant effects on DFTs acutely in response to intravenous bolus of procainamide (15 mg/kg) in the dog or the pig model.[85] It also has no effect on DFT in humans except occasionally with high doses.[80]

Guarnieri et al demonstrated that DFTs decreased in patients taking Class 1A agents at the time of the generator replacement relative to the DFTs at the time of the implant.[61] However, other factors may have been operative in these patients, for example, lead maturation, altered cardiac size, concomitant effects of other drugs or other, as yet poorly defined, clinical variables.

Contrasting results have been reported by Woolfolk[86] and Babbs[87] with respect to quinidine, demonstrating an increase in DFT. This discrepancy may be attributable to the high, probably toxic doses of quinidine used in these animal studies.

The effects of bretylium tosylate on DFT have been studied by a number of investigators.[83,86-88] Bretylium did not alter the relation between energy and the likelihood of successful defibrillation in dogs. Dorian et al found that bretylium (6-10 mg/kg) did not affect the relation between energy and the likelihood of successful defibrillation.[84] Similarly, no significant effect of bretylium on DFT was demonstrated by two other investigators.[88,89] On the other hand, Tacker et al found that DFT was lowered following intravenous bretylium tosylate (10 mg/kg IV), 15-90 min after injection in dogs.[90] These apparent differences in the results are most likely related to the differences in the methodology for measurement of DFTs

Drugs that Decrease DFT
A number of drugs have been shown to decrease DFT. Primary potassium channel blockers are agents with such an effect.[91] Clofilium is an antiarrhythmic drug that blocks outward potassium current in the cell membrane and produces clinical defibrillation. Tacker et al found that clofilium decreases the threshold current and energy following an intravenous bolus of the drug in the canine model.[90]

Other drugs, including D-sotalol and N-acetylprocainamide (NAPA), the metabolite of procainamide, have also been shown to decrease DFT.[92]

Catecholamines facilitate ventricular defibrillation in animals. Ruffy et al examined the effects of beta adrenergic stimulation and blockade on DFTs in anesthetized dogs. In that study beta adrenergic stimulation decreased DFT.[93] This effect was blocked by administration of propranolol.[93] However, Wang et al found a DFT increase with isoproterenol in dogs.[72]

Salutary effects on DFT also have been observed in response to aminophylline, an agent with sympathomimetic properties, due to the combined effects of catecholamine release from the sympathoadrenal system, blockade of adenosine receptors, and phosphodiesterone inhibition.[94]

The beneficial effect of catecholamines in lowering the DFT is important clinically, since their administration facilitates defibrillation during cardiopulmonary resuscitation. These effects should also be carefully considered during ICD implantation and administration of catecholamine infusions avoided when DFTs are assessed.

Anesthetic agents, such as fentanyl, can reduce the DFT as compared to pentobarbital or enflurane.[95] This could lead to a transient artifactual increase in the measured energy margin at implant.

Summary of Antiarrhythmic Drug Effects on DFT

Although the data with respect to antiarrhythmic drugs is incomplete and at times conflicting, some general observations may be derived from the available data. In general, those drugs that interfere with fast sodium transport tend to increase DFT. This may be due to the lowering of excitability which interferes with the effect of the defibrillating shock.[96] These effects appear to be dose dependent. In therapeutic doses, however, Type 1A antiarrhythmic drugs appear to have no significant effect on DFT. Drugs that alter repolarization velocity appear to have no consistent effect on the defibrillation requirements; whereas DFT appears to be higher on chronic oral amiodarone, defibrillation energy requirements appear reduced with sotalol. Drugs that have beta adrenergic stimulating properties facilitate defibrillation.

Consideration of potential effects of antiarrhythmic drugs on DFT should focus on drug metabolites as well as the parent compound, as in the case of amiodarone. Standardization of the methodology for testing DFT experimentally may shed additional light in cases where conflicting results appear to exist.

Effects of Cardiac Surgery

The impact of systemic and topical cooling, cardioplegia and ischemia from aortic cross-clamping on DFT was examined by Borbola et al.[97] Sensing parameters and DFTs did not significantly differ from those obtained one to two weeks post cardiopulmonary bypass.

Blakeman et al further examined the effect of coronary revascularization on DFT testing in 10 patients, five of whom were implanted with ICD immediately and five 1-week post-coronary revascularization.[98] They compared the DFTs with 20 patients who underwent ICD implantation without concomitant surgery. These investigations found no significant differences in DFTs between the two groups, suggesting that residual effects of cardioplegia, corecooling and operative ischemia may not have significant clinical effects on DFTs.

Approach to the Patient with High DFT

True incidence of high DFT, too high to permit a safe implantation of ICD, is unknown. In an earlier review of the literature, Troup[99] estimated the incidence of high DFTs at 0.4% of attempted implantations. In contrast, Epstein et al[70] in a more recent retrospective, multicenter study estimated the incidence of elevated DFTs at 4.6%, 10 times the incidence found by Troup[99] which may in part be accounted for by a selection bias inherent in a retrospective study design. Interestingly, greater than half these patients were taking amiodarone. It is the authors' opinion, that the "true" incidence is likely to be lower than that reported by Epstein et al even for that monophasic waveform era. The actual incidence, however, is difficult to ascertain, since absence of standardized testing protocols limits comparison of results between different clinical centers and investigators. Other clinical variables may preclude rigorous testing, e.g., hemodynamic instability or occurrence of myocardial or cerebral ischemia during the ICD implant and testing.

When confronted by a patient with elevated DFT, it should be noted that this parameter can be influenced by selection of different pulse waveform, duration, electrode polarity and multiple paths for defibrillation. (See Chap. 6 for a discussion of the last two issues.) The impact of these factors on the management of high threshold patients should be considered.[100]

In the current era of unipolar and biphasic waveform ICD systems, it has become fairly uncommon to encounter a situation in which DFT is elevated to an extent that encroaches on the energy margins desired for implantation. Given the concomitant trend towards lower energy and smaller devices, such a scenario may still arise despite these technological improvements. The following recommendations can then be considered for optimizing DFT.

1. Size and number of the defibrillation leads should be maximized whenever possible. Endocardial lead systems with longer right ventricular electrodes will lower the resistance to the current and increase the efficiency in delivering the shock to the heart. However, the optimal RV coil length may depend on the pathway used. For the unipolar approach a long RV coil is favored; for a purely transvenous system a long RV coil could direct too much current through the tricuspid valve region and too little through the apex. Hence the paradoxical (at first blush) result that when *all* leads are within the heart one wants to maximize the lead-to-lead resistance in order to maximize the amount of myocardium receiving the current.[101]

2. Optimize distribution of the defibrillation field to the cardiac mass. For *endocardial* lead systems, this may involve placement of the tip of the defibrillation catheter as deep in the right ventricular apex as possible. If lead alone (or with a possible unipolar system) defibrillation does not provide adequate energy margins, subcutaneous chest electrodes can be added to the endocardial system to improve efficiency of the system and distribution of the shock fields within the heart. An array of three long conductors (rather than the traditional "patch") placed in the left axillary region can provide low resistances and low DFTs.[102] One patient study reported an average threshold reduction of 40% over a pure transvenous approach.[103] The incremental advantage over a purely unipolar system remains to be investigated.

    For the rare patient with an *epicardial* patch electrode system, we place one patch electrode anterior to the right ventricle, the intraventricular septum and the anterior portion of the left ventricle. The other patch electrode is placed posterolateral, over the epicardial or extrapericardial aspect of the left ventricle. Patch orientation should be such that the anterior and the posterior patches are nearly parallel to one another. If this fails to achieve satisfactory DFT, then several alternative positions and orientations of the patches may be used. Alternative approaches have been described including placing one patch near the right atrium and the other over the cardiac apex or over the apicolateral left ventricular wall.[104,105] Other approaches have also been described, including an inferior-anterior[106] and inferior-posterior approach.[107]

If increasing the patch electrode surface area or orientation is unrewarding, then dual pathway epicardial defibrillation may be tried next. This may be accomplished by positioning a superior vena cava electrode at the junction of the right atrium and using that electrode and the left ventricular electrode in common, versus the right ventricular electrode. A reverse polarity may also be tried. Electrode geometry may be altered by connecting the superior vena cava electrode with the left ventricular patch electrode using a Y-adapter. Alternatively, superior vena cava electrode to left ventricular patch defibrillation may also be tried. See Chap. 6 for further discussion.

4. Consider converting to a higher output device. However, the higher output device must have a waveform of equivalent or improved performance. High energy biphasic waveforms generated from large capacitors[108,109] and with long pulse widths[110,111] have lower efficacies and hence the defibrillation success improvement desired with the higher energy may not actually occur. Higher energy shocks also require a proportional charge time (assuming equal battery capability—see Chap. 13) which can increase the acute DFT.

5. Finally, the role of myocardial ischemia and antiarrhythmic drugs should be considered in patients with high DFTs. Myocardial ischemia is difficult to assess during operative ICD testing. However, persistent ST elevation or hypotension should alert the implanting physician to the possibility of myocardial ischemia or infarction. In that case, further DFT testing should be postponed. In patients with high DFTs, antiarrhythmic drugs known to elevate DFTs should be either discontinued or the dose decreased. These drugs include amiodarone, Class 1C and Class 1B drugs (as discussed above).

What should be done with patients in whom despite all attempts at lowering DFTs, the energy margin remains < 10 J? Epstein's data[70] support implantation of ICD in such cases, anyway. Of 90 patients with DFTs > 25 J, 71 (82%) received an ICD. On followup, death occurred in 19 of the 71 patients (27%) with an ICD (eight arrhythmic) and 8 of the 16 (50%) without an ICD (four arrhythmic). Actuarial survival at 5 years for the ICD patients was 73%, whereas no patients without an ICD survived beyond 32 months. Although this study strongly argues for ICD implantation in such cases, it is possible that the clinical decision to implant or not to implant ICD differentiated clinical outcomes by biasing the "sicker" patients to the amiodarone group. Nevertheless, in the absence of prospective randomized studies, our practice currently concurs with that of Epstein.[70]

The rationale for this approach may be provided by the following arguments: First, the initial tachyarrhythmia in many ICD patients is ventricular tachycardia rather than ventricular fibrillation. Therefore, cardioversion may be effective even when defibrillation efficacy margin is inadequate. Second, despite an energy margin of < 10 J, probability of defibrillation, though less than 100%, is greater than zero and is most likely placed somewhere on the steep part of the defibrillation success curve. (Fig. 1) Hence, even if one cannot guarantee successful defibrillation, it is probable that the patient with a high DFT is more likely to survive an episode of ventricular tachyarrhythmia with an ICD.

Appendix A: Margins for Threshold Protocols

To estimate the magnitude of efficacy margins determined with threshold protocols, we must refer to data on the *width of the defibrillation success curve*. Davy et al[9] have reported a mean partial curve width (i.e., the difference between the energies at 80% and 20% success, E_{80}-E_{20}) of $[0.85 \pm 0.27] \cdot E_{20}$, in the canine model. Assuming a linear increase in energy between 20% and 80% (E_{50} = 1.4 E_{20}),[b] the partial width can also be expressed in terms of midpoint energy of the curve (E_{50}): partial width = E_{80} - E_{20} = (0.6 ± 0.2)·E_{50}.[c] By extrapolating the linear section of this curve to energies

---

b. Since E_{50} is midway between E_{20} and E_{80}, the value of E_{50} can be derived from E_{20} and the partial curve width (E_{80}-E_{20} = 0.85 E_{20}) as follows (by linear interpolation): E_{50} = E_{20} + (0.5 · partial curve width) = E_{20} + (0.5·0.85 E_{20}) = E_{20} + 0.4 E_{20} = 1.4 E_{20}.

c. Since E_{50} = 1.4 E_{20}, or E_{20} = E_{50}/1.4, the partial width from Davy et al.[16] can be expressed in terms of the mid-point energy as follows: partial width = 0.85 E_{20} =0.85 · (E_{50}/1.4)[b] = (0.85/1.4) · E_{50} = 0.6 E_{50}. Thus, the partial width measured in Davy's experiments can be expressed as E_{80}- E_{20} = (0.85 ± 0.27) · E_{20} = (0.85 ± 0.27) · [E_{50}/1.4][b] = (0.6 ± 0.2) · E_{50}.

at 1% and 99% success (E_1 and E_{99}), the full defibrillation success curve width in the dog (E_{99} - E_1) is approximately $(1.0 \pm 0.3) \cdot E_{50}$.[d]

Decreasing Step DFTs

The lowest $DFT_{MIN\ decr\ step}$ requires an increase of energy equal to three fourths of the defibrillation success curve to reach the 100% plateau. Therefore, the efficacy margin required to reach the top of the defibrillation curve from a $DFT_{MIN\ decr\ steps}$ of E_{25} is equal to $0.75 \cdot$ (full width) = $(1.0 \pm 0.3) \cdot DFT_{MIN\ decr\ steps}$.[e] If one used the DFT measured with the decreasing step protocol, one would have to deliver shock energies at (2.0 ± 0.3) $\cdot DFT$ to assure 100% defibrillation for all subjects: $E_{99} = DFT_{MIN}$ + largest efficacy margin = $DFT_{MIN} + (1.0 \cdot DFT_{MIN}) = 2.0 \cdot DFT_{MIN}$.

This closely agrees with the reported increase in energy needed above the decreasing step DFT to assure defibrillation success for test shocks in all animals $(1.7 \cdot DFT_{MIN\ decr\ steps})$.[8] This increment in energy was needed to move the lowest placed $DFT_{decr\ step}$ up the curve to reach the plateau for 100% probability of successful defibrillation.

Increasing Step DFTs

DFT protocols measured with an increasing step DFT protocol[a] require larger energy margins to guarantee defibrillation success in all patients. McDaniel and Schuder[6] predict that the average $DFT_{incr\ steps}$ is near E_{35}, and $DFT_{MIN\ incr\ steps}$ is near E_5. The efficacy margin to reach the top of the defibrillation curve corresponds essentially to the full curve width, which results in an energy margin of $2.7 \cdot DFT_{MIN\ incr\ steps}$.[f] Thus, with an increasing step DFT protocol,

---

d.   The full curve width of the defibrillation curve (E_{99} - E_1) can be defined by extrapolating the linear midsection of the defibrillation curve (E_{80} - E_{20}) to the upper and lower extremes of the curve, E_{99} and E_1. Since this full width spans a larger range of defibrillation percent probabilities (99% - 1% = 98%) than the partial width (80% - 20% = 60%), the full width will be proportionately larger: full width = (98%/60%) $\cdot$ partial width = $1.63 \cdot (0.6 \pm 0.2) \cdot E_{50} = (1.0 \pm 0.3) \cdot E_{50}$.

e.   The energy at E_{25} can be expressed in terms of the midpoint energy as follows: By linear interpolation, $E_{25} = E_{50} - 0.25 \cdot$ full width = $E_{50} - 0.25 \cdot [1 \cdot E_{50}]^d = 0.75 \cdot E_{50}$, or $E_{50} = E_{25}/0.75$. The energy required to reach the top of the curve from a $DFT_{MIN\ decr\ steps} = E_{25}$ is equal to $0.75 \cdot$ full width = $0.75 \cdot [(1.0 \pm 0.3) \cdot \{E_{50}\}]^d$ = $0.75 \cdot [(1.0 \pm 0.3) \cdot \{E_{25}/0.75\}^e] = (1.0 \pm 0.3) \cdot DFT_{MIN\ decr\ steps}$.

f.   The worst case position for $DFT_{incr\ steps}$ is at the 5% success point on the defibrillation curve; by linear interpolation, $E_5 = E_{50} - 0.45 \cdot$ full width = $E_{50} - 0.45 \cdot [(1.0 \pm 0.3) \cdot \{E_{50}\}]^d = 0.55 \cdot E_{50}$. The energy required to reach the top of the defibrillation curve from a $DFT_{MIN\ incr\ steps} = E_5$ is equal to $0.95 \cdot$ full width = $0.95 \cdot$

one would expect test shock energies to be at least (2.7 ± 0.3) · DFT before 100% defibrillation success is obtained for all patients.

This analysis of DFT energy margins agrees nicely with clinical work by Jones et al[11] Their study evaluated defibrillation success of test shocks above and below the DFT to determine energy margins for ICD implant. The DFT protocol used in this study involved increasing steps, since the initial shock energies were set below the average DFT energy. They found that 2.6 · DFT was required to achieve 100% success for all patients,[11] which is in close agreement with the predicted margin of 2.7 · DFT.

Enhanced DFT Protocols
For patients with DFTs ≥ 20 J, the variability of the DFT placement on the defibrillation success curve could have a significant impact on the efficacy and safety margins for devices. This may also be true if the ICD energy is programmed to a lower energy near the DFT value, so that the device energy margins are small.

Lang et al.[7] have proposed an enhanced DFT protocol to help obtain adequate energy margins in these situations. They recommended doing one or possibly two additional defibrillation trials at the measured DFT energy to determine where the DFT is located on the curve. If the first additional defibrillation test is successful, it is described as a DFT+. If two extra defibrillation tests are successful at the DFT, these are indicated as DFT++. If either DFT+ or DFT++ is encountered, there is a greater chance that the DFT is high on the curve. This would indicate that the efficacy margin needed to move all patients to the 100% success plateau is smaller.

Lang et al.[7] have shown that the minimum position for DFT+ on the defibrillation success curve is near E_{50}, while that for DFT++ is approximately E_{75}. The efficacy margins for these defibrillation threshold measures would be $1.5 \cdot DFT+$[g] and $1.2 \cdot DFT++$[h]. If the additional test fails (DFT-) or there is a mixed

---

$[(1.0 \pm 0.3) \cdot \{E_{50}\}]^d = 0.95 \cdot [(1.0 \pm 0.3) \cdot \{E_5/0.55\}^f] = (1.7 \pm 0.3) \cdot DFT_{MIN \text{ incr steps}}$. Thus, $E_{99} = DFT_{MIN} + \text{efficacy margin} = DFT_{MIN} + (1.7 \pm 0.3) \cdot DFT_{MIN} = (2.7 \pm 0.3) \cdot DFT_{MIN}$.

g. The energy required to reach the top of the defibrillation success curve from a $DFT_{MIN \text{ decr steps}} = E_{50}$ is equal to $0.5 \cdot \text{full width} = 0.5 \cdot [1.0 \ E_{50}]^d = 0.5 \ E_{50}$. Thus, $E_{99} = DFT_{MIN} + \text{efficacy margin} = DFT_{MIN} + 0.5 \cdot DFT_{MIN} = 1.5 \cdot DFT_{MIN}$.

h. The energy at E_{75} can be expressed in terms of the midpoint energy as follows: By linear interpolation, $E_{75} = E_{50} + 0.25 \cdot \text{full width} = E_{50} + 0.25 \cdot [1.0 \ E_{50}]^d = 1.25 \ E_{50}$, or $E_{50} = E_{75}/1.25$. The energy required to reach the top of the defibril-

outcome with multiple tests (one success and one failure, i.e. DFT+-), there is a high probability that the value is on the sloping portion of the curve within the bounds specified by the simple DFT protocol. If a failure is encountered when using an enhanced DFT protocol to justify a small energy margin for implant, it is recommended that the lead system or ICD be revised.

Appendix B: Margins for Verification Protocols

Step-Down Success Protocols
The step-down success (SDS) protocols define the upper limit for the decreasing step DFT, i.e., $DFT_{decr\ steps} \leq E_{SDS2}$, where E_{SDS2} is the second energy level in the SDS procedure. At worst case, E_{SDS2} equals the $DFT_{decr\ steps}$, so the energy margins for implant with the SDS protocol are the same as for the DFT: implant if $E_{ICD} \geq 2.0\ E_{SDS2}$ (see Appendix A).

Single-Energy Success Protocols
These protocols (1S, 2S or 3S) evaluate defibrillation efficacy at an energy that assures the desired energy margin for implant for the specific protocol. As with the SDS procedure, these single-energy success protocols do not locate the defibrillation curve, but only establish its upper boundary. Energy margin estimates are based on the *assumption that no failed defibrillation attempts have occurred at the test energy*. Each single-energy protocol has a different sized energy margin, since they have varying degrees of accuracy in defining the position of the defibrillation success curve.

1S Protocol
A one episode single energy protocol has limited accuracy in evaluating energy margins.[10] The energy yielding one defibrillation success (1S) may lie anywhere along the defibrillation curve above 5% success (corresponding to the 95% confidence interval). While a 1S testing outcome at a given energy (E_{1S}) may be consistent with a defibrillation curve far to the left, with E_{1S} out on the plateau, it is also consistent with a curve located completely to the right, with E_{1S} at the bottom of the curve. Assuming the worst case, $E_{MIN\ 1S} = E_5$, the 1S energy margins would have to be adjusted to allow for the full

---

lation curve from a $DFT_{MIN\ decr\ steps} = E_{75}$ is equal to $0.25 \cdot$ full width $= 0.25 \cdot [1.0$ $E_{50}]^d = 0.25 \cdot [1.0 \cdot \{E_{75}/1.25\}^h] = 0.2\ E_{75}$. Thus, $E_{99} = DFT_{MIN}$ + efficacy margin = $DFT_{MIN} + 0.2 \cdot DFT_{MIN} = 1.2 \cdot DFT_{MIN}$.

width of the defibrillation curve: 1S efficacy margin = 1.7 E_5.[i] These are the same margins as for the increasing step DFT protocol, thus, one would have to program a shock to 2.7 E_{1S} to guarantee defibrillation in all patients.

2S Protocol

If two successful defibrillations are required at a single energy, the 2S energy (E_{2S}) could lie far out along the defibrillation success curve on the plateau or on the curve slope somewhere above 25% success. Thus, the 2S has a similar worst case position as the decreasing step DFT. The energy associated with 25% success forms the lower boundary for the 2S confidence interval, since the probability of observing two consecutive defibrillations at a defibrillation probability of 25% is very low: $25\% \cdot 25\% \cong 6\%$. Because the 2S and $DFT_{decr steps}$ protocols have similar worst case positions on the defibrillation success curve, they have similar requirements for ICD energy margins: $E_{ICD} \geq 2.0\ E_{2S}$ for implant.

   If the first defibrillation attempt in the 2S protocol is successful, but the second trial failed (1S 1F), the test energy could lie anywhere on the defibrillation curve between E_5 to E_{95}. This forces the use of the larger ICD energy margins as specified for the 1S protocol. Energy margins for implant are then similar to the increasing step DFT protocols: 2.7 $E_{1S\ 1F}$.

3S Protocol

A greater precision could be obtained with three test shocks at one energy. While E_{3S} could lie out on the plateau, it could also be located as far down the curve as 40% (the 3S confidence interval extends down to 40%, since the probability of three successes at energies lower than E_{40} is $\leq 0.4^3 = 6\%$). With a higher $E_{MIN\ 3S}$ position on the curve, the 3S energy margin would be slightly less than that required for decreasing step DFTs: energy margin = $E_{3S} + 0.6 \cdot$ (full width) = 1.7 E_{3S}.[j]

---

i. The worst case position for 1S is at the bottom of the defibrillation success curve at E_5. This is the same worst case position as for the increasing step DFT protocol[f]. Thus the 1S protocol has the same worst case efficacy margin to reach the 100% defibrillation success plateau as the increasing step DFT: 1S efficacy margin = $(1.7 \pm 0.3) \cdot E_{MIN\ 1S}$.

j. The 3S efficacy margin equals the 60% of the width of the defibrillation success curve. Using the full curve width, we can obtain a relation between E_{40} and E_{50} that can be used to derive the 3S efficacy margin: By linear interpolation, $E_{40} = E_{50} - 0.1 \cdot$ full width = $E_{50} - 0.1 \cdot [1\ E_{50}]^d = 0.9\ E_{50}$, or $E_{50} = E_{40}/0.9$. Thus, the 3S efficacy margin which extends from the top of the curve down to E_{40} (i.e., 60% full curve width) has an efficacy margin slightly less than the DFT: efficacy

As more defibrillations are observed at the test energy (1S, 2S or 3S), the upper boundary for the defibrillation curve becomes more accurately defined, allowing smaller energy margins to be used for implant. This trend is also seen for the threshold methods. The adequacy of an ICD energy margin becomes more apparent as the amount of testing increases (DFT, DFT+ to DFT++). For both threshold and verification techniques, if energy margins are too small for a patient, a few extra defibrillation tests at the DFT or the test energy may be needed to assure adequate energy margins for implant. If adequate energy margins cannot be verified with the 3S or DFT+/DFT++ protocols, the lead system or waveform should be revised.

Appendix C: Variability of DFT Measurements

The curve width concept (Fig. 1) can help in understanding and estimating the variability of DFT measurements. The existence of a large curve width leads to the distribution of DFTs as seen in Fig. 3. In simplest terms, the gradual transition of the defibrillation success curve means that the DFT estimates are significantly affected by the "direction" from which one begins with a given measurement technique (protocol). For example, a decreasing step protocol will give a high estimate. Were the threshold sharp (i.e. no curve width) then this would not be the case. Specifically, the curve width is what leads to the lack of agreement among different DFT testing protocols.

In addition, the distribution of DFTs along the defibrillation curve for decreasing step DFTs (Fig. 3) can be used to estimate the variation expected with repeated DFTs *using the same protocol*. The probability of obtaining a specific difference between 2 DFT replicates is equal to the product of the probabilities for each individual DFT position on the curve. As an example, note that from Fig. 3 a $DFT_{decr\ step}$ has a 27% probability of being positioned near E_{82}, and an 8% chance of being near E_{40}. If these 2 DFT positions occurred during 2 successive DFT determinations (probability of happening = 27% · 8% = 2.2%), the difference between these repeated DFTs i.e., E_{82} and E_{40} would equal 42% of the defibrillation curve width. Extending this analysis to all possible replicate $DFT_{decr\ steps}$ combinations in Fig. 3, we find that approximately 58% of DFT replicates

---

margin = 0.6 · full width = 0.6 · $[1.0\ E_{50}]^d$ = 0.6 · $(E_{40}/0.9)^j$ = 0.7 $E_{MIN\ 3S}$. Adding this efficacy margin to the 3S energy, one obtains the implant energy margin: E_{ICD} ≥ E_{3S} + efficacy margin = 1.7 E_{3S}.

will differ by no more than ± 25% of the curve width. Eighteen percent of replicates will evidence a rise in DFT between 25-50% of the curve width, and another 18% will demonstrate a fall in DFT of the same magnitude. These changes constitute 94% of all possible DFT replicate combinations; *thus, we can expect that almost all repeated DFT_{decr step} measurements will differ from each other by no more than 50% of the defibrillation curve width.* Since a curve width equal to the E_{50} is not unusual, this means that the DFT_{decr step} measurements may vary nearly as much as the DFT itself!

The magnitude and direction of the DFT change will depend on the DFT location on the defibrillation success curve. Thresholds located high on the curve will tend to decrease on the next replicate, while thresholds low on the curve will tend to increase. For the decreasing step DFT, 70% of DFTs in Fig. 3 are located between E_{54} and the top of the curve. Thresholds within this upper group have an equal chance of increasing or decreasing upon a second DFT measurement. On average, those that increase will be located higher on the curve by an extra 10% of the curve width. Repeat DFTs in this group that fall will be located an average 26% further down the slope of the curve. The DFTs located on the lower part of the curve in Fig. 3 (located between E_{25} and E_{54}) constitute 30% of the total population. These thresholds have a 91% probability of increasing on a second threshold measurement, with an average increase of 24%. Conversely, 9% of these low thresholds (primarily those near the midpoint) will decrease on replicate, with an average decrease of 15% of the curve width. Given these trends, the 50% limit for maximum differences between DFT replicates will more directly apply to the DFT increases seen for low positioned thresholds and the DFT decreases for thresholds near the top of the curve. When pooling repeat DFT combinations from all sections of the curve, which weights the upper population more heavily, the average threshold increase was 16% of the curve width and average DFT decrease was 25%.

In the study depicted in Fig. 6, the majority of patients evidenced changes in DFT less than 50%, which is comparable to the variability inherent with the decreasing step DFT method. Since these small changes are within the error of the evaluation technique, threshold shifts of this magnitude are not clinically significant and might not even impact the safety margin obtained at implant. The defibrillation threshold changes greater than 50% in Fig. 6 cannot be attributed to replicate DFT variation alone, and probably also reflect contributions due to a rightward shift in the defibrillation success curve.

For any given change in threshold, it is not possible to identify exactly how much of this change is due to the repeated DFT and how much is due to a shift in the curve. Our estimates of the threshold changes expected for repeated $DFT_{decr\ step}$ indicate that the replicate factor could contribute no more than ± 50% of the curve width and probably contributes half of this amount on average. For DFTs that increase 50-100%, the replicate DFT factor may have contributed from one quarter to one half of the increase, possibly more. For thresholds that have increased more than 100%, the contributions of DFT variability are proportionally less, with most of the threshold change due to a shift in the position of the defibrillation success curve. Mechanisms for shifts in this curve could include microdislodgement of the lead,[28] changes in myocardial substrate,[23] or altered pharmacologic exposure.

ACKNOWLEDGMENTS:
Fig. 1 is modified and used with the permission of Futura Publishing.[4] Figs. 3 and 5 are derived from McDaniel and Schuder.[6] Fig. 4 is modified and used by permission of Futura Publishing.[5] Fig. 6 is derived from Tummala et al.[16]

1. Zipes DP, Fisher J. King RM, et al. Termination of ventricular fibrillation in dogs by depolarizing a critical amount of myocardium. Am J Cardiol 1975;36:37-44.
2. Jones JL, Jones RE. Improved defibrillator waveform safety factor with biphasic waveforms. Am J Physiol 1983;245:H60-65.
3. Mower MM, Mirowski M, Spear JF, et al. Patterns of ventricular activity during catheter defibrillation. Circulation 1974;49:858-861.
4. Singer I and Lang D. Defibrillation threshold, clinical utility and therapeutic implications. PACE 1992;15:932-949.
5. Lang D and KenKnight B. Implant Support Devices. In I Singer (ed.): Implantable Cardioverter Defibrillator. New York: Futura Publishing, 1994, p 223-252.
6. McDaniel WC, Schuder JC. The cardiac ventricular defibrillation threshold-inherent limitations in its application and interpretation. Med Instrum 1987;21:170-176.
7. Lang DJ, Cato EL, Echt DS. Protocol for evaluation of internal defibrillation safety margins. J Am Coll Cardiol 1989;13:111A. (abstract)
8. Rattes MF, Jones DL, Sharma AD, et al. Defibrillation threshold: A simple and quantitative estimate of the ability to defibrillate. PACE 1987;10:70-77.
9. Davy JM, Fain ES, Dorian P, et al. The relationship between successful defibrillation and delivered energy in open-chest dogs: Reappraisal of the "defibrillation threshold" concept. Am Heart J 1987;113:77-84.
10. Lang DJ, Swanson DK. Safety margin for defibrillation. In E Alt, H Klein JC Griffin (eds.): The Implantable Cardioverter/Defibrillator. Berlin: Springer-Verlag, 1992, p272.
11. Jones DL, Klein GJ, Guiraudon GM, et al. Prediction of defibrillation success from a single defibrillation threshold measurement with sequential pulses and two current pathways in humans. Circulation 1988;78:1144-1149.
12. Deeb GM, Griffith BP, Thompson ME, et al. Lead systems for internal ventricular fibrillation. Circulation 1981;64:242-245.

13. Guarnieri T, Levine JH, Veltri EP, et al. Success of chronic defibrillation and the role of antiarrhythmic drugs with the automatic implantable cardioverter/defibrillator. Am J Cardiol 1987;60:1061-1064.
14. Wetherbee JN, Chapman PD, Troup PJ, et al. Long-term internal cardiac defibrillation threshold stability. PACE 1989;12:443-450.
15. Frame R, Brodman R, Furman S, et al. Long-term stability of defibrillation thresholds with intrapericardial defibrillator patches. PACE 1993;16:208-212.
16. Tummala RV, Riggio DW, Weiss D, et al. Chronic changes in defibrillation parameters with a transvenous lead system. J Am Coll Cardiol 1994;February:112A. (abstract)
17. Winter J, Vester EG, Kuhls S, et al. Defibrillation energy requirements with single endocardial (Endotak) Lead. PACE 1993;16:540-546.
18. Vester EG, Kuhls S, Perings C, et al. Efficacy and long term stability of a single endocardial lead configuration for permanent implantation of cardioverter/defibrillators. PACE 1993;16:875. (abstract)
19. Pitschner H, Neuzner J, Huth C, et al. Long-term stability of nonthoracotomy lead defibrillation thresholds. PACE 1994;17:836. (abstract)
20. Neuzner J, Pitschner H, Stöhring R, et al. Implantierbare Kardioverter/Defibrillatoren mit endokardiaien Elektrodensystemen: Langfristige Stabilität der Defibrillationseffektivitat. Z Kardiologie 1995;84:44-50.
21. Hsia HH, Mitra RL, Flores BT, et al. Early postoperative increase in defibrillation threshold with nonthoracotomy system in humans. PACE 1994;17:1166-1173.
22. Bardy GH, Buono G, Troutman CL, et al. Subacute changes in defibrillation threshold following multiprogrammable defibrillator implantation in man. J Am Coll Cardiol 1991;17:344A. (abstract)
23. Venditti FJ, Martin DT, Vassolas G, et al. Rise in chronic defibrillation thresholds in nonthoracotomy implantable defibrillator. Circulation 1994;89:216-223.
24. Venditti FJ, Bowen S, John R, et al. Rise in defibrillation threshold in transvenous ICD using a biphasic waveform. PACE 1994;17:836. (abstract)
25. Schwartzman D, Mallavarapu C, Callans DJ, et al. Rise in defibrillation threshold early after implantation of non-thoracotomy defibrillation lead systems: incidence and predictors. J Am Coll Cardiol 1994;February:112A. (abstract)
26. Poole JE, Bardy GH, Dolack GL, et al. Serial defibrillation threshold measures in man: a prospective controlled study. J Cardiovasc Electrophysiol 1995;6:19-25.
27. Schwartzman D, Callans DJ, Gottlieb CD, et al. Early postoperative rise in defibrillation threshold in patients with nonthoracotomy defibrillation lead systems: attenuation with biphasic shock waveforms. J Cardiovasc Electrophysiol 1996;7:483-493.
28. Usui M, Walcott GP, KenKnight BH, et al. Influence on defibrillation efficacy of the malpositioning of transvenous leads with and without a subcutaneous array. PACE 1994;17:784. (abstract)
29. Echt DS, Barbey JT, Black NJ. Influence of ventricular fibrillation duration on defibrillation energy in dogs using bidirectional pulse discharges. PACE 1988;11;1315-1323.
30. Jones JL, Swartz JF, Jones RE, et al. Increasing fibrillation duration enhances relative asymmetrical biphasic versus monophasic defibrillator waveform efficacy. Circ Res 1990;67:376-384.
31. Tacker WA, Babbs CF, Parris RL, et al. Effect of fibrillation duration on defibrillation threshold in dogs using a pervenous catheter-electrode designed for use with an automatic implantable defibrillator. Med Instrum 1981;15:327. (abstract)
32. Fujimura O, Jones DL, Klein GJ. Effects of time to defibrillation and subthre-

shold preshocks on defibrillation success in pigs. PACE 1989;12:358-365.

33. Winkle RA, Mead RH, Ruder MA, et al. Defibrillation efficacy in man after 5 vs. 15 seconds of ventricular fibrillation. J Am Coll Cardiol 1988;11:18A. (abstract)

34. Bardy GH, Ivey TD, Allen M, et al. A prospective, randomized evaluation of effect of ventricular fibrillation duration on defibrillation thresholds in humans. J Am Coll Cardiol 1989;13:1362-1366.

35. Bardy GH, Ivey TD, Johnson G, et al. Prospective evaluation of initially ineffective defibrillation pulses on subsequent defibrillation success during ventricular fibrillation in survivors of cardiac arrest. Am J Cardiol 1988;62:718-722.

36. KenKnight BH, Johnson CR, Epstein AE, et al. Does the optimal biphasic waveform change with duration of ventricular fibrillation? PACE 1996;19:623. (abstract)

37. Troup PJ, Chapman PD, Wetherbee JN, et al. Do sub-threshold shocks increase energy requirement for subsequent defibrillation attempts? Circulation 1987;76:IV-311. (abstract)

38. CPI VENTAK PRx Clinical Report, PMA Panel for IDE #G900150, June 22, 1993.

39. Borbola J, Denes P, Ezri MD, et al. The automatic implantable cardioverter-defibrillator. Clinical experience, complications and followup in 25 patients. Arch Int Med 1988;148:70-76.

40. Meesmann M. Factors associated with implantation-related complications. PACE 1992;15(Pt. III):649-653.

41. Lehmann MH, Saksena S. Implantable cardioverter defibrillators in cardiovascular practice: report of the policy conference of the North American Society of Pacing and Electrophysiology. PACE 1991;14:969-979.

42. Strickberger SA, Brownstein SL, Wilkoff BL, et al. Clinical predictors of defibrillation energy requirements in patients treated with a nonthoracotomy defibrillator system: the Res-Q investigators. Am Heart J 1996;131:257-260.

43. Singer I, Edmonds HL, vander Lakern C, et al. Is defibrillation testing safe? PACE 1991;14:1899-1904.

44. Steinbeck G, Dorwarth U, Mattke S, et al. Hemodynamic deterioration during ICD implant: Predictors of high-risk patients. Am Heart J 1994;127:1064-1067.

45. Meyer J, Möllhoff, Seifert T, et al. Cardiac output is not affected during intraoperative testing of the automatic implantable cardioverter defibrillator. J Cardiovasc Electrophysiol 1996;7:211-216.

46. Konstadt SN, Blakeman B, Wilber D, et al. The effects of normothermic hypoperfusion on processed EEG in patients. Aneth Analg 1990;70:21.

47. Bruggeman T, Andresen D. Zerebrale Ischamie wahrend der Implantation automatischer Defibrillatoren. Z Kardiol 1995;84:798-807.

48. Ideker RE, Hillsley RE, Wharton JM. Shock strength for the implantable defibrillator: can you have too much of a good thing? PACE 1992;15:841-844.

49. Jones JL, Lepeschkin E, Jones RE, et al. Response of cultured myocardial cells to countershock-type electric field stimulation. Am J Physiol 1987;235:H214. (abstract)

50. Rubin L, Hudson P, Driller J, et al. Effect of defibrillation energy on pacing threshold. Med Instrum 1983;17:15-17.

51. Yabe S, Smith WM, Daubert JP, et al. Conduction disturbances caused by high current density electric fields. Circ Res 1990;66:1190-1203.

52. Cates AW, Wolf PD, Hillsley RE, et al. The probability of defibrillation success and the incidence of postshock arrhythmia as a function of shock strength. PACE 1994;17:1208-1217.

53. Pansegrau DG, Abboud FM. Hemodynamic effects of ventricular defibrillation. J Clin Invest 1970;49:282-297.

54. Dahl CF, Ewy GA, Warner ED, et al. Myocardial necrosis from direct current

countershock: Effect of paddle size and time interval between discharge. Circulation 1974;50:956-961.

55. Swerdlow CD, Ahern T, Kass RM, et al. Upper limit of vulnerability is a good estimate of shock strength associated with 90% probability of successful defibrillation in humans with transvenous implantable cardioverter-defibrillators. J Am Coll Cardiol 1996;27:1112-1118.

56. Swerdlow CD, Peter T, Hwang C, et al. Programming of implantable defibrillators based on the upper limit of vulnerability rather than the defibrillation threshold. PACE 1996;19:614. (abstract)

57. Chen P-S, Shibata N, Dixon EG, et al. Comparison of defibrillation threshold and the upper limit of ventricular vulnerability. Circulation 1986;73:1022-1028.

58. Kavanaugh KM, Harrison JH, Dixon EG, et al. Correlation of the probability of success curves for defibrillation and for the upper limit of vulnerability. PACE 1990;13:536. (abstract)

59. Chen P-S, Feld GK, Mower MM, et al. Effects of pacing rate and timing of defibrillation shock on the relationship between the defibrillation threshold and the upper limit of vulnerability in open chest dogs. J Am Coll Cardiol 1991;18:1555-1563.

60. Malkin RA, Pilkington TC, Ideker RE. Estimating defibrillation efficacy using combined upper limit of vulnerability and defibrillation testing. IEEE Trans Biomed Eng 1996;43:69-78.

61. Fabritz CL, Kirchhof PF, Behrens S, et al. Myocardial vulnerability to T wave shocks: relation to shock strength, shock coupling interval, and dispersal of ventricular repolarization. J Cardiovasc Electrophysiol 1996;7:231-242.

62. Chen P-S, Feld GK, Kriett JM, et al. Relation between upper limit of vulnerability and defibrillation threshold in humans. Circulation 1993;88:186-192.

63. Hwang C, Swerdlow CD, Kass RM, et al. Upper limit of vulnerability reliably predicts the defibrillation threshold in humans. Circulation 1994;90:2308-2314.

64. Singer I, Guarnieri T, Kupersmith J. Implanted automatic defibrillators: effects of drugs and pacemakers. PACE 1988;11:2250-2262.

65. Haberman RJ, Veltri, EP, Mower MM. The effect of amiodarone on defibrillation threshold. J Electrophysiol 1988;2:415. (abstract)

66. Fain ES, Lee JT, Winkle RA. Effects of acute intravenous and chronic oral amiodarone on defibrillation energy requirements. Am Heart J 1987;114:8-17.

67. Kentsch M, Kunze KP, Bleifeld W. Effect of intravenous amiodarone on ventricular fibrillation during out-of-hospital cardiac arrest. J Am Coll Cardiol 1986;7:82A. (abstract)

68. Fogoros RN. Amiodarone-induced refractoriness to cardioversion. Am Intern Med 1984;100:699-700.

69. Guarnieri T, Levine JH, Veltri EP. Success of chronic defibrillation and the role of antiarrhythmic drugs with the automatic implantable cardioverter/ defibrillator. Am J Cardiol 1987;60:1061-1064.

70. Epstein AE, Ellenbogen KA, Kirk K, et al. Clinical characteristics and outcome of patients with high defibrillation thresholds. A multicenter study. Circulation 1992;86:1206-1216.

71. Jung W, Manz M, Pizzulli L, et al. Effects of chronic amiodarone therapy on defibrillation threshold. Am J Cardiol 1992;70:1023-1027.

72. Wang M, Dorian P, Ogilvie RI. Isoproterenol increases defibrillation energy requirements in dogs. J Cardiovasc Pharmacol 1992;19:201-208.

73. Dorian P, Wang M, David I, et al. Oral clofilium produces sustained lowering of defibrillation energy requirements in a canine model. Circulation 1991;83:614-621.

74. Wang M, Dorian P. DL and D sotalol decrease defibrillation energy requirements. PACE 1989;12:1522-1529.

75. Fain ES, Dorian P, Davy JM, et al. Effects of encainide and its metabolites on

energy requirements for defibrillation. Circulation 1986;73:1334-1341.

76. Reiffel JA, Coromilas J, Zimmerman JM, et al. Drug-device interactions: clinical considerations. PACE 1985;8:369-373.

77. Frame LH, Sheldon JH. Effect of recainam on the energy required for ventricular defibrillation in dogs as assessed with implanted electrodes. J Am Coll Cardiol 1988;12:746-752.

78. Dorian P, Fain ES, Davy JM, et al. Lidocaine causes a reversible, concentration-dependent increase in defibrillation energy requirements. J Am Coll Cardiol 1986;8:327-332.

79. Marinchak RA, Friehling TD, Line RA, et al. Effect of antiarrhythmic drugs on defibrillation threshold: Case report of an adverse effect of mexiletine and review of the literature. PACE 1988;11:7-12.

80. Echt DS, Gremillion ST, Lee JT, et al. Effects of procainamide and lidocaine on defibrillation energy requirements in patients receiving implantable cardioverter defibrillator devices. J Cardiovasc Electrophysiol 1994;5:752-760.

81. Ujhelyi MR, Schur M, Frede T, et al. Differential effects of lidocaine on defibrillation threshold with monophasic versus biphasic shock waveforms. Circulation 1995;92:1644-1650.

82. Holt DW, Tucker GT, Jackson PR, et al. Amiodarone pharmacokinetics. Am Heart J 1983;106:840-847.

83. Barbieri E, Conti F, Zampieri P, et al. Amiodarone and desethylamiodarone distribution in the atrium and adipose tissue of patients undergoing short and long-term treatment with amiodarone. J Am Coll Cardiol 1986;8:210-213.

84. Dorian P, Fain ES, Davy JM, et al. Effect of quinidine and bretylium on defibrillation energy requirements. Am Heart J 1986;112:19-25.

85. Deeb GM, Hardesty RL, Griffith BP, et al. The effects of cardiovascular drugs on the defibrillation threshold and the pathological effects on the heart using an automatic implantable defibrillator. Ann Thorac Surg 1983;4:361-366.

86. Woolfolk DI, Chaffee WR, Cohen W, et al. The effect of quinidine on electrical energy required for ventricular defibrillation. Am Heart J 1966;72:659.

87. Babbs CF, Yim GKW, Whistler SJ, et al. Elevation of ventricular defibrillation energy requirements. Am Heart J 1986;112:19.

88. Koo CC, Allen JD, Pantridge JF. Lack of effect of bretylium tosylate on electrical ventricular defibrillation in a controlled study. Cardiovasc Res 1984;18:762-767.

89. Kerber RE, Pandian NG, Jensen SR, et al. Effect of lidocaine and bretylium on energy requirements for transthoracic defibrillation: Experimental studies. J Am Coll Cardiol 1986;7:397-405.

90. Tacker WA, Niebauer MJ, Babbs CF, et al. The effect of newer antiarrhythmic drugs on defibrillation threshold. Crit Care Med 1980;8:177-180.

91. Echt DS, Black JN, Barbey JT, et al. Evaluation of antiarrhythmic drugs on defibrillation energy requirements in dogs: sodium channel block and action potential prolongation. Circulation 1989;79:1106-1117.

92. Dawson AK, Steinberg MI, Shephard JE. Effects of Class I and Class III drugs on current and energy required for internal defibrillation. Circulation 1985;72:III-384.

93. Ruffy R, Schechtman K, Monje E, et al. B-adrenergic modulation of direct defibrillation energy in anesthetized dog heart. Am J Physiol 1985;248:H674-677.

94. Ruffy R, Monje E, Schechtman K. Facilitation of cardiac defibrillation by aminophylline in the conscious, closed-chest dog. J Electrophysiol 1988;2:450. (abstract)

95. Wang M, Dorian P. Defibrillation energy requirements differ between anesthetic agents. J Electrophysiol 1989;3/2:86-94.

96. Sweeney RJ, Gill RM, Steinberg MI, et al. Effects of Flecainide, Encainide, and Clofilium on ventricular refractory period extension by transcardiac shocks. PACE 1996;19:50-60.

97. Borbola J, Denes P, Ezri MD et al. The automatic implantable cardioverter/defibrillator: clinical experience, complications and follow-up in 25 patients. Arch Int Med 1988;148:70-76.
98. Blakeman BM, Pifarre R, Scanlon PJ, et al. Coronary revascularization and implantation of the automatic cardioverter/defibrillator: Reliability of immediate intraoperative testing. PACE 1989;12:86-91.
99. Troup PJ. Implantable cardioverters and defibrillators. In RA O'Rourke, MH Crawford (eds): Current Problems in Cardiology. St. Louis, MO, Yearbook Medical Publishers, Inc., 1989, Vol. XIV(12), p. 673-843.
100. Hillsley RE, Wharton JM, Cates AW, et al. Why do some patients have high defibrillation thresholds at defibrillator implantation? Answers from basic research. PACE 1994;17:222-239.
101. KenKnight BH, Eyuboglu BM, Ideker RE. Impedance to defibrillation countershock: does an optimal impedance exist? PACE 1995;18:2068-2087.
102. Jordaens L, Vertongen P, van Belleghem Y. A subcutaneous lead array for implantable cardioverter defibrillators. PACE 1993;16:1429-1433.
103. Higgins SL, Alexander DC, Kuypers CJ, et al. The subcutaneous array - a new lead adjunct for the transvenous ICD to lower defibrillation thresholds. PACE 1995;18:1540-1548.
104. Brodman R, Fisher JD, Furman S, et al. Implantation of the automatic implantable defibrillator by left subcostal thoracotomy. PACE 1984;7:1370. (abstract)
105. Thurer RJ, Luceri RM, Balooki H. Automatic implantable cardioverter defibrillator: Techniques of implantation and results. Ann Thorac Surg 1986;42:143-147.
106. Lawrie GM, Griffin JC, Wyndham CRC. Epicardial implantation of the automatic defibrillator by left subcostal thoracotomy. PACE 1984;7:1370-1374.
107. Echt DS, Armstrong K, Schmidt P, et al. Clinical experience, complication, and survival in 70 patients with the automatic cardioverter/defibrillator. Circulation 1985;71:289-296.
108. Block M, Breithardt G. Optimizing defibrillation through improved waveforms. PACE 1995;18:526-538.
109. Hahn SJ, Heil JE, Lin Y, et al. Improved defibrillation with small capacitance and optimized biphasic waveform. Circulation 1994;90:I-175. (abstract)
110. Swartz JF, Fletcher RD, Karasik PE. Optimization of biphasic waveforms for human nonthoracotomy defibrillation. Circulation 1993;88:2646-2654.
111. Natale A, Sra J, Krum D, et al. Relative efficacy of different tilts with biphasic defibrillation in humans. PACE 1996;19:197-206.

6

Pathways for Defibrillation Current

Michael J. Kallok, PhD

ELECTRICAL defibrillation of the heart is accomplished by the passage of current between two or more electrodes. Each electrode pair defines a pathway for current. The actual flow of current along a pathway is influenced by the electrode materials, surface dimensions and treatments, the conductivities and anisotropies of the tissues between electrodes, and the influence of shock strength on conductivity.

The objective of defibrillation is to restore orderly electrical activity to the myocardium that will result in effective pumping of blood. The precise mechanism of defibrillation is unclear, but at least two plausible theories exist. The first[1] states that fibrillation requires a *critical mass* of myocardium to be self sustaining. Effective defibrillation is accomplished when the electrical shock depolarizes a sufficient amount of tissue to reduce the fibrillating mass below the critical value. The second theory[2] proposes that a certain *critical voltage gradient* must be reached throughout the myocardium to depolarize the tissue, and that failed defibrillation results from re-initiation of fibrillation in areas of low gradient. The two theories are not incompatible, and may be complementary. (See Chap. 3 for a detailed discussion.) Both theories raise questions regarding the importance of pathways for defibrillation current, however.

If one accepts the critical mass theory, a common assumption is that a certain percentage of myocardium must be depolarized by the shock so the remaining tissue is below the critical mass for sustaining fibrillation. Another approach might be selective depolarization by pathway choice to divide the heart into a number of small masses, each below the critical mass and therefore incapable of sustaining fibrillation. In the first case, the challenge is to deliver a shock of sufficient strength to a large part of the myocardium using electrodes of finite area. Ideally, one wishes to achieve a uniform current density throughout the heart. In the second approach, the objective is to "electrically dissect" the heart by controlling current pathways. In this case the current density is not uniform throughout the heart, but rather varies from zero to a value high enough to cause depolarization in very carefully chosen areas of the heart. This concept of dissection has not been shown to be an effective method of defibrillation in well-controlled experiments.

The voltage gradient theory requires that a minimum voltage gradient be reached throughout most of the myocardium. The gradient is related to the shock strength and electrical field generated by the electrode system. As is the case for the critical mass hypothesis, a uniform gradient throughout the myocardium would result in the most efficient defibrillation. The challenge is to use electrode design and effective use of pathways to ensure an adequate voltage gradient throughout the heart.

Given the above theoretical reasons for selecting a certain defibrillation pathway, several practical factors must be considered when selecting a pathway for defibrillation. As described in Chap. 9, there are electrode systems that can be implanted completely within the heart and vascular system; systems that are implanted on the epicardial surface of the heart; systems that require intracardiac and epicardial or extracardiac electrodes; and systems that are entirely extracardiac. Additionally, one can use 2, 3 or more electrodes to create one or more pathways. Finally, shocks can be delivered simultaneously or sequentially on the pathways. For a complete discussion of electrode designs, per se, the reader is referred to Chap. 9, and to Chap. 7 for a discussion of waveforms.

The objective of this chapter is to describe the various pathways for defibrillation that have been proposed and tested. An attempt will be made to describe the advantages and limitations of each pathway system, and to explain the interdependence between pathways, waveforms, and electrodes.

Note: Although the biphasic has been clearly demonstrated to be superior to the monophasic waveform,[3,4] the literature covering various electrode systems is still dominated by monophasic studies, and these will emphasized here. Unless otherwise stated, thresholds should be assumed to be for monophasic waveforms.

Two-Electrode Systems

Two electrode pathways for ICDs were the first to evolve. Since transthoracic defibrillation was available before the concept of an implantable defibrillator emerged, some early systems were attempts to emulate the paddles used in external devices. When it

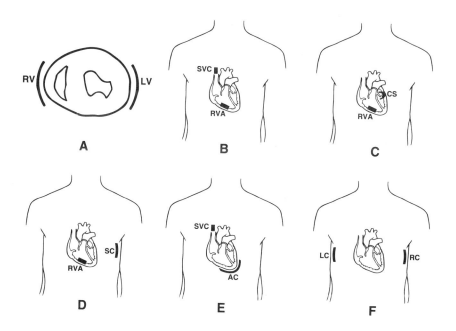

Figure 1. Most common 2-electrode pathways. SVC = superior vena cava; RVA = right ventricular apex; CS = coronary sinus; SC = subcutaneous; AC = apical cup; LC = left chest; RC = right chest.

became known that direct heart defibrillation (as in the paddles used for intraoperative defibrillation) required far less energy than transthoracic defibrillation, electrode systems that could be placed in contact with the heart were developed. Thus 2-electrode pathways include epicardial, intracardiac (transvenous), extracardiac and various combinations of these electrodes.

Epicardial Electrodes
Single pathway systems using epicardial electrodes have been used for some time (Fig. 1A). These systems resemble the hand-held paddles used to defibrillate intraoperatively. One advantage of these electrodes is that they can be implanted with direct visualization of the heart allowing accurate placement. They are generally large in surface area and produce relatively uniform electric fields throughout the heart. Finally, they can be firmly secured to the heart eliminating dislodgement and associated problems.

The disadvantages of epicardial electrodes include the need for thoracic surgery to implant the devices although techniques have been developed for limited exposure implantation.[5] The presence of large amounts of foreign material which predispose to infection (Chap. 18). There may be damage to underlying cardiac structures and decreased ability to transthoracically defibrillate in emergency situations due to the insulating nature of these electrodes.[6]

Despite the limitations associated with epicardial electrodes, these systems have proven efficacious. Various pathways have been tested, including apex-base, anterior-posterior, and left to right heart. The apex-base system was abandoned early due to difficulties in placing the basal electrode.[7] Chang demonstrated that defibrillation shocks that traverse the septum are more efficacious than those that do not.[8] Consequently, most clinical implants of defibrillators utilize a left-to-right pathway although this has not been shown to be superior in well-controlled studies. Typical defibrillation thresholds (DFTs) with this pathway are 10-20 J, and do not change with time after implantation.[9]

Most efforts to improve DFTs with the epicardial 2-electrode single pathway system involved surface area changes. Troup has shown that defibrillation thresholds in humans decrease with increasing surface area although this particular report combined results obtained with different pathways and different electrode systems.[10] In one animal study mean DFT in dogs was 4.1 J with a 20 cm^2 total epicardial patch surface area.[11] Mean DFT was reduced to 1.5 J when large contoured electrodes of 72 cm^2 were used. The reduction in DFT with increasing surface area is likely due to a decrease in impedance and a better current distribution.

A finite element analysis[12] has shown that increasing surface area beyond a certain point does not further reduce DFT. The reason is thought to be a shunting of current through low impedance pathways that exist between the edges of epicardial electrodes that are in close proximity to each other. This result was also demonstrated in an isolated heart preparation. Thus it appears that there is a limit to DFT reductions that can be accomplished with increasing the surface area of epicardial electrodes. Another practical limitation to patch surface area increases is the potential greater difficulty in transthoracic defibrillation due to the insulating effect of the patches on the heart.[13]

Intracardiac (Transvenous) Electrodes

The earliest report of an attempt to defibrillate with intracardiac electrodes was published by Hopps and Bigelow in 1954.[14] Alternating current shocks of 200 ms duration were unsuccessful in that experiment. In 1971 Mirowski described a catheter system, using

DC shock, that employed electrodes in the right ventricular (RV) apex and superior vena cava (SVC) (Fig. 1B).[15] This system was successful in terminating fibrillation in dogs with energies ranging from 10-25 J. A report by Schuder and colleagues in 1971 demonstrated similar results in dogs.[16] The first successful human defibrillation using a single pathway intracardiac system was published by Mirowski in 1972.[17] These limited acute results demonstrated successful defibrillation with shocks of 5-15 J. Various attempts to improve DFTs with a single pathway intravascular catheter included changing surface area, electrode spacing, and electrode surface characteristics.

Intuitively, the RV → SVC pathway would not appear to be a good choice for distributing current to the left ventricle. The need to depolarize tissue distant from the electrodes (e.g., the left ventricular free wall) requires an electrical overdose at the electrodes to compensate for the rapid decay of field strength with distance from the electrodes. One attempt to improve the current in the left ventricle involved implanting one electrode in the coronary sinus and one in the right ventricle (Fig. 1C);[18] mean DFT in 20 patients was approximately 17.5 J, and was less than 15 J in 9 patients. Despite the intuitive appeal of this pathway, the clinical data do not suggest that it offers much improvement over the RV → SVC pathway. Placing the "SVC" electrode up in the innominate vein may lower thresholds compared to the true SVC position.[19] A right sided insertion of a single lead (purely transvenous system with 2 electrodes) has significantly higher thresholds, in humans, than with a left sided insertion.[20]

Clinical acceptance of the transvenous (intracardiac) pathway awaited the dramatic influence of the biphasic waveform on thresholds.

Combination Electrodes

Combination electrode single pathway systems are defined as those with one intracardiac or intravascular electrode and one epicardial or extracardiac electrode. The number of possible pathways increases over those achievable with intracardiac systems. Historically, these pathways were among the earliest tested.

In the same study in which an intravascular electrode system was ineffective[21] Hopps and Bigelow demonstrated successful defibrillation with a right ventricular catheter and a large dispersive electrode on the anterior chest wall using a 200 ms alternating current shock (energy was not reported). Mirowski reported 100% successful defibrillation with 30-50 J shocks delivered between the right ventricular apex and a subcutaneous electrode implanted on the anterior chest (Fig. 1D). Schuder described a system that included a right atrial or SVC electrode paired with a subcutaneous (SubQ) anterior chest wall electrode.[22] Ninety percent successful defibrillation with 19 J was reported. The first implantable defibrillator clinical implantations utilized an SVC electrode paired with an apical epicardial cup electrode (Fig. 1E).[23] The apical cup was later replaced with a patch electrode. This pathway was reasonably successful in defibrillating patients with 24 J or less. However, the superiority of 2 epicardial patch electrodes for defibrillation eventually displaced the SVC - apical patch system in clinical use.

Historically, combination electrode pathways were developed to overcome some of the shortcomings of 2-electrode intravascular systems, including electrode dislodgement, suboptimal current distribution in the left ventricle, and electrode placement difficulties. Although some systems do solve these problems, several disadvantages are associated with the use of combination systems. If an epicardial electrode is used, the thoracic cavity must be entered. Subcutaneous electrodes usually require surgical incisions remote from the venous entry site and subsequent tunneling of electrode wires to the generator implant sites. Despite these disadvantages, combined pathways have demonstrated benefit in reducing DFTs.[24]

Extracardiac Electrodes
The concept for extracardiac electrodes with an implantable defibrillator likely evolved from transthoracic defibrillation (Fig. 1F). Schuder described a single pathway system in 1970[25] with a pair of electrodes implanted submuscularly one high on the right chest and the other over the cardiac apex . Dogs could be defibrillated with $\leq$ 37 J using this pathway. Although this is much less energy than that required for transthoracic defibrillation, this pathway was not as effective as those that included an electrode on or in the heart. There have not been any recent studies to re-examine this pathway.

Some advantages associated with this system include ease of implant and implantation outside the vascular system. However, since implantable defibrillators must detect fibrillation, this system might require an intracardiac electrode for sensing, although it might be possible to sense a "surface" electrocardiogram from subcutaneous electrodes.

Summary: Two-Electrode Systems

A variety of 2-electrode, single pathway systems have been proposed and tested. Although it is difficult to compare studies because different protocols, waveforms and electrode designs were used in various studies, the following generalizations can be made: Of all the pathways listed, the 2-epicardial patch system results in the lowest DFTs with demonstrated stability of thresholds with time. Intracardiac and combination electrode systems have great appeal because of the ease of implantation. DFTs achieved with these systems are quite variable: however numerous reports suggest values low enough to permit use of intracardiac and combination electrodes with permanently implantable defibrillators.

Note that these generalizations are derived from studies that utilized monophasic waveforms of various durations generated by different capacitor values. However, similar relative differences in DFT for these pathways would be expected were biphasic waveforms used exclusively.

Three-Electrode Systems

Since the objective of defibrillation is to provide an adequate distribution of current, or to achieve minimum voltage gradient throughout the ventricles, one method to improve defibrillation efficacy is to increase the number of electrodes. The addition of a third electrode creates a *second pathway* for defibrillation which theoretically allows one to better distribute current. As with 2-electrode pathways, epicardial, intracardiac, and combination systems have been tested. However, 2 shocks can be delivered either simultaneously or sequentially, thus increasing the number of possibilities for these systems.

The original reports of sequential pulse defibrillation hypothesized that both temporal and spatial separation of shocks contributed to the improvement over single pulse defibrillation.[26,27] However, conflicting results were subsequently reported that suggested only spatial separation is required.[28] These results will be discussed separately under each of the major electrode types.

Epicardial Electrodes

Three epicardial electrodes provide the simplest 2-pathway system (Fig. 2A). The advantages of this configuration are similar to those of the 2-electrode epicardial system and include accurate placement, secure fixation, and low, stable thresholds. The electrodes are generally placed at 120° intervals around the ventricles, corresponding to anterior and posterior septal, and left ventricular free-wall positions. The left ventricular electrode is the common cathode and the 2 pathways are anterior to left free wall and posterior to left free wall.

Other pathways are possible by using alternate electrode locations and changing the cathode, but these have not been systematically investigated. One animal study demonstrated lower DFTs when shocks were delivered sequentially compared to simultaneously through this type of electrode configuration, and sequential shocks resulted in lower DFTs than a single shock delivered on one pathway when total patch surface area and pulse duration were held constant.[29] Another animal study demonstrated no difference between sequential and simultaneous DFTs when patch position was optimized for each respective technique.[30] In both cases, however, mean DFTs were less than 4 J.

Although 2-pathway epicardial systems result in very low DFTs, the added surgical complexity of suturing an additional electrode to the heart has prevented more widespread clinical use. Also, they can require the implantation of a "Y-adapter" since some ICDs have only 2 high-voltage connections. Single pathway DFTs are currently low enough in the great majority of patients (since the advent of biphasic waveforms) to make implantation of another electrode generally unnecessary and only marginally contributory to reduced DFTs. This avoids the attendant increased risk of infection and possible reduced efficacy of transthoracic defibrillation.

Intracardiac (Transvenous) Electrodes
Two-pathway intracardiac electrode systems were developed to overcome some of the limitations of single pathway systems and to reduce DFTs closer to the level obtainable with single pathway epicardial electrodes. The only totally intracardiac 3-electrode system uses electrodes in the RV, SVC, and coronary sinus (CS) or great cardiac vein (Fig. 2B). In most reported uses, the RV electrode serves as the common cathode, with the 2 pathways being SVC→ RV and CS→ RV.[31] The CS catheter improves the distribution of current to the left ventricle and theoretically reduces the DFT. One animal study showed a 36% reduction in DFT when the CS electrode and sequential pulses were used, compared to the SVC→ RV single pathway.[32] Clinical trials have demonstrated moderate DFTs in patients receiving this 2-pathway system.[33] Although simultaneous shocks on the SVC→ RV, CS→ RV pathways have not been

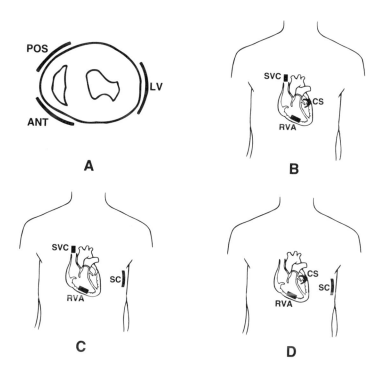

Figure 2. Most common pathways of 3 electrodes. ANT = anterior; POS = posterior; other abbreviations as in Fig. 1.

tested in humans, an animal study showed no difference between these pathways with a simultaneous shock compared to the CS→RV single pathway.[34] One clinical study found reasonable thresholds with one coil in the RV outflow tract (cathode) with the anodes being 2 of the following choices: SVC, CS, or SubQ.[35] Configurations using another electrode as the cathode in this 3-electrode system have not been tested.

Combination Electrodes
If one adds an extracardiac electrode to the possible electrode locations described above, several other 2-pathway systems can be achieved. The most common extracardiac location is a *subcutaneous electrode* which can be positioned virtually anywhere on the thorax. The most common position is on the left anterolateral thorax to help distribute current to the left ventricle. The subscapular location also produces good results.[36] Only 2 different configurations have

been tested, since from a practical standpoint, the right ventricular electrode is virtually always needed for sensing and pacing.

The first combination-electrode, 2-pathway system that was described included the SVC and RV electrodes and a SubQ electrode on the left thorax (Fig. 2C). The RV electrode was the common cathode with sequential shocks delivered from SVC → RV followed by SubQ → RV.[37] Both sequential and simultaneous shocks result in DFTs less than that obtained via either single pathway.[38] Attempts to use the SVC electrode as the common cathode have not been systematically investigated. The SVC electrode appears to improve on the SubQ → RV pathway if the resistance of this pathway is high.[39]

The second combination electrode system includes the CS, RV, and SubQ electrode sites (Fig. 2D). The only data reported had the CS electrode as the common cathode with RV → CS, and SubQ → CS as shock pathways. The mean DFTs measured in 12 patients using sequential, simultaneous, and single shocks were 14.8, 18.0, and 16.1 J, respectively, but were not statistically different from each other.[40]

Summary: Three-Electrode Systems

When a third electrode is added to conventional single pathway systems, a second pathway is available. Shocks can be delivered either sequentially or simultaneously over the pathways. The objective of the third electrode and second pathway is to improve the current distribution to the left ventricle. The results from both animal and human studies suggests that 2-pathway shocks are more efficacious than single pathway shocks. The data comparing sequential with simultaneous shocks is conflicting. It appears that there is no universally best electrode configuration for defibrillation, but in an individual patient one pathway may result in lower DFTs than all other pathways regardless of waveform.

Four-Electrode Systems

The use of a third electrode to provide an additional pathway for defibrillation appears to result in sufficient benefit to offset the disadvantage incurred due to a particular electrode configuration. Whether this benefit extends to more than 3 electrodes has not been established. Although very few multiple electrode systems have been described in the literature, and the fact that the biphasic waveform largely obviates the need for these more elaborate systems, they are discussed here only for completeness. These systems may become more relevant for DFT reduction with the present trend towards reductions in ICD energy capability with the trend towards ICD size reduction.

Multiple shock, multiple pathway defibrillation was described by Wiggers[41] in 1940 and by Kugelberg[42] and Resnekov[43] in the late 1960's. The basic premise was that the fibrillating myocardium includes cells in various stages of refractoriness, randomly distributed throughout the myocardium. When multiple pathways are used for shock delivery, and the shocks are separated in time, cells that were in their absolute refractory period during one shock will be depolarized by a later shock. Thus, by delivering multiple pathway shocks, the amount of energy required per shock could be reduced. In the limit (as the number of pathways is increased), one might speculate that the energy per pathway would be reduced to that required for pacing. This has never been demonstrated experimentally , however, and remains an intriguing possibility.

A 4-electrode, 2-orthogonal-pathway epicardial system was tested in animals and exhibited reduced DFTs compared to single pulse shocks.[44] The reduction in DFT compared to 2 large well placed electrodes is probably not sufficient to warrant the extra surgery required to implant the system. A 4-electrode nonthoracotomy system can be implemented by combining RV, CS, SVC, and SubQ electrodes. Such a scheme using a biphasic shock from the SubQ $\rightarrow$ SVC pathway followed a biphasic shock from the RV $\rightarrow$ CS route may show fairly low thresholds in humans.[45] The Active Can approach (next section) can also facilitate a 4-electrode implementation.

Current Issues

The Unipolar Approach
A new electrode approach, now very popular, is the Hot Can (Active Can or unipolar) system.[46] "Hot Can" is an Angeion trademark while "Active Can" is a Medtronic trademark; "unipolar" is the generic term. With this system, the ICD is implanted pectorally and the ICD housing serves as an electrode as shown in Fig. 3. A conventional coil is used in the right ventricular apex.[47] Average DFTs with biphasic waveforms are about 10 J. Thresholds can be lowered by adding electrodes in the SVC and SubQ (left axillary subcutaneous) location and delivering a simultaneous shock using the RV as common.[48] Adding electrodes in line with the RV $\rightarrow$ ICD

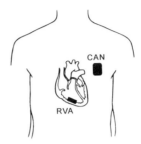

Figure 3. Unipolar electrode system. The ICD is implanted pectorally and the housing (CAN) serves as one electrode. The other electrode is the right ventricular apex (RVA).

housing vector (e.g. an electrode at the CS) do not seem to further lower thresholds.[49]

The size of the ICD housing does not appear to affect the unipolar defibrillation thresholds.[50]

Subcutaneous Array

A SubQ array of 3 long conductors (rather than the traditional "patch" electrode) placed in the left axillary region has provided low resistances and low DFTs.[51] One patient study reported an average threshold reduction of 40% over a pure transvenous approach.[52] While the array is usually implanted through a left chest incision, it can also be implanted via the same infraclavicular incision as used for the transvenous lead system.[53] The long term performance of the array in large numbers of patients is still being defined.

Preferred Polarity

The preferred polarity for endocardial lead systems was traditionally RV coil as cathode (negative). This may have been based on the pacemaker experience which found that cathodal stimulation was far less likely to cause fibrillation. However, it has been shown that using the RV coil as an anode, with monophasic shocks, reduces energy thresholds by about 30%.[54] No advantage was found, in general, for this polarity using sequential monophasic shocks.[55] Another study showed a DFT reduction with the RV as anode for both monophasic and biphasic waveforms.[56] Several other studies have shown that, for biphasic shocks, the RV anode polarity is better[57] or at least no worse[58] than the traditional RV cathode polarity. An animal study considered both monophasic and biphasic waveforms and found that only the monophasic benefited from the RV anodal polarity; the biphasic case was unaffected.[59] A human study using the Ventritex biphasic waveform (with RV cathode) found that its thresholds were equivalent to the Ventritex monophasic waveform with the RV as anode.[60]

Summary

Defibrillation requires depolarization of a critical mass of myocardium, or reaching a critical voltage gradient throughout the heart. Current is delivered to the heart along pathways that are created by sets of electrodes. Electrodes can be implanted in the heart and vascular system, on the epicardial surface of the heart, or subcutaneously on the thorax. Several factors must be considered when selecting an electrode system that defines pathways for defibrillation current. These factors include ease of implantation, defibrillation efficacy, and capability of the ICD to accommodate the electrodes and pathway(s) chosen.

For a given waveform, the most effective defibrillation pathways reported to date are 2- and 3-patch epicardial systems. DFTs are, for most patients, consistently and reproducibly under 20 J, even with monophasic waveforms, with these systems. It is not clear why some patients require significantly more energy for defibrillation than others, and defibrillation energy is not clearly related to type and extent of cardiac disease, infarction, heart size, body size, etc. The great interpatient variability in DFT prevents investigators from establishing a universally "best" pathway for defibrillation. Until a better understanding of the mechanism of defibrillation is available, physicians may have to test a number of pathways to establish the best defibrillation modality for individual patients.

The biphasic waveform has revolutionized the field by reducing DFTs by up to 40% permitting much greater flexibility in choice of defibrillation pathway—allowing especially for the widespread use of purely transvenous systems.

1. Mower MM, Mirowski M, Moore EN. Patterns of ventricular activity during catheter defibrillation. Circulation 1974;49:858-861.
2. Ideker RE, Tang ASL, Frazier DW, et al. Ventricular defibrillation: basic concepts. In El-Sherif N, Samet P (eds): Cardiac Pacing and Electrophysiology. Philadelphia, WB Saunders Co., 1991, pp 713-726
3. Block M, Hammel D, Böcker D, et al. A prospective randomized cross-over comparison of mono- and biphasic defibrillation using nonthoracotomy lead

configurations in humans. J Cardiovasc Electrophysiol 1994;5:581-590.

4. Schwartzman D, Concato J, Ren J-F, et al. Factors associated with successful implantation of nonthoracotomy defibrillation lead systems. Am Heart J 1996;131:1127-1136.
5. Watkins L, Mirowski M, Mower MM, et al. Implantation of the automatic defibrillator: the subxiphoid approach. Ann Thorac Surg. 1982;34:515-520.
6. Pinski SL, Arnold AZ, Mick M, et al. Safety of external cardioversion/defibrillation in patients with internal defibrillation patches and no device. PACE. 1991;14:7-12.
7. Langer A, Heilman MS, Mower MM, et al. Consideration in the development of the automatic implantable defibrillator. Med Instrum 1976;10:163-167.
8. Chang MS, Inowe H, Kallok MJ, et al. Double and triple sequential shocks reduce defibrillation threshold in dogs with and without myocardial infarction. J Am Coll Cardiol 1986;8:1393-1405.
9. Wetherbee JN, Chapman DP, Troup PJ, et al. Long-term internal cardiac defibrillation threshold stability. PACE 1989;12:443-450.
10. Troup PJ, Chapman PD, Olinger GN, et al. The implanted defibrillator: relation of defibrillating lead configuration and clinical variables to defibrillation threshold. J Am Coll Cardiol 1985;6:1315-1321.
11. Dixon EG, Tang ASL, Wolf PD, et al. Improved defibrillation thresholds with large contoured epicardial electrodes and biphasic waveforms. Circulation 1987;76:1176-1184.
12. Mehra R, DeGroot P, Norenberg S. Three dimensional finite element model of the heart for analysis of epicardial defibrillation: effect of patch surface area. PACE 1989;12:652. (abstract)
13. Lerman BB, Deale OC. Effect of epicardial patch electrodes on transthoracic defibrillation. Circulation 1990;81:1409-1414.
14. Hopps JA, Bigelow WG. Electrical treatment of cardiac arrest: a cardiac stimulator-defibrillator. Surgery 1954;36:833-849.
15. Mirowski M, Mower M, Staewen WS, et al. Ventricular defibrillation through a single intravascular catheter electrode system. Clin Res 1971;19:328. (abstract)
16. Schuder JC, Stoeckle H, West JA, et al. Ventricular defibrillation with catheter having distal electrode in right ventricle and proximal electrode in superior vena cava. Circulation 1971;43:44:11-99.
17. Mirowski M, Mower M, Gott VL, et al. Transvenous automatic defibrillator-preliminary clinical tests of its defibrillating subsystems. Trans Am Soc Artif Intern Organs 1972;18:520-525.
18. Bardy GH, Allen MD, Mehra R, et al. Transvenous defibrillation in humans via the coronary sinus. Circulation 1990;81:1252-1259.
19. Stajduhar KC, Ott GY, Kron J, et al. Optimal electrode position for transvenous defibrillation: a prospective randomized study. J Am Coll Cardiol 1996;27:90-94.
20. Epstein AE, Kay GN, Plumb VJ, et al. Elevated defibrillation threshold when right-sided venous access is used for nonthoracotomy implantable defibrillator lead implantation. The Endotak investigators. J Cardiovasc Electrophysiol 1995;6:979-986.
21. Hopps JA, Bigelow WG. Electrical treatment of cardiac arrest: a cardiac stimulator-defibrillator. Surgery 1954;36:833-849.
22. Schuder JC, Stoeckle H, Gold JH, et al. Ventricular defibrillation with unipolar catheter electrode positioned in the right atrium and superior vena cava. Circulation 1973;47:48:IV-13.
23. Mirowski M, Reid PR, Mower MM, et al. Termination of malignant ventricular arrhythmias with an implanted automatic defibrillator in human beings. N. Engl J Med 1980;303:322-324.
24. McCowan R, Maloney J, Wilkoff B, et al. Automatic implantable cardioverter-

defibrillator implantation without thoracotomy using an endocardial and submuscular patch system. J Am Coll Cardiol 1991;17:415-421.

25. Schuder JC, Stoeckle H, Gold JH, et al. Experimental ventricular defibrillation with an automatic and completely implanted system. Trans Am Soc Artif Int Organs 1970;16:207-212.
26. Bourland JD, Tacker WA, Wessale JL, et al. Reduction of defibrillation threshold by using sequential pulses applied through multiple electrodes: a preliminary report. Proc AAMI 19th Annual Meeting, April 14-18, 1984:13.
27. Jones DL, Klein GJ. Improved internal ventricular defibrillation with twin pulse energy delivery. Proc. AAMI 19th Annual Meeting, April 14-18, 1984:40.
28. Mehra R., Marcaccini S. Comparison of sequential and simultaneous pulse defibrillation threshold with a non-epicardial electrode system. Circulation 1986;74:II-185. (abstract)
29. Kallok MJ. Sequential pulse defibrillation with a 3-patch system. Circulation 1986;74:II-185. (abstract)
30. Mehra R., Norenberg MS, DeGroot P. Comparison of defibrillation thresholds with pulsing techniques requiring three epicardial electrodes. PACE 1988;11:527. (abstract)
31. Bardy GH, Allen MD, Mehra R, et al. An effective and adaptable transvenous defibrillator system using the coronary sinus in humans. J Am Coll Cardiol 1990;16:887-895.
32. Kallok MJ, Tacker WA, Jones DL, et al. Transvenous electrode systems and sequential pulse stimulation for reduced implantable defibrillator thresholds. J Am Coll Cardiol 1985;5:456. (abstract)
33. Yee R, Klein GJ, Leitch JW, et al. A permanent transvenous lead system for an implantable pacemaker cardioverter-defibrillator. Circulation 1992;85:196-204.
34. Kadish AM, Childs K, Levine J. An experimental study of transvenous defibrillation using a coronary sinus catheter. J Cardiovasc Electrophysiol 1989;3:253-260.
35. Tang ASL, Hendry P, Goldstein W, et al. Nonthoracotomy implantation of cardioverter defibrillators: preliminary experience with a defibrillation lead placed at the right ventricular outflow tract. PACE 1996;19:960-964.
36. Swartz JF, Fletcher RD, Karasik PE. Optimization of biphasic waveforms for human nonthoracotomy defibrillation. Circulation 1993;88:2646-2654.
37. Kallok MJ, Marcaccini S. Efficacy of two transvenous electrode systems for sequential pulse defibrillation. In Gomez FP (ed): Cardiac Pacing: Electrophysiology Tachyarrhythmias. Madrid, Editorial Grouz, 1985, pp 1497-1504.
38. Moore SL, Maloney JD, Edel TB, et al. Implantable cardioverter-defibrillator implanted by nonthorocotomy approach. PACE 1991;14:1865-1869.
39 Swerdlow CD, Davie S, Kass RM, et al. Optimal electrode configuration for pectoral transvenous implantable defibrillator without an active can. Am J Cardiol 1995;76:370-374.
40. Bardy GH, Allen MD, Mehra R, et al. A flexible and effective three electrode non-thoracotomy defibrillation system in man. J Am Coll Cardiol 1989;13:65A. (abstract)
41. Wiggers CJ. The physiologic basis for cardiac resuscitation from ventricular fibrillation - method for serial defibrillation. Am Heart J 1940;20:413.
42. Kugelberg J. Ventricular defibrillation - a new aspect. Acta Chir Scand 1967;372:1-93.
43. Resnekov L, Norman J, Lord P, et al. Ventricular defibrillation by monophasic trapezoidal-shaped double pulses of low electrical energy. Cardiovasc Res 1968;2:261-264.
44. Bourland JD, Tacker WA, Jr, Wessale JL, et al. Sequential pulse defibrillation for implantable defibrillators. Med Instr 1986;20:138-142.

45. Exner D, Yee R, Jones DL, et al. Combination biphasic waveform plus sequential pulse defibrillation improves defibrillation efficacy of a nonthorocotomy lead system. J Am Coll Cardiol 1994;23:317-322.
46. Bardy GH, Johnson G, Poole JE, et al. A simplified, single-lead unipolar transvenous cardioversion-defibrillation system. Circulation 1993;88:543-547.
47. Gold MR, Shorofsky SR. Transvenous defibrillation lead systems. J Cardiovasc Electrophysiol 1996;7:570-580.
48. Saksena S, Krol R, Kaushik R, et al. Endocardial defibrillation with dual, triple, and quadruple nonthorocotomy electrode systems using biphasic shocks. PACE 1994;17:743. (abstract)
49. Kudenchuk PJ, Bardy GH, Dolack GL, et al. Efficacy of a single-lead unipolar transvenous defibrillator compared with a system employing an additional coronary sinus electrode. Circulation 1994;89:2641-2644.
50. Newby KH, Moredock L, Rembert J, et al. Impact of defibrillator-can size on defibrillation success with a single-lead unipolar system. Am Heart J 1996;131:261-265.
51. Jordaens L, Vertongen P, van Belleghem Y. A subcutaneous lead array for implantable cardioverter defibrillators. PACE 1993;16:1429-1433.
52. Higgins SL, Alexander DC, Kuypers CJ, et al. The subcutaneous array - a new lead adjunct for the transvenous ICD to lower defibrillation thresholds. PACE 1995;18:1540-1548.
53. Kall JG, Kopp D, Lonchyna V, et al. Implantation of a subcutaneous lead array in combination with a transvenous defibrillation electrode via a single infraclavicular incision. PACE 1995;18:482-485.
54. Strickberger SA, Hummel JD, Horwood LE, et al. Effect of shock polarity on ventricular defibrillation threshold using a transvenous lead system. J Am Coll Cardiol 1994;24:1069-1072.
55. Block M, Hammel D, Böcker D, et al. Transvenous-subcutaneous defibrillation leads: effect of transvenous electrode polarity on defibrillation threshold. J Cardiovasc Electrophysiol 1994;5:912-918.
56. Thakur RK, Souza JJ, Chapman PD, et al. Electrode polarity is an important determinant of defibrillation efficacy using a nonthoracotomy system. PACE 1994;17:919-923.
57. Natale A, Sra J, Deshpande S, et al. Effects of the initial polarity of biphasic pulses on defibrillation efficacy. Circulation 1994;90:I-228. (abstract)
58. Shorofsky SR, Foster AH, Gold MR, et al. The effect of polarity reversal on biphasic defibrillation threshold with an integrated transvenous lead system. Circulation 1994;90:I-228. (abstract)
59. Usui M, Walcott GP, Strickberger SA, et al. Effects of polarity for monophasic and biphasic shocks on defibrillation efficacy with an endocardial system. PACE 1996:19:65-71.
60. Strickberger SA, Daoud E, Goyal R, et al. Prospective randomized comparison of anodal monophasic shocks versus biphasic cathodal shocks on defibrillation energy requirements. Am Heart J 1995;131:961-965.

7

The Defibrillation Waveform

Susan M. Blanchard, PhD, Raymond E.
Ideker, MD, PhD, Randolph A. S. Cooper,
MD, and J. Marcus Wharton, MD

T HE EFFICACY of the shock used for internal defibrillation depends upon the shape of the defibrillation waveform as well
as the placement of the defibrillation electrodes and the sequence in which shocks are delivered. The waveform shape also
has a direct bearing on the lifetime of the battery used in an ICD
since battery and capacitor size are the main determinants in the
development of small, efficient devices.[1] Much work is being done
to diminish the energy requirements for defibrillation without reducing the effectiveness of the ICD by using more effective waveforms. Reducing the energy required for defibrillation could also
lead to fewer instances of adverse effects, such as conduction disturbance,[2] ventricular dysfunction,[3] and myocardial necrosis,[4,5]
which occur when myocardium is exposed to high energy shocks.

Historical Perspective

Many different waveforms have been tested for use in defibrillation.
Some of the earlier work used large transformers to generate the
shock from alternating current that was applied transthoracically.[6-8]
This was followed by the work of Lown et al[9] in which a damped
sinusoidal waveform was generated by capacitor discharge through
a series inductor and the "resistor" formed by the paddles and thorax. This waveform is employed in most portable defibrillators today and is known as the Lown waveform. Lown et al showed that
DC shocks had fewer side effects in experimental animals—
including post shock arrhythmias, myocardial injury, and deaths—
than AC shocks. Straight capacitor discharges without truncation
and square wave pulses have also been tested,[10-13] but the former
tend to have high peak currents associated with myocardial de-

pression and a greater incidence of post shock arrhythmias[12,13] while the latter require large capacitors that waste a great deal of energy.[14,15] A major contribution from the early work was the suggestion that shorter duration waveforms required less energy for defibrillation than did longer pulse durations.

The effects of polarity and capacitance size are well covered in the review article of Block et al[16] and will not be discussed here.

Monophasic Waveforms

Several groups have found monophasic truncated exponential waveforms (Chap. 4) to be superior to untruncated capacitor discharges for defibrillation in implantable devices.[17,18] Truncation avoids the refibrillatory effects caused by the low voltage tail of straight capacitor discharges.[12,13] Wessale et al[19] used a bipolar catheter with electrodes in the apex of the right ventricle and superior vena cava of dogs to demonstrate that peak current dose (peak current divided by body weight) increased with increasing tilt (with tilt defined as the difference between initial and final currents—expressed as a percent of the initial current: <5%, 50%, 65%, 80%) and decreasing pulse duration (20, 15, 10, 5, and 2 ms). They also showed that total delivered energy per unit of body weight increased with increasing pulse duration but was not related to tilt. Waveform tilt is also defined as: $1 - e^{-d/RC}$ and thus depends upon the pulse duration (d), the capacitance in farads of the defibrillator (C), and the total resistance in ohms of the defibrillator-electrode-heart circuit (R). The capacitance of present ICDs is in the range of 95-150 µF.[1] Kroll[20] reported that the optimum pulse duration, i.e. that which produces a maximum effective current that can satisfy the largest rheobase requirement (Chap. 4) needed to defibrillate, is given by d = 0.58 RC + 0.58 d_c, where d_c is the average chronaxie duration of 2.7 ± 0.9 ms based on the evaluation of results from several studies in different animals. For a capacitance of 140 µF and a resistance of 50 Ω, the optimum duration would be 5.6 ms = 0.58 · 50 · 0.14 + 0.58 · 2.7. This is equivalent to a tilt of 55% = {1 - $e^{-5.6/(50· 0.14)}$} · 100%.

Chapman et al[21] used a transvenous catheter in the right ventricle to subcutaneous patch system in dogs to show that lower defibrillation energy requirements were associated with shorter pulse durations in truncated exponential monophasic waveforms with fixed pulse width and variable tilt. They also demonstrated that the shortest (2.5 ms) and longest (20 ms) pulse width durations were associated with higher threshold voltages than were durations in the middle of this spectrum. For the catheter-patch electrode system used by Chapman et al, pulse durations of approximately 5-15 ms were associated with the best combination of low initial voltage (596-632 V), low delivered energy (18-25 J), and low average current (5-7 A).

The effect resulting from applying sequential shocks of monophasic waveforms has also been investigated, but only modest improvements were found for 2 pulses of the same magnitude, duration, and polarity that were separated in time.[22] To explain the modest improvement which obtained, it was postulated that the first pulse depolarized all non-refractory cells while the second pulse depolarized cells which were refractory at the time the first pulse was given.[23] Work by Sweeney et al[24] indicated that the optimum time separation between 2 (sequential monophasic) shocks is approximately 85% of the activation rate (i.e. cycle length) during fibrillation.

Bourland et al[25] introduced the concept of reducing defibrillation energy requirements with temporal and spatial summation of energy by separating pulses in both time and space to achieve a more uniform field. Several groups have supported this theory by using various monophasic waveforms with at least 2 different current pathways and have shown that significant reductions in defibrillation threshold resulted for sequential pulses given through different lead systems as compared to single pulses given through each separate lead system.[26-29] The optimal separation in time for shocking from 2 different lead systems seems to be 0.2-1 ms with any advantage disappearing when the shocks are given more than 10 ms apart.[30]

Biphasic Waveforms

Another approach to dividing the shock into more than one phase was taken with the introduction of the biphasic waveform in which the polarity of the second phase is opposite to that of the first (Fig. 1). The polarity of the first phase, e.g. negative as shown in Fig. 1, is often shown as positive but this is merely a consequence of the choice of reference electrode. Several groups have demonstrated that some biphasic waveforms can defibrillate with considerably lower voltage and energy than monophasic waveforms of the same or half the same duration.[31-34] Schuder et al[32] showed in calves that certain symmetric biphasic waveforms could defibrillate at lower

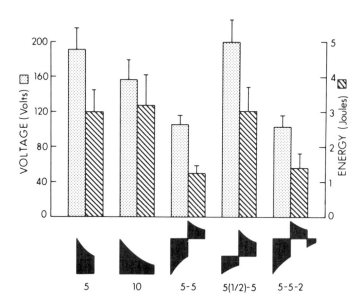

Figure 1. Defibrillation threshold voltage and energy values for 5 waveforms. Diagrams of the waveforms (2 monophasic, 2 biphasic, and 1 triphasic) with corresponding phase durations (in milliseconds) are shown below the bar graphs. See text for additional explanation.

energies and lower currents than monophasic waveforms of similar durations and that asymmetric biphasic waveforms, with the amplitude of the second phase lower than that of the first, defibrillated at lower energies than those with larger second phases.

Dixon et al[33] used large epicardial patches in dogs to show that biphasics in which the second phase was equal to the first phase in duration but reduced by half in leading edge voltage were more effective than monophasics of the same total duration (116 ± 19.4 V and 1.6 ± 0.5 J for a waveform with 5 ms first and second phases versus 165 ± 26.9 V and 3.1 ± 1.2 J for a 10 ms monophasic waveform). Note Fig. 1. The first 2 waveforms from the left are monophasic truncated exponential waveforms while the next 2 are biphasic and the last is triphasic; numbers below waveforms indicate pulse phase durations (in ms).

In the 5(1/2)-5 ms biphasic waveform, the leading edge voltage of the first phase was one-half that of the second phase. The shocks were delivered from a 175 µF capacitor except for the first phase of the 5(1/2)-5 ms shock, which was delivered from a 350 µF capacitor. For the shocks delivered from the 175 µF capacitor through a 40 Ω impedance, the waveform tilt was 50% for a 5 ms shock and 75% for a 10 ms shock. The left ventricular patch electrode was anode for the monophasic shocks, cathode then anode for the biphasic shocks, and cathode, anode, cathode for the triphasic shocks. The switch time between phases of multiphasic shocks was 0.12 ms.

For the full voltage biphasic and triphasic waveforms, the energy of each shock was calculated from the measured leading and trailing edge voltages of the shock and from the impedance at the beginning of the phase for which the left ventricular electrode was the anode. The mean values and standard deviations are shown. The 5-5 ms biphasic and 5-5-2 ms triphasic waveforms had significantly lower leading edge voltage and energy requirements than the 3 other waveforms tested. The 10 ms monophasic required significantly lower leading edge voltage (but not energy) to defibrillate than did the 5 ms monophasic or the 5(1/2)-5 ms biphasic waveform. They also showed that those biphasics with second phases longer than the first required more voltage and energy for defibrillation (221 ± 38.8 V and 5.0 ± 1.6 J for a waveform with a 3.5 ms first phase and 6.5 ms second phase versus 97 ± 15.7 V and 1.1 ± 0.3 J for a waveform with a 6.5 ms first phase and 3.5 ms second phase).

Additional studies by Tang et al[35] demonstrated that the improved effectiveness of single capacitor biphasic waveforms is dependent on both the amplitudes and the durations of the 2 phases. These investigators used large contoured defibrillation patches on the hearts of open chest dogs and found that the peak current at the defibrillation threshold was similar for waveforms with 3.5 ms first phases and 1.0, 2.0, and 3.5 ms second phases (2.2 ± 0.7, 2.0 ± 0.5, and 2.2 ± 0.5 A, respectively) but was significantly higher for a monophasic waveform of 3.5 ms duration (3.2 ± 0.5 A) and for biphasic waveforms with a longer second phase (6.0 and 8.5 ms; 2.7 ± 0.7 and 4.0 ± 0.5 A, respectively—Fig. 2). As the duration of the second phase (T_2) increases, with a first phase (T_1), the threshold current is stable until $T_2 = T_1$, then increases sharply for $T_2 > T_1$.

Tang et al[35] also showed that biphasic waveforms with the second phase longer than the first had significantly higher voltage requirements for defibrillation (Fig. 3). The dose-response curves for the 3.5-2 (first and second phase durations, respectively, in ms) and 6-6 waveforms are almost superimposed, but the 3.5-8.5 curve is shifted to the right indicating a higher leading edge voltage re-

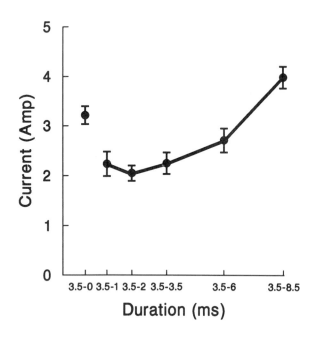

Figure 2. Plot of peak current at defibrillation threshold versus duration of second phase. The threshold current for the monophasic 3.5 ms waveform (3.5-0) is also shown.

quirement for defibrillation when the duration of the second phase exceeds that of the first phase. Thus, the improved efficacy of biphasic waveforms depends upon both the amplitudes and the durations of the 2 phases. Cooper et al[36] found that the optimum separation between the 2 phases of a biphasic waveform was 5 ms or less and that defibrillation requirements increased when the separation between the 2 phases was 50 ms, but improved again as the separation approached 100 ms.

Kavanagh et al[37] used cathodal catheter electrodes in the right ventricular apex and outflow tract and an anodal electrode over the left side of the chest in dogs that had not undergone a thoracotomy to demonstrate that single capacitor biphasic waveforms, delivered from a 150 μF capacitor, required less energy and lower leading edge voltages to defibrillate than did monophasic or double capacitor biphasic waveforms. Single capacitor biphasic waveforms have the leading edge voltage of the second phase equal to the trailing edge voltage of the first phase. Two capacitors are re-

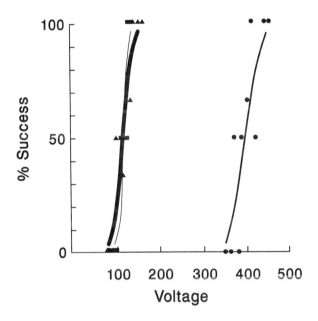

Figure 3. Data points and fitted dose-response defibrillation curves for 3 biphasic waveforms: 3.5-2 ms (▲, thick line), 6-6 ms (■, thin line), and 3.5-8.5 ms (●, medium line) in a dog.

quired to produce a waveform with the leading edge voltage of the second phase equal to the leading edge voltage of the first phase.

Kavanagh et al found that a 6-6 ms single capacitor biphasic waveform required 6.4 ± 1.6 J to defibrillate while the double capacitor biphasic waveform of the same durations in which the leading edge voltage of the 2 phases was equal required 18.0 ± 8.0 J, and a 12-ms monophasic waveform required 17.4 ± 8.0 J. The leading edge voltage required for the first phase of the single capacitor biphasic waveform (266 ± 51 V) was also significantly less than that required for either the double capacitor biphasic (336 ± 6 V) or the monophasic waveform (427 ± 117 V).

Two human studies[38,39] that used biphasic waveforms have supported the experimental findings that biphasics with a second phase of shorter duration and smaller amplitude than the first phase appear to be more effective than monophasic waveforms. Human studies also appear to confirm that a single capacitor biphasic waveform is more effective than monophasics of the same or half the total duration.[38] These findings suggest that effective biphasic waveforms could be generated from a single capacitor. The decreased energy requirements for a single capacitor biphasic waveform could result in longer battery life in ICDs while the single versus double capacitors could result in smaller devices.

Perhaps not all biphasic waveforms are strongly advantageous over the monophasic. A study of 18 patients compared the biphasic waveform which used a 150 µF capacitor and a second phase whose leading edge voltage was only half that of the first phase trailing voltage. No difference was found compared to the monophasic of the same capacitance value.[40]

Additional work has also been done to determine whether it is beneficial to use sequential biphasic waveforms. Guse et al[41] reported that 2 sequential biphasic shocks delivered through 2 different sets of electrodes defibrillated with less energy and voltage than did 2 sequential monophasic shocks delivered through the same leads. However, Jones et al[42] have recently reported that monophasic waveforms delivered sequentially through 2 pathways via 3 epicardial patches in pigs required less delivered energy to defibrillate (9.9 ± 1.5 J vs. 14.2 ± 1.6 J) than did biphasic waveforms in which the first and second phases were delivered through the same pathways that were used for the first and second monophasic waveforms. Johnson et al[43] found that giving the successive biphasic shocks through 2 separate lead systems improved defibrillation efficacy over a single biphasic shock when the separation between the shocks was either less than 10 ms or greater than 75 ms. As was the case for a single lead system, defibrillation energy requirements increased markedly for a delay of 50 ms and even exceeded the thresholds for the single lead system.

Saksena et al[44] compared biphasic and monophasic shocks for ICDs using a triple electrode system in patients that included 2 catheter electrodes (one in the right ventricle and one in the right atrium) and a left thoracic patch. They found that simultaneous biphasic shocks were more effective and reduced the energy requirements of bi-directional shocks when compared to simultaneous monophasic shocks (9 ± 5 J vs. 15 ± 4 J) and that both were significantly more effective than sequential monophasic shocks. In 82% of the patients tested (9 of 11), biphasic shocks were successful at identical energy levels at which simultaneous monophasic shocks had failed to successfully terminate the polymorphic VT or VF. There was no patient for whom sequential monophasic shocks worked but simultaneous biphasic shocks did not.

Hypotheses for the Success of Biphasic Waveforms

The mechanisms underlying the improved success of biphasic waveforms as compared to monophasics for defibrillation remain unclear although several theories have been developed. One possibility is that biphasic waveforms defibrillate better than monophasics due to effects on the refractory period of cells. Cranefield et al[45] demonstrated that giving a hyperpolarizing pulse during phase 2 of the action potential shortened the refractory period so that a depolarizing pulse applied after the hyperpolarizing pulse was effective even though the strength and timing of the pulse had been previously ineffective. Thus, the first phase of a biphasic waveform either depolarized the cells directly or shortened their refractory periods due to hyperpolarization of the transmembrane potential. If the latter was the case, then the second phase of the waveform occurred when the cells were less refractory and caused them to depolarize.

Another possible mechanism is that the first phase of the biphasic waveform "conditions" the cells to make it easier for the second phase to excite them. Jones et al[46] demonstrated in cultured chick embryo myocardial cells that biphasic pulses resulted in lower excitation thresholds than did monophasic pulses. They postulated that the first phase of the biphasic waveform acts as a "conditioning" pulse by causing hyperpolarization of some parts of the heart. The transmembrane potential of the "conditioned" portions was thus brought closer to the resting potential, and sodium channels were reactivated. The second phase could then more easily excite these portions, and lower excitation and defibrillation thresholds resulted.

Ideker et al[47] have reported that the critical point, where shock strengths of a critical value of potential gradient intersect with vulnerable tissue with a critical degree of refractoriness to form the center of a reentrant pathway, is different for biphasic versus monophasic waveforms. They suggest that their finding is related to the likelihood that a reentrant circuit that leads to the reinitiation of fibrillation will be created by the shock. Zhou et al[48] found that a one capacitor biphasic waveform with each phase lasting 5 ms required 2.7 ± 0.3 V/cm for 80% probability of success while a 10 ms monophasic truncated exponential waveform required 5.4 ± 0.8 V/cm for the same success rate. In addition, monophasic waveforms can induce conduction block at a lower potential gradient than biphasic waveforms.[2]

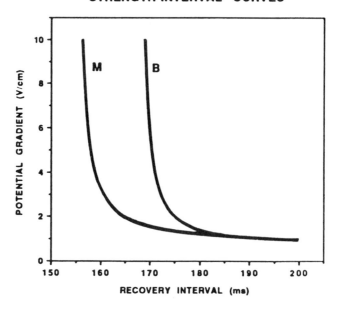

Figure 4. Monophasic and biphasic strength-interval plots in 1 dog.

Daubert et al[49] found that the strength-interval curve for a 3 ms monophasic waveform was situated to the left of the curve for a 2-1 ms biphasic waveform (Fig. 4). Curves which misclassified the fewest total points into directly excited, i.e. activated during the stimulus, (right and above curves) and not directly excited (left and below curves) were fitted to the potential gradient (V/cm) versus recovery interval (ms) for monophasic and biphasic waveforms. The biphasic curve is to the right of the monophasic indicating that the biphasic waveform is less able to directly excite partially refractory myocardium. Absolute refractory period (ARP) is the y asymptote of the strength-interval curve, whereas the diastolic threshold is the x asymptote. ARP values were 155 ms for the monophasic curve and 168 for the biphasic curve. Diastolic thresholds were 0.7 and 0.6 V/cm for the monophasic and biphasic waves respectively.

The biphasic waveform defibrillated better but the monophasic shock excited refractory, non-fibrillating tissue more effectively. The biphasic waveform was less able to stimulate (i.e. directly excite) partially refractory tissue than was the monophasic waveform. Daubert et al[49] postulated that the biphasic shocks defibrillated better because they initiated fewer new activation fronts which could recreate fibrillation rather than because they directly activated a critical mass of tissue during the shock. For longer waveforms (10 ms total duration for the monophasic waveform and 10 ms for each phase of the biphasic waveform), Swartz et al[50] found that the biphasic waveform had a greater ability to stimulate the myocardium and produce prolonged refractoriness than the monophasic.

Another explanation for the mechanism of the biphasic shock is the "burping" theory. This theory suggests that the function of the first phase is to act as a monophasic shock; the function of the second phase is to then remove (or "burp") away the residual charge on the membrane.[51,52] A fundamental hypothesis is that the first phase functions similarly to a monophasic shock. However, an additional hypothesis of this biphasic model is that the first phase leaves a residual charge on the cell membrane which can then reinitiate fibrillation. The second phase (of appropriate shape) will diminish this residual charge thus reducing the opportunities for refibrillation. To protect from this potential refibrillation, a monophasic shock must be strong enough to synchronize a critical mass of nearly 100 per cent of the myocytes and generate a significant extension of the refractory period. Since the biphasic waveform performs this protection function by removing the residual charge (with its second phase), its first phase may be of significantly lower strength than a monophasic shock of equivalent performance. Thus, the second phase "burping" of the deleterious residual charge of the first phase (which reduces the synchronization requirement and hence the amplitude requirements of the first phase) may explain the effectiveness of the biphasic waveform.

This theory is indirectly supported by experiments with chopped waveforms demonstrating that the heart cells appear to show a charge holding time constant of about 3.7 ms.[53] The theory is also supported by a study confirming the most radical prediction of the burping model—that phase 2 should be longer than phase 1 for short time constant shocks.[54]

Other Waveforms

Triphasic Waveforms
Some work has also been done with waveforms in which a third phase is added that has the same polarity as the first phase.[55,56] Early work by Dixon et al[33] (Fig. 1) did not demonstrate any im-

provement of the triphasic waveform (5-5-2) over that of the biphasic (5-5). Chapman et al[52] have recently reported that triphasic waveforms (2.5-5-2.5) required significantly less energy (14.3 J) than 10 ms monophasic waveforms (21.1 J) but more energy than biphasic waveforms with 5 ms phases (10.1 J) when used for internal defibrillation in dogs.

However, Jones et al[53] have shown that the safety factor, i.e. the ratio between the shock level that stimulated cultured chick myocardial cells and the shock level that caused dysfunction, improved when triphasic waveforms were used. They postulated that the 3 phases each have a different effect with the first phase acting as the "conditioning prepulse," the second phase as the "exciting" or "defibrillating" phase, and the third phase as the "healing" post pulse. It is possible that less dysfunction will result from triphasic waveforms at the suprathreshold shock strengths likely to be used in ICDs. However, the burping theory for the biphasic mechanism of operation predicts that the triphasic waveform would have no advantage over an optimized biphasic.[51]

Multiple Capacitance Waveforms

It is possible to make practical biphasic waveforms which take advantage of electronic switching to vary the connections of the high energy capacitors. For example, the first phase could have the capacitors in parallel—giving low tilt—while the second phase had the capacitors in series—giving a high voltage.[57] This gives another degree of freedom for the optimization of the biphasic waveform.[58]

Summary

Defibrillation waveforms have changed markedly since alternating current was first used to generate transthoracic shocks. Damped sinusoidal waveforms, generated by capacitor discharge through a series inductor and the body's resistance, have become the waveform used by most external portable defibrillators but cannot be used internally due to physical size requirements. Early work with implantable devices focused on monophasic truncated exponential waveforms which avoided the refibrillatory effects of straight capacitor discharges. Biphasic truncated exponential waveforms were introduced and found to defibrillate with lower energy requirements and fewer adverse side effects than monophasic waveforms. Much work remains to be done to explain the mechanisms responsible for the superiority of the biphasic over the monophasic waveform. Once the mechanisms are understood, it should be possible to select the optimal waveform for individual patients with fewer fibrillation and defibrillation tests at the time of implantation.

ACKNOWLEDGMENTS:

This work supported in part by the National Institutes of Health research grants HL-42760, HL-44066, HL-28429, and HL-33637, and National Science Foundation Engineering Research Center Grant CDR-8622201. Fig. 1 is based on Dixon et al.[33] Fig. 2 and 3 first appeared in Tang et al.[35] Fig. 4 first appeared in Daubert et al.[50]

1. Troup PJ. Implantable cardioverters and defibrillators. Curr Probl Cardiol 1989;14:675-843.
2. Yabe S, Smith WM, Daubert JP, et al. Conduction disturbances caused by high current density electric fields. Circ Res 1990;66:1190-1203.
3. Lerman BB, Weiss JL, Bulkley BH, et al. Myocardial injury and induction of arrhythmia by direct current shock delivered via endocardial catheters in dogs. Circulation 1984;69:1006-1012.
4. Jones JL, Lepeschkin E, Jones RE, et al. Response of cultured myocardial cells to countershock-type electric field stimulation. Am J Physiol 1978;235:H214-H222.
5. Doherty PW, McLaughlin PR, Billingham M, et al. Cardiac damage produced by direct current countershock applied to the heart. Am J Cardiol 1979;43:225-232.
6. Hooker DR, Kouwenhoven WB, Langworthy OR. The effect of alternating currents on the heart. Am J Physiol 1933;103:444-454.
7. Beck CS, Pritchard WH, Feil HS. Ventricular fibrillation of long duration abolished by electric shock. JAMA 1947;135:985-986.
8. Zoll PM, Linenthal AJ, Gibson W, et al. Termination of ventricular fibrillation in man by externally applied electric countershock. N Engl J Med 1956;254:727-732.
9. Lown B, Newman J, Amarasingham R, et al. Comparison of alternating current with direct current electroshock across the closed chest. Am J Cardiol 1962;10:223-233.
10. Gurvich NL, Yuniev GS. Restoration of regular rhythm in the mammalian fibrillating heart. Bulletin of Experimental Biology in Medicine 1939;8:55-58.
11. Peleška B. Optimal parameters of electrical impulses for defibrillation by condenser discharges. Circ Res 1966;18:10-17.
12. Geddes LA, Tacker WA. Engineering and physiological considerations of direct capacitor-discharge ventricular defibrillation. Med Biol Eng 1971;9:185-199.
13. Schuder JC, Stoeckle H, Keskar PY, et al. Transthoracic ventricular defibrillation in the dog with unidirectional rectangular double pulses. Cardiovasc Res 1970;4:497-501.
14. Koning G, Schneiger H, Hoelen AJ. Amplitude-duration relation for direct ventricular defibrillation with rectangular current pulses. Med Biol Eng 1975;13:388-395.
15. Bourland JD, Tacker WA, Geddes LA. Strength-duration curves for trapezoidal waveforms of various tilts for transchest defibrillation in animals. Med Instrum 1978;12:38-41.
16. Block M, Breithardt G. Optimizing defibrillation through improved waveforms. PACE 1995;18:526-538.
17. Schuder JC, Stoeckle H, Gold JH, et al. Experimental ventricular defibrillation

with an automatic and completely implanted system. Trans Am Soc Artif Intern Organs 1970;16:207-212.

18. Mirowski M, Mower MM, Reid PR, et al. The automatic implantable defibrillator. PACE 1982;5:384-401.

19. Wessale JL, Bourland JD, Tacker WA, et al. Bipolar catheter defibrillation in dogs using trapezoidal waveforms of various tilts. J Electrocard 1980;13:359-366.

20. Kroll MW. A minimal model of the monophasic defibrillation pulse. PACE 1993;16:769-777.

21. Chapman PD, Wetherbee JN, Vetter JW, et al. Strength-duration curves of fixed pulse width variable tilt truncated exponential waveforms for nonthoracotomy internal defibrillation in dogs. PACE 1988;11:1045-1050.

22. Tacker WA, Geddes LA. The automatic implantable defibrillator (AID). In: Electrical Defibrillation. Boca Raton. Florida: CRC Press, Inc., 1980 pp 167-178.

23. Orias O. Possible mecanismo de la defibrilación miocárdica por contrachoque eléctrico. Acta Physiol Pharmacol Lationam 1953;3:147-150.

24. Sweeney RJ, Gill RM, Reid PR. Characterization of refractory period extension by transcardiac shock. Circulation 1991;83:2057-2066.

25. Bourland JD, Tacker WA, Wessale JL, et al. Sequential pulse defibrillation for implantable defibrillators. Med Instrum 1986;20:138-142.

26. Jones DL, Klein GJ, Guiradon GM, et al. Internal cardiac defibrillation in man: Pronounced improvement with sequential pulse delivery to two different lead orientations. Circulation 1986;73:484-491.

27. Jones DL, Klein GJ, Guiradon GM, et al. Prediction of defibrillation success from a single defibrillation threshold measurement with sequential pulses and two current pathways in humans. Circulation 1988;78:1144-1149.

28. Bardou AL, Degonde J, Birkui PJ, et al. Reduction of energy required for defibrillation by delivering shocks in orthogonal directions in the dog. PACE 1988;11:1990-1995.

29. Jones DL, Klein GJ, Kallok MJ. Improved internal defibrillation with twin pulse sequential energy delivery to different lead orientations. Am J Cardiol 1985;55:821-825.

30. Jones DL, Sohla A, Bourland JD, et al. Internal ventricular defibrillation with sequential pulse countershock in pigs: Comparison with single pulses and effects of pulse separation. PACE 1987;10:497-502.

31. Gurvich NL, Markarychev VA. Defibrillation of the heart with biphasic electrical impulses. Kardiologilia 1967;7:109-112.

32. Schuder JC, McDaniel WC, Stoeckle H. Defibrillation of 100-kg calves with asymmetrical, bidirectional, rectangular pulses. Cardiovasc Res 1984;18:419-426.

33. Dixon EG, Tang ASL, Wolf PD, et al. Improved defibrillation thresholds with large contoured epicardial electrodes and biphasic waveforms. Circulation 1987;76:1176-1184.

34. Holley LK, McCulloch RM. Comparison of biphasic and monophasic defibrillation waveforms in an isolated rabbit heart preparation. Cardiovasc Res 1991;25:979-983.

35. Tang ASL, Yabe S, Wharton JM, et al. Ventricular defibrillation using biphasic waveforms: The importance of phasic duration. J Am Coll Cardiol 1989;13:207-214.

36. Cooper RAS, Guse PA, Dixon-Tulloch EG, et al. The effect of phase separation on biphasic waveform defibrillation. PACE 1991;14:667. (abstract)

37. Kavanagh KM, Tang ASL, Rollins DL, et al. Comparison of the internal defibrillation thresholds for monophasic and double and single capacitor biphasic waveforms. J Am Coll Cardiol 1989;14:1343-1349.

38. Bardy GH, Ivey TD, Allen MD, et al. A prospective randomized evaluation of

biphasic versus monophasic waveform pulses on defibrillation efficacy in humans. J Am Coll Cardiol 1989;14:728-733.

39. Winkle RA, Mead RH, Ruder MA, et al. Improved low energy defibrillation efficacy in man with the use of a biphasic truncated exponential waveform. Am Heart J 1989;117:122-127.
40. Dutinth V, Schwartzman D, Callans DJ, et al. Defibrillation thresholds with monophasic versus biphasic shocks delivered through a single-lead endocardial defibrillation system. Am Heart J 1996;131:611-613.
41. Guse PA, Walcott GP, Rollins DL, et al. Defibrillation electrode configurations developed from cardiac mapping that combine biphasic shocks with sequential timing. Am Heart J 1992;124:1491-1500.
42. Jones DL, Klein GJ, Wood GK. Biphasic versus sequential pulse defibrillation: A direct comparison in pigs. Am Heart J 1992;124:97-103.
43. Johnson EE, Walcott GP, Melnick S, et al. Defibrillation efficacy for various delays between two successive biphasic shocks. PACE 1991;14:715. (abstract)
44. Saksena S, An H, Mehra R, DeGroot P, et al. Prospective comparison of biphasic and monophasic shocks for implantable cardioverter-defibrillators using endocardial leads. Am J Cardiol 1992;70:304-310.
45. Cranefield PF, Hoffman BF. Propagated repolarization in heart muscle. J Gen Physiol 1958;41:633-349.
46. Jones JL, Jones RE, Balasky G. Improved cardiac cell excitation with symmetrical biphasic defibrillator waveforms. Am J Physiol 1987;253:H1418-H1424.
47. Ideker RE, Tang ASL, Frazier DW, et al. Ventricular defibrillation: Basic concepts. In El-Sherif N, Samet P, (eds) Cardiac Pacing and Electrophysiology. Orlando, Florida: W. B. Saunders Co., 1991 pp 713-726.
48. Zhou X, Daubert JP, Wolf PD, et al. Epicardial mapping of ventricular defibrillation with monophasic and biphasic shocks in dogs. Circ Res 1993;72:145-160.
49. Daubert JP, Frazier DW, Wolf PD, et al. Response of relatively refractory canine myocardium to monophasic and biphasic shocks. Circulation 1991;84:2522-2538.
50. Swartz JF, Jones JL, Jones RE, et al. Conditioning prepulse of biphasic defibrillator waveforms enhances refractoriness to fibrillation wavefronts. Circ Res 1991;68:438-449.
51. Kroll MW. A minimal model of the single capacitor biphasic waveform. PACE 1994;17:1782-1792.
52. Walcott GP, Walker RG, Cates AW, et al. Choosing the optimal monophasic and biphasic waveforms for ventricular defibrillation. J Cardiovasc Electrophysiol 1995;6:737-750.
53. Sweeney RJ, Gill RM, Jones JL, et al. Defibrillation using a high-frequency series of monophasic rectangular pulses: observations and model predictions. J Cardiovasc Electrophysiol 1996;7:134-143.
54. Swerdlow CD, Fan W, Brewer JF. Charge-burping correctly predicts optimal ratios of phase duration for biphasic defibrillation waveforms. Circulation in press 1996/1997.
55. Chapman PD, Wetherbee JN, Vetter JW, et al. Comparison of monophasic, biphasic, and triphasic truncated pulses for non-thoracotomy internal defibrillation. J Am Coll Card 1988;11:57A. (abstract)
56. Jones JL, Jones RE. Improved safety factors for triphasic defibrillator waveforms. Circ Res 1989;64:1172-1177.
57. Walcott GP, Rollins DL, Smith WM, et al. Effect of changing capacitors between phases of a biphasic defibrillation shock. PACE 1996;19:945-954.
58. Fujiyama, Tchou P, Brewer JE, et al. Defibrillation thresholds with parallel series waveforms. Circulation 1996; (in press)

8

The System

C. G. "Jerry" Supino

THE ICD is more than just a device that is implanted in the patient. It is a part, albeit the central element, of a collection of electrical and mechanical components — a System. In fact without the other parts of the system, it would be impossible to properly implant ICDs.

It goes without saying that the ICD has become more complicated due to the demand for more sensitive and specific tachyarrhythmia detection, tiered therapy (antitachycardia pacing, cardioversion and defibrillation), in situ recording capabilities (patient tachycardia episode history and stored intra-cardiac signals), and diagnostic aids in the form of continuous telemetry transmission (real-time telemetry) of device events (commonly called markers) and intra-cardiac signals (electrograms). With the ever growing need for the improvement and evolution of these, and newer, functions and features, it is apparent that the associated electronic equipment is getting more complex. We will identify and examine the parts of the system (Table 1) and look at their basic functionality with emphasis on the ICD itself.

Table 1. The components of an ICD system.

Leads
Test instruments
External Cardioverter Defibrillator (ECD)*
Pacing System Analyzer (PSA)
ICD
Programmer

* Some manufacturers use other synonymous terms: Defibrillation System Analyzer (DSA), Defibrillation Test System (DTS).
† The PSA function is usually included in the programmer/ICD system.

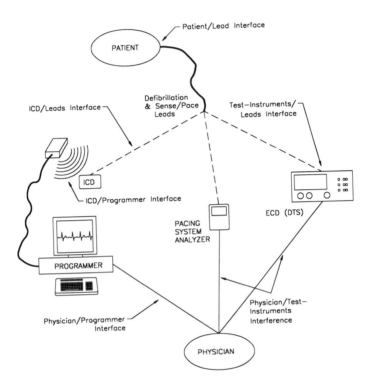

Figure 1. The ICD System and its interfaces

Ancillary Components of the System

One way to approach the identification of the various components of the ICD system is from the perspective of the various system interfaces between the ICD, per se, and its ancillary components.

The Leads

Generally, the implanted lead configuration will be composed of an arrangement of one or more of the following leads:

1. Transvenous defibrillation lead with integrated sense/pace electrodes. The sense/pace electrodes are used for rate sensing and bradycardia and antitachycardia pacing.
2. Subcutaneous defibrillation patch or array to be used with the transvenous defibrillation lead.
3. Transvenous defibrillation lead without sense/pace electrodes. Using this lead, a separate sense/pace lead would be required.

4. Transvenous sense/pace lead.
5. Epicardial defibrillation patches
6. Epicardial sense leads. This pair of leads, attached to the myocardium, is utilized in thoracotomy implants where epicardial defibrillation patches are used.

For a thorough description of the various types of defibrillation leads and lead configurations see Chaps. 6 and 9.

The External Cardioverter Defibrillator (ECD)

This instrument was originally used primarily to determine the defibrillation threshold. Synonyms are Defibrillation System Analyzer (DSA) and Defibrillation Test System (DTS). Current units can perform other significant roles such as providing an impedance measurement for the defibrillation leads, current and voltage measurement of the defibrillation pulse, mimic the detection algorithm of the implanted unit, provide access to the rate sense and defibrillation leads for monitoring, and print reports. The ECD can be a stand alone instrument or it may be an integral part of a more complex system that includes the programmer and possibly EP (electrophysiology) testing support.

The user interface can vary considerably from no display of information (i.e., instrument settings are made using switches and appropriate buttons activated to defibrillate during threshold determination) to a full computer screen display of instrument functions and operational selections. The ECDs are generally battery powered to provide the required patient electrical isolation, but with suitable designs they may be AC powered.

Not all manufacturers provide ECDs at present but rather have the DFT testing features included in the programmer. This approach is referred to as *device based testing* so that both VF induction and test shock delivery are pefromed via the ICD at the time of implantation. The advantages of the device based testing approach are that it minimizes equipment and lead reconnections. The disadvantage is that it occasionally requires, in a high threshold patient, the use of a transthoracic rescue shock and possible disposal of the ICD.

The Pacing System Analyzer (PSA)

This instrument would not immediately be considered part of today's ICD system. However, the same PSA that is used for pacemaker implants can be used to evaluate the sense lead for an ICD implant; measure R-wave amplitude and lead impedance; de-

termine pacing capture threshold; ICD systems now typically incorporate the functions and features of a PSA. For example, the
programmer (in conjunction with the ICD) allows semiautomatic
pacing threshold measurements.

The Programmer

The programmer is the physician's window to the operation and
settings of the ICD. The presentation of information and the
method of interaction with this information will vary considerably
from manufacturer to manufacturer. One of the reasons that computer displays are used is due to the greater volume of information
associated with these implanted devices versus the information related to pacemakers. Not only are there many more parameters for
the ICD, but the ICD also stores extensive information (therapy history) about tachyarrhythmia detection and subsequent therapy delivery in the form of a data history and a stored, digitized electrogram associated with the tachyarrhythmias. This information, predischarge or for a followup procedure months later, is extracted by
the physician when interrogating the ICD. (Chap. 20)

   The programmer should format all information in such a
fashion as to make it useful to the physician in determining the cor-
rectness of the detection and treatment of the patient's tachyarrhythmias by the ICD. It has been demonstrated that this information is invaluable in analyzing the occurrence of tachyarrhythmias
and the performance of the ICD especially with regard to suspected
abnormal device behavior. (Chap. 21)

   Modern ICD programmers include additional features to
facilitate the pre-implant, implant, and post-implant activities. A
printer is provided for hard copy output for patient files or for the
purpose of analysis. At any time, the user can print the programmed ICD settings for the implant and, after the implant,
interrogate and print any therapy history and stored electrogram
data. The programmer has one or two signal outputs that can be
connected to a chart recorder or monitor for recording real-time
electrogram and event markers that are (when this feature is selected by the user) continuously transmitted by the ICD to the programmer and in turn reflected on these outputs. In some cases,
where the programmer has a surface ECG input channel, the programmer can print a real-time ECG and at the same time annotate
the recording with telemetry, real-time event markers from the ICD
on another channel of the recording. Another feature is a signal input channel that can be connected to an EP stimulator to provide
noninvasive programmed stimulation (NIPS) via telemetry. For each

pacing pulse in a train of pacing pulses output by the stimulator, the programmer, upon detecting the pulse, will convert that into a telemetry command that is immediately sent to the ICD. The ICD decodes the command and instantly (within a few milliseconds) delivers a pacing pulse to the patient.

The ICD as a Component of the System

We can approach the ICD in the same manner with which we investigated the overall system, that is, by starting with the device interfaces and, in this case, working our way into the device. The interfaces to be explored are the telemetry interface, the sense input interface, the high-voltage output interface, the pace output interface, the audio transducer (beeper) interface, and the magnet interface. (Fig. 2) Not all ICDs have the beeper interface.

We will begin with the *telemetry interface*. When, via the programmer, the physician desires to communicate with the ICD the programming head must be within approximately 10 cm of the ICD. Implementation of the telemetry communication in the form of the actual data transmitted and the rate of data transmission will vary from manufacturer to manufacturer. Generally speaking, however, communication between the two devices consists of messages sent by the programmer to the ICD and a corresponding response on the part of the ICD.

Even though the link is referred to as the "RF link" it is actually not a radio transmission as the two antennas are too close together for radio waves to be developed. It is rather an inefficient (in terms of power transfer) transformer coupling with one winding in the ICD and the other in the programming wand. (See Chap 13, "Charging Circuit" for a discussion of transformer operation.) A high frequency (~100 kHz) "carrier" signal is modulated by the information (data) through a variety of techniques. These include using the data bits (1 or 0) to turn the carrier on or off, to shift the carrier frequency, or to change the gap between on/off cycles.

It is of paramount importance that the information intended for the ICD (i.e., the message sent by the programmer) and the information that the ICD receives be one and the same, that is, one or more means must be employed by the programmer and the ICD to check and maintain the integrity of the transmitted data. Different manufacturers have different mechanisms to accomplish this. In some cases the programming head may contain, in addition to the telemetry circuitry, a *magnet* such that within the ICD a magnetic

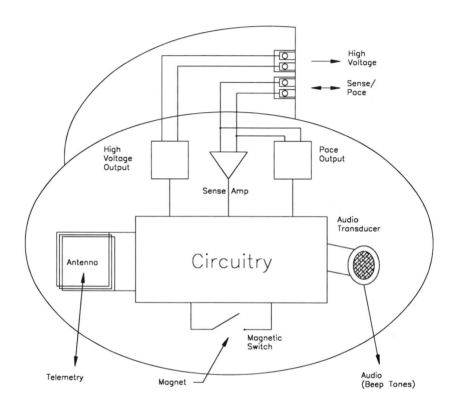

Figure 2. The ICD and its interfaces.

reed switch must be closed before the device will even begin to as-
semble the incoming telemetry message.

This *magnetic reed switch* is the same type of device which
was used in the earlier nonprogrammable devices to inhibit/enable
therapy or to enable the beeper. (See Appendix to Chap. 20,
"Magnet Function Table.") A thin magnetic strip (resembling a
woodwind reed) and another conducting strip are sealed within a
slender glass cylinder. A sufficiently strong magnetic field will cause
the strips to touch thus making an electrical circuit.

As a supplement to the magnet, or even in place of the magnet, elaborately generated *check characters* are transmitted as part of
the message. Mathematical formulas from number theory (the study
of the properties of integers) are used to generate a distinctive
matching "check sum" code in order to verify the authenticity and

reliability of the message. With these checksum codes, the ICD can check the information in the message for errors and, if found, reject the message (i.e., take no action) and so inform the programmer of the error. The programmer, receiving a return message (there are also checks in this direction) with information that an error occurred, can then either inform the user of the telemetry failure or automatically try it again one or more times before notifying the user of a telemetry problem.

A message from the programmer might be to change one or more of the programmable parameters within the ICD. Such parameters may include tachycardia detection criteria, tachycardia therapy, and bradycardia pacing parameters. In addition, the programmer may be requested to transmit what can be classified as immediate directives: e.g., enter real-time electrogram transmission mode (continuously transmit the digitized intra-cardiac signal), stat shock (immediately charge the capacitors to maximum voltage and deliver the shock), abort therapy (immediately terminate the ongoing therapy), or start bradycardia pacing.

The incoming message may be assembled by the microcomputer or it may be acquired by a custom digital circuit; in any case, once the incoming message has been accumulated in the ICD and checked for error, the program will interpret the message and take the appropriate action.

Internal ICD System

With this opening excursion into the ICD we can now begin to identify the major internal components and functions. Fig. 3 provides a block diagram of a typical device. The sense input interface is joined to an *amplifier circuit* that accomplishes R-wave detection. (Chap. 14) In all current devices, the amplifier is either of the automatic gain control or of the automatic threshold control variety. These automatic adjustment functions can be purely hardware circuits or can be partly implemented in software by the microprocessor. Sensing is required not only for tachycardia detection but also for bradycardia pacing. Designs will vary from one amplifier for both functions to separate amplifiers for each function. For tachycardia (or bradycardia) detection the intervals between detected R-waves may be monitored by the custom digital circuitry in the block diagram or directly monitored by the microcomputer program.

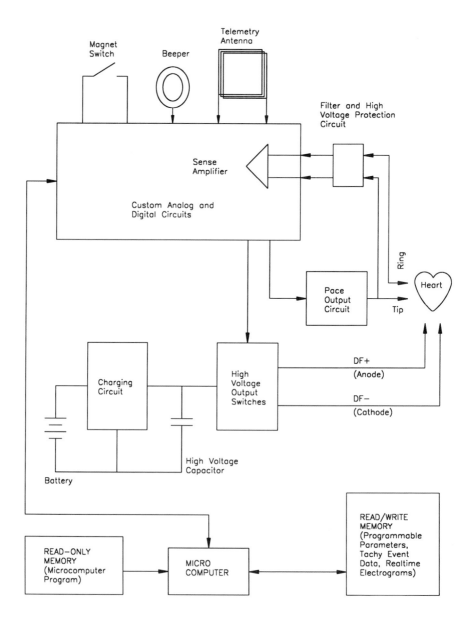

Figure 3. The internal ICD system

The next interface, and the reason for the ICD's existence, is the *high-voltage output circuit*. (Chap. 13) For our discussion, this includes the charging circuit, the high voltage storage capacitors (Chap. 11), and the high-voltage output switches. After a tachyarrhythmia detection or when requested via the programmer, and initiated by the ICD microcomputer program, the charging circuit converts the battery voltage (approximately 6 V) to a much higher voltage in order to charge the capacitors. For a maximum energy defibrillation shock the capacitors will be charged to around 750 V in about 10 seconds. Once the capacitors are charged and it is decided by the microcomputer program to deliver a shock to the patient, the high-voltage output switches are activated. Again, the initiation of this action is by the program and may be entirely controlled by the microcomputer or by custom digital circuitry.

The *pacing output circuit* interface delivers the pacing therapy for bradycardia or tachycardia therapy. In any case, the microcomputer is the decision maker with regard to tachyarrhythmia detection and ensuing therapy delivery, and, if not in total control (custom digital circuitry could automatically control the delivery of an antitachycardia pacing sequence), at least the initiator of such activity. Also, bradycardia pacing could be either entirely under the control of the microcomputer or it could be autonomous via digital circuits. In either case the microcomputer, in response to programmer messages, would control the bradycardia parameters (rate, pulse width, etc.) and turning bradycardia pacing on and off.

Some devices have an *audio transducer* (or beeper) built into them. This feature can be used for several purposes. One use is to provide a means to quickly evaluate R-wave sensing in the ICD. The ICD could be programmed to beep with each sensed R-wave by simply applying a magnet to the device, or by a programmer command. However it is accomplished (i.e., however the manufacturer designs it), the beeps can be compared to an ongoing surface ECG chart recording or display monitor for over, under, or just normal sensing. In some cases a stethoscope or even an audio amplifier is required to hear or record the beeps.

Another use for the beeper has been to quickly, (and in the absence of a programmer), indicate if the ICD is enabled or not for tachyarrhythmia therapy delivery. This has been done by applying a magnet and listening for R-wave sensing (therapy enabled) or for a continuous tone (therapy disabled). Still another use is to have the device periodically beep when it has detected the battery ERI (Elective Replacement Indicator) level and so inform the patient of this event. Also, the beeper could be used to indicate some abnormal activity in the device, again beeping periodically after the problem occurred.

Aside from its earlier mentioned use in the programming head of the programmer, a *magnet* can be used in an emergency situation, and in the absence of a programmer, to temporarily disable tachyarrhythmia therapy delivery. For some ICDs, placing the magnet over the device and holding it in place for a specified period of time (e.g., 30 s) will indefinitely disable therapy if it was enabled before placing the magnet. Conversely, if the therapy was disabled when the magnet was placed over the device and held there for the specified period of time, therapy will be re-enabled. As mentioned above the beeper can reflect the state of the device and its operation in the case of R-wave sensing in conjunction with the use of a magnet. (See the appendix of Chap. 20 for model-specific details.) Magnet deactivation of the ICD should be considered during testing of a separate implanted pacemaker.[1] Inadvertent deactivation of the ICD due to stray magnetic fields is a frequent occurrence.[2] (See Chap. 21) Magnetic resonance imaging can also activate the magnetic reed switch.[3]

As we have seen, there is much more to the ICD than the device itself. The elements constitute an integrated system of electronic components.

1.   Kim SG, Furman S, Matos JA, et al. Automatic implantable cardioverter/defibrillator: inadvertent discharges during permanent pacemaker magnet tests. PACE 1987;10:579-582.
2.   Bonnet CA, Elson JJ, Fogoros RN. Accidental deactivation of the automatic implantable cardioverter defibrillator. Am Heart J 1990;120:696-697.
3.   Erlebacher JA, Cahill PT, Pannizzo F, et al. Effect of magnetic resonance imaging on DDD pacemakers. Am J Cardiol 1986;57:437-440.

9

Leads for the ICD

Randall S. Nelson, Byron L. Gilman, J. Edward
Shapland, PhD, and Michael H. Lehmann, MD

FTER OVER a decade of research and development, much has been learned about the factors that influence defibrillation, the nature of the underlying arrhythmias, and their interactions. Factors that influence the success of a defibrillation shock include the underlying physiologic substrate of the heart, the associated characteristics of the tachyarrhythmia, the magnitude and profile of the defibrillation waveform, and the lead/electrode system used to deliver the shock to the heart.

The lead system and electrodes employed for defibrillation are especially critical. Leads are the components of the ICD system that must deliver the shock in an environment that flexes and twists millions of times (over 40 million times per year at 75 beats per minute). The electrodes may also become encapsulated by fibrotic tissue, thereby isolating the electrical shock from the surrounding tissue and resulting in defibrillation threshold rises. The lead is potentially in place for use with multiple replacement pulse generators. It is therefore the component of the defibrillation system that is most chronic as well as most abused by the body.

For clarity, electrodes will be distinguished from leads according to the following definitions: The *lead* is that portion of the implanted device that conducts electrical impulses between the pulse generator and the patient and is composed of the electrode(s), conductors, insulating coating, a connector and, typically, a fixation mechanism. The *electrode* is that portion of the lead that is intended to be in electrical contact with the body for pacing or defibrillation pulse therapy as well as sensing of the cardiac activity.

Leads are designed to allow the positioning of the electrode(s) in an epicardial, endocardial, or extrathoracic location. The first ICD lead systems used two *epicardial* patches (similar to that shown in Fig. 1) or an epicardial patch with a transvenous spring electrode for defibrillation.

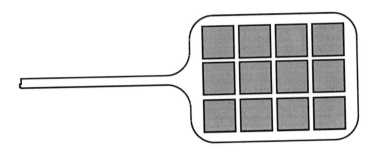

Figure 1. Epicardial patch electrode

For sensing (no pacing was available), two epicardial screw-in leads (similar to standard epicardial pacing leads) were typically implanted. All commercially available patches are designed for defibrillation only, even though integrated pacing, sensing and defibrillating patch leads have been investigated. Large and small epicardial patches are available, with larger patches generally providing lower defibrillation thresholds, particularly in patients with large hearts. Later, transvenous leads were used for pacing and sensing with a pair of epicardial patches for defibrillation.

Development then turned to a *purely transvenous* electrode system. Continuing development has resulted in three types or categories of transvenous leads to provide pacing, sensing and defibrillation electrodes:

Type I.   A single lead providing all defibrillation and pace/sense electrodes (Fig. 2). A current example of this type is the CPI Endotak.

Type II.   A pair of leads, one of which has the right ventricular (RV) defibrillation electrode and the pace/sense electrode(s), the second has the superior vena cava (SVC), coronary sinus (CS), or right atrial (RA) defibrillation electrode (Fig. 3). Current examples of this type are the Medtronic Transvene, Ventritex TVL, Intermedics transvenous lead system, and the Telectronics EnGuard.

Type III.   A pair of leads, one of which contains both RV and SVC/RA defibrillation electrodes, the second containing the pace/sense electrodes (Fig. 4). A current example of this type is the Angeion AngeFlex.

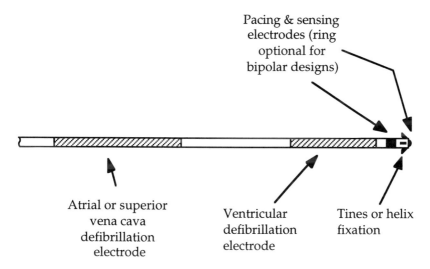

Pacing & sensing
electrodes (ring
optional for
bipolar designs)

Atrial or superior
vena cava
defibrillation
electrode

Ventricular
defibrillation
electrode

Tines or helix
fixation

Figure 2. Type I transvenous lead system: All defibrillation and pace/sense electrodes in one lead.

Each lead type may be implanted in various configurations based on the manufacturer's recommendations and implanting physician's preferences. Configurations may include the can of the ICD as an electrode in conjunction with a transvenous lead. This "hot" or "active" can electrode may be used with the RV electrode alone or as part of a split electrical vector using the RA/SVC electrode. Configurations are discussed in more detail in Chap. 6.

A drawback of completely transvenous defibrillation electrode systems is that they may have higher defibrillation thresholds due to a less favorable distribution of voltage gradients throughout the heart (Chap. 6) and higher resistances (Chap. 4). In some patients it may be necessary to add an additional electrode to the transvenous lead system to obtain acceptable thresholds. To avoid the thoracotomy required with an epicardial patch lead, three methods have been developed. In one, a subxyphoid approach has been used to place a standard epicardial patch lead. In another method, a patch is placed outside the thoracic cavity, subcutaneously or submuscularly in the left lateral chest wall. The third alternative to the thoracotomy is the subcutaneous electrode array lead. The electrode of this lead consists of coiled electrodes attached in parallel and tunneled subcutaneously across the chest wall. Currently, the problem of potentially higher defibrillation thresholds associated with completely transvenous lead systems

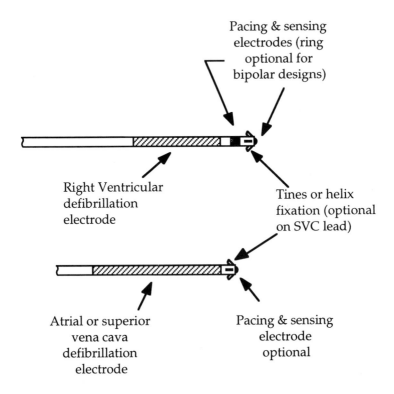

Figure 3. Type II transvenous lead system: RV electrode with pace/sense electrode(s) on one lead. The RA/SVC electrode is positioned on a second lead with optional atrial pace/sense electrodes.

has been largely obviated through the use of biphasic shock waveforms.

Physiological Requirements and Considerations

The electrodes must provide a voltage gradient or current density in excess of some minimal value to over 90% of the heart, as explained in detail in Chap. 3. They must not only deliver energy, but must also sense intrinsic cardiac electrical activity under varying conditions and provide this critical information to the defibrillator. Coupled with the implanted device, the sensing electrodes must permit the ICD to rapidly detect and, ideally, distinguish poten-

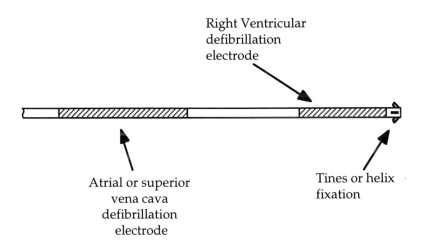

Right Ventricular
defibrillation
electrode

Atrial or superior
vena cava
defibrillation
electrode

Tines or helix
fixation

Figure 4. Type III transvenous lead system: RV and RA/SVC electrodes on one lead. Pace/sense electrodes are located on a second lead.

tially life-threatening ventricular tachyarrhythmias from supraventricular tachyarrhythmias.

Sensing and Detection

The determination of the heart rate is the primary component of the arrhythmia detection schemes in all present ICDs. The sensing leads and ICD must be sensitive enough to interpret heart rates over a 10:1 range (40-400 beats per minute). For this reason, closely-spaced bipolar electrodes have been found to provide optimal sensing waveforms for rate counting compared to unipolar sensing. Such an electrode configuration provides discrete localized sensing, required for accurate rate counting, with relatively little far field interference. By contrast, unipolar sensing is more susceptible to far field interference including remote cardiac electrical signals, myopotentials or environmental electrical interference.

Early implanted systems primarily incorporated two epicardial screw-in leads for rate sensing, placed no further than 1 cm apart. Transvenous leads, using a bipolar configuration with either the RV electrode or an independent ring, have become natural replacements for rate sensing. Because signal characteristics change with electrode size, spacing and location,[1] it is important that signals be properly matched to ICD device circuitry.

In addition to rate counting, detection and discrimination criteria may require a morphological or other analysis of the cardiac electrograms.[2,3] Such techniques often require a more global picture of the heart's electrical activity. Some systems use a probability density function or other morphological analysis detection scheme in which signals are taken from the same patch electrodes used for delivering the defibrillation shocks. To allow these types of morphological analysis, different types of electrodes and lead systems may be needed.

A well documented problem involves sensing immediately following the defibrillating shock. (See Chaps. 14, 21, and 23) Several researchers have shown temporary cellular dysfunction after high energy shocks. Jones[4] demonstrated that chick cell aggregates were temporarily stunned following defibrillation shocks. Ideker's group[5] (then at Duke University) reported conduction delays in myocardial tissue receiving high energy shocks, greater than 64 V/cm. Thus, for sensing electrodes close to the shocking electrodes, defibrillation may cause significant changes in electrogram amplitude and slew rates in tissue near the shocking electrodes, potentially causing difficulties in post-shock sensing.[6] The clinical significance of this phenomenon is dependent on the sensing characteristics of the ICD and on the spacing between the sensing electrodes and the RV shocking electrode. A true bipolar sensing electrode has also been shown to potentially minimize the post-shock R-wave amplitude reduction when compared to an integrated bipolar sense electrode.[7]

The Defibrillation Electrodes

Early studies indicated that ventricular fibrillation conversion was achieved when shocks depolarized a critical mass of the heart.[8,9] Later studies by Wharton et al further revealed a minimum voltage gradient in excess of 6 V/cm, with a monophasic waveform, is necessary for defibrillation to occur.[10] Uniformity of current density is desirable because (1) low voltage gradient areas contribute to the continuation or reinitiation of the ventricular fibrillation, and (2) high current areas may induce temporary damage that then may cause sensing difficulties, produce areas of reinitiation of fibrillation, or even potentially cause permanent tissue damage.

When two patches are used, the heart is located between the large electrodes, so most of the current goes directly into the heart tissue, making this one of the most efficient means of applying current to the heart. In this case, defibrillation can occur with relatively low energy. The size, number, shape, and position of epicardial patch electrodes will also influence defibrillation energy requirements.[11,12] These myocardial electrodes, however, have the potential to reduce ventricular function, especially when large patch electrodes are implanted intrapericardially.[13]

A key advantage for any defibrillation lead system is the ability to implant the electrodes without the need for a thoracotomy or other major surgical procedure. A variety of multi-polar transvenous lead systems have been developed. Although their ease of implant is a major advantage, these transvenous lead systems also have disadvantages. Defibrillating electrodes, which are incorporated onto the transvenous lead body, are usually positioned in the right heart or great veins. Due to the relatively small electrode surface area and the position within the heart, highly nonuniform current densities or gradients can be produced. Since the blood surrounding the electrodes, in the veins and heart, has a lower electrical impedance than the myocardial tissue (against the grain of the myocytes), some of the current may be shunted away from the myocardium. This current shunting can cause further nonuniformity of the defibrillation electrical fields. The requirement to provide more uniform current densities and lower the energy requirements for defibrillation can be enhanced by transvenous systems that incorporate three or more defibrillating electrodes.[14,15] (Chap. 6)

Transvenous lead systems must not only deliver the defibrillation shocks but also must provide sensing capability. Such combination systems can be designed in several ways, but have their own unique problems. A single lead, whether with one or two defibrillation electrodes, can be used for both sensing and defibrillating. Having the sensing and defibrillating electrodes on the same lead may result in the sensing electrodes being located near the high current density areas associated with the defibrillating electrodes. As previously described, these high gradient areas and the resulting tissue dysfunction may cause sensing problems. In addition, for a single lead incorporating both defibrillation electrodes and pace/sense electrodes (type I), several conductors are required which increases the lead diameter and may make handling and positioning more difficult. The single lead may also be more difficult to extract due to its size which may cause additional mechanical trauma to the heart. The separate SVC defibrillation electrode lead configuration (type II) may also be susceptible to the same post shock sensing problems due to the RV electrode proximity to the sensing tip. A type III system with separate leads for pace/sensing and defibrillating may circumvent these problems. This system would allow the passage of two thinner, more supple leads and facilitate the placement of the pace/sense lead outside the traumatized area. However, the additional lead necessitates a second lead through the tricuspid valve, and care in placement for effective sensing and pacing. If the outer insulation of both leads is silicone, there may also be a problem of chronic abrasion or of passing the second lead during implant due to the propensity of silicone to stick to itself. Manufacturers are investigating surface treatments and modifications to the silicone to address this issue.

Table 1 shows the variations between current lead models with regards to tip to electrode distance, which affects sensing performance, and electrode length and surface area, in turn, affecting defibrillation efficacy. As the understanding of defibrillation advances, length and surface areas of the electrodes can be expected to become similar. Even now, there are more similarities than differences.

Current ICD systems not only detect and treat a tachyarrhythmia, but are being called upon for backup bradycardia pacing support. Such therapy may be necessitated by post-shock dysfunction of the sinus node, atrio-ventricular node, or various conduction disturbances, or by nonrelated disease conditions. Increases in pacing thresholds have been reported immediately after delivery of a defibrillation shock.[16,17] The rise in threshold is most likely due to the cellular dysfunction induced by the high energy field of the defibrillation shock. Therefore, the pacing electrode must be far enough away from the shocking electrodes to avoid high current density areas and thus reduce the potential for temporary pacing exit block. Increases in chronic pacing threshold may also result from the increased stiffness of current single pass transvenous defibrillating leads that also incorporate pacing electrodes.

Time Dependent Changes in Lead Function

Sensing and therapeutic functions (pacing and defibrillation) of a lead system may not remain constant during the chronic implant life of the device. Sensing and pacing thresholds may increase due to fibrotic changes at the electrode and tissue interface.[18] For pacemakers, steroid eluting tips have buffered the sharp increase in thresholds.[19] For ICD use, these changes may be minimized by the utilization of lead designs that provide the greatest lead flexibility and adequate separation between the shocking and sensing/pacing electrodes. Energy requirements for defibrillation may also change over time.[20] These changes may be due to changes in the myocardial substrate or to the lead system.

The leads and electrodes, especially in transvenous systems, may shift slightly or migrate, causing significant changes in defibrillation threshold.[21] As with sensing and pacing electrodes, fibrosis at

Table 1. Comparison of transvenous defibrillation systems.

Model	Lead Type	Tip→RV spacing	RV length	RV surface area[†]	SVC/RA length	SVC/RA surface area[†]
Angeion						
AngeFlex 4020	III	0.7 cm	5.0 cm	268 mm²	6.5 cm	347 mm²
CPI						
Endotak DSP	I	1.2 cm	4.5 cm	450 mm²	6.7 cm	660 mm²
Endotak 70	I	1.2 cm	4.7 cm	531 mm²	6.9 cm	826 mm²
Endotak 60	I	0.5 cm	3.6 cm	406 mm²	6.9 cm	826 mm²
Intermedics						
	II	0.6 cm	5.0 cm	440 mm²	5.0 cm	440 mm²
Medtronic						
Transvene	II	2.4 cm	5.0 cm	448 mm²	5.0 cm	361 mm²
Pacesetter						
1536/ 1559	II	2.4 cm	5.0 cm	459 mm²	8.0 cm	523 mm²
Telectronics						
EnGuard	II	2.1 cm	6.0 cm	600 mm²	6.0 cm	600 mm²
Ventritex						
TVL	II	1.1 cm	5.0 cm	470 mm²	7.2 cm	550 mm²

* Dimensions courtesy of the manufacturers.
† Surface area is measured as *shadow area*—the superficial cylinder surface of the electrode; mathematically referred to as the area of the convex hull.
RV is right ventricular electrode; SVC/RA is superior vena cava (or right atrial) electrode.

the interface of the defibrillating electrode,[18,22] or other changes on the electrode surface, such as oxidation, may also decrease electrode efficiency and change the energy needed for defibrillation.

Considering these factors when designing new lead systems may help reduce chronic threshold changes. Nevertheless, thorough testing at the time of implant will help to ensure that appropriate safety margins are established to compensate for potential threshold changes. (Chap. 5)

Engineering Requirements and Considerations

The functional engineering requirements of a defibrillator lead system can be divided into three categories: defibrillation, pacing, and sensing. Requirements for defibrillation are to provide a low resistance current path to the heart, to isolate the high voltage defibrillation pulse from the body, and to shape the electric field in the heart for minimum defibrillation thresholds. For pacing, the lead must provide a low threshold pacing electrode and a flexible lead body to minimize myocardial trauma, thus minimizing the potential for significant threshold increase over time. For sensing, the lead must provide electrodes to sense and an isolated path for transmitting millivolt intracardiac electrogram signals. Finally the lead system must perform all these tasks while exerting minimal impact on the pumping efficiency of the heart.

In considering the engineering aspects of defibrillator lead design, it is useful to think of the lead as having five distinct areas, a connector, conductor, insulator, fixation mechanism and electrodes. Implantable defibrillator leads and pacemaker leads are very similar but with notable differences. For a comprehensive review of the engineering aspects of pacemaker leads the reader is referred to Timmis.[23] Only those aspects of defibrillator leads that differ will be addressed in detail in this chapter.

Connectors

The connector must ensure that the lead is secured mechanically and electrically to the pulse generator for the life of the device, provide electrical isolation to the surrounding tissue, and provide strain relief at the pulse generator so that stress on the lead is not concentrated at one site of the conductor. In transvenous defibrillator leads, at least one of the connectors must have a lumen through which to pass a stylet used for placement.

Early connectors used with implantable defibrillator leads looked superficially like the 5 mm pacemaker lead connectors. However, they were designed with a smaller diameter connector pin and a larger diameter sealing surface (6.1 mm diameter) to prevent a pacemaker lead from being inserted into a defibrillator receptacle. Considering that most defibrillators have four receptacles, those connectors are cumbersome. As pulse generators have become smaller, the use of a smaller connector has become necessary. The current defibrillation lead connector standard ISO-11318, is commonly referred to as "DF-1." The objective of this standard, modeled after the "IS-1" pacemaker connector standard, is to ensure physical interchangeability of DF-1 leads and pulse generators from different manufacturers. However neither standard guarantees that complying products from different manufacturers will provide electrical, and therefore therapeutic, compatibility. The standards also do not ensure that all manufacturers' designs are equally reliable. The use of specific leads and pulse generators is validated by manufacturer's testing as well as clinical performance, subject to regulatory approval.

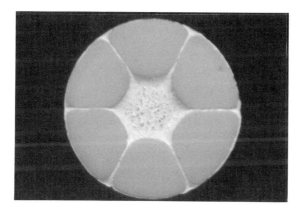

Figure 5. Cross-sectional photograph (500x) of 0.0059" diameter DBS composite wire showing six stainless steel strands and silver in the center, between the strands, and on the outer surface.

Conductors

Note: The abbreviation "DFT" in this chapter refers to a type of wire construction (described below) and not defibrillation threshold as used elsewhere.

Defibrillator conductors must have the corrosion resistance, flexibility and fatigue resistance of pacemaker lead conductors. In addition, they must carry very high peak currents. While the peak current expected in a pacemaker conductor may be approximately 15 mA, a defibrillator conductor must deliver up to 40 A. To deliver this current efficiently with minimal voltage losses, low resistance conductors must be used.

The required low resistance has generally been achieved using a *composite wire* of Drawn Brazed Strand (DBS) or Drawn Filled Tube (DFT) construction. These sophisticated wires combine the conductivity of silver, or other low resistance metals with Stainless Steel (SS), MP35N (an alloy of Nickel, Cobalt, Chromium and Molybdenum), Titanium (Ti) or other high strength metal to obtain strong low resistance wire. In the case of DBS wire conductors, six (as shown in the example of Fig. 5) or seven wires of high strength are combined with a single strand of a relatively soft and low electrical resistance metal. The strands are then drawn through a series of dies forcing the silver between and around the other strands. This results in a single composite strand of wire having low electrical resistance and high strength and fatigue life.

DFT is made from a high strength shell such as SS, MP35N, or Ti that is filled with a low resistance metal. This combination is then drawn through a series of dies to produce a bimetal composite.

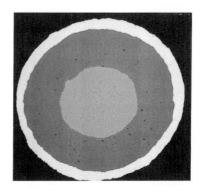

Figure 6. Cross-sectional photograph (500x) of 0.0064" diameter Drawn Filled Tube (DFT) composite wire showing the low resistance inner conductor (silver); a high strength shell (MP35N); and an optional noble metal outer layer (platinum iridium) for use as an electrode.

The DFT can be further modified for electrode use by adding a third layer of a noble electrode material such as platinum or platinum/iridium (Fig. 6). The selection of metals and the positioning of them in a DFT allows one to adjust the trade-offs of strength, fatigue life, conductivity, mass, biocompatibility, and electrochemical resistance to the specific requirements of the application.

To improve flexibility and fatigue resistance, the wires are further formed into coils (for DFT) or twisted into small diameter cables (for DBS wire). Coiling enhances both the fatigue life and the flexibility but increases the length of wire and thus its resistance. By using multiple filaments, as in Fig. 7, coils can be made with lower resistance and with redundant current pathways as a guard against a single wire fracture. Coils also provide a lumen for the passage of a stylet for use during lead placement. When three filaments are used the coil is referred to as *trifilar,* while four filaments are used in the *quadrafilar* configuration.

When a lumen for a stylet is not required, as for a patch or parallel path conductor, a twisted cable made of 49 strands of DBS wire provides a very low resistance and perhaps more fatigue resistant alternative to the coil.[24] Electrical resistance as low as 0.01 Ω/cm have been achieved with the silver/MP35N DBS pacemaker cable shown in Fig. 8. This cable is used with and without a Teflon-like coating. Several companies are using the coated cable to provide additional electrical insulation between conductors.

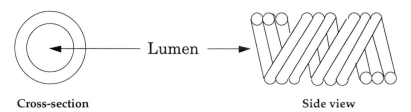

Cross-section   **Side view**

Figure 7. Trifilar coil constructed from three DFT wires. Quadrafilar coil construction uses four wires coiled in a similar manner. Pitch, spacing between filars, and constant coil diameter of the wires are all important for lead longevity.

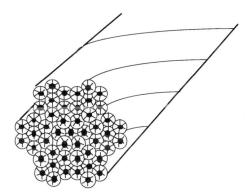

Figure 8. DBS cable, also called "pacemaker cable". Forty-nine DBS wires are wound into seven cables which are then wound into a single cable. This is also known as 7 x 7 construction.

To obtain the two, three, and four conductive paths needed for integrated transvenous defibrillation, pacing, and sensing, lead coils can be arranged concentrically or in parallel paths as shown in Fig. 9. With more than two or three conductors, a parallel path arrangement must be used to prevent the lead body from becoming too large and stiff. As of this writing, there are no leads comprised of four or more conductors on the market. This could change if sensors were introduced to the lead.

Transvenous, epicardial and subcutaneous leads all require the low electrical resistance, high strength and high fatigue life provided by the sophisticated wires described above. In addition, they all benefit from the added fatigue life offered by coiling or cabling. The only constraint is that in transvenous leads using current design and implantation techniques, the conductor connected to the distal electrode must be a coil to provide a lumen for stylet insertion.

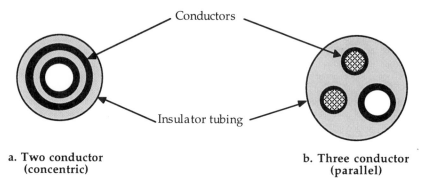

a. Two conductor
(concentric)

b. Three conductor
(parallel)

Figure 9. Concentric and parallel lead conductor configurations. *a.* a typical concentric lead construction. *b.* a parallel construction of two DBS cables and a DFT coil. The DFT coil contains a center lumen for stylet passage.

Insulators

The insulating tubing must provide a minimum of 50,000 Ω resistance (isolation) to any leakage current. Below this resistance, sensing signals are attenuated and a loss of sensing can occur. Isolation of the defibrillator pulse of over 700 V is ensured primarily by avoiding microscopic pinholes in the insulation wall. With commonly used insulators having dielectric strengths in the 1,000-2,000 V/mil (1 mil=0.001 inch) range, the minimum wall thickness is determined by the need for mechanical and material biostability more than the requirements of electrical isolation. For both defibrillation and pace/sense leads, implantable grade *silicone rubber* or *polyurethane* has been used for electrical insulation between conductors within the lead and between conductors and the body. Either material may be extruded as tubing for the lead body and molded for connectors or tines (if required). Silicone is also used as the backing material for epicardial and subcutaneous patches.

Polyurethane has been used extensively for pacemaker leads and is also used for defibrillation leads. It provides a thin walled insulation with a high tensile strength and good dielectric strength (approximately 2,000 V/mil). Polyurethane based leads are also more "slippery" than silicone based leads, allowing easier passage of multiple leads. Although there is still no conclusive evidence proving an increased long term failure rate higher than for silicone,[25,26] degradation factors have been recognized for a specific polyurethane (Pellethane 80A). These factors include metal ion oxidation and environmental stress cracking, both time dependent failure modes that harden and crack the polyurethane insulation.[27] Another polyurethane (55D) that is stiffer has a good reliability record for pacing leads. New polyurethane formulations are being evaluated that may provide the thinness and slipperiness that polyurethane provides without the loss of durability.

Silicone rubber has also been used extensively for pacemaker and defibrillator leads. It requires a greater wall thickness due to its lower tensile strength, but provides an insulation barrier with no known long term degradation. Silicone also has good dielectric strength (approximately 1,000 V/mil). It may abrade when in constant contact with an edge of the pulse generator, eventually wearing through to the conductor. As mentioned previously, silicone will stick to itself, which creates difficulty in passing one lead aside another. Coatings or surface treatments are becoming available that will allow smoother multiple lead passage.

Recently, the major suppliers of implantable grade silicone rubber and polyurethane have stated that they will no longer make their materials available in the future. The reason stated for this action is a concern for the potential liability incurred with implantable products. In some cases, the larger device manufacturers have entered into specific contracts with the suppliers addressing this concern. Implementation of this action has been distressing to the leads business, but alternative suppliers have evolved to focus on the medical market requirements. Even so, efforts by engineers, physicians, policy makers and lawmakers must be made and coordinated to ensure the continued availability of proven implantable materials.

Fixation Mechanisms

Endocardial leads typically use either flexible tines or a rigid or retractable metallic helix on the distal tip for fixation at the selected site. Tines for fixation are commonly used for a lead (defibrillation or pacing) fixated in the apex of the right ventricle. Screw-in mechanisms (metallic helix) are also commonly used in defibrillation leads[28] because they are known to provide more secure acute fixation, while tined leads develop maximum holding power after the fibrotic tissue response has matured. The screw-in type (active fixation) also allows a greater choice of fixation sites in the ventricle or atrium. Epicardial and subcutaneous patch type leads often have suture sites with holes, dimples and/or mesh reinforcements designed to facilitate suturing the lead in place. If patches are not sutured in place, crinkling of the electrode may occur, causing decreased tissue contact and reduced efficacy.

Electrodes

The electrode position and characteristics have the greatest impact on defibrillation thresholds. This fact has resulted in a wide diversity of electrode designs. These designs differ most obviously by their placement in endocardial, epicardial or subcutaneous positions. In addition, there are a variety of metals, configurations and surfaces being used as electrodes.

Implanted defibrillation electrode systems have *system impedances* ranging from a low of 20 Ω to a high of 100 Ω. Two epicardial patch leads exhibit impedances at the low end of this range, transvenous to epicardial or extrathoracic patch systems are in the midrange; an occasional completely transvenous system will be in the high impedance range but most are 40-60 Ω. Impedance readings outside these ranges may indicate a problem with the lead system.

As described earlier, *transvenous* leads can have pacing, sensing, and defibrillation electrodes in one multipolar lead, or can be single or double electrode defibrillation leads. If included on the defibrillation lead, pacing and sensing electrodes differ very little (if at all) from those on a standard pacing lead. In contrast, the defibrillation electrode(s) must provide a large electrode surface area distributed over a large portion of the heart while maintaining the flexibility of the lead. Several novel designs for achieving a larger surface area electrode for a transvenous lead have been tested, including a flat ribbon helix, a fine wire helix,[29] a series of rings,[30] and a braided fine wire electrode.[31]

Epicardial, subcutaneous and *submuscular* leads generally have a single electrode made of a flexible mesh or coils molded into a "patch" configuration. These leads generally allow the active electrode surface to be distributed over a larger area than an endocardial electrode and consequently, can usually provide lower defibrillation thresholds than transvenous leads alone. Novel systems have been evaluated including those with single or multiple fingered coil electrodes (array)[32] and folded coil electrodes for extrathoracic placement.[33] A three fingered coil electrode system is currently available and has been shown to provide reduction in defibrillation thresholds.[34]

The defibrillator electrode material has been the subject of much study. Solid platinum and platinum/iridium wire, solid titanium ribbon and wire, platinum coated wires and ribbons, and carbon fibers[35] have been studied. Platinum/iridium wire, platinum coated wire or ribbons, and titanium wire (patches) are in current use. Surface enhancements such as platinizing, carbon and nitride coating, and sintered microspheres have been effective in reducing pacing thresholds but have not conclusively shown a corresponding reduction of defibrillation thresholds. Work on titanium nitride coated coils and patches indicates a potentially lower defibrillation threshold with electrodes so treated.[36] Coatings or surface treatment of electrodes will continue to be an area of fruitful research for the near future.

Adapters, etc.

Use of terminal adapters, extenders, etc. is required to mate replacement pulse generators to existing lead implants, mate lead/pulse generator combinations not designed by the same company nor intended to work together, or tie electrode combinations (e.g. SVC and subcutaneous patch) together as a common electrode. These unintended combinations often work well for individual patients or the population in general but may not be long enough or have a matching port-to-pin interconnect. These adapters and extenders must be designed and manufactured to the same reliability and performance requirements as the leads and use similar materials. Older adapters have used an uncured medical adhesive to seal the setscrew in the port end of the device while newer adapters use the setscrew seal similarly used in the pulse generator. While adapters, etc., are typically reliable, they require extra attention in application to ensure the setscrew is properly tightened and a suture is tied around the port connection of the adapter if required. This suture may be important to ensure a fluid seal between two flexible pieces (port and connector sleeve) whereas the fluid seal for the pulse generator is a flexible piece (connector sleeve) to a rigid piece (header), providing better structural support for the seal.

Testing

All lead types undergo rigorous testing by the companies to ensure reliability during the stresses of a long-term implant. Typically, leads are placed under durability tests that mimic stresses in use, for example, flexing and pulling. In addition, leak tests, thermal cycling, and various electrical conductivity and insulation tests are performed to prove design integrity. In manufacturing, specific processes are constantly verified and each lead is tested for compliance to performance criteria. Until recently, there have been no common test criteria established and companies have set their own standards, subject to approval by the regulatory agencies. There is presently a leads test task force, made up of representatives of the implantable pacemaker and defibrillator industry, actively working toward standardized test criteria and methodologies. These internationally recognized standards, when established and applied, will help promote reliable leads design.

Potential Complications

As noted above, leads are the most chronic component of the defibrillation system. While they are a less complex construction than the pulse generator to which they are connected, leads are subject to greater stresses which may lead to various complications. Incidence of lead failure can vary between manufacturers, lead type, and implant center. Lead-related complication rates of 5-36% have recently been reported for transvenous and non-transvenous lead systems.[37-50] (Table 2) While complications for leads are well documented, many of the same complications may be exhibited by adapters,[45,38] producing similar manifestations and requiring the same resolution. Some lead adapter models have failure rates as high as 21%.[38]

Dislodgement
Lead dislodgement or migration has occurred primarily for transvenous leads, but has also been reported for patches[48] and subcutaneous wire electrode leads.[39] For the transvenous leads, dislodgement may occur for both screw-in or tined fixation and may be attributed to the extension and contraction of the torso tending to tug the relatively free distal end of an lead tunneled to an abdominal implant site. If there is a case of dislodgement, it is most likely to occur shortly after implantation, before fibrosis has taken place to fully anchor the lead (transvenous) or before ingrowth has occurred (patches). Dislodgement of transvenous leads may also be caused by *"twiddler's syndrome"*, whereby the patient manipulates the pulse generator in a manner that can dislodge the lead and possibly remove the lead from the heart entirely.[40,41] (See Fig. 7, Chap.12 for an example) The pectoral ICD location may actually increase the risk of this syndrome.[42]

Manifestations of lead dislodgement include increased pacing or defibrillation threshold; possible loss of capture or failed defibrillation; or loss of sensing. The problem is usually identifiable radiographically (Chap. 21), highlighting the importance of periodic chest X-rays during ICD followup. A dislodged lead can generally be repositioned if diagnosed shortly after implant. Preventive measures may include the use of extra suture sleeve(s) for added

Table 2. Incidence of ICD lead complications in 9 studies.

Paper	Winkle[43]	Grimm[44]	Stambler[45]	Pfeifer[37]	Kleman[46]	Nunain[47]	Mattke[48]	Jones[49]	Schwartzman[50]	Total[*] (%)
Year	1989	1993	1994	1994	1994	1995	1995	1995	1995	
No. Pts.	273	241	343	140	212	154	130	159	170	1822
Lead Types	E/T	E/T	E/T	E/T	E/T	E/T	E/T	T	T	
Lead migration	5	9	6	2	4	5		11	6	2.6%
Patch migration					5				2	
Crinkled patch	1			4						
Insulation break	1	2	7	4		3	1			1.0%
Conductor fracture	13		5	1	2		2	10	6	2.1%
Conn/adap failure			16	1						
Electrode fracture				2			2		1	
Infection	5	13		14	8	1	1	2	7	2.8%
Thrombus		10		20		1		1	3	1.9%
RV perforation						1	1			
Septal perf.		1								
Frozen shoulder								1		
Seroma				1						
Dressler's syndrome				1						
Total	25	35	34	50	19	11	6	26	25	231
% Complications	9.2%	14.5%	9.9%	35.7%	9.0%	7.1%	4.6%	16.4%	10.6%	12.7%

* Percentages are shown when ≥ 1.0%. No. Pts. = number of patients; E=epicardial; T=transvenous; Conn/adap = connector or adapter. Failures of sensing or pacing are not listed if no frank lead defect was listed as found which could exonerate the electronics (e.g., AGC) or programming.

fixation of the lead body near the venous entry site or, for patches, additional sutures. With the advent of pectorally implanted ICDs, dislodgement may become less frequent due to the diminished need to accommodate motion of the torso.

Conductor/Insulator Fracture

Conductor and insulator fractures are a widely reported failure mode (3.1% of lead systems; Table 2). A conductor fracture is a break in the wire of the lead while an insulation fracture (or erosion) refers to an opening in the surrounding polymer. A defibrillator *conductor fracture*, that is initially partial (i.e., involving only 1 of the 3 or 4 conductors strands), will continue to deliver the shock (with

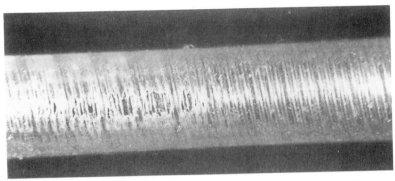

Figure 10. Insulation break exposing the conductor coil in an endocardial sensing lead. This break was encountered 14 months post implant and may be attributed to rubbing against the pulse generator can.[51]

increased electrical resistance) to the electrode due to the redundant nature of the multifilar construction. (Such an increased resistance would not be a problem for sensing and pacing as they require very little current.) The initial fracture will, however, establish a weak point in the lead and potentially accelerate additional wire fractures at the same spot. Occurrence of a *complete* fracture in a given lead, of course, would totally impair its expected function (be it defibrillation, sensing, or pacing). A broken wire also has sharp ends and could possibly penetrate the insulation over time and become exposed to the body or another conductor in the lead body. In general, however, a conductor fracture does not imply a coexisting insulation failure. A fracture to the conductor will be generally due to stretching or crushing of the conductor, making it susceptible to damaging flexural stresses.

To minimize the occurrence of fractures of DFT constructed conductors, the wire is coiled as in a tension spring to absorb and diffuse the flexural energy over a longer distance of wire. The cabling of DBS wire, as described earlier, allows the use of extremely small diameter wire, which reduces flexural stresses. For each construction, there will be a fatigue point, determined by the material, construction of the conductor, and frequency/displacement of the flex at which fracture will occur.

Insulation erosion or fracture will expose the lead's outermost conductor to the body (Fig. 10) and will shunt current from the defibrillation electrode, reducing efficacy of the shock. (With concentric lead designs [Fig. 9] a defibrillation conductor is outermost.) Causes of insulation fracture may include scalpel or suture damage

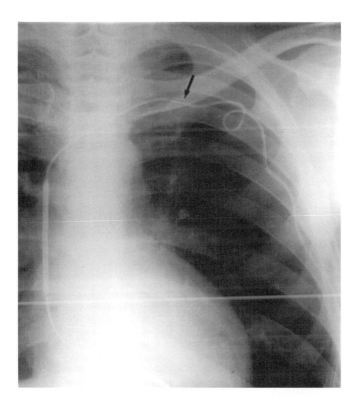

Figure 11. Chest X-ray showing separation of a CPI-Guidant Endotak lead (arrow) in the clavicle-first rib "crush" zone.[55]

during implant and material erosion due to rubbing against the pulse generator body.[51]

While smaller diameter leads may help minimize insulation failure, implants via the cephalic vein[52] or a modified subclavian venipuncture procedure[53] have been suggested as preferred insertion methods. There is some indication that polyurethane insulation may lead to a higher incidence of lead failure in the clavicle-first rib area.[54] Defibrillation leads have predominantly used silicone insulation and there is little evidence to reach a conclusion of which material is more durable. Additionally, some pacemaker leads manufacturers have used different polyurethane grades, and data are not available on the alternatives.

For transvenous defibrillation leads, a predominant failure mode has been fracturing of the conductor or insulator in the

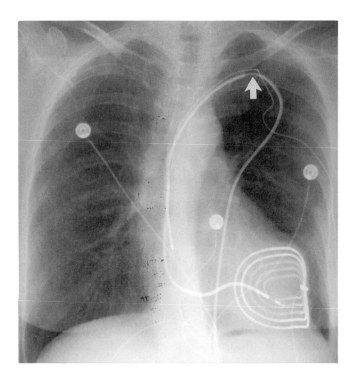

Figure 12. Chest X-ray showing a conductor fracture in the clavicle-first rib "crush" zone, in a patient with a Medtronic Transvene lead (arrow). A similar fracture subsequently developed in the replacement lead. (Shown in Fig. 13)

clavicle-first rib region — not limited to any one lead model and capable of recurring at the same site. (Figs. 11-13)   Lead fracture in this location is often attributed to frequent upper arm motion in physically active patients or in association with particularly repetitive activities, e.g., a weight lifter doing bench presses, a softball player pitching, or someone painting with a constant up and down movement.

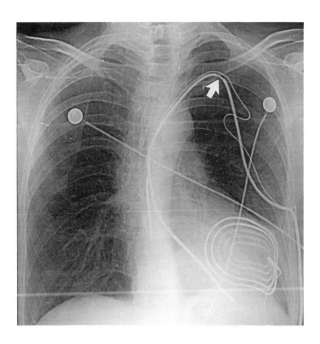

Figure 13. Chest X-ray showing a recurrent conductor fracture in the clavicle-first rib "crush" zone, involving a replacement Medtronic Transvene lead (arrow)[60] in the same patient as in Fig. 12.

Cadaver and cineradiography studies have shown the potential for lead entrapment in the subclavius muscle when subclavian venipuncture lead placement is used.[56] The cephalic approach, while technically more difficult, may reduce the incidence of this problem.[57] This entrapment creates a fixed pivot point for the conductor to focus the flexural energy, causing either elongation of the conductor[58] or fracture due to fatigue. Large lead diameter is believed to contribute to this fracture mode[58] but smaller diameter pacemaker leads have also fractured. A more unusual possibility for lead entrapment is an instantaneous entrapment in the superior rim of the tricuspid valve.[59]

Patch lead fracture may occur either in the mesh structure or conductor wire.[44,61] Fracture of a coiled patch or the conductor wire(s) would be caused by flex fatigue similar to the fracture mechanism for the transvenous leads. A woven mesh patch is also subject to flex fatigue[49] or possible rubbing interference between two patches if they are implanted on a small heart. To date, however, these have been much less frequent complications than for the transvenous leads, per se.

Manifestations of a complete (all strands) conductor fracture include increased pacing thresholds or failed defibrillation.[43,48,49] For pace/sense leads (or conductors in multifunctional leads), conductor fracture commonly present as inappropriate delivery of a shock due to inappropriate sensing (from electrical noise at the fracture site) and, less often as failed antitachycardia (or brady-cardia backup) pacing therapy. Identification of a pace/sense conductor fracture can sometimes be achieved radiographically, but is more commonly documented by direct visual observation post-explantation, a high lead impedance ($>1000 \Omega$), or a significant in-crease in pacing threshold after lead maturation. A pace/sense in-sulation failure may show a lowered impedance or inappropriate sensing. An insulation failure for a defibrillation conductor may show increased DFT. (See Chap. 21 for further details on diagnos-ing lead fractures.) Resolution of the complication typically re-quires replacement or repair of the affected lead. (See "Extraction and Repairs" below.) In the infrequent case of concomitant insula-tion and conductor fracture the manifestations of the conductor break—being the most dramatic—will dominate the clinical presen-tation.

Perforation/Infection/Thrombogenicity

With the introduction of non-thoracotomy implant systems, other lead complications similar to those seen with pacemakers have oc-curred. Perforation of the right ventricle has been noted[46,49,62] as have infection[46,49,50,63] and thrombosis.[49,50] Infection, a complication that usually necessitates ICD system explantation in addition to antibiotic therapy, may occur with variable frequency at different implant centers. (Chap. 18) Besides thrombus formation resulting from the presence of a lead (as a foreign body), thrombus may also be attributable to delivery of a therapeutic shock.[64]

Pericardial constriction has been reported as a complication of epicardial patches.[65,66]

Pulse Generator Connection

Connection of the lead to the pulse generator is typically free of complications. However, *loose setscrews,* a known pacemaker prob-lem, can also occur with defibrillators. This problem will present as a broken conductor and is not identifiable without reopening the pocket. Resolution requires opening the pocket and retightening the screw.

Extraction and Repair

As discussed above, leads may require *extraction* due to fracture (conductor or insulation), infection or (rarely) thrombosis; or *repair* due to proximal insulation damage.

One to 2 months post-implant, the transvenous lead becomes more difficult to remove due to the fibrotic tissue that envelops the lead body, especially at the defibrillation lead-cardiac interface.[18] There are established methods for pace/sense lead extraction (percutaneous and open intracardiac),[67] but no generally accepted technique for the larger diameter, longer electrode defibrillation leads has been developed. Even with the development of smaller diameter defibrillation leads, there is expected to be increased extraction complications compared to pacing leads because of the longer defibrillation electrodes promoting fibrous tissue over and around the electrode wires for abdominal ICD implants.[68] The trend towards pectoral implants (and thinner transvenous leads) should bring the difficulty and risk of ICD lead extraction down to that of pacing leads.

Repair of a lead may be attempted on the proximal end (near the pulse generator) where a nick or erosion of the insulation has been observed,[69] but this is not a generally recommended practise. Repair may be made using medical adhesive and a section of slit tubing placed over the damaged area. Compared to actual lead replacement, however, attempted repair may not always provide adequate durability over years of flexure.

With the advent of multifunctional leads, it is possible to have a lead with a fractured conductor for the defibrillation electrode or the pace/sense tip. If this conductor is not a multifunction (defibrillation, pace/sense) conductor, it is theoretically possible to leave the damaged lead in place, saving an extraction, while inserting another lead to handle the function (defibrillation or pace/sense) of the damaged conductor. One recent study has shown good sensing performance using independent pace/sense leads with the multifunctional (Type I) lead in place.[70] While these studies are short-term, they open up the possibility of the same positive results chronically. Arguing for complete multifunctional lead replacement is the possibility of the same fracture source (e.g.,

Table 3. Acute and latent lead complications.

Acute complications (typically presenting within 2 months of implantation)
- ◆ loose setscrew
- ◆ infection
- ◆ thrombosis
- ◆ dislodgement
- ◆ migration

Long-term complications
- ◆ conductor fracture (e.g., clavicle-first rib lead site)
- ◆ adapter failure
- ◆ insulation erosion
- ◆ insulation breaks from suturing directly onto the lead body
- ◆ general insulation failure.

subclavian crush) subsequently causing fracture of the other con-
ductor(s) within the already damaged lead.

Clinical Surveillance of Lead Function and Integrity

Routine followup is necessary to anticipate potential problems with
ICD lead function and integrity.   Post-implant testing of the
pace/sense lead or section of a multifunctional lead may be tested
through impedance measurements. (See Chap. 20, "Lead Integrity.") Post-implant routine testing of the defibrillation lead, however, is more difficult because of the lack of indicators available.
(High voltage impedance of last delivered shock is available, but
would not be helpful if a defibrillation lead conductor fracture occurred in the interim.) One might argue, therefore, that late elective
VF testing of an ICD be considered in patients who have not had a
spontaneous shock for some prolonged interval (say, ≥ 1 year post
implantation or since last shock). No systematic data are as yet
available evaluating the utility of such an approach, however.

Based on the usual time course of presentation, complications may be loosely categorized as acute (<2 months) or latent.
(Table 3) However, it must be noted that occasionally acute complications may be observed after 2 months and latent complications
may occur shortly after implant. The occurrence of complications
are not only design related, but also patient and procedure dependent. These various factors, in addition to time following implantation, may serve to guide clinical surveillance and increase the index
of suspicion for certain potential complications.

With earlier devices, detection was limited to chest X-rays,
"beep-o-grams," notation of inappropriate device discharges, and
intraoperative exploration. Current models contain stored electro-

grams and/or marker signals that help a physician to determine device efficacy upon shock discharge.

Chest X-rays continue to provide useful surveillance information on lead integrity, especially to aid in detecting unsuspected problems (e.g., fracture or migration of defibrillation electrode in a patient who has not yet had tachyarrhythmia recurrence). It is generally advisable that chest X-rays should be made on some regular basis during followup[50,71,72] or, more immediately if stored electrograms/marker signals suggest a problem. A loose setscrew may be difficult to identify on an X-ray and ultimately requires re-opening the pocket for definitive diagnosis.

Future Systems

While the ICD has proven successful, future lead systems will provide improved arrhythmia detection and discrimination while allowing more efficient defibrillation capability. Advanced sensing techniques and multiple electrode configurations plus the desire for uncomplicated implantation will greatly increase the demands and complexity of future cardioverter defibrillator lead systems.

Future ICD systems may increasingly provide dedicated *bipolar sensing leads* for obtaining discrete, localized rate counting. In addition, these same leads may be used to obtain additional morphological information or *atrial sensing* to discriminate various rhythms. *Steroid eluting tips* will be incorporated similar to those used for pacemaker leads. New designs will likely prevent potential sensing problems caused by localized tissue trauma due to high current density near the defibrillating electrodes. These same designs will avoid the potential for increases in post-shock pacing thresholds.

Advanced arrhythmia discrimination algorithms will not only examine the heart's electrical activity but other physiological parameters. The ability to monitor a patient's hemodynamic condition will provide valuable information to the implanted device. *Hemodynamic sensors* are being evaluated that would be integral to the lead system. These could monitor cardiac pressures, volumes or other hemodynamic variables for discriminating unstable from stable ventricular tachycardias that could not otherwise be determined by rate or other electrical analysis. The resulting data would be used to select the most appropriate therapy. For example, patients with hemodynamically unstable tachycardias would be treated aggressively with a high energy shock, while hemodynamically stable patients would be treated less aggressively with antitachycardia pacing.

Multi-electrode systems to optimize current distribution, combined with new defibrillation waveforms will continue to reduce defibrillation energy requirements. Future electrode materials and geometries should allow more efficient charge transfer across the bioelectrical interface between the electrode and tissue. Patch electrodes may also incorporate concepts to shape electric fields across the electrode surface.[73,74] This will allow more field uniformity and lower defibrillation energy requirements.

As the pulse generator becomes smaller, *connector miniaturization* is an area which needs to be addressed. The increasing use of multipolar leads and sensor based systems will also make the size of the connector a significant portion of the pulse generator's volume. With the advent of the "DF-1" connector standard, it will become more difficult for companies to develop smaller connectors independently. To this end, a proactive effort by the manufacturers would serve the medical community well in establishing a down-sized standard connector.

The single biggest challenge for designers of defibrillator lead systems is the continued development of improved lead configurations and implant procedures that provide reliably *lower defibrillation thresholds*. All future defibrillator implants will continue to include transvenous lead systems and the active electrode pulse generator is expected to become a predominant implant choice. A number of patients, however, will still require subcutaneous, or, rarely, even subxiphoid or epicardial electrodes as part of the lead system.

The future challenge for *multifunction transvenous defibrillation leads* is to incorporate the optimized features of pacing leads to provide low pacing thresholds while continuing to improve defibrillation performance. Improvements are needed to increase the lead body flexibility and reduce the mass of the distal portion of the lead. These features are necessary to minimize trauma to the pacing site, thus maintaining low chronic pacing thresholds. A key to improving lead flexibility and providing multiple conductive paths is an innovation in multiple conductor technology. One approach to this is to individually insulate the filaments of a multifilar coil. This has met with problems of inadequate isolation, crosstalk, abrasion, fatigue of the filament insulator, and difficulty in passing stylets. Further improvements in design and materials may yet lead to a suitable multiconductor-multifilar coil.

"Tougher" insulation that will provide long term durability, a thinner profile, high lubricity (slipperiness) as well as smaller diameter conductor wires that maintain their impedance and fatigue resistance will be critical to future improvements. *Advancements in extrusion* of the insulator materials, coiling, or stringing of the conductor wire through the insulator may also provide smaller profile leads that implant easier, are more comfortable for the patient, and, if necessary, will explant easier.

ACKNOWLEDGMENTS
Figs. 10 and 11 are used with the permission of PACE. Figs. 12 and 13 are used with the permission of Journal of Interventional Cardiology. We thank the following individuals for their technical review and comments: Ben Pless (Ventritex), Stuart Chastain (Guidant-CPI), Eliot Ostrow (Intermedics), Rita Theis (Pacesetters), John Helland (InControl), and Tim Holleman (Medtronic).

1. Irnich W. Intercardiac electrograms and sensing test signals: electrophysiological, physical, and technical considerations. PACE 1985;8:870-888.
2. Jenkins J, Kriegler C, DiCarlo L. Discrimination of ventricular tachycardia from ventricular fibrillation using intracardiac electrogram analysis. Pace 1991;14-II:718. (abstract)
3. Camm AJ, Davies DW, Ward DE. Tachycardia recognition by implantable electronic devices. PACE 1987;10:1175-1190.
4. Jones JL, Jones RE. Decreased defibrillator-induced dysfunction with biphasic rectangular waveforms. Am J Physiol 1984;247:H792. (abstract)
5. Yabe S, Daubert JP, Wolf PD, et al. Effect of strong shock fields on activation propagation near defibrillation electrodes. Circulation 1988;78:154. (abstract)
6. Jung W, Manz M, Moosdorf R, et al. Failure of an implantable cardioverter-defibrillator to redetect ventricular fibrillation in patients with a nonthoracotomy lead system. Circulation 1992;86:1217-1222.
7. Schwartzman D, Gottlieb CD, Callans DJ, et al. Comparative effect of shocks on the endocardial rate-sensing signals from transvenous lead systems. JACC 1995;25:15A. (abstract)
8. Mower MM, Mirowski M, Spear JF, et al. Patterns of ventricular activity during catheter defibrillation. Circulation 1974;49:858-861.
9. Zipes DP, Electrophysiological mechanisms involved in ventricular fibrillation. Circulation 1975;52:120-123.
10. Warton JM, Wolf PD, Chen PS, et al. Is an absolute minimum potential gradient required for ventricular defibrillation? Circulation 1986;74:342. (abstract)
11. Nogami A, Takahashi A, Nitta J, et al, Comparative efficacy of subcutaneous mesh and plate electrodes for nonthoracotomy canine defibrillation. PACE 1991;14:1402-1410.
12. Chen PS, Wolf PD, Claydon FJ, et al, The potential gradient field created by epicardial defibrillation electrodes in dogs. Circulation 1986;74:626-636.
13. Auteri JS, Jeevanandam V, Bielefeld MR, et al. Effect of AICD patch electrodes on the diastolic pressure-volume curve in pigs. Ann Thorac Surg 1991;52:1052-1057.
14. Chang MS, Inoue H, Kallock MJ, et al. Double and triple sequential shocks reduce ventricular defibrillation thresholds in dogs with and without myocardial

infarction. J Am Coll Cardiol 1986;8:1339-1405.

15. Bardy GH, Allen MD, Mehra R, et al. Transvenous defibrillation in humans via the coronary sinus. Circulation 1990;81:1252-1259.

16. Rubin L, Hudson P, Driller J, et al. Effect of defibrillation energy on pacing threshold. Med Instrum 1983;17:15-17.

17. Yee R, Jones DL, Klein GL. Pacing threshold changes after transvenous catheter countershock. Am J Cardiol 1984;53:503. (abstract)

18. Epstein AE, Anderson PG, Kay GN, et al. Gross and microscopic changes associated with a nonthoracotomy implantable cardioverter defibrillator. PACE 1992;15:382-386.

19 Mond HG, Stokes K. The electrode-tissue Interface: the revolutionary role of steroid elution. PACE 1992;15:95-107.

20. Venditti FJ, Martin DT, Vassolas G, et al. Rise in chronic defibrillation thresholds in nonthoracotomy implantable defibrillator. Circulation 1994; 89:216-223.

21. Stanley M. Bach, Jr., personal communication.

22. Stokes K, Bornzin G. The electrode bio-interface, In Modern Cardiac Pacing, Berold SS (ed), Mount Kisco, NY, Futura Publishing Company Inc.,1985:33-77.

23. Timmis GC. The electrobiology and engineering of pacemaker leads, Chapter 4, In: Electrical therapy for cardiac arrhythmias: Pacing antitachycardia devices, catheter ablation, Saksena S and Goldschlager N (eds), Saunders, Philadelphia, PA, 1990 pp 35-90.

24. Moore SL, Maloney JD, Edel TB, et al. Implantable cardioverter defibrillator implanted by nonthoracotomy approach: initial clinical experience with the redesigned transvenous lead system. PACE 1991;14:1865-1869.

25. Mugica J, Daubert J, Lazarus B, et al. Is polyurethane lead insulation still controversial? PACE 1992;15:1967-1969.

26. Sweesy M, Forney C, Hayes D, et al. Evaluation of an in-line bipolar polyurethane ventricular pacing lead. PACE 1992;15:1982-85.

27. Coury AJ, Slaikeu PC, Cahalan PT, et al. Factors and interactions affecting the performance of polyurethane elastomers in medical devices. J Biomater Appl 1988;3:130-179.

28. Yee, R, Klein GJ, Leitch, et al. A permanent transvenous lead system for an implantable pacemaker-cardioverter-defibrillator: nonthoracotomy approach to implantation. Circulation 1992;85:196-204.

29. McCowan R, Maloney J, Wilkoff B. Automatic implantable cardioverter-defibrillator implantation without thoracotomy using an endocardial and submuscular patch system. J Am Coll Cardiol 1991;17:415-421.

30. Bourgeois I, Smits K, Kallok MJ. New low energy transvenous cardioverting and pacing electrode. PACE 1983;6:475-481.

31. Saksena S, Ward D, Krol RB, et al. Efficacy of braided endocardial defibrillation leads: acute testing and chronic implant. PACE 1991;14:II-719. (abstract)

32. Swanson DK, Lang DJ, Dahl R, et al. Improved defibrillation efficacy with separated subcutaneous wires replacing a subcutaneous patch. Eur. J.C.P.E.,1992;2:A106. (abstract)

33. DeGroot P, Mehra R, Norenberg MS., inventors, Medtronic Inc., assignee. Transvenous defibrillation lead and method of use. US patent No. 5,144,960. 1992 Sep 8.

34. Higgins SL, Alexander DC, Kuypers CJ, et al. The subcutaneous array - a new lead adjunct for the transvenous ICD to lower defibrillation thresholds. PACE 1995;18:1540-1548.

35. Alt E, Theres H, Heinz M, et al. A new approach towards defibrillation electrodes: highly conductive isotropic carbon fibers. PACE 1991;14:677. (abstract)

36. Stroetmann B, Siemsen G. TiN—A suitable coating for defibrillator electrodes? Eur J.C.P.E. 1994;4: 514. (abstract)

37 Pfeiffer D, Jung W, Fehske W, et al. Complications of pacemaker-defibrillator devices: Diagnosis and management, Am Heart J 1994;127:1073-1080.

38. Sgarbossa EB, Shewchik J, Pinksi SL. Performance of implantable defibrillator pacing/sensing lead adapters. PACE 1996;19:811-814.

39. Munsif A, Liem L, Lauer M, et al. Initial experience with 71 patients undergoing non-thoracotomy defibrillator system implantation using the new subcutaneous array. J Am Coll Cardiol 1994;21:204A. (abstract)

40. Robinson LA, Windle JR. Defibrillator twiddler's syndrome. Ann Thorac Surg 19;58:247-249.

41. Mehta D, Lipsius M, Suri RS, et al. Twiddler's syndrome with the implantable cardioverter-defibrillator. Am Heart J 1992;123:1079-1082.

42. Crossley GH, Gayle DD, Bailey JR, et al. Defibrillator twiddler's syndrome causing device failure in a subpectoral transvenous system. PACE 1996;19:376-377.

43. Winkle RA, Mead RH, Ruder MA, et al. Long-term outcome with the automatic implantable cardioverter-defibrillator. J Am Coll Cardiol 1989;13:1353-1361.

44. Grimm W, Flores B, Marchlinski F. Complications of implantable cardioverter defibrillator therapy: follow-up of 241 patients. PACE 1993;16:218-222.

45. Stambler BS, Wood MA, Damiano RJ, et al. Sensing/pacing lead complications with a newer generation implantable cardioverter-defibrillator: Worldwide experience from the Guardian ATP 4210 clinical trial. J Am Coll Cardiol 1994;23:123-132

46. Kleman JM, Castle LW, Kidwell GA, et al. Nonthoracotomy- versus thoracotomy-implantable defibrillators: intention-to-treat comparison of clinical outcomes. Circulation 1994;90:2833-2842.

47. Nunain SO, Roelke M, Trouton T, et al. Limitations and late complications of third-generation automatic cardioverter-defibrillators. Circulation 1995;91:2204-2213.

48. Mattke S, Müller D, Markewitz A, et al. Failures of epicardial and transvenous leads for implantable cardioverter defibrillators. Am Heart J 1995;130:1040-1044

49. Jones GK, Bardy GH, Kudenchuk PJ, et al. Mechanical complications following implantation of multiple lead nonthoracotomy defibrillator systems: Implications for management and future system design. Am Heart J 1995;130:327-333.

50. Schwartzman D, Nallamothu N, Callans DJ, et al. Postoperative lead-related complications in patients with nonthoracotomy defibrillation lead systems. J Am Coll Cardiol 1995;26:776-786.

51. Peters R, Foster A, Shorofsky S, et al. Spurious discharges due to late insulation break in endocardial sensing leads for cardioverter defibrillators. PACE 1995;18: 478-481.

52. Jacobs DM, Fink AS, Miller RP, et al. Anatomical and morphological evaluation of pacemaker lead compression. PACE 1993;16:434-444.

53. Magney J, Staplin D, Flynn D, et al. A new approach to percutaneous subclavian venipuncture to avoid lead fracture or central venous catheter occlusion. PACE 1993;16:2133-2142.

54. Freedman R, Marks M, Chapman P. Subclavian crush lead failure compared in polyurethane versus silicone leads in a single implanting center. PACE 1994;17:867. (abstract)

55 . Renzulli A, Vitale N, D'Onofrio A. Implantable cardioverter defibrillator malfunction due to transvenous lead insulation break. PACE 1994;17:245-246.

56. Magney JE, Flynn DM, Parsons JA, et al. Anatomical mechanisms explaining damage to pacemaker leads, defibrillator leads, and failure of central venous catheters adjacent to the sternoclavicular joint. PACE 1993;16:445-457.

57. Magney JE, Parsons JA, Flynn DM, et al. Pacemaker and defibrillator lead entrapment: case studies. PACE 1995;18:1509-1517.

58. Tullo N, Saksena S, Krol R, et al. Management of complications associated with

a first-generation endocardial defibrillation lead system for implantable cardioverter-defibrillators. Am J Cardiol 1990;66:411-415

59. Parsonnet V, Bernstein AD, Omar AM, et al. Instantaneous lead entrapment: an unusual complication of nonthoracotomy implantation of an endocardial defibrillation lead. PACE 1995;18:2100-2102.

60. Lindsay BD. Troubleshooting new ICD systems. J Interv Cardiol 1994;7:473-485.

61. Almassi G, Olinger G, Wetherbee J, et al. Long-term complications of implantable cardioverter defibrillator lead systems, Ann Thorac Surg 1993;55: 888-892.

62. Molina JE. Perforation of the right ventricle by transvenous defibrillator leads: prevention and treatment. PACE 1996;19:288-292.

63. Epstein AE, Kay GN, Voshage L, et al. Probability of implantable defibrillator system survival: comparison of systems implanted by nonthoracotomy versus other routes. PACE 1994;17:851. (abstract)

64. Benedini G, Marchini A, Curnis A, et al. Implantable defibrillation and thromboembolic events. PACE 1994;18:199-202.

65. Almassi GH, Chapman PD, Troup PJ, et al. Constrictive pericarditis associated with patch electrodes of the automatic implantable cardioverter-defibrillator. Chest 1987;92:369-371.

66. LeTourneau T, Klug D, Lacroix D, et al. Late diagnosis of pericardial constriction associated with defibrillator patches and deformation of the left ventricle. J Cardiovasc Electrophysiol 1996;7:539-541.

67. Niederhäuser U, vonSegesser L, Carrel T, et al. Infected endocardial pacemaker electrodes: Successful open intracardiac removal. PACE 1993;16:303-308.

68. Wilkoff B, Smith H, Goode L. Transvenous extraction of non thoracotomy defibrillator leads. European JCPE 1994;4:132. (abstract)

69. Dean DA, Livelli FD, Bigger JT, et al. Safe repair of insulation defects in implantable cardioverter defibrillator leads. PACE 1996;19:678. (abstract)

70. Tummala RV, Weiss DN, Feliciano Z, et al. The effects of defibrillation on endocardial rate-sensing leads. Circulation 1994;90:I-498. (abstract)

71. Drucker EA, Brooks R, Garan H, et al. Malfunction of implantable cardioverter defibrillators placed by a nonthoracotomy approach: frequency of malfunction and value of chest radiography in determining cause. Am J Roentgenol 1995;165:275-279.

72. Korte T, Jung W, Spehl S, et al. Incidence of ICD lead related complications during long-term followup: comparison of epicardial and endocardial electrode systems. PACE 1995;18:2053-2061.

73. Kim Y, Fahy JB, Tupper BJ. Optimal electrode design for electrosurgery, defibrillation, and external cardiac pacing. IEEE Trans Biomed Eng MBE 1986;33:845-853.

74. Ksienski DA. A minimum profile uniform current density electrode. IEEE Trans Biomed Eng MBE 1992;39:682-692.

10

The Battery

Curtis F. Holmes, PhD

THE ICD presents a significant challenge to the battery designer. The battery must be capable of operating at low current drains (for monitoring) for long periods of time, and then be capable of providing high-current pulses (for capacitor charging) when the patient requires defibrillation. As discussed in the Appendix, a typical requirement for monitoring is the delivery of $10\,\mu A$ (microamperes) for 5 years. A typical requirement for capacitor charging is that the battery provide a current in excess of 2 A, at voltages above 2 V, for periods as long as 10 s. The cell must therefore exhibit high energy density, high current-delivery capability, and low self-discharge (loss of energy due to internal leakages). It must also meet the high standards of safety and reliability required of all implantable power sources. In addition, it is desirable that the battery's discharge curve provide a state of charge indication which can signal the need for device replacement.

The following sections will present a brief discussion of the battery system used in the first implantable defibrillators. This will be followed by a detailed description of the system used in ICDs today, i.e., the lithium/silver vanadium oxide solid cathode, liquid organic electrolyte battery. For historical reasons, battery manufacturers use the *ampere hour* (Ah), as opposed to the coulomb (C), to measure charge. The Ah is merely 3600 C since there are 3600 seconds in an hour. To convert to *energy capacity* one must then also multiply by the average voltage of the cell. (Table 1, Chap. 4)

The Lithium/Vanadium Oxide System

The first battery system used in implantable defibrillators was a high-rate lithium/vanadium pentoxide battery designed by the Honeywell Corporation.[1] The cell was designed to deliver up to 150 pulses of 10 s duration at a current of 2 A. The nominal capacity was 800 mAh. This converts to an energy capacity of about 8000 J. The chemical system consisted of a high surface area lithium anode, a cathode of vanadium pentoxide mixed with carbon, an organic separator material, and a mixed salt electrolyte dissolved in methyl formate.

The cell design was a rectangular parallelepiped configuration of nominal dimensions 4.1 × 2.2 × 1.2 cm. The interior construction provided a high surface area which provided the needed pulse capability. These cells were used in early defibrillators produced by the Intec Corporation and in later versions produced until mid-1989.

The Lithium/Silver Vanadium Oxide System

Practically all ICD's being manufactured since 1992 use the lithium/silver vanadium oxide system. This lithium battery chemistry was first developed by Liang and coworkers.[2,3] This system was first implanted in 1987, and to date over 70,000 cells have been used in this application.

The active cathode material is silver vanadium oxide. Silver vanadium oxide belongs to a class of nonstoichiometric compounds known as vanadium oxide bronzes. These compounds are of interest because they are semiconductors and exhibit tunnel-line crystal structures which provide diffusion paths for metal ions.[4] It has been demonstrated[5] that the optimum composition of the cathode material is $Ag_2V_4O_{11}$. Cell discharge takes place in multiple steps. The first two steps, which occur simultaneously, are the reduction of vanadium (V) to vanadium (IV) and the reduction of silver (I) to silver (O). The final step is the reduction of vanadium (IV) to vanadium (III).[6] (The Roman numerals refer to the valence state of the elements.) Because of the reduction of silver to the metallic state, the conductivity of the cathode increases during discharge. One mole of $Ag_2V_4O_{11}$ can react with a total of 7 moles of lithium.

Over eight different cell models are currently in use. They differ in size and shape but share certain common design features. Cells are typically of a cuboid (rectangular parallelepiped) form factor, although cells with a rounded dimension are now routinely designed. The anode is pure lithium metal pressed onto a nickel current collector. The cathode material is a mixture of silver vanadium oxide a Teflon binder, and a conductive carbon material. Individual cathode plates are formed by pressing the cathode material onto a metal current collector to produce a structurally sound

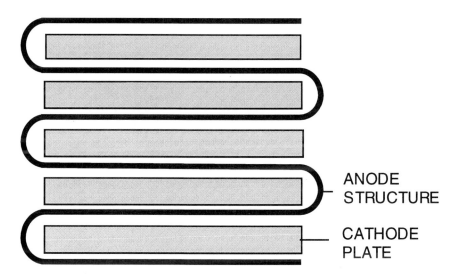

Figure 1. Conceptual sketch of cell design. The cathode plates are connected in parallel in another plane which is not shown here.

pellet. The pellet contains 95% live cathode material. The anode is folded into an "accordion" design, and individual cathode plates are placed between each "fold" of the anode.[7] Fig. 1 shows a conceptual diagram of the basic cell design. Both the anode and the cathode plates are enclosed in an organic separator for redundancy.

The surface area of the anode is designed to provide the current-delivery capability necessary to meet the pulse requirements. The dimensions of the electrodes are driven by two requirements - the current-carrying capability and the total energy capacity requirement of the cell. Even if a cell is designed to deliver a few pulses (say 50 vs. several hundred pulses throughout its life), the surface area of the electrodes will need to be large enough to deliver the required current. Thus a cell designed to deliver fewer pulses will still require a minimum volume in order to deliver pulses of the required amplitude. The electrolyte solution consists of a lithium salt dissolved in a mixed organic solvent. Materials have been chosen carefully to insure long-term stability. The design is case-negative, and the enclosure is made of grade 304L stainless steel.

The cell is hermetically sealed, and the positive electrode lead is brought out through a glass-to-metal seal. The glass composition has been chosen to be resistant to corrosion by the components of the cell. A redundant polymeric internal seal prevents the glass from being contacted by liquid components of the battery.

Discharge Characteristics

The chemical reactions discussed above result in a constantly changing chemical composition of the cathode as the cell reaction proceeds, with a resultant change in the energetics of the reaction. This phenomenon leads to a *discharge curve* which exhibits plateaus at various voltages and a general gradual decline in the voltage over time. This discharge curve determines the *beginning-of-life* (BOL) and *end-of-life* (EOL) for the ICD battery and makes possible an assessment of the state of discharge of the cell by interrogating the cell voltage during discharge. The decline in voltage is not caused by an increase in cell resistance in general; hence, the cell's current delivery capability is retained throughout the discharge process. (The phenomenon of "voltage delay," discussed later, is an exception.)

Fig. 2 illustrates the voltage change with the discharge of a cell. Shown is a typical discharge curve for a cell of nominal dimensions $43 \times 27 \times 9$ mm and a volume of 10.3 cm^3. The curve demonstrates the results of a 1-year test in which the cell was subjected to a constant background load of 17.4 KΩ. (This load is a more severe load than the typical ICD monitoring circuitry provides; the 1-year test period is correspondingly much shorter than the typical ICD lifetime.) Every 2 months the cell is required to produce a train of 4 pulses of 2 A each, simulating charge cycles for 4 defibrillation shocks. Each pulse is of 10 s duration with a 15 s pause between pulses to accurately model ICD charge and redetection times.

The top curve in Fig. 2 shows the measured voltage under the 17.4 KΩ background (monitoring) load. This quantity is referred to as the *open circuit voltage,* as it measures the voltage while the cell is under a small or nonexistent load. (The monitoring current is very small compared to the load during capacitor charging; see Appendix.) The bottom curve, referred to as the *loaded voltage,*[a] shows the minimum voltage of the fourth pulse train of the 4-pulse sequence.

The loaded voltage is less than the open circuit voltage by about 0.6 V, since the *equivalent series resistance* (ESR), i.e. internal impedance, of the cell is about 0.3 Ω yielding a voltage drop of 0.6 V = 2 A $\cdot$ 0.3 Ω (by Ohm's law). Representing the battery voltage during a hypothetical charging of the high voltage capacitors, the loaded voltage is relatively constant throughout the simulated 4 shock therapy regimen.

---

a.   The loaded voltage is referred to as the *charging voltage* by some ICD manufacturers, as this is the most significant load that the battery ever sees.

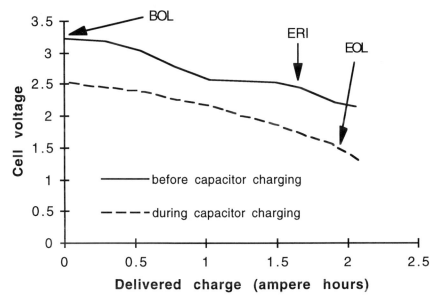

Figure 2. Discharge test of a battery in a simulated ICD application which includes an exaggerated steady monitoring (or background) current and a defibrillation regimen of 4 shocks delivered every 2 months. This simulates 100% pacing with a very high output (15 V and 1 ms). The top (solid) trace shows the *open circuit voltage* decay (measured before capacitor charging begins, i.e. just prior to each 4 pulse test sequence). The bottom (dashed) trace is the *loaded voltage* (measured at the end of the fourth shock charging cycle). The voltage is plotted versus the cumulative charge delivered in ampere hours. Typical voltages for BOL (beginning of life) and ERI (elective replacement indicator) are shown on the top trace. The EOL (end of life) point is shown on the lower curve as this is often specified by a minimum voltage regardless of the condition under which it is measured (with charging being the harshest condition).

The ICD electrode "load" (i.e., 25 Ω or 85 Ω) is not relevant to battery function since the shock energy drawn from the battery to the capacitors is determined by the stored energy setting alone. The curve showing the "background voltage," i.e., voltage under the 17.4 KΩ constant resistive load, decreases as charge is delivered over time, because the open circuit voltage is decreasing as the chemical composition of the cathode material changes. The horizontal axis of the curve shows the charge delivered by the battery in ampere hours (Ah).

A voltage of 2.5 V (range is 2.38-2.55 V across manufacturers) on the top curve is a typical value for the *elective replacement indicator* (ERI); this corresponds to a system voltage of 5.0 V in a typical 2 cell ICD. (Table 1, Chap. 20) A voltage of 1.5 V on the

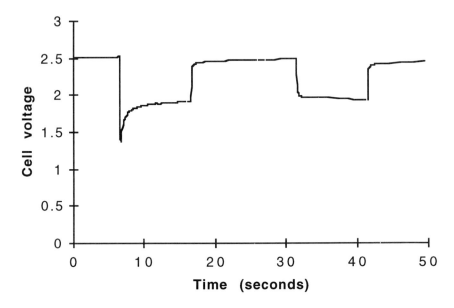

Figure 3. Cell voltage during two simulated charging cycles in a case of severe voltage delay. The cell had an open circuit voltage of 2.51 V which immediately decreased to 1.35 V at the start of charging. During the charging, the voltage recovered to 1.91 V. After a 15 s rest period, another charging cycle was initiated which had an initial voltage of 2.00 V. Thus the battery had recovered to normal operation for the second shock charging cycle. The lowest voltage of 1.35 V was below the typical end-of-life voltage of 1.5 V and thus could cause significant circuitry malfunction.

bottom curve is a representative value for end-of-life (EOL) also termed end-of-service.

An important phenomenon, exhibited in Fig. 3, known as *voltage delay* is present under certain pulsing conditions. With voltage delay the cell voltage at the start of a capacitor charging cycle is lower than at the end. During the first 10 s charging cycle of Fig. 3, the voltage rises from an initial minimum voltage during the first 2 or 3 s of the pulse and then continues at the typical pulse voltage throughout the rest of the 10 s interval. This phenomenon can begin to occur during the time in which the cell is in the plateau region of the discharge curve, i.e., when the background voltage shown in Fig. 2 is at approximately 2.6 V and "flat."

Since voltage delay occurs near the half-life region of the silver vanadium oxide cells, it has earned the sobriquet of "battery mid-life crisis." This phenomenon occurs only if the time between pulses is longer than approximately 3 months. In other words, if the battery has not been pulsed during an interval of at least 3 months and if the cell is in the "flat" portion of the discharge curve, the voltage delay phenomenon is observed. This problem is due to a chemical buildup on the battery cathode which increases the equivalent series resistance (ESR). If the battery is pulsed monthly or more frequently, the phenomenon is inconsequential. For this reason also, the voltage delay is not present beyond the first shock.

Voltage delay can lead to a significant voltage decrease during the start of charging, and a consequent prolongation of capacitor charge time. This is because the power output of the battery is equal to the product of the battery current and voltage (Chap. 4); so the charge time is thus inversely proportional to battery voltage. (See "Efficiency Limitations" in Chap. 13.) The combined effect of voltage delay and capacitor deforming can be dramatic. In one chronic animal study (unpublished observations), an ICD without automatic reforming was allowed to go 4 years without operation. At the end of the 4 years, a charging cycle was initiated. The charge time was 45 seconds!

The effect of voltage delay on the performance of the defibrillator depends on many factors, including pulse amplitude, time interval between pulses, and manner in which the circuitry draws energy from the battery. If, for example, the circuitry ramps up to a maximum current drain from an initial low current, the effect may be minimal regardless of the time between pulses. If, however, the circuitry requires an initial high current from the battery, and if the resulting low voltage adversely affects the circuitry, therapy could be blocked by the voltage delay. Thus, it may be necessary to require that the battery be pulsed from time to time during that portion of the discharge in which voltage delay manifests itself. This is somewhat analogous to the requirement that the capacitors in the defibrillator be reformed at certain intervals between pulses.

Advanced modeling experiments are underway, at the Wilson Greatbatch battery company, to assess the effects of these parameters, and a clearer understanding of the behavior of the battery under a variety of pulse conditions under long-term testing conditions is being gained and will eventually be published.

Safety and Qualification Testing

Because of the critical nature of this application, extensive safety and environmental testing must be performed on these high-rate lithium cells. An extensive design qualification program is conducted for each new defibrillator battery model. This testing includes design-phase safety testing, environmental qualification testing and abuse testing.

In the design/development phase, safety testing is done to establish proper design limits for such design characteristics as separator thickness, surface area, electrolyte composition and concentration, and cell size. During the early stages of the development of defibrillator batteries, tests were conducted on candidate cell designs. Special cells using intentionally thin separators were constructed and tested under normal and abusive conditions to determine proper design limits. The intentional induction of internal short circuits in test cells was instituted to assess the consequences of such defects as separator failure. Cells employing various concentrations and compositions of electrolyte were tested under high-rate discharge and short-circuit conditions to establish proper formulations. The results of this testing experience provided guidelines valid for the design of newer shapes and sizes of cells in the current era.

A formal environmental qualification test is conducted for each new defibrillator battery model.[8] The purpose of this test program is to demonstrate the fitness of the cell for use under "normal" conditions to be encountered during handling, transportation, storage, device fabrication, and final use in the patient.

The *environmental qualification* tests (along with some justifications) are as follows:

1. Thermal cycling from 70 °C to -40 °C with 1 minute transition time.
2. High pressure testing at 90 and 120 PSI.
3. Low pressure testing in vacuum equivalent to 4,500, 12,030, and 15,000 meters altitude. (Required by US Department of Transportation for air shipping.)
4. Low and high temperature exposure. (To represent the extremes seen from an ICD being left in a car during winter and summer.)
5. Short circuit at room temperature and at 37 °C.
6. Forced overdischarge by negative power supply. (This test and #7 represent the possible discharge of one cell by another with which it is connected in series. Such a cannibalistic discharge could theoretically occur through a major circuitry failure.)
7. Forced overdischarge of a depleted cell by a fresh cell.

8. Shock testing with a 1,000 g force. (Represents a drop to a hard floor.)

9. Vibration testing at frequencies of 5-5,000 Hz, peak acceleration 5 g.

Cells are subjected to these tests in three states of discharge: beginning of life, half-depleted, and fully depleted. After each test the cells are visually inspected, measured for dimensional changes, examined by X-ray, and submitted to pulse testing. Often multiple tests are performed on the same cells in order to evaluate the effects of combining several tests. None of the above tests have led to cell leakage, rupture, or the creation of an internal short circuit. Short-circuit testing causes cells to swell and results in a peak temperature rise of approximately 100°C in fresh cells. Fig. 4 shows a flow chart of the environmental qualification test program.

In addition to the above tests, a formal program of abusive testing is conducted to document the response of cells to abusive conditions and to demonstrate the inherent forgivability of the system under abuse. The following *abuse tests* are performed:

1. *Slow Dent and Puncture* — Cells are subjected to a sharp metal rod, powered by a hydraulic press, which dents and subsequently punctures the cell.

2. *Crush Test* — A hydraulic press is used to power a hemispherical ram which crushes the cell until an internal short circuit is induced. Cell temperature and electrical characteristics are monitored.

3. *Recharge* — Cells are subjected to a recharge current for 24 hours.

4. *High Rate Forced Overdischarge* — Cells are subjected to a demand current of 1.6 A, by a negative voltage load, for a minimum of 1.5 times the expected capacity. (See rationale under environmental qualification test #6 above.)

The crush test is an informational test to demonstrate the reaction of the cell to a massive internal short circuit. The cell does not normally rupture as a result of this abusive test, indicating that a massive internal short will not lead to dangerous consequences. The results of all of this testing are presented in a formal qualification report which can be used by device manufacturers as part of a submission package for regulatory agencies.

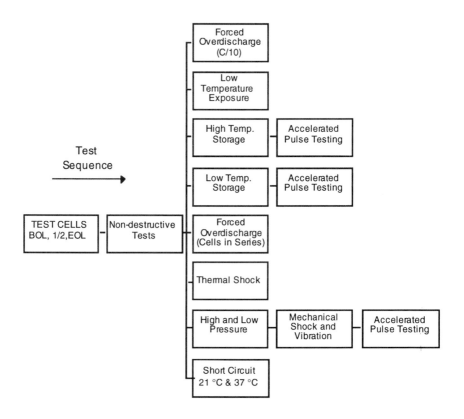

Figure 4. Environmental qualification program for ICD cells. The terms BOL, 1/2, and EOL in the box labeled "Test Cells" refer to the fact that the tests are conducted on cells in the beginning of life, half-depleted, and end-of-life conditions, respectively.

Electrical Testing of Cells

Cells are routinely subjected to a variety of electrical tests in order to assess electrical performance and document discharge characteristics under use conditions. Tests vary in duration from an accelerated test which occurs over a three day period to life tests lasting several years.

A standard *accelerated test* is routinely performed on a running sample of 1% of all production. This test consists of a train of four high-current pulses of 10 s in duration, separated by a 15 s time period, administered every 30 minutes until the cell is depleted. These high-current pulses vary from 1.2 to 2.0 A in current depending on the application requirements of the particular cell model being tested. A cell of nominal dimensions $43 \times 27 \times 9$ mm can deliver 300 pulses while always keeping its voltage above 1.5 V under this regime.

Life testing is routinely carried out on a running sample of 2% of all cells manufactured. All testing is conducted at 37 °C. Cells are divided into 2 groups for life testing. The first group is subjected to a constant resistive load corresponding to a typical background current, i.e., 100 or 300 KΩ. This is to simulate an ICD implant in which no shocks and few or no pacing pulses are delivered. Note that this more realistic load is significantly lower in current (higher in resistance) than that used to generate Fig. 2. Cell voltages are measured monthly. In the second test, cells are placed under the same constant resistive load and are pulsed once per month with the 4-pulse regime described above. This is to simulate the other extreme, namely, an ICD from which a 4-shock therapy regimen is delivered every month. (By contrast, the discharge test shown in Fig. 2 represents a higher but more steady load—it has only 4 shocks every 2 months but the background current is set very high—simulating 100% pacing at about a 15V output.) A typical response to the regimen in cell group 2 is seen in Fig. 5; no plot is shown for the test results for group 1. The top curve represents the background voltage, and the points below it represent the minimum voltage of the fourth pulse of the 4-pulse train administered monthly. This particular sample has been on test for over 3 years and is discharging normally. The decreasing voltage levels (both open circuit voltage and loaded voltage) can be used to estimate end-of-life and elective replacement times. This cell is still in its mid-life voltage plateau region.

Cells are tested until a predefined end-of-life (or end-of-service) voltage is observed. (For this test, end-of-life is defined as the point at which the voltage during any of the 4 pulses falls below 1.5 V.) Regular reports of life test results are compiled and distributed to users of the cells. These reports give histograms of the voltage at 4 points during a simulated therapy regimen: (1) voltage before start of charging, (2) the lowest voltage during the first shock, (3) the voltage at the end of the first shock, and (4) the lowest voltage during the fourth shock. A summary of life test results for the Wilson Greatbatch silver vanadium oxide cells has been published.[9]

Over 2500 cells are currently on this life test regime in a testing program in the laboratories of Wilson Greatbatch. To date, there have been no observations of cell failure while some early cells

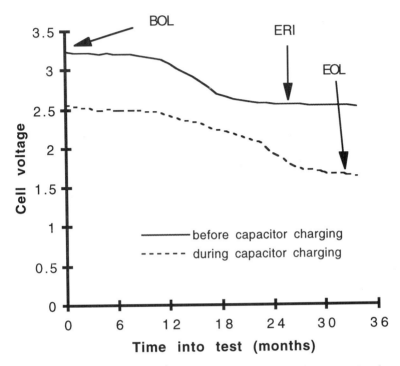

Figure 5. Life test discharge results for a defibrillator battery in a simulated ICD application which includes the steady low-level monitoring current and monthly 4-shock defibrillation regimens. (This is the testing for the second group discussed under *Life Testing*.) The top trace shows the voltage decay before capacitor charging begins and the bottom trace is the minimum voltage at the end of the fourth charge.

have attained their end-of-service voltage as expected (i.e. not prematurely).

Performance in Devices

It is difficult to assess longevity in actual devices, since the frequency of pulsing is highly dependent on the condition of the patient's medical condition. Over 70,000 lithium/silver vanadium oxide cells in clinical applications have shown high reliability to date, with no catastrophic failures having been reported to Wilson Greatbatch. Cells have attained end-of-life under some clinical conditions to date due to failure to replace an ICD.

It is impossible to state the "longevity" of a particular cell without careful specification of the regime under which the cell is used. For example, the cell whose performance is illustrated in Fig. 5 above, can remain in clinical service for approximately 44 months if the unit defibrillates 4 times per month (assuming a 2 A pulse of 10 s duration for each defibrillation charging cycle) and otherwise operates drawing a 20 μA background current drain. For the typical ICD, using only silver vanadium oxide cells, the background current is the main component of battery depletion. If the same battery is required to provide a pulse only once per month, the expected longevity would be approximately 75 months. If defibrillation occurred only twice yearly, the longevity might be closer to 100 months. (See Appendix.) None of these estimates includes test pulses which are performed clinically or pulses required to reform capacitors.

Continuous VVI pacing represents a significant load on the battery. The average current for pacing (with a high threshold patient) at 6 V into a 500 Ω load at a rate of 70 BPM with a pulse width of 500 μs is about 7 μA. While this is not as great as the traditional 20 μA monitoring current of ICDs before 1996, it is nearly as great as that of the newest ICDs which use lower current monitoring circuitry which requires < 10 μA. (These estimates highlight the fact that in pacemaker dependent patients, VVI pacing by the ICD is suboptimal from an energy consumption standpoint vs. implantation of a concomitant permanent pacemaker.)

Tiered therapy further complicate the estimation of longevity, since a wide variety of current-drawing requirements may be utilized in a specific patient. Determination of the approaching *elective replacement time* (ERI) of the battery (with the entire ICD pulse generator) involves an estimate of the remaining time before the pulse voltage drops below a level which can achieve defibrillation. Several methods are available for performing this estimate, and different manufacturers use different parameters for this. The open circuit voltage, the minimum pulse voltage, or some related (albeit indirect) parameter, such as capacitor charge time, may all be used to signal the need for device replacement. The CPI Mini uses a combination of voltage and charge time to declare the ERI, i.e., if either the open circuit or "monitoring" voltage is low or the charge time is excessive then an ERI is declared.

The temporal "safety margin" for acceptable battery function prior to end-of-life, i.e., the time between the signaling of elective replacement and the point past which the device will no longer operate correctly, depends not only on the discharge characteristics of the battery, but also on other factors such as the energy required to achieve defibrillation, the performance characteristics of the capacitors, the charging current waveform, and the time between shock delivery. In most cases, the ICD manufacturers include a 3 month safety margin if no additional shocks are delivered. Other factors can influence battery longevity. For example, exposure to radiation at levels typically used in radiation therapy (50 grays) can destroy battery capacity.[10]

Specific ICDs have well-characterized elective replacement protocols which are explained in the manufacturers accompanying manuals. The methods used to determine elective replacement points depend not only on the battery performance but also on the manner in which the circuitry interacts with the battery and the properties of the capacitors. Elective replacement criteria and their measurement methodology are thus determined by device manufacturers using data provided from battery testing as well as parameters associated with the electronic circuitry.

Batteries which might be returned to the manufacturer after explantation are routinely put through a standard fault-tree analysis if there is a suspicion of premature depletion. This analysis includes a review of all manufacturing history of the cell, a review of life test performance of cells made during the same time frame, complete electrical characterization of the cell, microcalorimetric assessment of self-discharge to determine if an internal short circuit exists, and radiological and visual examination. Finally, a destructive analysis of the cell is performed to examine internal components for potential defects.

Summary

The ICD presents challenging requirements for a power source. The cell must exhibit low self-discharge and must be able to deliver high-current pulses on demand to charge the capacitors of the device. The cell must exhibit the safety and reliability requirements demanded of implantable devices and must have a predictable discharge characteristic which can indicate the onset of the elective replacement time.

ICDs today use lithium/silver vanadium oxide batteries as power sources. These cells have been used since 1987 and have exhibited reliable field performance. The cells have been subjected to extensive safety and qualification testing, and a program of accelerated and real-time discharge tests has provided information necessary to understand the performance of this system in the device.

Research and development work continues both in the further characterization of the lithium/silver vanadium oxide system and in optimization of electrode fabrication techniques and cell design, in order to further reduce battery size and optimize performance and longevity. Work is also in progress in the development and testing of alternate cathode materials. The ultimate goal of this ongoing effort is the development of well-characterized batteries with optimum energy density, safety, and reliability to meet the needs of future ICDs.

Appendix: Sizing The Battery

For a given battery technology, the size of the battery is directly proportional to its energy content.[b] The three main energy requirements are:

1. *Number of shocks.* Consider the defibrillation capability goal of 200 shocks each of 30 J. Assume a charging efficiency of 75% (Chap. 13) and a pair of LiSVO cells yielding 6 V total. The charging circuit must draw 40 J = 30 J/75% from the 6 V battery. The total energy is then 8,000 J = 200 · 40 J. This is equivalent to 0.37 ampere hours (Ah) = 8,000 J/(3600 s)/ 6 V. (For historical reasons, batteries are rated in Ah instead of J or C.)

2. *Monitoring current.* This is the overhead (or background) current being consumed even when there are no defibrillation shocks and no pacing stimuli. Sometimes this is called *sensing current.* It is a continuous drain on the battery every second of every minute of every day, and is approximately 10 μA (microamperes). *This continuous drain is usually the main reason why the battery gets depleted and requires replacement* (rather than shocks having depleted the battery). For example, the total monitoring current charge required over 5 years is approximately 0.43 Ah = 5 years · 3.1 × 10^7 s/year · 10 μA/3600 s/hour. This is more than the 0.37 Ah that might be expected to be consumed by a total of 200 shocks delivered, as calculated above. So, more energy is needed for monitoring than for defibrillation. Advances in integrated circuit technology continue to lower the monitoring cur-

---

b. This is not exactly true in all cases. A very low energy (e.g. 5 shock capacity) battery will not be any smaller than a 50 shock battery since there is a minimum cell plate area required to produce the current output for acceptable charge times.

Table 1. Battery budget for a typical ICD to meet the worst case energy requirement.

Function	Capacity	Assumptions
5 years background (monitoring)	0.43 Ah	10 µA drain (idle)
5 years pacing	0.30 Ah	100% pacing
200 shocks	0.37 Ah	75% efficiency 30 J shock
Total	1.10 Ah	

rents but the benefit is somewhat overshadowed by the modern desirable feature of continuous electrogram recording.

3. *Pacing energy.* Pacing can extract considerable energy from an ICD. For example, with a pacing impedance of 500 Ω and a high amplitude of 6 V, the current during the pulse will be 12 mA. For pacing 100% of the time at a rate of 70 pulses/minute (equals 857 ms interval) and a 500 µs pulse width, the *average current* drain due to pacing will be about 7 µA = 12 mA · 500 µs/857 ms. This requires 0.3 Ah = 7 µA · 3.1×10^7 s/year · 5 years/ 3600 s/hour.

The energy budget incorporating these examples is summarized in Table 1. A 1.1 Ah battery (actually 2 cells) meeting these demanding energy requirements will occupy a considerable portion of the pulse generator, approximately 15 cm^3 for the cells themselves, plus 3-6 cm^3 to insulate and cradle them. The LiSVO batteries require about 10 cm^3 per Ah. Two important notes are in order. The first is that some ICD manufacturers power their devices from one large cell rather than two smaller cells in series. While this doubles the Ah capability, it halves the voltage of the battery and thus the energy and battery size requirements are little changed. This design choice, therefore has no significant impact on device size. Second, by using the dual energy sources (LiSVO for defibrillation shocks and lithium iodide for the monitoring), it is possible to draw the heavy monitoring energy requirements from the more energy dense lithium iodide cell. This results in a smaller overall battery volume.

ACKNOWLEDGMENTS

Thanks to Ken Anderson (Medtronic) for the battery sizing appendix and to Esther Takeuchi (Wilson Greatbatch) for the voltage delay example.

1. Horning RJ, Viswanathan S. High rate lithium cell for medical application, Proc. 29th Power Sources Symp., 1980:64-66.
2. Liang CC, Bolster ME, Murphy RM, inventors. Wilson Greatbatch Ltd., assignees. Metal oxide composite cathode material for high energy density batter

ies; heat treatment. U.S. Patent No. 4,391,729. 1983 Jul 5.

3. Liang CC, Bolster ME, Murphy RM, inventors. Wilson Greatbatch Ltd., assignees. Metal oxide composite cathode material for high energy density batteries. U.S. Patent No. 4,310,609. 1982 Jan 12.

4. Casalot A, Pouchard M, New nonstoichiometric phases of the silver oxide-vanadium pentoxide-vanadium dioxide system. Chemical and crystallographic study. Bull. Soc. Chim. Fr. 1967;10:3817-3820.

5. Takeuchi ES, Piliero P. Lithium/silver vanadium oxide batteries with various silver to vanadium ratios, J Power Sources 1987;21:133-141.

6. Takeuchi ES, Thiebolt WC. The reduction of silver vanadium oxide in lithium/silver vanadium oxide cells. J Electrochem Soc 1988;135:2691-2694.

7. Keister P, Mead RT, Muffoletto BC, et al , inventors. Wilson Greatbatch Ltd., assignees. Non-aqueous lithium battery; implantable cardiac defibrillator. U.S. Patent No. 4,830,940. 1989 May 16.

8. Visbisky M, Stinebring RC, Holmes CF. An approach to the reliability of implantable lithium batteries, J Power Sources 1989;26:185-194.

9. Holmes, CF, Visbisky M. Long-term testing of defibrillator batteries. PACE 1991;14:341-345.

10. Rodriguez F, Filimonov A, Henning A, et al. Radiation-induced effects in multiprogrammable pacemakers and implantable defibrillators. PACE 1991;14:2143-2153.

11

The High Voltage Capacitor

Joel B. Ennis and Mark W. Kroll, PhD

ONE OF the most critical components of the ICD is the high voltage capacitor, which stores the electrical pulse just before delivery to the heart. This capacitor also represents an increasing fraction of the total physical volume of the ICD. In fact, the capacitor (as it will be referred to below, for simplicity) is the primary reason that an ICD is so much larger than an implantable pacemaker.

This chapter will cover the various capacitor technologies to provide an understanding of the size limitations of the capacitor. It is also important for the clinician to understand the reasons for capacitor maintenance and the consequences of failing to do maintenance in certain applications. A final and important topic is the meaning and accuracy of the device capacitance specification.

Role of the Capacitor

Whereas the battery is the prime power source for the entire ICD, the capacitor is a temporary energy storage component. The function of the capacitor is to store the energy provided by the high voltage charging circuitry (Chap. 13) over a period of seconds and deliver that energy to the heart, as a high voltage countershock, over a period of a few milliseconds. Whereas the capacitor is charged to over 700 V with typically 10 mA of current, it may be required to deliver a pulse well over 30 A in current. This represents about a 3000 : 1 increase in the current level between the capacitor charging circuit and the capacitor discharge circuit.

An analogy often used is that of a bucket which is slowly filled with water from a garden hose, and then quickly dumped out. The amount of water moved per second corresponds to the current, while the volume of water is analogous to the total electrical charge stored by the capacitor.

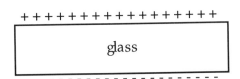

Figure 1. The simplest capacitor is merely an insulator separating different charges.

The value of the capacitance, measured in farads (F, or — more typically — microfarads, μF), describes the amount of charge and energy stored at a given voltage, and also plays a major role in determining the shape of the shock pulse which is delivered. A common parameter for the shape is the "tilt" or voltage decay percentage at the time of truncation or polarity shift. (Eq 7, Chap. 4) The greater the capacitance, the more time the capacitor requires to discharge completely into a given resistance load. Thus, for a given tilt a larger capacitance increases the duration of the discharge waveform.

A secondary role that the capacitor plays is to store the energy for a defibrillation pulse until the precise instant that the discharge is triggered. This permits the timing of the pulse to be synchronized to a ventricular depolarization or to be delayed pending reconfirmation of the tachyarrhythmia.

In summary, the capacitor provides the means for storing energy from the battery for delivery at a voltage and for a duration appropriate for defibrillation.

Basic Principles of Capacitor Operation

Consider the piece of glass in Fig. 1. It has positive charges on the top and negative charges on the bottom. The negative charges are attracted to the positive charges due to their polarity difference. However, due to the insulating glass the charges cannot combine and must stay separated.[a] In this way the piece of glass stores charge. Note that there are no conductors involved in this paradigm capacitor. The metal conductors in a practical capacitor are only necessary to deposit and remove charge.

This is very similar to the first recorded capacitor which was made in the Dutch town of Leyden around 1740. The "Leyden

---

a. Assuming that the voltages are moderate so that the air around the edges does not "arc over" and allow the passage of current.

jar" was a jar with one metal sheet on the outside and one on the inside.

On an electrical circuit schematic, an ideal capacitor is represented by two parallel lines perpendicular to the connecting wiring. (Chap. 13) The lines are a two dimensional representation of conducting plates, or electrodes, while the gap between them represents an insulating material or "dielectric". When current is forced into the capacitor negatively charged electrons accumulate (or condense, as in "Kondesator", the German term for capacitor) on one plate while positive charges condense on the opposite plate. As the charges accumulate, the potential energy associated with the attractive force between positive and negative electrical charges results in a voltage across the capacitor which eventually becomes equal and opposite to the applied voltage of the current source. At this point, current will no longer flow through the circuit (assuming that the capacitor insulator is perfect); the capacitor is said to be charged.

The charge (Q), in coulombs, on a capacitor is given by the capacitance value (C) and the voltage (V) by:

Eq. 1 $Q = C V$

For example, a 100 μF capacitor at 1000 V stores 0.1 coulomb. The coulomb is about 0.00001 mole of electron charges or about 6×10^{18} electron charges. The potential energy (E) associated with this storage of charge is given by

Eq. 2 $E = 0.5 C V^2$

where E is measured in J (joules). Note that the potential or stored energy increases as the square of the voltage.

To discharge the capacitor, a second circuit pathway is used. With the closing of a switch, this circuit is completed and the charge stored on the capacitor plates will rush out of the capacitor, seeking to return to an equilibrium condition having zero potential energy. The voltage across the capacitor decreases as the charge escapes, until the capacitor voltage and charge are both zero. Intuitively, the positive and negative charges reunite through the pathway of the switches and load.

Work is accomplished by putting a resistive load in the discharge circuit. In the case of the ICD, the load is the heart tissue between the electrodes, which has a characteristic electrical resistance. As the capacitor discharges through this resistance, the voltage pulse generates a current through the tissue, according to Ohm's law. (Chap. 4)

Capacitor Design Fundamentals

The capacitance value of a capacitor depends upon the area (A) of the plates on which the charge accumulates, the spacing (s) created by the insulator separating the plates, and the dielectric constant or relative permittivity (k) of the insulating material according to the equation:

Eq. 3 $$C = \varepsilon\, k\, \frac{A}{s}$$ (C in farads)

where ε is a constant known as the permittivity of free space, which has the value 8.854×10^{-14} F/cm. The capacitance unit, the farad, is named in honor of Michael Faraday who did pioneering work with capacitors and coined the term "dielectric constant."

The physical size of a capacitor depends first upon the volume of the dielectric material (equaling the plate area times the spacing of the plates—or thickness of the dielectric), then on the volume occupied by the plates, and finally on the volume of the package. For comparing the physical size of capacitors of different voltage or capacitance ratings, it is useful to calculate their energy density in J per cubic centimeter or J per gram.

The photo-flash capacitor of a present ICD has an energy density of about 1.7 J/cm³ as a cylinder. Due to the often unusable space around the cylinder the (lower) density of the circumscribing cuboid is also calculated.[b] This value is about 1.3 J/cm³.

The electric field (F) (Chap. 4) represents the stress on the insulator and is given by:

Eq. 4 $$F = \frac{V}{s}$$ (F in volts per unit of distance)

The maximum stress which can be applied to an insulating material is known as its *dielectric breakdown strength* (F_{max}). At the breakdown point, the voltage gradient will result in an electrical break-

---

b.   As the capacitors can be placed in the rounded edge of the ICD housing, not all of the cuboid volume is wasted. (Chap. 12) Thus the effective density of the photo-flash capacitor lies between the two numbers of 1.3 and 1.7 J/cm3.

down and a sudden localized rush of current will flow through the dielectric. The values of breakdown strength of different materials vary as widely as do the mechanical strengths of materials. In fact, the two strengths appear to be correlated. For example, ceramics, which are mechanically brittle, have an F_{max} of about 40,000 - 400,000 V/cm, while familiar strong plastics such as polypropylene have breakdown strengths of 2,000,000 - 8,000,000 V/cm.

If we consider only the dielectric material itself, the ultimate energy density (D) in J/cm^3 can be calculated based on knowing only the permittivity (k) and dielectric breakdown strength, F_{max}, of the material, using

Eq. 5 $$D = 0.5 \ \varepsilon \ k \ F_{max}^2$$

The ultimate energy density of a capacitor may be increased by: (1) changing the insulating material to one with a higher value of k, or (2) changing to one with a higher breakdown strength (and then using the appropriate higher voltages).

Capacitors are not operated at electrical stresses very close to their breakdown strengths. As one might expect based on mechanical analogy, if one stresses a dielectric material near its ultimate strength for a period of time, it gradually fatigues and eventually breaks down. The lower the applied stress, the longer the capacitor will endure. The lifetime, L, of a capacitor depends inversely upon the electrical stress level applied according to a power law:

Eq. 6 $$L \propto \frac{1}{F^n}$$

where the exponent, n, depends upon the dielectric material as well as a variety of other factors, but is typically in the range of 2-15. Most capacitors intended for general use are designed to be operated at a stress level which is < 50% of their breakdown strength capability. Capacitors designed for a specific use and having a defined, limited life may be operated at up to 90% of their breakdown strength. For example, external defibrillation capacitors are typically operated well above the 50% level as they are only charged for brief periods of time.

Types of Capacitors

There are a wide variety of capacitors categorized by their dielectrics and their electrodes. The three primary "orders" in the capacitor class are: electrostatic, electrolytic, and double layer. *Electrostatic capacitors* have a permanent dielectric and two metallic electrode plates. *Electrolytic capacitors* have a permanent dielectric formed on the surface of a metal electrode, while the opposing electrode is an electrolyte. *Electrochemical capacitors* have (at least for part of their charge storage) no permanent dielectric.

The Electrostatic Capacitor: Films and Ceramics
Electrostatic capacitors are manufactured using a wide variety of different dielectric materials. The most interesting types for possible future use in implanted defibrillators are metallized film and ceramic dielectric capacitors. These types are the highest energy density electrostatic capacitors in the present ICD operating voltage range (under 1000 V), but still have lower energy density than the electrolytic (specifically the aluminum photo-flash capacitor) in this range. Thus, their usage, at least with present technologies, would make ICDs prohibitively large.

Metallized film capacitors are composed mostly of insulator material. Metallized film capacitors have a thin plastic film (typically 20 μm thick) for their dielectric, and the film is metallized (deposited with metal of about 1000 Å or 0.1 μm thickness) on one side to create an electrode. Two metallized films are wound together in a spiral to form a laminated structure or stacked with dielectric layers with alternating electrodes. Most plastics have low permittivities (k = 2-4) but very high dielectric breakdown strength. Thus the key to achieving a high energy density with this technology is the use of high voltages or very thin films. For example, capacitors developed for missile defense purposes have densities of $4\,J/cm^3$ which is triple the useful (cuboid) density of present ICD photo-flash capacitors. However, these military-use capacitors are charged to many thousands of volts to generate the high internal electrical fields to attain this energy density.

Consider instead a hypothetical 800 V metalized film ICD capacitor. In order to attain the high F_{max} of 4,000,000 V/cm which a polyester film needs to achieve high energy density the film would have to be only 2 μm = 800 V/4,000,000 V/cm. (Eq. 4) While films of a few μm thickness have been experimented with, their reliability is limited by local defects such as pinholes. Thus, for lower voltage

ICD applications, the density requirement translates into the need for very thin, defect-free films so that a high electric field is developed.

Ceramic dielectrics can have very high dielectric constant (k), but their dielectric strength (F_{max}) is relatively low. Dielectric constants are typically in the range of 100-10,000, but formulations with k over 100,000 have been described. These high-k materials often exhibit nonlinear characteristics and the value of k generally falls as the voltage is increased. A drawback for the ICD is that ceramics have high mass densities (~ 7 g/cm^3), so that capacitors which are volumetrically compact may still be relatively heavy compared to other types of capacitors. It is theoretically possible to match the size of the present photoflash capacitors but the capacitor would weigh over 3.5 gm/J giving a weight of 105 gm for the capacitor alone in a 30 J ICD!

The Electrolytic Capacitor

Present ICDs use the electrolytic capacitor. In this technology, a high surface area metallic electrode is made from either a thin foil or powder. The surface is thinly coated with an insulating metal oxide layer via an electrochemical oxidation process, known as "forming". The structure is impregnated with an electrolyte which covers the outside surface of the oxide coating, acting as a second electrode. While the metalized film capacitor is mostly insulator, the electrolytic is mostly conductor. The two major types of electrolytic capacitors are defined by the metal oxide, which are the aluminum and the tantalum varieties.[1] The aluminum electrolytic is used in present ICDs and will be emphasized here.

To achieve high energy storage one must achieve either a high voltage or a high capacitance. (Eq. 2) While the film capacitor allows high voltages, the electrolytic achieves its high energy density by providing a very high capacitance value with only moderate voltages (under 400 V).

Recall Eq. 3 for the capacitance value. The permittivity of free space (ε) is a universal constant and thus not manipulable. The aluminum electrolytic achieves its impressive capacitance by improving on all three remaining factors, namely the dielectric constant (k), the surface area (A), and the layer spacing (s). To increase the surface area, an aluminum foil is deeply etched. The etching is accomplished by inserting the foil into a chloride solution and passing a small electrical current through it. A highly stylized (for ease of visualization) cross-sectional view is shown in Fig. 2A. In reality, depending on the process, the etching results in tangled

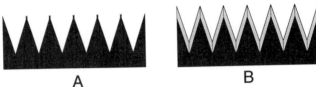

Figure 2. Metal (anode) and oxide layer of aluminum electrolytic capacitor (stylized cross section). On the left (A) is the aluminum anode foil cross section after chemical microscopic etching. On the right (B) is the cross section after the addition of the oxide layer.

tunnels[2] or a cratered surface resembling the lunar landscape.[3] The surface area multiplication is referred to the "foil gain" and ranges from 10-150. For the high voltage ICD capacitors the etching results in about 10,000,000 pits per square centimeter.[4]

The etched foil (the "anode") is then placed in an anodizing solution (for example - ammonium borate) and a voltage is applied. This causes a buildup of Al_2O_3 on the foil (Fig. 2B). This oxide becomes the capacitor insulator (dielectric) and accomplishes three important things. First, it allows for a dielectric which follows the drastic unevenness of the etched foil. Secondly, it provides a very thin spacing ("s" in Eq. 3) of about 10,000 Å or only 1 μm. (This thickness is proportional to the anodization voltage at 14 Å/V.) Finally (and rather fortuitously), it provides a fairly high (compared to films) dielectric constant (k) of about 8-10.

This leaves one major problem. How does the other "conductor" of the capacitor get placed up against the oxide? The answer (reminiscent of current conduction in the human body) is to use dissolved ions. An electrolyte solution is formed by dissolving an ionic solute in a solvent. A classical approach was to dissolve ammonium borate in an ethylene glycol (automobile antifreeze) solution. The electrolytic solution (hence the name of the capacitor type) carries the current to another foil which is the cathode. (Fig. 3A) Finally, to prevent the cathode foil from damaging the thin oxide a porous paper separator is inserted as shown in Fig. 3B. The paper also provides a convenient means of delivering the electrolyte solution during manufacturing.

Another separator is inserted "over" the cathode to separate it from the anode of the next layer in a winding. The layers are then wound as shown in Fig. 4. Present ICD capacitors were originally developed for the photo-flash application. The photo-flash capacitor has a "double anode." This is created by deeply etching both sides of the anode foil.

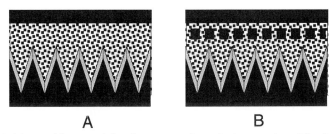

A   B

Figure 3. Additional layers of the aluminum electrolytic capacitor. The left side (*A*) depicts the electrolyte (stippled area) filling in the microscopically etched gaps. The cathode foil (dark band) is shown on the top. The right side (*B*) shows the addition of the porous paper separator (dashed band).

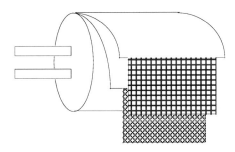

Figure 4. Winding of the electrolytic capacitor. The four layers from the top are: anode, porous separator, cathode, and porous separator. Connection electrodes are attached to the anode and cathode on the side of the package.

An alternative approach involves stacking the aluminum foils like sheets of paper, again with porous paper separators. A variant on the electrolytic involves electrically forming (building an oxide layer on) both foils. The capacitor can now store voltages of either polarity and is said to be a "nonpolarized" electrolytic. In other words, there is neither a fixed anode nor a fixed cathode.

The aluminum electrolytic capacitor has a maximum practical voltage of about 450 V. To attain the popular 750 V used in today's ICDs requires the use of two photo-flash aluminum electrolytic capacitors (each of 375 V) in series. As mentioned earlier, this variety of aluminum electrolytic capacitor has energy densities of nearly 2 J/cm^3.

Electrolytic capacitors may also be based on tantalum.[5] These may be subdivided into three types: foil, sintered powder with a liquid electrolyte (known as wet slug tantalum), and sintered powder with a solidified conforming electrode (known as solid tantalum). Solid tantalum capacitors are generally manufactured for operation at 100 V or less, whereas wet slug tantalums may be rated at up to 125 V, and foil tantalums at up to 200 V. To achieve voltages useful for the ICD would require the use of four such capacitors in series.

The Electrochemical Capacitor

The electrochemical capacitor category includes the double-layer and the pseudo-capacitor. *Double-layer capacitors* are similar to electrolytic capacitors in that there is a high surface area conductor for one electrode, and an electrolyte for the other. In this case, however, there is no permanent dielectric coating on the solid electrode. Instead, the dielectric is created as the capacitor is charged by the polarization of electrolyte molecules at the electrode surface, forming what is referred to as the "double layer". This phenomenon was first described by Helmholtz in 1879.[6] The double layer is only about 4 Å thick, and despite its high dielectric strength, it can sustain a voltage of only 1-4 V. Higher voltage capacitors must be constructed by series-connection of these low voltage cells.

In order to maximize the energy density of double layer capacitors, very high surface area materials are used, such as carbon powders, which have effective surface areas measured in the hundreds of square meters per gram. The energy densities available today are impressive—on the order of 10 J/cm^3. Unfortunately, defibrillation voltage needs would require hundreds of the double-layer capacitors be connected in series which presents a packaging nightmare and a reliability problem. Also, the equivalent series resistance (Table 1) of present double layer capacitors is extremely high and would limit the shock current to about 1 A which is insufficient for defibrillation, regardless of the energy delivered. (Chap. 4).

The push for an electric car has led to a great deal of research with these capacitors and thus further progress is expected. Some devices are now being tested with extremely low equivalent series resistances (sufficiently low for defibrillation).[7]

The *pseudo-capacitor* stores charge with a Faradic charge transfer (as well as in the double layer at the electrode surface—as above).[8] These capacitors are also referred to as mixed-metal oxide electrochemical capacitors. In Faradic charge transfer an adsorbed monolayer of a given species is formed on an electrode surface. With RuO_2 (on titanium) electrodes it appears that a proton (as opposed to electron) condenser obtains.[9] Hence, these devices have been described exotically as "proton injection" capacitors. A hybrid capacitor using a tantalum anode and a RuO_2 cathode may offer promise for the ICD application.[10]

Table 1. ICD energy storage capacitor specifications.

Parameter	Desired Value
Capacitance	80-200 μF
Operating voltage	700-1000 V
Energy stored	25 -40 J
Active life	200 -500 pulses
Shelf life	> 10 years
Volume	< 30 cm³
Weight	< 60 g
Internal parallel resistance	> 5 MΩ
Equivalent series resistance (ESR)	< 2.0 Ω

Selecting the Capacitor for the ICD

The most critical issues for the high voltage capacitor used in the ICD are the operating voltage, capacitance, size and weight, and the high reliability required for a relatively small number of charge and discharge cycles. Also important are the *internal parallel resistance* , which causes the leakage current (that can increase charge times), and the *equivalent series resistance* (which can decrease delivered voltage and current). There are several other variables. Table 1 shows typically specified values.

The product of a 100 μF capacitance and an internal parallel (leakage) resistance of 5 MΩ gives a time constant (Chap. 4) of 500 s. Thus, during a 3 s reconfirmation delay in "noncommitted" ICDs, such a capacitor will lose only 3/500 or 0.6% of its charged voltage.

Limitations of the Aluminum Electrolytic

Double anode aluminum electrolytic capacitors have been selected for use in ICDs because they have the highest energy density of any type of capacitor available in this voltage range.

The aluminum electrolytic capacitor, however, suffers from a number of shortcomings for which manufacturers of ICDs have learned to compensate. Aluminum electrolytic capacitor manufacturers do not offer a medical grade component, so that the ICD manufacturer must do considerable testing and screening to assure the level of reliability required for this application. The maximum energy density capacitors available are designed for operation at less than 375 V, so that two capacitors must be connected in series to create a 750 V capacitor. An electrolytic capable of operation over 500 V is not available. Another limitation of these capacitors is that their cylindrical geometry is not ideal for the packaging of an ICD. (Customized package designs are not yet available.)

Moreover, aluminum electrolytic capacitors, as supplied to the ICD manufacturer, are not hermetically sealed. All aluminum electrolytic capacitors develop hydrogen gas at the cathode due to electrolysis.[11] Consequently, another issue is that the electrolytic capacitor can generate hydrogen gas under overstress conditions, and the commercial versions have been designed with a pressure relief vent to minimize the hazard of explosion under extreme overvoltage conditions not possible in the ICD application. While this gas evolution follows Faraday's laws, a "depolarizer" is added to the electrolyte to promote its absorption. The net hydrogen generated is minimal at moderate temperatures such as 37 °C.[12]

The relief vent also represents a source of outgassed moisture from the electrolyte which could affect the surrounding electronics inside the ICD. The loss of moisture from the capacitor represents a long-term failure mechanism for the capacitor as well. However this effect is minuscule at body temperature (on the order of a milligram over a device lifetime).[13] Some ICD manufacturers have encased the capacitor in a hermetically sealed enclosure to eliminate the outgassing problem. However, this increases the total size of the packaged capacitor and limits the volume for expansion of the hydrogen gas.

Two other limiting factors are the capacitance variability and reforming, as will now be discussed.

When a Farad is not a Farad

The capacitance value of the ICD capacitor is of paramount importance. First, it determines the maximum stored energy. (Eq. 2) Also, in tilt based devices, the capacitance determines the pulse duration (Chap. 4, Eq. 8) which, in turn, significantly affects the defibrillation efficiency.[14] Smaller capacitance values have been shown to significantly reduce defibrillation energy thresholds[15] (but not voltage thresholds[16]) especially in cases with high impedance pathways.[17] Finally, the ICD capacitance value must be known with some degree of accuracy in order to transfer threshold readings from an external test device with a presumably known capacitance value.

In spite of the importance of an accurate capacitance measurement, some ICDs have their capacitance value specified with a significant error. A typical example is a 135 µF capacitance specified as being 120 µF. This error may arise from misapplying the conventional electronic capacitance measurement. The primary (i.e., non-medical) use of electrolytic capacitors is for absorbing alternating current in order to smooth power supply voltages. Thus, the capacitance measurement is traditionally made with a low voltage ($\approx$1 V) alternating current (typically 1 KHz) and at room temperature (25 °C). Unfortunately, these conditions are at odds with the ICD application given that: capacitance increases with high voltages[18,19] (such as 750 V), with low frequencies[20,21] (such as a single DC pulse), and with higher temperatures[19,22] (such as the 37 °C body temperature).

Thus, a "120 µF" capacitor tested at 25 °C and 1 V alternating current becomes a 135 µF capacitor when tested at 37 °C and a 750 V DC pulse. We strongly recommend that ICD manufacturers rate their capacitors at values measured according to their intended use. This will ensure that the capacitance, energy storage capability, and pulse durations are accurately known.

One manufacturer uses a 132 µF capacitor (with the appropriate room temperature measurement) but calculates all energies as if the value was actually 120 µF. The calculation of electrode resistance (from shock waveform duration—see Eq. 8, Chap. 4) is, however, based on the more accurate value of 132 µF. If this was not done then all reported resistances would be overstated by 10 %. Even the 132 µF value is lower than that which occurs once the ICD is implanted and achieves body temperature.

Reforming

Perhaps the greatest complaint with the aluminum electrolytic capacitor is that it degrades when not in use. The degradation results, among other things, in considerably greater energy being required to charge the capacitor the first time after a period of storage than is normal immediately after use. (See Chap. 20, "Capacitor Reforming") This means that it takes longer for the power supply to charge the capacitor, and that more of the energy stored in the battery is consumed in the process. In order to control this degradation and limit the maximum charge time to an acceptable number of seconds, the capacitor is usually "reformed" on a regular schedule. (Table 2, Chap. 20)

The reader who has a photoflash unit is familiar with the reforming process, in which the capacitor will charge at a slower rate for its first usage in a given setting. In the reforming process, the capacitor is effectively repaired electrochemically, so that the capacitor behavior returns to normal. However, the battery must be designed to deliver the extra energy required for these reforming cycles throughout the life of the implant. Capacitor reforming is generally not necessary if only submaximal voltage (e.g. < 600 V) shocks will be delivered.

The exact etiology of the degradation process is not perfectly understood (at least not publicly) and probably involves multiple mechanisms. Free oxygen which had helped to cover defects in the oxide (after being attracted during the forming process) can diffuse into the electrolyte thus increasing the leakage through the oxide layer.[23] Residual water in the electrolyte may attack the oxide and form hydrides[24] such as $Al(OH)_3$. This theory is supported by the empirical finding that older capacitors have thicker and more porous oxides.[25] (On the other hand, some water is probably required to provide oxygen for the healing of oxide defects.[26]) These processes can increase the leakage current and hence increase the charge time. Reforming should ameliorate this problem.

Another aspect of degradation is the decrease in the capacitance value itself.[27] This is due to the electrolyte slowly drying out which increases the average effective charge separation[28] ("s" in Eq. 3). Another cause is the gradual buildup of oxide on the *cathode* film. This allows a competitive charge storage which decreases the overall capacitance.[29] The first problem (drying) is not helped by the reforming, while the cathode oxide problem probably is. Ironically, this decrease in capacitance reduces charge times (but not enough to offset the increase from the oxide degradation); but, of course, it also reduces energy storage.

One popular reforming regimen involves charging the capacitor to maximum voltage and then dumping the charge into an internal load (which generates an extremely high current with a 2-4 Ω load - Chap. 13; Fig. 5). This is in stark contrast to the ideal technique which allows the capacitor to slowly "bleed off" its charge over a period of hours. In fact, the high reverse polarity (compared to the charging or forming) current caused by the sharp discharge during charge dumping actually promotes buildup of oxide on the cathode. (The discharge of a therapy shock into a lower current heart load, say 50 Ω, should not promote such a buildup.) Nevertheless, dumping the charge into an internal load (or the heart) still does a reasonable job of reforming. If time (and programmer software) permits, it is preferable to allow the capacitor charge to slowly bleed off.

The issue of ICD capacitor reforming is further complicated by other issues. First, the need for reforming varies significantly with the capacitor manufacturer. Some brands suffer unrecoverable damage from a reforming delay. The most popular brand of capacitor used in ICDs today (Rubycon of Japan) seems to require little reforming. It degrades slightly after a few weeks so that charge times are increased by about 1/3 over a freshly reformed capacitor. Also, after one full energy shock the capacitor is effectively re-formed. Thus, in a multiple shock therapy regimen the increased charge time will only affect the first shock delivery time.

Since the present ICD batteries require reforming (or—more accurately— periodic usage) to maintain a low internal impedance, the ICD reforming schedule is perhaps independent of the capacitor. (See Chap. 10 discussion of "voltage delay").

Future Possibilities

Research into capacitor technology is underway at many capacitor manufacturing and dielectric materials manufacturing companies. Some of this research is aimed at developing electrostatic capacitors based on either polymer film or ceramic dielectrics which could be superior to the aluminum electrolytic in the ICD application. A major driving force for this work is the desire to eliminate the capacitor reforming requirement and to allow a cuboid shape.

The film capacitor approach requires a thin film with high dielectric strength. Depending on the dielectric constant of the film, the film thickness would need to be in the range of 1-4 μm and yet the film must still be able to withstand a voltage of 700 V or more. Today's commercially available polymer films do not have the combination of dielectric constant, dielectric strength, and small thickness required to achieve the energy density of the electrolytic at this voltage. The lack of a suitable material is a difficult hurdle to clear, especially where the potential market for a new material is relatively small.

The problem for ceramic capacitors is slightly simpler in that the dielectric thickness is not an issue. A combination of high dielectric constant and high (relative to currently utilized ceramics) dielectric strength is still required to meet the energy density needed for the ICD. The mass density of ceramic materials makes the gravimetric energy density (J/g) goal more difficult to achieve than the volumetric energy density (J/cm^3) goal. Thus far, ceramic capacitors have not matched the aluminum electrolytics for this application, again because of the absence of a suitable material.

Other types of capacitors, including double layer capacitors, have been considered for the implantable defibrillator application. A hybrid technology using a tantalum anode and a RuO_2 cathode is being evaluated for the ICD application.

Summary

The high voltage capacitor represents the single largest component in the ICD. Of the many types of capacitors manufactured today, the aluminum electrolytic capacitor has been selected for use in the ICD because it is the smallest available which meets the ICD operational requirements. Unfortunately, this type of capacitor may require regular reforming to maintain its electrical properties. The exact cause of the capacitor degradation and the precise requirements for reforming are not perfectly understood and vary with the process and manufacturer. Development of compact versions of other types of capacitors, which do not suffer this drawback, is on-going.

ACKNOWLEDGMENTS:

We thank Bennie Barker (Barker Microfarads), Jack Keimel (Medtronic), John Greenwood (Critical Medical Components), Ben Pless (Ventritex), Jim Causey (Pacesetter) and Rolie Hron (Angeion) for help with this chapter.

1. Moynihan JD. Theory design and application of electrolytic capacitors. Component Technology Institute, 1982.
2. Albella JM, Hornillos A, Sanz JM, et al. A mathematical approach to the CV product in aluminum electrolytic capacitors. Electrochemical Science & Tech. 1978;125:1950-1954.
3. Terryn H, Vereecken J, de Jaeger N. Characterization of aluminum surface treatments by means of gas adsorption measurements. Colloids & Surfaces 1993; 80:171-179.
4. Wakino K, Tsujimoto Y, Morimoto K, et al. Technological progress in materials application for electronic capacitors in Japan. IEEE Electrical Insulation Magazine, 1990;6:29-43.
5. Nakata T, Ohi M. Tantalum dielectrics open tantalizing potential in capacitor field. J Electronic Eng 1993;30:74-78.
6. Bockriz JO, Drazic DM, Electrochemical Science. 1972 Taylor & Francis, London.
7. Yoshida A, Imoto K, Nishino A, et al. An electric double-layer capacitor with high capacitance and low resistance. IEEE Proc 41st Electronic Components Technology Conf 1991:531-536.
8. Oxley JE. High rate solid state electrochemical capacitors. IEEE Proc 34th Intl Power Sources Symp 1990:346-350.
9. Ardizzone S, Fregonara G, Trasatti S. Inner and outer active surface of RuO_2 electrodes. Electrochem Acta 1990;35:263-267.
10. Evans DA. High energy density electrolytic-electrochemical hybrid capacitor. Carts' 94 Proceedings 1994:
11. Buczkowski GJ. Hydrogen evolution in aluminum electrolytic capacitors. IEEE Proc 37th Electronic Components Conf 1987:440-448.
12. Gomez-Aleixandre C, Albella JM, Martinez-Duart JM. Gas evolution in aluminum electrolytic capacitors. J Electrochem Soc 1984;131:612-614.
13. Nakata T. Long life low impedance aluminum electrolytic capacitors overcome

many problems. J Electronic Eng 1989;26:46-49.
14. Swartz JF, Fletcher RD, Karasik PE. Optimization of biphasic waveforms for human nonthoracotomy defibrillation. Circulation 1993;88:2646-2654.
15. Rist KE, Tchou PJ ,Mowrey K, et al. Smaller capacitors improve the biphasic waveform. J Cardiovasc Electrophys 1994;5:771-776.
16. Matula MH, Brooks MJ, Pan Q, et al. Can capacitance be lowered without affecting defibrillation requirements using biphasic waveforms? Circulation 1994;90:I-228. (abstract)
17. Swerdlow CD, Kass RM, Chen PS, et al. Effect of capacitor size and pathway resistance on defibrillation threshold for implantable defibrillators. Circulation 1994;90:1840-1846.
18. Albella JM, Gomez-Aleixandre G, Martinez-Duart JM. Dielectric characteristics of miniature aluminum electrolytic capacitors under stressed voltage conditions. J Applied Electrochem 1984;14:9-14.
19. Bora JS, Short-term and long-term performance of electrolytic capacitors. Microelectron Reliab 1978;18:237-240.
20. de Wit HJ, Crevecoeur C. The CV product of etched aluminum anode foil. J Electrochem Soc 1983;130:770-776.
21. Morley AR, Campbell DS. Electrolytic capacitors: their fabrication and the interpretation of their operational behaviour. Radio and Electronic Engineer 1973;43:421-429.
22. Harper CA. Handbook of Components for Electronics. McGraw-Hill. New York 1977.
23. Aluminum electrolytic capacitors. Rubycon Technical Note REB G88-03. Rubycon Corporation, Japan.
24. Kadaba PK, Dobbs W. Dielectric study of anodized foils of aluminum electrolytic capacitors. Material Sci & Eng 1982;54:279-283.
25. Kadaba PK, Dobbs W. TEM and SEM analysis of the anode layer of aluminum electrolytic capacitors. J Materials Sci Letters 1982;1:203-206.
26. Bernard WJ, Florio SM. The oxide forming role of water in aluminum electrolytic capacitors. ElectroComponent Sci Tech 1984;11:137-145.
27 Kiuchi K, Yanagibashi N. Operating life of aluminum electrolytic capacitor. Fifth Intl Telecommunications Energy Conf 1983. IEEE 83CH 1855-6:535-540.
28. Greason WD, Critchley J. Shelf-life evaluation of aluminum electrolytic capacitors. IEEE Trans Components, Hybrids, and Mfg Tech 1986;CHMT-9:293-299.
29. Harris KW, McDuff G, Burkes TR. Evaluation of electrolytic capacitors for high peak current pulse duty. IEEE Trans Electron Devices 1991:38:758-766.

12

The Pulse Generator

Randall S. Nelson

THE FIRST ICDs, implanted in 1980, were large (162 cm^3, 292 g)[1] compared to the most current devices that are about 60 cm^3 and 110 g. Since that time, emphasis on packaging of current ICDs has focused on the continual increase of device functions, whether it be therapies (pacing, different defibrillation modes) or features (telemetry, electrocardiogram storage, etc.), with continuing emphasis on decreasing the package size. Until recently, most devices have required abdominal implantation because of their size, as was the case with early pacemakers. Whereas pacemaker development had definite leaps in technology to allow the downsizing of that device (lithium batteries, integrated circuits, hermetic enclosures), size reduction of the ICD has been a net result of paying close attention to detail and making small reductions that have added up to the overall package efficiency.

Much of the technology for the ICD is an extension of that which has been developed for the pacemaker over the past 30+ years. Due to this available technology, as well as technology advancements from the aerospace industry, the defibrillator has enjoyed a rapid size reduction which has allowed the smaller devices to achieve a major design goal: pectoral implant of the ICD. Fig. 1 shows the size (volume) reduction since the first ICD to those implanted in 1996. This volume decrease can also be seen between the early CPI Ventak, based on the original Intec AID-C, and the Medtronic Jewel, one of the smaller currently released ICDs. (Fig. 2) The Jewel, as with all current designs, is smaller while providing more therapies, programmability, a more comfortable profile for the patient, and potentially a longer device life. One may expect ICDs to continue this downward trend in size with some slowing.

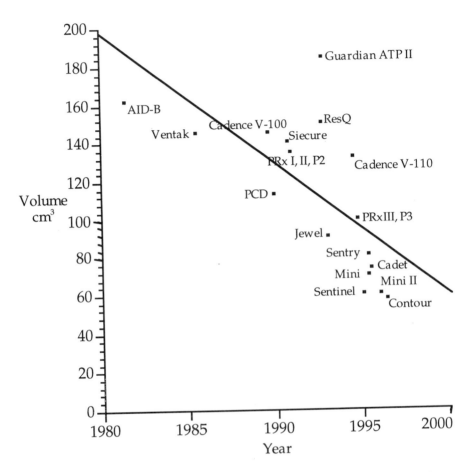

Figure 1. The ICD pulse generator volume has decreased an average of 7 cm³ per year since 1981.[1,2] The linear regression line has r²= .48 and p = .0014. As the volume has decreased below 90 cm³, the number of pectoral implants has increased. At 60 cm³ and below, pectoral implants comprise ≥ 95% of all implants.

General Description

The ICD package may be divided into two sections. One, the hermetic enclosure, provides environmental protection (physical, fluid) to the internal electrical components. Hermeticity of the ICD is required to prevent fluid passage into the electronic assembly, thereby eliminating corrosion of the circuitry and components as was common with epoxy potted pacemakers. Devices are expected

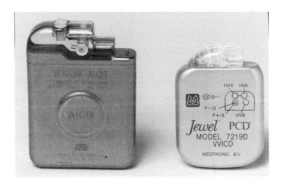

Figure 2. An early CPI Ventak (Model 1500), based on the original Intec AID-C and a current Medtronic Jewel (Model 7219D).

to be sealed to a leakage resistance of greater than 1×10^{-8} atm ml/s helium . The leakage is quantified using a mass spectrometer which measures, for a pressure differential of 1 atmosphere, the rate (milliliters per second) at which helium, an element of the internal can atmosphere, escapes the enclosure.

The enclosure of the hermetically sealed portion of a typical device consists of two formed titanium can halves, welded (typically by laser) so as to provide a smooth, unobtrusive seam that provides a high reliability seal for the internal components. *Titanium* has three characteristics that make it a preferred enclosure material. It is compatible with the human body (although there have been rare, isolated cases of adverse reaction) as well as corrosion resistant. It is also very lightweight. Titanium is 2/3 the weight of stainless steel, a material that has been used in the past for pacemaker housings.

To provide electrical conduction from the internal circuitry to the header and leads, *ceramic feedthrus* are typically used. Fig. 3 depicts a common feedthru structure. A ceramic feedthru uses alumina (ceramic) for the hermetic barrier as well as electrical isolation between conductors and the can. Platinum or platinum/iridium wire is brazed through the ceramic to provide the conductive path from internal circuitry to header. To provide the hermetic seal between feedthru and can, the feedthru is typically laser welded into the can.

These feedthrus may also integrate a capacitor into the ceramic as a filter before the internal circuitry. The feedthru

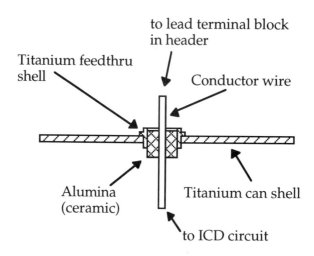

Figure 3. Cross section of a typical feedthru without integral capacitor. The optional feedthru capacitor would live in the ceramic region with one capacitor electrode (See Chap. 11) connected to the conductor wire and the other capacitor electrode connected to the titanium can shell.

capacitor is critical to eliminating potential problems with cellular phone compatibility. (See Chap. 14 for further discussion.) The feedthru capacitor does this by conducting the high frequency signal of the cellular phone interference (about 900 MHz) directly to the ICD housing and preventing its entrance into the device. The electrogram signal (less than 100 Hz (Chap. 14) are not affected. Theoretically, the pacing and defibrillation pulses are affected slightly but the effect is practically unmeasureable.

Enclosed within the hermetic enclosure is, for all practical purposes, a self powered computer. Batteries and defibrillator capacitors occupy a majority of the space. The operational circuitry—resistors, capacitors, transformers, microprocessors, antenna, diodes, etc.—occupy the bulk of the remaining space while a molded polymer frame is used to provide structural integrity. The circuitry is generally laid out with the low power (sensing, pacing) circuit components mounted on printed circuit board or ceramic substrate and the high power (defibrillation) circuit components mounted on a polyimide "flex tape" or ceramic material. More specific size considerations are described in detail later in this chapter.

The second major section of the pulse generator, the *header*, provides an electrical interface between the internal electronics and the implanted leads as well as electrical isolation to the surrounding tissue. Throughout the life of the pulse generator, it must remain biocompatible; provide electrical isolation between leads, the can, and the surrounding tissue; and maintain electrical contact from the internal circuitry to the leads. The body of the header is made of either an implantable grade polyurethane or epoxy. To the implanter and patient, there is no advantage of one compared to the other and use of one material over the other may be regarded as a manufacturer's processing preference. Both materials have provided highly reliable headers in chronic implants. Even so, the manufacturer of the implantable grade polyurethane has opted to discontinue its material as an implantable grade due to potential liability issues. Fortunately, other companies have stepped in to provide high quality material for this application.

The header is the source of most design related pulse generator implant complications.[3] The lead ports—defibrillating, pacing, and sensing—must maintain resistance to fluid penetration. As with pacemakers, this is accomplished with *silicone sealing rings* located on the lead. The header must also allow use of a tool, typically a *setscrew wrench*, to tighten the fastening mechanism onto the lead tip or ring. Molded *silicone seals* are most commonly used to provide the fluid barrier in the setscrew access port. These seals have a slit through which the wrench may pass with ease and, after the wrench has been removed, the slit will close against fluid penetration. An alternative, used in older devices, has been a cap which is attached after tightening of the setscrew. This cap will seat against the header to prevent fluid penetration.

Inside the header are located *terminal blocks* for lead contact. They are machined of either stainless steel or titanium and use a setscrew machined of the same metal to anchor the lead pin. It may be expected that "toolless" connectors will be available in the future to provide an automatic or semiautomatic electrical and mechanical connection to the lead. These continue to be developed for pacemakers and, due to the increased number of lead interconnects for an ICD, would be an advantage at implant. For a such a toolless lead connection to work reliably with an ICD the much higher voltages must be taken into account.

A header also provides a suture hole to tie down the pulse generator as a preventive measure against migration and erosion. Some devices include the radiologic identification (manufacturer, model) labeling in the header while others include it inside the titanium housing.

Unique to ICDs is the requirement to isolate large voltages (700-800 V) from shorting to surrounding components. This is typically provided by a nitrogen gas atmosphere inside the hermetic enclosure. This gas provides a dry, high breakdown voltage barrier to components in close proximity to other high or low voltage components. An alternate method is to coat the internal electronics with a high dielectric strength, semi-hermetic coating such as parylene. If the titanium can is used as an electrode, it is charged at the defibrillation voltage during the defibrillation pulse and is capable of inappropriately transferring the high voltage back into the internal circuitry. In these situations, the can must be treated as an electrical component and be isolated by nitrogen gas, a coating, or a high dielectric strength film (or a combination of these). In some cases, a thin shield is also inserted between the can and the electronics.

Reliability

In order to provide a reliable device, the pulse generator is tested to both satisfy design and process requirements. Design requirements are performed upon completion of the design to verify the integrity of the design. Process requirements are performed on every device being manufactured or on each production lot (depending on the test required) to verify the integrity of the individual device. In the broader scope, the new ISO 9000 requirements[a] have brought a focus to the importance of uniform compliance and auditing (inspections) by outside sources.[4]

Over the past five years, *international design standards* have begun to evolve, driven by the need to provide uniform reliability or compatibility. Compatibility standards include the ISO 5841-3 (commonly referred to as the IS-1 standard) for pacing/sensing lead interconnects and a comparable standard, ISO 11318 (commonly referred to as the DF-1 standard), for defibrillation lead interconnects. These standards have established criteria to verify that standardized leads and pulse generators will physically interconnect and provide a reliable seal against fluid penetration through the lead port. These standards help to ensure a reliable fit whereas previous voluntary standards (VS-1 pacing) or attempts to

---

a.   These requirements help to define design and manufacturing general policies and procedures to promote the development of high quality devices.

match a nonstandard termination (6.1 mm defibrillation) have not always been reliable.

General reliability standards have been drafted to provide uniform minimum durability of the device, labeling, and packaging regardless of manufacturer. The two draft standards, Cenelec[5] prEn45502-1 and prEn45502-# (numerical designator not assigned as of this writing), respectively define requirements for general implantable devices and ICDs. For the pulse generator, the primary requirements for packaging are shock, vibration, and thermal stress. The objectives of these requirements are twofold: (1) to ensure the integrity of the device from final testing by the manufacturer until it is implanted in the patient, and (2) to identify any weak physical characteristics within the device that may deteriorate over time and render the device ineffective. After implant, the human body protects the ICD from long term physical stresses.

In addition to these requirements, a manufacturer will internally develop tests and requirements to verify the processes required to build a device. Mil-Std 883 is a military standard for high reliability electronics that is often referenced and modified, if necessary, to meet the specific processes and uses of the device. Tests may include accelerated life tests to verify reliability of an electronics design, thermal shock to identify any long term stress failures within the circuit, and stabilization bake and burn-in testing to identify early failures during the build of the pulse generator.

Size and Weight

As noted above, size is a major consideration in the design of the pulse generator. Larger devices requiring *abdominal implant* can be uncomfortable for many patients, are prone to erosion or irritation, and are more likely to migrate. Pacemaker complications have been reported to be negatively correlated with device size with a leveling out at about 25 cm^3 in volume.[6] This would suggest that we should strive to continue to reduce the volume of the ICD to this approximate level.

Implanted in the abdominal area, a device is physically obvious in thinner patients and impairs various physical work or leisure activities that require bending and twisting at the waist. Even with the advent of transvenous defibrillation leads, the larger device requires an abdominal implant and tunneling of the lead(s) into the vein entry site. A *pectoral implant*, in contrast, requires only local anesthesia (except for threshold tests—and even that is not

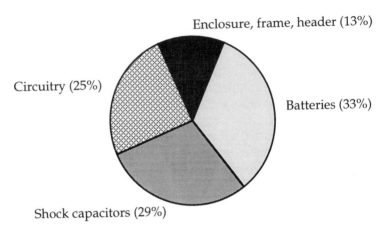

Figure 4. Typical volume distribution of a current ICD. Variations between manufacturers will be due to power output, longevity, and circuit efficiency.

universally accepted), and is quicker and less costly for the patient. The maximum size for a pectoral implant will depend on the physical size of the patient. Current devices in the 60-83 cm^3 range (Medtronic Jewel, CPI Mini, Ventritex Contour, and Angeion Sentinel) are commonly implanted pectorally. Smaller sized devices being developed can be expected to have higher rates of pectoral implants, leaving the abdominal procedure as the rare instance.

Design of the pulse generator begins as an evaluation of three factors: functionality, longevity, and size. All three are important to the patient and the physician and the proportions allocated for each factor are critical to the success of any particular model ICD. Unfortunately, increases in functionality or longevity offer only an increase in size. More efficient power utilization helps buffer the longevity vs. size issue, but battery size is the ultimate trade-off. Increased functionality, due to the increased number of components and power requirements, also works against size. This is true to a limit; much functionality, such as fancier antitachycardia pacing schemes require primarily an increase in software. The increase in physical volume to hold a much more complex software component is insignificant. After defining the requirements for each of the three factors, the requirement becomes singular: *pack as much performance into as small a volume as possible while maintaining reliability for the patient.*

As newer devices have been developed, each of these categories have contributed to device downsizing in specific ways. (See Fig. 4)

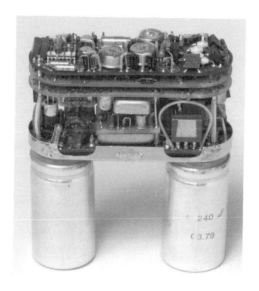

Figure 5. The Intec AID-C (162 cm^3) internal structure showing two defibrillation capacitors under three printed circuit boards full of discrete electrical components. The batteries (removed in photo) would be located between the defibrillation capacitors. This device was not programmable and provided only a maximum output shock, but no pacing.

The components of an ICD may be roughly divided into four categories:

1. Enclosure, internal frame, and header
2. Batteries
3. Defibrillation capacitors
4. Electronics other than defibrillation capacitors and batteries

Compare the internal construction of the early Intec AID-C (162 cm^3), shown in Fig. 5, with the construction of the newer (Jan. 1995 first implant), fuller functioning Angeion Sentinel (about 58 cm^3—including header) which is shown in Fig. 6. These two models demonstrate the evolution in packaging design over the past 14 years. In general, the enclosure, internal frame, and header of ICDs have been carefully redesigned for size reduction: thinner can material, smaller lead ports for the DF-1 leads, smaller internal frame.

Battery chemistry was modified from a Lithium Vanadium Pentoxide (LiVO) to the current Lithium Silver Vanadium Oxide

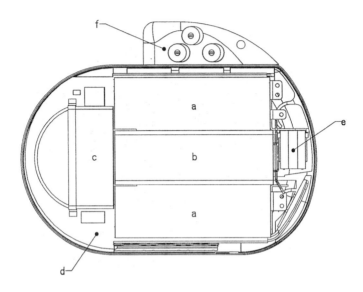

Figure 6. Example of a current ICD internal structure (Angeion Sentinel, volume 58 cm³). Components are: (*a*) high voltage capacitors, (*b*) high power batteries, (*c*) low power battery, (*d*) low power circuitry, (*e*) high power circuitry, and (*f*) header (for lead attachment— shown on top).

(LiSVO) with the first CPI device in the mid 1980's. (Chap. 10) Since then, the batteries have not significantly changed chemically, but more efficient packaging parameters have produced a higher energy density (J/cm³). Some designs have used dual battery sources (LiSVO for defibrillation pulses, lithium iodide for pacing/sensing) to optimize battery usage.[7] The dual battery optimization takes advantage of the fact that the SVO cells—while offering high current for quick capacitor charging—have about half the energy density of a conventional pacemaker lithium iodide cell. I.e., the SVO cells have great strength but low stamina. This dual source design promises to have great longevity advantages if the circuit can be designed to optimize the characteristics of each battery over the lifetime of the ICD.

Defibrillation capacitors have been reduced in physical size because more efficient defibrillation waveforms have allowed lower energy capacitors. Higher energy density capacitor technology is also helping to reduce the physical size of the capacitors. A typical energy density today is 1.8 J/cm³. (See Chap. 11) The electronics subsystems have grown smaller even while functionality—and reliability—have increased due to the continued rapid progress in silicon microelectronics. Smaller high voltage components have become available, integrated circuit density has increased, and denser circuit layout is available.

Future size decreases will be derived from both therapy and technology advances. As more efficient defibrillation leads and waveforms are developed, the defibrillation capacitors and other high voltage components may be expected to become smaller since energies will be reduced. Continual advances are made in further miniaturizing integrated circuits, discrete components, and the circuitry paths. Efforts continue to develop more advanced capacitors. Most of the technology advances in high power capacitors are focused toward military or electric car use and adaptation of these technologies for use in ICDs will require significant time and resources. (Chap. 11)

Battery technology can be expected to make moderate advances using the existing LiSVO chemistry. (Chap. 10) Alternate chemistries will be evaluated as will rechargeable batteries. Rechargeable battery technology is currently being driven by consumer and military usage. Significant research has developed polymer based rechargeable batteries, but use in an implantable product has yet to be achieved. In addition to the technology issues, the medical community and the patient would need to become comfortable with the recharging procedure.

Potential Complications

The pulse generator, in comparison to the lead, is implanted into a relatively protective environment. The device operates at a tightly controlled temperature range and the body structure protects it from extreme shock or vibration levels. It is expected to be a non-deformable structure, whereas the lead is expected to be highly deformable. Materials in contact with the body are biocompatible (as are lead materials) and the hermetic sealing of the can prevents fluid penetration and corroding the electronics, as was common in earlier epoxy potted pacemakers. Most complications are very similar to those seen with pacemakers. ICD specific complications are size related and as the device becomes smaller, these size related complications will diminish. Complications for the pulse generator may be categorized as procedure related or post-implant related.

Header Related Complications

Complications associated with the ICD generator can involve the header-lead interface and include lead port or setscrew port leakage, infection, a loose setscrew, and damage to the setscrew or setscrew wrench. These problems occur or begin at the time of implantation. Lead port leakage is uncommon and, with the DF-1 standard, may be expected to be even more uncommon. *Upon insertion of the lead into the pulse generator, it is important to verify complete insertion by observing that the lead tip has passed through the terminal block.* This will provide assurance that the lead seals are within the seating zone and the conductor pin or ring is within the setscrew contact zone. To prevent leakage at implant, the seals on the lead must be protected from cuts or nicks.

On replacement of the pulse generator, the seals on the existing lead should be examined for damage and resiliency before inserting into the new device. Setscrew port leakage is generally due to a coring out of the seal by the setscrew wrench against the screw. This is uncommon, however, due to much effort on the part of the device companies. It is also easy to identify prior to inserting the device into the patient by looking for a small hole in the center of the seal. If a hole is noted, a gentle wipe of medical adhesive across the seal will seal it. Failure to identify and seal these leak paths will permit current shunting to the surrounding tissue, thereby inhibiting sensing, pacing, or defibrillation.

Loose setscrews have been reported over the years and continue with present day devices.[8] The cause or causes have not been clearly identified, but discussions have focused on the setscrew wrench-to-setscrew interface. There have been instances of loose setscrews discovered post implant, but there is no method of loosening available after the pocket is closed and it must be assumed to be a latent presentation of an implantation complication. Identification of a loose setscrew is not possible without opening the pocket. Symptoms are identical to that of a conductor fracture, and include increased thresholds or loss of capture for a defibrillation lead or inappropriate delivery of a shock or inappropriate pacing or sensing for a pace/sense lead.

A precaution that may help reduce the potential of the setscrew loosening is to remove the wrench straight out of the pulse generator. If the wrench feels stuck in the screw, twisting or wiggling the wrench may jar the screw loose. Torque limiting wrenches have a noticeable click to identify when the screw is secured. Some torque wrenches, however, can be overdriven if they are not held perpendicular to the device. A straight shaft wrench may have no indication of excessive force and an implanting physician must be aware of the force being applied. With either wrench, if excessive force is applied, the wrench will tend to jam or stick in the setscrew socket.

Stripped setscrews or broken wrench shafts (typically below the seal) are caused by excessive force or shallow insertion of the wrench into the screw socket. Either will prevent further operation of the setscrew and render the pulse generator useless as the lead cannot be securely attached. The device must then be replaced.

Other Complications

Additional generator-related complications include migration, erosion, twiddler's syndrome, and infection. (Some of the uncommon electronics failures are mentioned at the end of Chap. 13.) Pulse generator *migration* has been noted with abdominally implanted devices[9], potentially causing additional complications to surrounding abdominal organs. Erosion has been found, particularly with the older squarer-cornered devices in thinner patients. With the relatively large mass of the older devices, it is considered important to anchor the device with nonabsorbable sutures through the suture hole located in the header and attach it to the surrounding muscle fascia.

Twiddler's syndrome is defined as a patient digitally manipulating (or "twiddling") the implanted device in such a way as to produce a force on the lead. This force can fracture a lead conductor whether transvenous lead or patch,[10,11] or retract and distort a transvenous lead from its implanted position. (Fig. 7) Twiddler's syndrome may accompany pulse generator migration if the patient is aware of the movement of the device and attempt to reposition it. The syndrome may be more common in obese women with an overly large ICD pocket.[12] Rectification of this problem requires opening the pulse generator pocket and suturing the enlarged pocket tighter with possible use of a Parsonnet pouch to completely anchor the device.

Infection of the pulse generator pocket is a known complication and may occur at certain implant centers more frequently than others. Some implanting physicians give the device an antibacterial wash prior to implant and then flush the pocket with an antibacterial solution. (See Chap. 18 for a detailed discussion of infection control.)

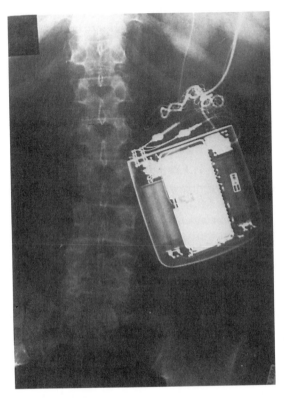

Figure 7. Example of lead insulation failure due to twiddler's syndrome.[13] Note the knotting of the leads close to the pulse generator.

Future Pulse Generators

As ICD technology matures, it is not unreasonable to foresee 30 cm^3 pulse generators. To accomplish this goal, therapy requirements will be redefined by advanced waveforms (beyond the, now conventional, biphasic waveform) and lower energy shocks. These advances will be accompanied by technical advances in circuitry, batteries, and the defibrillation capacitors. Additional gains will be made with smaller, more efficient pulse generator-to-lead connection mechanisms, a potential only delayed by the need for a new standard to be created. As devices grow smaller and provide more functionality, whether it be therapy or additional features, implant procedures will continue to become less traumatic for the patient and less complicated for the physician. The devices will become increasingly more comfortable and provide better therapy for the patient while providing more information for the physician.

ACKNOWLEDGMENTS

Special thanks to Dick Reid (Medtronic) for Fig. 2 and to Lyle Ware for his technical review and comments. Fig. 7 is used by permission of PACE.[13]

1. Mirowski M. The automatic implantable cardioverter-defibrillator: An Overview. J Am Coll Cardiol 1985;6:461-466.
2. Sassouni C. An industry overview of the market for implantable cardioverter-defibrillators. Raymond James & Ass., St. Petersburg, Florida, 1995.
3. Hief C, Podczeck A, Frohner K, et al. Cardioverter discharges following sensing of electrical artifact due to fluid penetration in the connector port. PACE 1995;18:1589-1591.
4. International Organization for Standardization
5. CEN/CENELEC Joint Working Group on Active Implantable Medical Devices
6. Cazeau S, Ritter P, Lazarus A, et al. Pacemaker miniaturization: a good trend? PACE 1996;19:1-3.
7. Adams TP, Brumwell DA, Perttu JS, Supino CG, inventors. Angeion Corp., assignee. Improved dual battery power system for an implantable cardioverter defibrillator. US Patent No. 5,372,605. 1994 Dec 27.
8. Kleman JM, Castle LW, Kidwell GA, et al. Nonthoracotomy versus thoracotomy implantable defibrillators. Circulation 1994;90:2833-2842.
9. Dougherty AH, Wolbrette D. Implantable defibrillator generator migration. Circulation 1994;90:1557
10. Robinson LA, Windle JR. Defibrillator twiddler's syndrome. Ann Thorac Surg 19;58:247-249.
11. Mehta D, Lipsius M, Suri RS, et al. Twiddler's syndrome with the implantable cardioverter-defibrillator. Am Heart J 1992;123:1079-1082.
12. de Buitleir M, canver CC. Twiddler's syndrome complicating a transvenous defibrillator lead system. Chest 1996;109:1391-1394.
13. Beauregard LM, Russo AM, Heim J, et al. Twiddler's syndrome complicating automatic defibrillator function. PACE 1995;18:735-737.

13

High Power Circuitry

Stan M. Bach, Jr., BSEE, MD
and Paul Monroe, PE

THE ICD must have two high power circuits in order to function. First, charging circuitry must convert the 6 V typically available from the battery to the much higher voltage (usually up to 750 V) necessary for successful defibrillation. Secondly, after this high voltage energy is concentrated in the capacitor, output switching circuitry then transfers this energy to the heart.

The nature of the output switching circuitry determines the types of waveforms which are practical with present ICDs. Since the waveform has a significant influence on the efficiency of the energy used for defibrillation (see Chaps. 4 and 7) these circuits have a major influence on the effectiveness of ICD therapy.

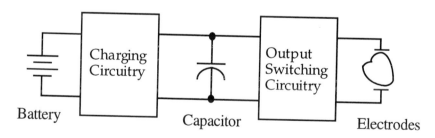

Figure 1. Block diagram of high power components in an ICD.

In addition to the two circuits mentioned above, there are three other power components—the battery, capacitor, and electrodes. Fig. 1 shows these five high power components of an ICD. These are, from left to right: the battery, charging circuitry, capacitor, output switching circuitry, and electrodes. The battery, capacitor, and electrodes are discussed in Chaps. 10, 11, and 9 respectively.

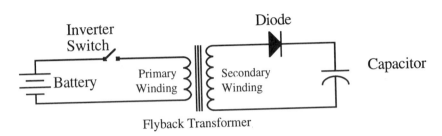

Figure 2. Simplified charging (inverter or DC/DC converter) circuit. The 6 V battery transfers energy to the capacitor via the transformer, repetitively and in a cumulative fashion through the rapid on-off cycling of the inverter switch.

The Charging Circuit

The basic charging circuit, also known as a DC/DC converter, or *inverter* is shown in Fig. 2. The circuit consists of the battery, a transformer, an inverter switch, a diode and the energy storage capacitor. Since capacitor technology currently provides capacitors that are capable only of about 375 V, two must be connected in series in order to achieve a 750 V voltage. For simplicity, in this circuit and all following, the capacitor is shown as a single device. The emphasis of this section is on the basic operation of the transformer and the charging circuit as a whole.

Interconvertability of Electrical and Magnetic Energy

To fully understand the charging circuit, one must first understand the relationship between electricity and magnetism. A current in a wire creates a magnetic field proportional to the current; conversely, a varying magnetic field near a wire causes a current. A familiar example in which a current causes a magnetic field is a junkyard electromagnet. The magnet suspended from a crane used to lift automobiles is simply a wire wrapped around an iron core with a current passing through it. In this case of the electromagnet, the electrical energy is converted to magnetic energy. This works with either DC or AC current. In a transformer, the magnetic energy is converted once again to electrical energy, typically at a different voltage. This conversion works only with AC, as only a varying magnetic field will induce a voltage into a wire. (If this were not the case then the earth's steady magnetic field would wreak havoc on our utility power distribution system.)

The transfer of energy between electricity and magnetism is the basis for the most important part of the charging circuitry, the transformer. A transformer has two separate wire windings, a primary and a secondary, that are wrapped around a (typically ferrous) core. The transformer in the ICD charging circuit simply transfers electrical energy from its primary (battery side) to magnetic energy in its core which, in turn, transfers electrical energy to the secondary (capacitor side). This magnetic field energy is proportional to the square of the current (I):

$$\text{Energy} = \frac{1}{2} \cdot L \cdot I^2$$

The proportionality constant, L, is referred to as the inductance of the transformer (in henries). The inductance, L, is a property of both the geometry of the circuit and the materials near the coil. A given length of wire when wound in the shape of a coil will concentrate the magnetic field and have many times the inductance of that same wire in a single loop. Furthermore, if the same coil is wound over a core consisting of a magnetic material, the inductance will be anywhere from 10-20,000 times greater than if the core were air or a non-magnetic material. This is why conventional power transformers contain steel cores and are heavy.

The Capacitor Charging Process
The operation of the capacitor charging circuit commences when the inverter switch is closed. This initially results in a primary current that increases approximately linearly with time as the transformer is being "charged up" with magnetic energy. At a point at which the transformer is nearly saturated (with magnetic energy storage) the switch is opened. This is done automatically by the inverter control circuitry. The saturation point is either estimated by monitoring the time since switch closure or by measuring the actual primary current.

When the inverter switch opens, the current loses its original path. Recall that the energy in the magnetic field is proportional to the current squared. Energy must be conserved in a closed system such as the transformer. Thus a new current must appear through a new path, to conserve the original energy. The only remaining path is through the secondary winding, the diode, and into the capacitor. (Fig. 2) The magnetic field energy provides the voltage necessary to "push" the current into the capacitor. The current continues to flow until the magnetic energy in the collapsing magnetic field has been

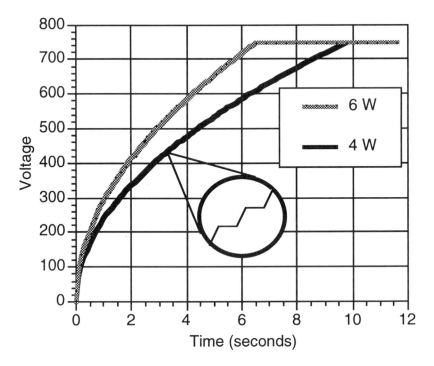

Figure 3. Voltage as a function of time in a typical ICD capacitor charging circuit. Results of charger output power of 4 W and 6 W are depicted for a typical 140 μF capacitor. The magnified area has dimensions of about 0.1 ms and shows how the capacitor is "pumped up" in small voltage steps. Charge times are 6.5 s and 9.5 s.

converted to electrical energy stored in the capacitor—supplementing any pre-existing stored energy.

The diode prevents the flow of the capacitor charge back into the transformer secondary. This is analogous to the operation of the aortic valve preventing retrograde flow from the (pressure charged) compliant aorta and arterial tree back into the ventricle after the ventricle returns to a lower pressure. Thus with each on-off cycle of the inverter switch the transformer repetitively and cumulatively "pumps up" the voltage in the capacitor.

Note the voltage accumulation curves in Fig. 3. They are proportional to the square root of time. The energy in the capacitor, however, increases linearly over time, during charging. As discussed later (under "Efficiency Limitations") the linear increase of the energy is equal to the power of the inverter. That is, a 4 W inverter will charge the capacitor at the rate of 4 joules per second since a joule is precisely a watt-second. However, since the capacitor energy is proportional to the voltage squared (Chap. 4,

Eq. 12) the voltage increases as the *square root* of time. This is seen for a 140 µF capacitor being charged at rates of 6 W and 4 W in the two curves of Fig. 3.

Note the magnified portion of the 4 W curve. Here one sees the flat regions during which time the magnetic field is being charged (current through primary) and the upslope regions during which time the capacitor is being charged (current through secondary). Thus, on a microscopic level, the capacitor voltage does not increase smoothly but rather "ratchets" up to its maximum.

In its simplest form, the inverter switch is controlled by a high-frequency (e.g., 50 kHz) oscillator. The microprocessor (Chap. 8) turns on the oscillator after a tachycardia (for which a shock is indicated) is detected and turns it off after the capacitor attains the desired voltage for the programmed energy.

The Flyback Transformer

The transformer used in an ICD charging circuit is called a "flyback" transformer. A conventional power transformer continuously transfers power from the primary to the secondary winding. In contrast, the flyback transformer gets its name from the fact that it delivers power through the secondary winding only during the collapse of the magnetic field—which occurs when the primary current is removed. When this happens, the secondary voltage abruptly changes polarity—or "flies back".

The flyback transformer used in ICDs is quite small for the power levels involved (5-10 W). This is allowable due to the high frequency at which it is operated (see next section). The transformer wire is of small diameter, which increases its resistance, and hence, the circuit power lost as heat. This is, again, allowable since the circuit need operate only intermittently (when a shock is required), Likewise, the core itself can be of smaller size than if the circuit were designed to operate continuously. These two factors cause the transformer to begin to heat up (in some ICDs) when the circuit is operating, but the temperature rise is not significant due to the short charge time (5-15 s). This heating can lower the charging efficiency and increase charge times slightly for the last shocks in a multi-shock full energy therapy regimen.

Efficiency Limitations

Ferro-magnetic materials within the transformer core allow a tremendous increase in energy density. However, they do have some disadvantages that must be taken into consideration when designing a transformer. The primary one is *hysteresis*. The magnetic field in a ferro-magnetic material depends not only on the coil current, but on the past history of the field. Suppose a ferro-magnetic coil current is alternated by increasing it in one direction, decreasing it to zero and then increasing it in the opposite direction and again returning it to zero. A plot of the resulting magnetic field strength verses the applied current intensity will produce a curve known as a hysteresis loop which looks like two probability-of-success sigmoid curves (with different DFTs) connected at the ends. The value of the energy lost per current cycle is represented by the area inside the hysteresis loop.

As a result, in a defibrillator circuit, more battery energy must be applied to the coil to make up for the energy lost. This "hysteresis loss" decreases the charging circuit efficiency. Equally important efficiency losses arise from the inverter switch (typically a MOSFET—see next section) and the transformer windings.

Closely related to hysteresis loss is the important choice of a switching rate for the charging circuit. A typical circuit will deliver a charge of 30 J to the capacitor over a period of 5 s. With a switching frequency of 50 kHz there will be 5 s · 50 kHz = 250,000 switching cycles. Thus the transformer must store a magnetic energy of 30 J / 250,000 cycles = 120 µJ per switching cycle.

The magnetic energy storage requirement, small in this case, essentially determines the size of the transformer. Thus, the high switching frequency allows the transformer to be very small (on the order of 1 cm^3). Contrast this to the size of a wall-plug transformer for an electronic device. Even though these also deliver about 30 J/ 5 s = 5 W, they are much larger since they must operate at the lower 60 Hz utility power frequency and thereby store 5 W/ 60 Hz = 83,333 µJ per cycle. These transformers must also be larger since they are operated continuously.

High frequency switching, however, increases hysteresis losses. The inverter switch also introduces some losses with each switching cycle. Thus, the choice of switching frequency must achieve a compromise between transformer size and charging efficiency. Efficiency is also influenced by winding techniques, number of "turns," and the wire diameter; attempts to enhance these factors, here too, must be balanced against the desire to minimize transformer size.

The charging circuit efficiency has a major impact on charge times and, hence, therapy delay. A typical overall efficiency for the charging circuit is about 75%. Thus, if the battery is capable of supplying 8 W of power, the inverter will be able to supply only 6 W (i.e., 75% of 8 W). The charging time for a 30 J stored energy shock is thus 5 s = 30 J/ 6 W, as opposed to 3.75 s = 30 J/ 8 W, if 100% charging efficiency could be attained. Of course, the primary concern in the charging circuit design is reliability and thus some design approaches, which could increase efficiency at the expense of reliability, are not used.

The Discharge Circuit

After the charging circuit has done its job to fill the capacitor with energy, another circuit must deliver that energy to the heart. Over the years, this "discharge circuit" has used many different switching components, circuitry designs, and timing approaches. The large voltages and extreme currents involved introduce important reliability considerations. This section will hence be broken up into parts covering the switches, the circuit designs, the timing, and the reliability issues.

Electronic Switches

The energy transfer to the heart is accomplished by high power electronic switches which operate either completely on or completely off. These components reduce energy loss, while carrying a high current, since "fully on" devices generally have a resistance of $0.5 \, \Omega$ or less. This is about 1% of the value of the combined heart and electrode resistance which is typically $50 \, \Omega$. Since energy transfer is proportional to resistance, nearly 99% of the energy delivered from the capacitor is dissipated outside the electronic switch, most of it in the tissue-electrode interface and bulk resistance of the heart.

The high power switches must control a very high peak current. For example, with a unipolar transvenous electrode system resistance of $45 \, \Omega$ and a peak voltage of 750 V, the peak current is 18.8 A. This represents a peak power of 14,100 W. The electronic switch capabilities and output circuit design challenge may be appreciated by comparing this to the typical stereo amplifier of 200 W output; or to the peak power delivered during cold weather car starting which is only about 5,000 W.

There are four common types of high power electronic switches. The schematic symbols for these are shown in Fig. 4. The switches are all three terminal devices. In each case shown, the control terminal is on the left, and the current flows from the top to the bottom terminal. The Metal Oxide Semiconductor Field Effect Transistor (MOSFET) is turned on by the application of a voltage

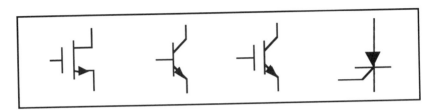

Figure 4. The schematic symbols for the common three terminal electronic switches used in ICDs. Left to right: MOSFET, BJT, IGBT, and SCR. The first three are transistors. For each switch, the control terminal (or "gate") on the left, modulates current flow from the top to the bottom terminal. The "gate" of the BJT is referred to as the "base" for historical reasons.

to the gate. This is also known as the Insulated Gate FET (IGFET) since DC current cannot pass through the gate to the other terminals.

The common classic Bipolar Junction Transistor (BJT) is not used in ICD output circuitry and is shown only for continuity. It has a very low output on-resistance but requires a current injected into the base in order to be turned on. As one might infer from the symbols, the IGBT is a hybrid of the BJT and the MOSFET, combining the desirable input characteristics of the MOSFET with the output characteristics of the BJT. It is commonly used in biphasic bridge circuitry. It requires only a voltage (no DC current) for turn-on (like the MOSFET/IGFET) and yet has the low output on-resistance of a BJT, hence its name. The Silicon Controlled Rectifier (SCR) was used in monophasic circuits and is still used in parts of some output bridges for generating biphasic waveforms.

The high power switches must be carefully mounted in order to minimize the electrical resistance to the substrate (connections of circuit). Any excessive connection resistance can lead to huge peak power losses and temperature rises which can destroy the device when it is passing large currents. For example, a solder joint with a resistance of only 1 Ω will generate 900 W of power when passing a current of 30 A. (Chap. 4) Imagine the heat of a 900 W light bulb concentrated on the tiny dot of solder or the attached electronic switch, and it will be appreciated that this extra resistance can generate enough of a temperature rise to destroy the solder joint or the switch.

Wire connections to the device must also be rugged. Because there are large voltage differences and small distances between the terminals of the device, arcing of high voltages can be a problem. Providing a surrounding gas environment of 100% dry nitrogen (a good insulator) is one method used to overcome the arcing problem.

Specific electronic switches will now be discussed in more detail.

The Silicon Controlled Rectifier

The silicon controlled rectifier (SCR) was the first electronic high power switch to be used in an ICD. SCRs have a number of desirable characteristics. One very useful characteristic is that they are easy to turn on. Injecting a current into the gate of only 0.1% of the switched current is all that is required. This turn-on, or "trigger," current need only be present for about 1 μs. Because SCRs are so easy to turn on, care must be taken in the design of their gate circuitry in order to eliminate false triggering. Also, once the SCR is turned on, it stays on until its current is reduced below a very low level known as its "holding" current. This feature is a disadvantage for biphasic circuitry since the switches must be turned off between the positive and negative phases. (See next section.)

The SCRs used in ICDs are capable of briefly passing currents as high as 400 A. This is ten times the current the device is expected to deliver to the heart. Thus there are no concerns about the current capability of these devices. However, these SCRs are generally operated close to their maximum rated voltage in order to reduce size, since higher voltage devices are necessarily physically larger. For instance, devices rated for 1000 V by the manufacturer will be required to switch 750 V. Due to the relatively low frequency of shock delivery, however, this level of voltage *safety margin* is very adequate.

Insulated Gate Devices: MOSFETs and IGBTs

For multiphasic output pulse designs, the most important electronic switches are the MOSFETs and the IGBTs (Insulated Gate Bipolar Transistor). These high power devices were developed to replace SCRs in industrial motor control applications. The IGBT and new power MOSFET have nearly ideal switching characteristics: low on resistance at high current, high rated voltage (up to 1000 V), and high input (gate) resistance. The insulated gate means that the device which provides the signal to the high power switch need supply no DC current. This low current requirement allows the "driving" device circuitry to be smaller and less complex.

The MOSFET terminals are: drain, source, and gate. The IGBT terminals are: collector, emitter, and gate. The terms drain, source, collector, and emitter were chosen historically to refer to inputs and outputs of charge carriers. No other significance need be attached to them.

Switching on is accomplished by application of a positive voltage to the gate terminal. While no DC current is required, 10-15 V is necessary to turn these devices on. This is a complication since ICD batteries are typically only 6 V. A low power DC/DC converter is used to boost the 6 V to a level useful in switching the IGBT or MOSFET (e.g. 15 V). When the gate voltage is removed, the devices turn off almost immediately. This is in sharp contrast to SCRs which remain on until their current is reduced below their holding current. It is this feature, rapid turn on and turn off at 1000 V, which makes MOSFETs and IGBTs useful in generating biphasic defibrillating waveforms. (See below.)

IGBTs and power MOSFETs for implantable devices are not as rugged as SCRs. Their peak current handling capability is only about 100 A vs. 400 A (or more) for the SCR. However, it is impractical to design output waveforms which reverse polarity using only SCR devices. For this reason, combined use of SCR and IGBT devices in the same circuit (or a pure IGBT circuit) is popular for biphasic devices.

Output Circuit Designs

The high voltage output circuitry of an ICD transfers the energy stored in the high voltage capacitor(s) to the heart. It should perform this function with minimal wasted energy, since implantable batteries and capacitors have limited energy capacity. The time course of energy delivery is also critical. Only a few voltage waveforms that can be generated by implantable circuitry are also currently known to be useful for internal defibrillation of the heart. These are the monophasic truncated exponential, the sequential monophasic truncated exponential, and the biphasic truncated exponential.

The Schuder Monophasic Circuit

The famous "Schuder" circuit (Fig. 5) has been the standard for the delivery of monophasic truncated exponential defibrillation pulses. (Chap. 4, Fig. 3) This circuit was used in all of the original CPI Ventak devices. Schuder demonstrated, in the 1960's, that discharging a capacitor into the heart and then abruptly truncating the applied current could accomplish defibrillation.[1]

The voltage applied to the heart is approximately that of the capacitor stored voltage. As with any capacitor, the voltage decays with a time course defined by the equation:

$$V(t) = V_{init} \cdot e^{-t/RC}$$

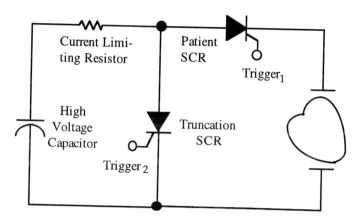

Figure 5. Schuder circuit. The patient SCR is first turned on by application of the trigger$_1$ pulse to its gate. The high voltage capacitor then discharges until truncation is desired. At this point, the trigger$_2$ pulse is applied to the truncation SCR gate. This provides a low resistance path (i.e., high current detour), which reduces the current though the patient SCR to less than its "holding current" allowing it to turn off.

where R is the circuit resistance, C is the high voltage capacitor value, t is time, and V_{init} is the initial capacitor voltage. (See Chap. 4 for detailed discussion of these parameters.)

In the Schuder circuit the high voltage switching to the heart is accomplished by the "patient" SCR. In order to truncate the pulse, Schuder added a second SCR in parallel with the high voltage capacitor and current limiting resistor.[2] This device is known as the "truncation" SCR. At the time that pulse truncation is desired, the truncation SCR is turned on. This "steals" enough current from the patient SCR so that its current drops below the "holding current" value so that it turns off. The current to the heart then abruptly drops to zero.

Since SCRs are rugged devices, very high currents can flow in the truncation SCR enabling it to reliably take most of the capacitor current.   However, some current limiting (i.e., resistance) is necessary so that the current rating of the device and its connections is not exceeded. This current limiting resistor (2-4 Ω) also helps to protect against a short on the patient leads (as might occur with an internal insulation failure on a 2-electrode transvenous lead—a type III lead in Chap. 9). Additionally, the current limiting resistor provides the load for "dumping" the capacitor charge after an unconfirmed episode (in a noncommitted device) or possibly after capacitor reforming. In this case the

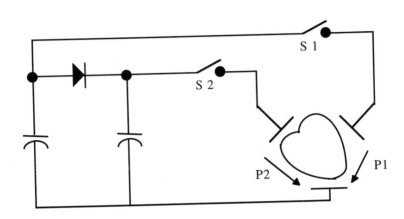

Figure 6. Sequential pulse circuitry employs two different cardiac current pathways. The method uses two separate high voltage storage capacitors. For clarity, the switches in this circuit, and in those of the following figure, are shown here only as ideal switches. In the 7217 PCD they are MOSFETs. P_1 and P_2 are the first and second pathways, respectively.

truncation SCR is used to discharge the capacitor after it has been charged.

Sequential Pulse Circuitry
The Schuder output circuit delivers a monophasic shock between two terminals and over one fixed set of defibrillating pathways simultaneously. Another approach uses three output terminals. (Fig. 6) The defibrillating current passes between two of the terminals for the first pulse and the other two terminals for the second pulse. This is known as *sequential monophasic pulse* defibrillation and is the approach used in the Medtronic 7217 PCD.[3] This method requires the use of two separate storage capacitors.[3] The time between the pulses is less than 1 ms. Alternatively, the switches can be programmed to deliver their shocks simultaneously if desired.

"H"-Bridge Biphasic Waveform Circuitry
Schuder also discovered that reversal of the direction of the voltage and current through the heart during the pulse delivery improved defibrillation efficacy[4]. This method could not be applied to implantable devices until suitable solid state electronic switches operating at 1000 V were developed. Fig. 7 shows the most popular circuit for producing the waveform. This circuit is referred to as an

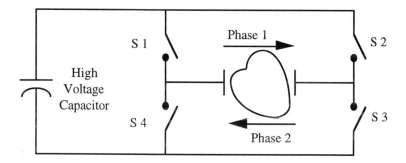

Figure 7. The "H" bridge used to develop a biphasic waveform. Switches 1 and 3 are first turned on. This results in a left to right current through the heart. At the appropriate time, switches 1 and 3 are turned off and switches 2 and 4 are turned on, reversing the current through the heart.

"H" bridge due to the shape of the four switches and heart connections.

Note that the heart and leads are connected horizontally. The circuit functions as follows: At the start of shock delivery, switches 1 and 3 are turned on by application of suitable gate voltage to each. This causes the high voltage capacitor to discharge through the heart with the first polarity and current direction. At a designated time during the discharge, switches 1 and 3 are turned off.

After a brief delay period of about 1 ms, switches 2 and 4 are turned on. The voltage polarity and current to the heart now reverses and the capacitor continues its discharge until switches 2 and 4 are turned off. If two switches in the same leg (e.g., S2 and S3 in Fig. 7) are on at the same time, there is a virtual short circuit across the capacitor and the current would be such that the switches would be destroyed. Recall that each of these switches is actually one of the high-voltage devices shown in Fig. 4. The delay period between the two "phases" of the waveform is necessary to ensure that switches 1 and 3 are both off before switches 2 and 4 are turned on.

Since SCRs are so reliable and easy to turn on, it would be tempting to use them for the biphasic bridge. Recall that the SCR must have its current removed in order to turn off. This is done in the monophasic Schuder circuit by discharging the capacitor. If this same trick was used to truncate the first phase of a biphasic circuit, there would be no charge remaining for the second phase. Thus any practical bridge must include at least one switching device which

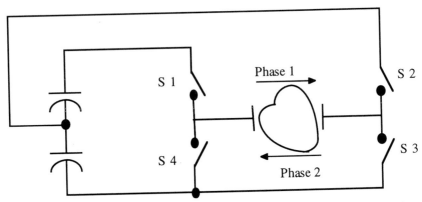

Figure 8. A variant on the "H" bridge. Switches 1 and 3 are first turned on. This results in a left to right current through the heart. At the appropriate time, switches 1 and 3 are turned off and switches 2 and 4 are turned on, delivering a reverse current of *only one of the two* capacitors through the heart.

can be turned off at the end of phase one (without the need to completely discharge the capacitor). The bridge may be constructed with all MOSFETs,[5] SCRs with IGBTs,[6] or SCRs with MOSFETs.[7]

Other Biphasic Waveform Circuitry
One interesting variant on the H-bridge is a circuit which delivers a biphasic waveform in which the phase two initial voltage is equal to *half* of the trailing voltage of phase one.[8,9] Recall that the capacitor shown in the above schematics is actually two photo-flash capacitors connected in series so as to achieve 750 V. In order to deliver the reduced voltage of phase two, this biphasic circuit only reverses the voltage of one of the two capacitors. Its phase one delivery is conventional. The circuit is shown in Fig. 8. Such an output is used by the Ventritex Contour and its predecessors.

Output Circuit Timing
Turn-on and turn-off times of the electronic switches used to deliver the truncated exponential waveforms are controlled by either a timing circuit, which begins with pulse delivery, or a voltage monitoring circuit, which measures the voltage on the capacitor and causes a turn-off when it falls to a specified percentage of the initial voltage. This latter method is known as the "tilt method" whereas the former is known as the "fixed duration" method. (See Chap. 4, "Specification of the Duration" section).

For example, consider the Schuder circuit (Fig. 5) operating with a tilt duration specification of 65%. After the voltage on the capacitor is charged to the required level for the programmed shock energy (say 500 V), and tachycardia reconfirmation is made, then the microprocessor will generate a signal (trigger$_1$) to enable the patient SCR. The voltage on the capacitor is continuously monitored during the pulse. When this voltage has decayed by 65% (i.e. to 105 V) then the microprocessor will generate a signal (trigger$_2$) to enable the truncation SCR thus terminating the shock pulse.

For a fixed duration specification (e.g. 8 ms) the time since the start of the shock pulse is monitored instead of the capacitor voltage. Such a method is used in the Ventritex Contour and its predecessors. The trigger$_2$ signal is then generated at the end of the programmed time. A final approach is a composite of tilt and fixed duration. With this method of specifying the duration, the capacitor is monitored for a fixed decay (say 44%) and then the microprocessor timer is started. Only after the microprocessor times out a fixed duration extension (of, for example, 2 ms) is the pulse finally truncated. That is how the first phase duration is generated in the Angeion Sentinel and Pacesetter Aegis. The second phase is set at a fixed 2.5 ms.

For biphasic shocks using other circuit designs, the control signals will be different but the basic choices remain similar. There are some hybrid timing specification methods. For example, the Guidant/CPI Mini and its biphasic predecessors have a timing technique which uses a 60% tilt specification for the first phase and then records the resulting duration (ms). The second phase is then set to a "fixed" duration of 2/3 of the duration of the first phase.

Output Circuit Malfunctions

Because of the high voltages and currents involved in the high power circuits there are many plausible opportunities for complete output failure. However, due to the extreme care taken in the design, construction, and testing of these circuits, therapy delivery failures are rare. Nunain et al reported 3 circuitry failures (2 capacitors and 1 battery) out of a series of 154 patients.[10] All of these problems were detected on routine followup and there were no adverse clinical outcomes. In the clinical trials for the CPI Ventak P2 involving 1044 patients, there were only 2 failures in the digital circuitry and a failure of the output bridge from a short between the patch leads; no deaths were attributed to these problems.[11] In general, deaths due to therapy delivery failure are extremely rare and are statistically insignificant compared to the other opportunities for mortality in the arrhythmia patient. (See Chap. 23, especially Tables 3 and 6)

In theory, there are also some partial failures which are possible. These will be discussed in the context of the charging circuit in Fig. 2 and the biphasic circuit in Fig. 7.

Extended Charge Times.
Besides the well known battery and capacitor degradations, (Chaps. 9, 10) there are other circuit characteristics which could extend charge times. These include reverse leakage in the charging diode (analogous to aortic regurgitation) which can occur as a partial failure mechanism. Similarly, forward leakage through combinations of two switches in the H-bridge circuitry could extend charge times. In such scenarios, it is possible for lower energy shocks to be stored and delivered while higher programmed energies never are reached.

Reduced Shock Efficacy
For a monophasic device scenario, consider the Schuder circuit of Fig. 5. If the truncation SCR were to fail "open" (i.e., be permanently open, thus never close or "turn on") then the monophasic shock would be untruncated. Animal studies suggest that this would significantly decrease defibrillation efficacy.[1,12]

For a biphasic scenario, consider the H-bridge circuit in Fig. 7. If switch S2 were to fail open then the device would only deliver the first phase of a biphasic waveform. Thus the ICD would be degraded to a monophasic device with possibly lower defibrillation efficacy.

If switch S1 failed in a biphasic scenario, depending on the type of phase 1 duration specification, there might be no shock delivered. If phase 1 was tilt specified then the lack of a current path would mean that the capacitor never achieved its required tilt and the system could not progress to phase 2. However, if the device had a fixed duration specification for phase 1 then, after the appropriate delay for the phantom phase 1, the capacitor charge would actually be delivered during phase 2. This would then be a reversed polarity monophasic shock.

This type of rare failure might be suspected with the failure of a delivered shock despite documented adequate DFT at implant and during repeat testing. The delivered waveform can be monitored by attaching conventional ECG electrodes to the patient's skin surface and feeding the signal into an oscilloscope.

ACKNOWLEDGMENTS

We thank Ben Pless (Ventritex) and Jack Keimel (Medtronic) for their contributions to this chapter.

1. Schuder JC, Stoeckle H, West JA, et al. Transthoracic ventricular defibrillation in the dog with truncated and untruncated exponential stimuli. IEEE Trans Bio-Med Eng 1971;18:410-415.
2. Schuder JC, Gold JH, Stoeckle H, et al. Transthoracic ventricular defibrillation in the 100 kg calf with untruncated and truncated exponential stimuli. IEEE Trans Bio-Med Eng 1980;27:37-43.
3. Keimel J, inventor. Medtronic Inc., assignee. Apparatus for delivering single and multiple cardioversion and defibrillation pulses. US Patent No. 5,163,427. 1992 Nov 17.
4. Schuder JC, McDaniel WC, Stoeckle H. Transthoracic defibrillation of 100 kg calves with bidirectional truncated exponential shocks. Trans Am Soc Artif Intern Organs 1984;30:520-525.
5. Bocchi DE, Laackman JT, Bach Jr SM, inventors. Cardiac Pacemakers Inc., assignee. Implantable N-phasic defibrillator output bridge circuit. US Patent No. 4,998,531. 1991 March 12.
6. Bach Jr SM, inventor. Cardiac Pacemakers Inc., assignee. Biphasic pulse generator for an implantable defibrillator. US Patent No. 4,850,357. 1989 July 25.
7. de Coriolis PE, Batty Jr JR, Shook BJ, inventors. Telectronics Pacing Systems Inc., assignee. Method and apparatus for applying asymmetric biphasic truncated exponential countershocks. US Patent No. 5,083,562. 1992 Jan 28.
8. Winstrom WL, inventor. Intermedics Inc., assignee. Apparatus for generating multiphasic defibrillation pulse waveform. US Patent No. 4,800,883. 1989 Jan 31.
9. Pless B, Ryan JG, Culp JM, inventors. Ventritex, assignee. System configuration for combined defibrillator/pacer. US Patent No. 5,111,816. 1992 May 12.
10. Nunain SO, Roelke M, Trouton T, et al. Limitations and late complications of third generation automatic cardioverter-defibrillators. Circulation 1995;91:2204-2213.
11. Cardiac Pacemakers Inc. Ventak P2 AICD summary of safety and effectiveness data. St. Paul, Minnesota, CPI/Guidant 1995.
12. Schuder JC, Stoeckle H, Gold JH, West JA, Keskar PY. Experimental ventricular defibrillation with an automatic and completely implanted system. Trans Am Soc Artif Intern Organs 1970;16:207-212.

14

The Amplifier: Sensing the Depolarization

Dennis A. Brumwell, BSEE, Kai Kroll, BSEE, and Michael H. Lehmann, MD

THE ROLE of the sense amplifier in an ICD is to register the occurrence of successive cardiac depolarizations, and, thereby allow measurement of the consecutive time intervals demarcated by these events. This is accomplished in a similar fashion to the familiar external heart monitor that relies on electrocardiogram waveforms. Depolarization of heart muscle is the source of the electrical signals for both the ICD and the external heart monitor, but the waveforms are slightly different due to the location and size of the sense electrodes. Surface electrodes sense voltage waveforms (ECG) of a far-field average of the dynamic voltages from the heart muscle. In contrast, typical intracardiac bipolar electrodes sense a waveform generated by the passage of a depolarization wave through a nearby region of the heart. The intracardiac ventricular electrogram (EGM), as recorded by the ICD, shows a much reduced P-wave amplitude and a narrower QRS complex (R-wave) compared to the surface ECG. The sense amplifier must detect this R-wave and mark each occurrence with a digital pulse suitable for rate counting by other circuitry.

In common ICD parlance, the term "sensing" is reserved for the noting of a depolarization; "detection" is the processing of these sensed depolarizations and noting the presence of an arrhythmia.

The Ideal Sense Circuit

Ideally, the incoming cardiac waveform simply would be compared to a fixed reference voltage by a *comparator*, which outputs a digital pulse when the input signal exceeds its reference voltage. (Fig. 1)

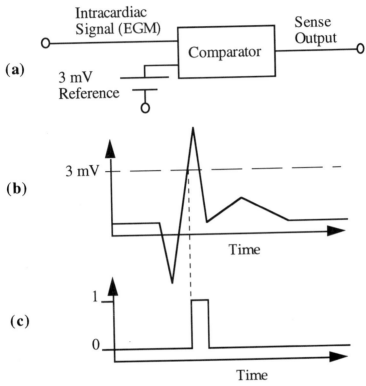

Figure 1. The ideal comparator and output: (a) simplified schematic; (b) a portion of an electrogram (EGM) signal; (c) the comparator's digital output pulse. A 3 mV reference voltage is used in the schematic and shown on the waveform graph.

The reference voltage would be set at a level which is only exceeded by the R-wave.

In actuality, however, besides the fundamental variability of the input waveform (as discussed below), there are technological limitations in practical electronic circuitry for such an ideal comparator. For example, the ideal threshold reference voltage would be on the order of 3 mV (in order to be exceeded by most intra-cardiac R-waves). This is a relatively small voltage level, however; one which is difficult for semiconductor devices to accurately create with low current drain budgets.[1,2]

Additionally, real comparators have a random error associated with them that is often greater than 3 mV, making reliable comparison, of millivolt levels, impossible. Because of these and other reference and comparator related problems, the input signal

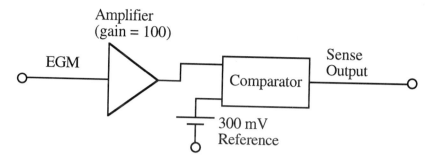

Figure 2. Amplifier connected to comparator to boost EGM signals by a factor of 100. The amplified signals will now be at levels more compatible with good comparator performance.

must first be amplified up to a range closer to practical comparator capabilities.

Amplifier Basics

An amplifier is a circuit that is capable of increasing the amplitude of a given signal. In general, the signal can be either a voltage or a current (See Chap. 4 for definitions.) All electrogram (EGM) amplifiers are voltage amplifiers. Many parameters, such as *gain, noise, dynamic range,* and *bandwidth* are used to characterize an amplifier. In the case of a voltage amplifier, gain is simply the ratio of the output voltage (V_o) to the input voltage (V_i):

$$gain = \frac{V_o}{V_i}$$

An amplifier is connected to the comparator as shown in Fig. 2. As is typical for ICDs, the depicted sense amplifier has a gain of 100 (thereby boosting input signal voltage a hundred-fold); the comparator may now use a more realistic reference voltage of 300 mV rather than the lower 3 mV value shown in the "ideal" circuit of Fig. 1.

Amplification is not without limit, however, as the output signal cannot be greater than the amplifier's supply voltage (i.e. the battery), which may be only 3 V. For example, consider an ICD amplifier with gain of 100 and a supply voltage of 3 V. Such an amplifier is limited to a 30 mV maximum input signal (since maximum output is 3 V = 100 · 30 mV). Input signals greater than this

30 mV value will cause the output signal to be limited or "clipped" at 3 V, resulting in distortion.

Amplifiers also have intrinsic noise due to quantum mechanical and thermal effects in their components.[3] A typical pacing or ICD amplifier has an intrinsic noise level on the order of 30 µV. This level is referred to as the "noise floor," as input signals below this level are masked by the noise and hence effectively invisible.

The ratio of the maximum input level to the minimum input level is termed the "dynamic range" of an amplifier. In a typical ICD sense amplifier with a 30 µV noise floor, a 3 volt supply, and a gain of 100, the dynamic range is $1000 = 30 \, mV/30 \, µV$. In comparison, a typical audio amplifier has a dynamic range of 100,000. The relatively low dynamic range of sense amplifiers requires the use of automatic signal adjustment to maintain detection. The two methods used for dealing with this problem are automatic gain control (AGC), and automatic threshold control (ATC). (See AGC/ATC section.)

"Bandwidth" is the parameter which specifies the range of frequencies over which the amplifier can accurately reproduce the signal. (See Filtering section.)

Even with the addition of the amplifier, many real-world factors further complicate the task of the sensing circuitry. The R-wave amplitude would have to be consistently over 3 mV—even during fibrillation. Further, the T-wave and other noise sources would have to be less than 3 mV to guarantee that every R-wave—but nothing else—is detected. In addition, a sense amplifier has to contend with other electrical anomalies such as direct current (DC) electrode offset voltage,[4] baseline voltage drift, electromyogram interference, and electromagnetic interference due to other electronic equipment operating nearby. Throughout all of this the amplifier must continue to accurately count the heart rate even as the waveform degenerates into the "noisy" low amplitude waveform characteristic of ventricular fibrillation.

Further complicating the sense amplifier system, as well as the rest of the implantable device circuitry, is that it must run on a small battery for as long as 5 years. Clearly the circuitry must draw as little current as possible from the battery which is constrained by severe space limitations. (Appendix of Chap. 10) Typical ICD current budgets are on the order of 10 µA for all monitoring circuitry.

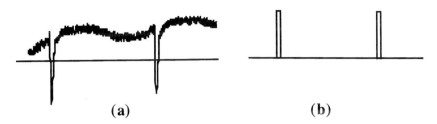

(a)   (b)

Figure 3. Real world input vs. desired amplifier output. (*a*) Sample raw ECG waveform; (*b*) the ideal amplifier output signal.

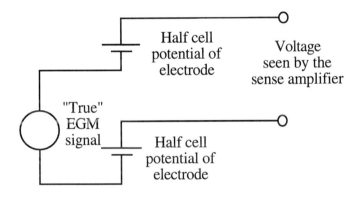

Figure 4. Equivalent circuit showing the effect of electrode half cell potentials, interpreted as extraneous DC voltage offsets.

Electrical Filtering

The raw (unfiltered) electrogram shown in Fig. 3a highlights the problems mentioned above; it has high frequency noise, DC offset, baseline drift and a noticeable T-wave. The goal of filtering is to achieve a signal similar to that of Fig. 3b, i.e., a clean noise-free waveform suitable for rate counting. The filtering circuitry components are physically located throughout the amplifier chain; some filtering occurs before any amplification and some occurs after amplification. These implementation details are not critical to understanding the function and effects of the filtering.

High-pass Filtering

Constant (or background) DC signals are always present to some extent when metallic electrodes are in contact with physiologic electrolytes as shown in Fig. 4. Each metal-electrolyte interface has a characteristic half-cell potential that varies with the type of metal used.[5] Titanium, platinum, and stainless steel are typical metals used in implantable devices. Since a pair of electrodes is always necessary to sense a voltage in the body tissue, the resulting voltage is a combination of the desired signal along with two half cell potentials, one from each electrode. If both electrodes are constructed of the same material (usually they are), a near-perfect cancellation occurs, leaving only the electrogram voltage and a small residual DC offset due to electrode size differences and other second-order effects.

When the electrodes are constructed of different materials, the residual offset can be several hundred mV due to the different half-cell potentials with each electrode. This can occur with unipolar sensing from a titanium ICD housing to a platinum pacing tip. In effect the electrode pair becomes a battery, albeit a poor one. (Commercial batteries are intentionally made from electrode materials with dramatically different half-cell potentials to provide a useful output voltage.)

Adding to the complexity, the DC voltages produced are not constant and vary with time due to physical motion of the electrodes and electrolyte changes at the electrode sites. High-pass filtering is used to deal with these DC voltages and reduce baseline variations.

A high-pass electrical filter passes the high frequency and blocks the low frequency components of a signal.[6] High-pass filtering helps with the problems of DC offsets, baseline drift, and T-wave detection. T-wave detection is also referred to as double counting as it results in two events being sensed for each R-wave. When the signal from the electrodes is passed through a high-pass filter, the DC voltages are eliminated. Slowly varying baseline voltages are also effectively removed. Finally, the filter also significantly reduces the amplitude of the T-wave as the T-wave has lower frequency components than does the R-wave. Fig. 5 shows the low frequency components in a typical EGM signal and the gain reduction of these components due to the filter. The lowest frequency components are reduced the most as shown by the filter gain curve.

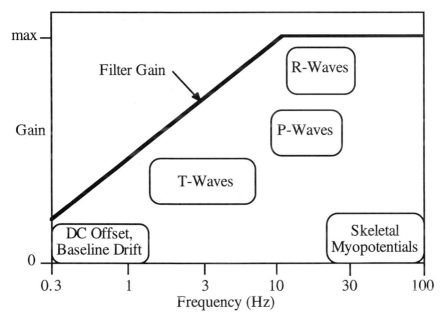

Figure 5. Gain versus frequency for a high pass filter. The high pass filter attenuates the frequencies below the filter's "cutoff" (about 10 Hz in this example).

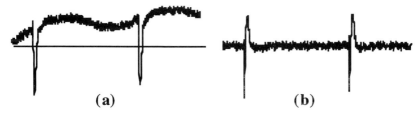

Figure 6. Action of a high-pass filter. (a) The raw EGM waveform and (b) the same
waveform after passing through a high-pass filter with a cutoff frequency of 10 Hz.
Note virtual elimination of low frequency noise components of EGM.

Fig. 6 shows the raw EGM waveform and the same waveform after high-pass filtering. Note that the DC offset, baseline
drift, and T-wave sensing have nearly disappeared.

The side effect of this process is that filtering inevitably re-
moves some of the information in the electrogram by attenuating
portions of the R-wave. The filter cutoff frequency is chosen as a
compromise between "cleaning up" the signal and losing the desired
information. This is reminiscent of the classical clinical diagnostic
dilemma of choosing between sensitivity and specificity. Filtering

characteristics are carefully considered design parameters. A typical ICD high-pass filter cutoff frequency is about 10 Hz, as illustrated in Fig. 5.

High Frequency Interference

Electronic equipment and machinery emit a variety of electric and magnetic fields which can create voltages on electrode systems and corrupt the EGM signal. Chest wall myopotentials[7] and television (horizontal sweep frequency) noise also interfere with signal sensing. These are examples of high frequency noise sources. Fortunately, the majority of these interference sources are at frequencies which are far above the part of the frequency spectrum occupied by the EGM and therefore can usually be filtered out without significant information loss.

However, some signal sources are strong enough, and reside close enough in frequency to the electrogram spectrum, to require that the high frequency response be limited. Even then, some interference cannot be filtered out and could cause sensing problems. External medical devices, for example, are a concern.[8] Magnetic resonance scanners can cause a high sensed rate in pacemakers—not from the magnetic field—but rather from the pulsed radio frequency (RF) signal which is part of the imaging technique.[9] The magnetic field is strong enough to trip magnetic reed switches.[10] For ICDs (e.g. Ventak series) in which the therapy enable is toggled by the magnetic reed switch one should verify that the ICD is left toggled on. In the Mini series the magnet therapy toggling can be disabled. (See Chap. 20 for discussion of the role of the reed switch.) In general MRI should not present a problem for ICD patients.[11]

Lithotripsy can cause false sensing in pacemaker patients.[12] The general contraindication for lithotripsy is perhaps overly conservative, as ICD patients have received the procedure without complication.[13] TENS (Transcutaneous Electrical Nerve Stimulator) units are probably not a problem for sensing.[14] There is one report of a patient (with a Medtronic PCD 7217) tolerating arc welding.[15] There have also been reports of nonmedical device RF interference causing false sensing e.g., a hand held radio control transmitter caused an ICD to inappropriately deliver a shock.[16]

The unipolar sensing mode is less resistant to interference, as a virtual antenna is created of the straight line from the sensing tip to the pulse generator can. (This is not the case with bipolar sensing, as the return path of the ring conductor bypasses this virtual antenna.) The unipoar virtual antenna effect is not normally of concern with ICDs (as opposed to pacemakers) since ICDs are designed to always sense in a bipolar fashion. However, there is a published report of a patient that had an ICD lead insulation defect defeating the normal ring signal conduction path and hence accidentally developing a de facto unipolar sensing mode.[17] This allowed the sensing of his electric razor and resulted in an inappropriate shock.

Some store security systems can cause false sensing in pacemaker patients as the patient walks through.[18] The impact of such a phenomenon in the ICD patient should only be an extra sensed beat which should not trigger any therapy. The only reported case of a patient receiving a shock from a security system involved a man that leaned on such a system while chatting with the cashier.[19] Slot machines, in contrast, apparently do present a high risk of inappropriate shock delivery.[20]

Low-Pass Filtering

Most sources of high frequency can be attenuated by the use of closely spaced (bipolar) sensing electrodes; these theoretically only sense the signals between the endocardial electrodes while unipolar sensing picks up the myopotential signal generated between the heart and the generator itself. Bipolar sensing also can reduce other types of interference as it reduces the effective size of the interference sensing "antenna." Low-pass filtering still remains necessary to ensure that the myopotential noise will not be sensed.

A low-pass filter passes low frequency and blocks high frequency components of a signal. High frequency components of an EGM signal are shown in Fig. 7. The effects of low-pass filtering are shown in Fig. 8. As in the case of high-pass filtering, the choice of a low-pass cutoff frequency is a critical design parameter. A typical low-pass cutoff frequency is about 30-100 Hz. By combining circuitry for both high-pass and low-pass filters, a typical ICD has a sense amplifier "passband" from 10 Hz (high-pass) to 30-100 Hz (low-pass).[a] This range includes the majority of signal energy in the electrogram while rejecting as much interference as possible.

---

a.   Electrogram storage has different filtering than the sense amplifier. To provide maximum accuracy and diagnostic power (to the physician) electrograms are generally stored with broader bandwidths. A typical high-pass value is 0.5 Hz and a typical low-pass value is 200 Hz.

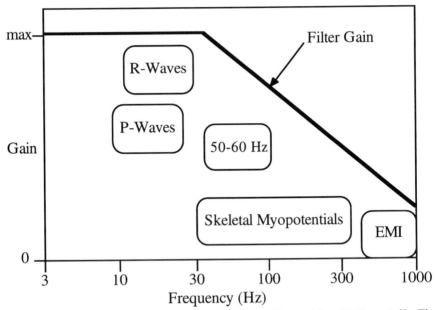

Figure 7. Gain versus frequency for a low-pass filter with a 30 Hz cutoff. The figure shows the high frequency components of an EGM signal, their relative amplitude compared to P- and R-waves, and how they are affected by the filter. EMI is electromagnetic interference and includes RF interference as a subset.

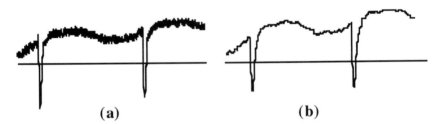

Figure 8. Action of a low-pass filter. (a) The raw EGM waveform; (b) the same waveform after passing through a low-pass filter with a 30 Hz cutoff. The high frequency noise is sharply reduced.

Radio frequencies, per se, are well above the intracardiac EGM frequency band—by a factor of thousands or millions in frequency—but the modulation signals carried may reside in the EGM band. The modulation signals control the amplitude or some other feature of the RF signal. For example a radio control device may have a 30 MHz main frequency ("carrier") but is modulated at 25 Hz. The 25 Hz may be recovered inadvertently (demodulated) from the RF signal by the ICD amplifier. If—in an attempt to deal with this signal—the low-pass filter were set to reject all signals above 15 Hz then the QRS complex would be significantly attenuated and distorted.

As another, increasingly common example, consider the cellular telephone. The European GSM standard carrier of 900 MHz is not a problem per se. However, its 2.2 Hz (132 beats/min) switching component can interfere with pacemakers.[21] Cellular interference with pacemakers is most commonly found with unipolar sensing[22] and this is not used with ICDs. In fact, ICD interference is not seen with North American digital cellular phones.[23,24] There also appears to be no problem with European analog phones.[25] However, the European digital phones can even interfere with pacemakers in the bipolar sensing mode.[26] It remains to be seen if the European digital phones will interfere with ICDs.

Other Filtering

One interference source which is particularly troublesome falls right in the middle of the 10-100 Hz electrogram signal band This is the 60 Hz AC power line frequency pervasive in homes and work sites in North America (or 50 Hz outside North America). Power lines, lights and equipment generate electric and magnetic fields at 60 Hz. Fortunately, the electric fields are largely "shorted out" by the conductive mass of the patient's body. The magnetic fields do penetrate the body but are not usually converted into detectable voltages unless they are very strong.

One of the electronic methods for dealing with 60 Hz interference, if it does appear at the sense electrodes, is a "notch filter." This frequency selective filter strongly attenuates a particular frequency while passing all others. Notch filters must be carefully tuned to the interference frequency and therefore require great stability to be practical. They also can cause distortion of the electrogram. Consequently, notch filters are considered somewhat troublesome circuits. Although common in electrophysiology laboratory equipment, they are losing popularity in surface ECG units and are rarely used in implantable devices.

Another technique for dealing with AC power line interference, which has been used in practical ICD systems, takes advantage of the fact that R-waves are similar to spikes, while power line interference is inherently sinusoidal and continuous or at least slowly varying. By designing the R-wave detection comparator described above to respond only to the "bumps" in the signal rather than directly to its absolute peak voltage, it is possible to reject continuous interference to some extent.

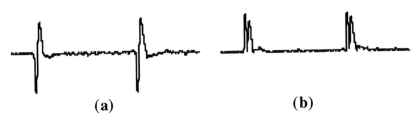

(a)   **(b)**

Figure 9. Action of the full wave rectifier. *(a)* The filtered EGM waveform (pass band = 10-30 Hz), and *(b)* after passing through a rectifier.

Rectification

The polarity or direction of the R-wave signal is unpredictable. This necessitates designing the sense amplifier to respond equally in both directions. Once the signal has been filtered and amplified, therefore, it is common to perform a full-wave rectification, which is algebraically equivalent to an absolute value function. This allows the detector to sense both positive and negative going R-waves. Fig. 9a shows the waveform after both high and low-pass filtering; Fig. 9b shows the same waveform after it has passed through a rectifier. Note that the portion of the signal that is below zero volts is mirrored or flipped onto the positive side. This allows the sense circuitry to use a single positive voltage as a reference threshold. It is this rectified waveform that is fed into the comparator for comparison to the threshold.

Comparator Output and the Initiation of the Refractory Period

The amplified, filtered, and rectified signal is fed to the comparator, and then compared with a voltage reference threshold. When the signal exceeds the threshold, a digital pulse is created. Beginning at the start of the output pulse, a *refractory period* (during which sensed signals are ignored) is imposed to minimize double and triple counting. Typical refractory periods are (in ms): Angeion, 115; CPI, 135-140; Intermedics, 135-165; Medtronic, 120; Telectronics, 70-100; and Ventritex, 135. The refractory period function may be implemented (to varying degrees) by software. It may also be implemented in part by *pulse stretching* which is the use of a long (e.g. 100 ms) output pulse from the comparator.

Some manufacturers distinguish that first part of the refractory period which is controlled by the electronics and call it the "blanking" period. Others refer to the entire refractory period after a sensed event as the blanking period. Chap. 15 refers to this period as the "tachyarrhythmia sense refractory period." These distinctions are not generally relevant clinically. None are to be confused with the hardware "input blanking" discussed under "Post-Shock Sensing." (See Chap. 19, Fig. 8.)

Automatic Gain and Threshold Control

Signal amplification and filtering idealize a cardiac signal for many applications. This is sufficient for a heart monitor or a pacemaker, but an ICD must deal with a wider range of signal amplitudes in order to sense fibrillation from both pre- and post-shock signals. Also, to prevent false shocks the amplifier must reliably detect the reduced amplitude post-shock normal sinus rhythm signals.

The fixed, but programmable, threshold of the typical pacemaker would be too high to detect the reduced signals present during fibrillation.[27] The problem is illustrated in Fig. 10a. The magnitude of R-waves during ventricular tachycardia or fibrillation can be as small as 20% of the magnitude of normal sinus rhythm R-waves.[28] In addition, the normal sinus rhythm R-wave amplitude typically varies over a ± 12% range and can drop much more at the end of a short coupling interval.[29] Unfortunately, the threshold cannot simply be lowered, because then T-waves might be detected (Fig. 10b). This risk of sensing T-waves may be especially of concern in long QT syndrome patients[30] and in patients with concomitant ventricular pacemakers. Therefore the solution lies in the application of an automatic adjustment to maintain reliable sensing.

There are two basic techniques for accomplishing this task. The first is *automatic threshold control* (ATC). In such a system the comparator threshold level is decreased when the electrogram signal amplitude falls. (Fig. 10c) The second is *automatic gain control* (AGC), in which the amplifier gain is increased when the signal amplitude falls. (Fig. 11)

The CPI Mini, the Intermedics Res-Q, and the Ventritex Contour devices, (and their predecessors) use the AGC technique. The ATC approach is used by the Angeion Sentinel, the Medtronic PCD 7217 and Jewel (called "autoadjusting sensitivity threshold"), the Pacesetter Aegis, and the Telectronics Sentry 4310 (called "automatic sensitivity tracking"). Both of the automatic adjustment methods accomplish the same goal of adapting the sensitivity of the system to changing signal levels.

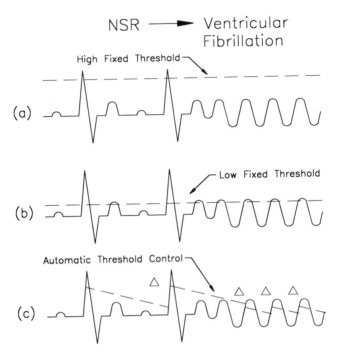

Figure 10. Action of automatic threshold tracking. (*a*) A fixed threshold device may not sense low level fibrillation if the threshold is too high; (*b*) If the threshold is set to a low level, T-waves as well may be counted; (*c*) Automatic threshold control (ATC) can track the lower level signals during fibrillation, while avoiding the detection of T-waves (double counting) during sinus rhythm. Resets of the threshold are designated by △. NSR = normal sinus rhythm.

Fig. 12 shows how the different sensitivity levels correspond to the actual signal components present in an electrogram. Fig. 12 also shows the effect of the filtering on the threshold sensitivity.[31] The amplitude of high or low frequency signals must be very large to cause the amplifier to sense them.

Circuitry Operation
The AGC and ATC approaches, while different electronically, are mathematically related. In an AGC system with a fixed threshold of 1 V the gain would have to vary from 100-1000 to sense an input varying from 10 mV to 1 mV, respectively. In an ATC system, the gain is fixed and the voltage reference varies. For the same input signal and a fixed gain of 100, the voltage reference must vary from 1 V to 0.1 V to sense the signal. In other words, for both systems the effective threshold, called the *input referred threshold* is equal to the comparator voltage reference divided by the gain.

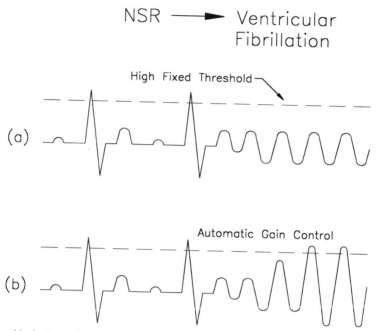

Figure 11. Action of automatic gain control (AGC). With this system, the threshold is fixed, *(a)* but the amplitude of the fibrillation waveform is quickly boosted *(b)* to match that of the sinus rhythm by increasing the gain.

$$\text{input referred threshold} = \frac{\text{comparator reference threshold}}{\text{gain}}$$

The input referred threshold can be controlled either by changing the amplifier gain (AGC technique) or the internal voltage reference (ATC technique). Due to the inherent similarities, many components of the two systems are the same.

The amplitude of the electrogram signal level is usually estimated by a peak detector circuit as shown in Fig. 13. Since the signal is at or near the baseline most of the time between R-waves, the information about signal amplitude is only available at the peak of the wave. The peak detector creates a stored, but slowly decaying, signal which represents the peak amplitude of the previous R-wave. The information is most often stored as a voltage on a capacitor. Both ATC and AGC systems require some memory of the signal amplitude to set current levels of sensitivity. For ATC systems the threshold is then derived from this stored voltage. (The actual

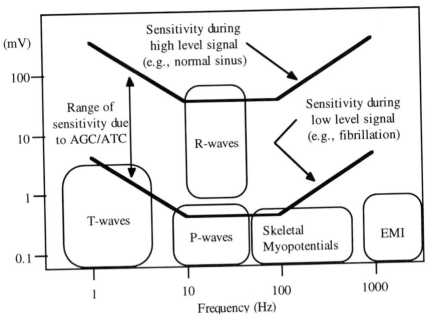

Figure 12. Interaction of AGC/ATC system with filtering. In an AGC or ATC system, the sensitivity level will move up or down depending on the last R-wave sensed. The sensitivity is lower outside the pass band due to the filtering. During fibrillation, the curve would move down to account for the lower level signals; note, however, that the reduced threshold also makes sensing of other signals more likely.

threshold produced will be some fraction of this voltage.) For AGC systems the gain will be determined from this same stored signal.

There are two important design issues involved with the peak detector. The first is setting the fraction of the last R-wave level to be used for the present threshold. A typical setting might be 0.5. In other words, the threshold for the next R-wave will be 50% of the stored peak of the last R-wave. The second issue involves setting the time constant of the peak detector. It is important that the time constant (inverse of the decay rate) of any such memory system be appropriately chosen. If the time constant is too long, then the sensitivity will be based mostly on old events and will not respond quickly enough to changes in signal amplitude.[32] Also the AGC or ATC will miss small fractionated depolarizations preceded by larger ones. (Chap. 14) (These occasional signal "dropouts" result in cycle lengths falsely interpreted as long.) Alternately, if the memory period is too short, then any brief signal disturbance will throw off the threshold to an inappropriate value.

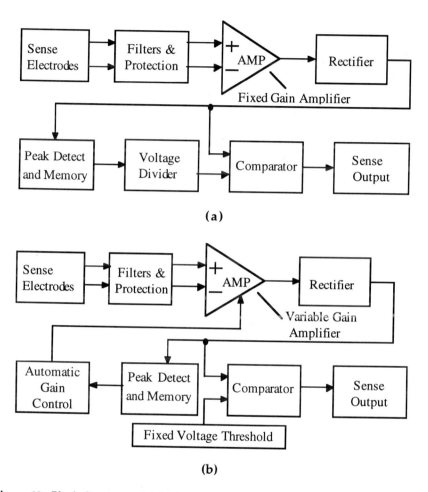

Figure 13. Block diagrams of AGC/ATC systems. (*a*) Automatic Threshold Control (ATC) sense amplifier system (*AMP* is a fixed gain amplifier); (*b*) an Automatic Gain Control (AGC) sense amplifier system (*AMP* is a variable gain amplifier).

The optimum AGC/ATC time constant is a careful compromise between these two extremes.

The dashed line in Fig. 10c shows the ATC system lowering the threshold to detect fibrillation in a system with an appropriate time constant (about 1 s). A typical AGC time constant is 300 ms (CPI Mini and predecessors). A typical ATC time constant is 560 ms (Medtronic PCD 7217 and Jewel). The ATC system used in the Angeion Sentinel and Pacesetter Aegis uses a large time constant for the period immediately after the detection (to "hop" over T-waves) and a shorter time constant after that.[33] Block diagrams of the two basic sense amplifier systems are shown in Fig. 13. The time constant is set by a memory capacitor and a decay resistor in the "Peak Detect and Memory" box. It is interesting to compare the two amplifier design methods. The ATC system is easier to implement but may suffer from limited dynamic range, that is, it can only accommodate a limited range of signal strengths. The AGC system has a wider dynamic range, but it is difficult to describe what the detection threshold of the system is at any given time since the closed loop behavior can be rather complex. In practice, both approaches work and are used in ICDs.

It is also possible to build an AGC system which sets the gain through microprocessor control. Such an approach is used in the Ventritex Cadence, Cadet, and Contour. A software implemented algorithm decides which of 8 different gain settings should be used based on the previous 3-5 sensed beats. (The Cadet and Contour also allow a lower minimum sensing threshold to be programmed; this is called the "Brady AGC mode".) Note that the adjustments are not based on time (and hence related to a time constant) but rather require a certain number of paced or sensed beats for a gain adjustment. An advantage of this approach is that the AGC response can be made very intelligent. A disadvantage is that the response may be slow and detection could possibly fail.[34,35]

There have been some fixed gain devices produced, but these have suffered from undersensing during fibrillation.[36,37] Even with AGC or ATC approaches up to about 20% of patients have rate sensing problems which require reprogramming.[38]

Sensing Limitations

The ICD pacing function can interfere with sensing, requiring reprogramming or the implantation of a separate pacemaker to prevent recurrence.[39] The AGC function is a major offender in this regard, as the increased amplifier gain during ventricular pacing in some ICD systems has been reported occasionally to result in sensing of spurious noise or respiratory artifact that could either mimic tachyarrhythmia or act to inhibit the ICD pacing function.[40,41]

The implantation of a separate pacemaker may itself lead to both undersensing and oversensing problems. Careful separation of pacing and ICD leads may alleviate this problem.[42] Also, the use of "true" bipolar ICD sensing appears to minimize the sensing of pacing artifact.[43] See Fig. 14 for an example of peaceful coexistence between an ICD and an existing pacemaker.[44] It has been reported recently that an ICD with AGC may also allow the detection of atrial pacing spikes in patients with a concomitant DDD pace-

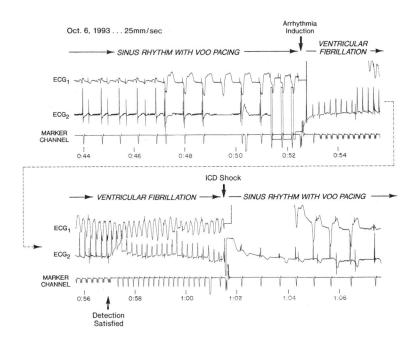

Figure 14. Surface ECG leads and ICD (Medtronic Jewel) marker channel during defibrillation testing. A concomitant VVI pacemaker is temporarily programmed to VVO operation. While pacing artifact is seen on the ECG lead, it never appears on the sensing Marker Channel.

maker, especially in the case of an integrated bipolar lead which will have a larger electrode area for sensing atrial signals; this problem may necessitate reprogramming the pacemaker to VDD mode.[45] Another problem is that a regular VT may cause the pacemaker to go into noise reversion mode which could then prevent the detection of the VT.[46]

There are limits to the sensitivity of a sense amplifier. Even with the best filtering there is a minimum signal level for reliable sensing. This minimum threshold is dictated by an overall noise floor, including all possible sources of interference. A practical minimum threshold, for present electronic technology and current limitations, is approximately 0.15 mV (150 μV). Hence AGC and ATC circuits will tend to have a designed sensitivity limit on this order. This "sensitivity floor" is also necessary to prevent continuous false sensing in the case of signal loss, e.g., with sinus arrest.

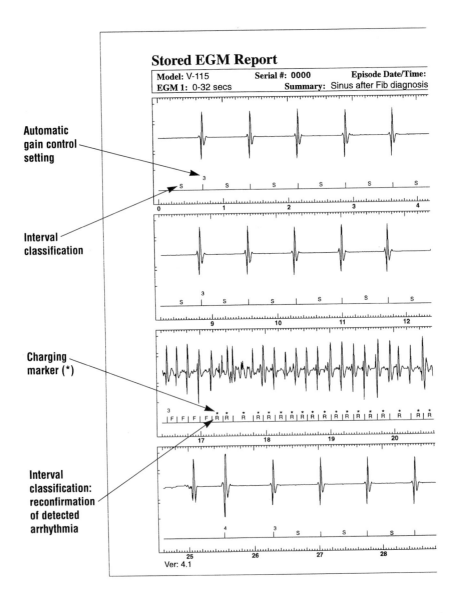

Figure 15. AGC amplifier sensing response. (Ventritex Cadet) Tracings are read left-to-right across the two pages.

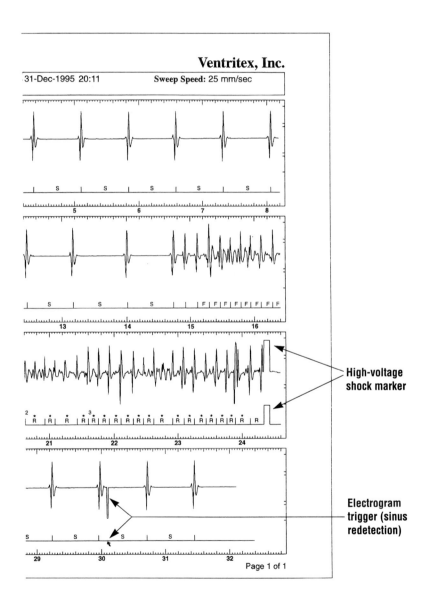

Figure 15. (ctd.) S = sinus; T = tachycardia; F = fibrillation; R = reconfirmation; * = charging.

This sensitivity limit is programmable on the Intermedics Res-Q and the Medtronic Jewel.[47] The Medtronic Jewel has a programmable sensitivity limit of 0.15-2.10 mV. This limit is used in an algorithm to make the ATC less affected by exogenous pacemaker activity. After a sensed beat, the sense threshold is set to the lesser of 75% of the peak amplitude and 10 times the sensitivity limit.[b] For example, if the sensitivity limit were set at 0.2 mV, and a 20 mV R-wave were sensed, the new threshold would be set to: min(0.75×20 mV, 10×0.2 mV) = min(15 mV, 2 mV) = 2 mV. (The threshold would then decay exponentially as is standard). In this way the large amplitude R-wave (possibly caused by pacing) does not render the ATC circuit unduly insensitive. A disadvantage of this approach, however, is the possibly increased likelihood of T-wave oversensing.[48]

Post-Shock Sensing

The sense amplifier must be protected from up to a 750 V defibrillation pulse. Recovery from this massive transient, and from the pacing pulse, must be rapid. (See Fig. 15, preceeding pages.) The design of the electrode interface electronics (to accomplish pacing, sensing, high voltage pulse output in multiple polarities, and protection from defibrillation pulses from externally applied electrodes) is a significant challenge in itself. A network of current limiting resistors and voltage limiting diodes is often combined with the input filters to accomplish this function.

The inputs to the amplifier are also blanked in most systems during these pulses. Hardware *input blanking* involves temporary shorting of the inputs together to prevent disruption of the internal amplifiers. Note that this blanking is implemented only in hardware and stops signals from entering the amplifier. This has no relation to the (much longer) sensing refractory periods discussed earlier.

The problems of ICD system recovery in the post-shock period are particularly acute when coupled with the increasingly popular integrated transvenous lead systems. One such lead system (CPI Endotak series) senses from a small tip to the distal defibrillation coil. The manufacturer refers to this as "integrated bipolar." Since the defibrillation coil is used as one of the sensing electrodes, the defibrillation shock may leave a residual charge

---

b.   The PCD 7217 uses a 6× multiplier rather than 10×, but an otherwise similar sensing algorithm.

(*polarization*) on the coil for some time in this system.[49] The other problem is that the myocardium nearest the shocking electrode is stunned and thus produces a significantly attenuated R-wave.[50] (The AGC and ATC approaches are incompletely protective of such drastic and sudden reductions in signal amplitude.) These effects can complicate post-shock sensing, particularly in cases of failed defibrillation with the first shock, resulting in signal "dropout" and delayed redetection of fibrillation.[51-53] In one study involving the Endotak 60 lead system (6 mm from tip to RV coil) the EGM signals were not back to normal for over a minute and R-waves were typically < 5 mV for 20 s following a successful shock.[57] Although these phenomena have been most extensively studied with respect to the Endotak 60 lead system due to its early and wide usage, similar post-shock behavior might be expected with other brands of integrated defibrillation/sensing leads, depending on the interelectrode distance.

One (electrode) solution to this problem involves using a completely separate sensing electrode pair (i.e., true bipolar sensing).[54,55] Another approach is to completely separate the defibrillation and sensing electrodes.[56] However, good results are usually obtained with integrated bipolar systems (tip to RV coil sensing) when the tip is moved further away from the coil (e.g., 12 mm, as in the Endotak 70 lead[57,52] or 11 mm in the Ventritex TVL lead).[58] One study, however, found no benefit in the increased distance.[59] (For further discussion on leads, see Chap. 9.) It may, however, be possible to design the amplifier to filter out polarization effect (as is done to a lesser extent with Autocapture pacing), thereby minimizing post-shock R-wave attenuation.   Such an approach would eliminate the need for more complicated (or multiple) lead systems. This would not necessarily help with the post-shock myocardial stunning problem, itself.[50]

The magnitude of reported redetection delays following deliberate delivery of a failed defibrillation shock via an integrated transvenous lead system is variable[53,60,61] even rarely necessitating external defibrillation.[52,53] It is not clear, however, whether this is a clinically significant problem, since first shock energies are typically programmed to a high enough energy to assure defibrillation success.[61] From the available data, it would appear prudent to obviate this potentially serious problem altogether by programming the first shock energy to the maximum value. This is especially suggested if the integrated transvenous lead and ICD are from different manufacturers[62] although recent published data gives increased comfort with such "hybrid systems."[63] (A subtlety which arises is that the higher energy shocks are those with the greatest propensity for electrogram attenuation.[64]) Defibrillation testing (at least at maximal shock energy) predischarge and at 1-2 months post-implantation may be helpful in screening more extensively for post-shock undersensing. The precise role of redetection testing following deliberately failed defibrillation, however, remains to be defined.

Final Thoughts

The design of the sense amplifier of an ICD presents a formidable electronic design challenge. The battery current budget for monitoring circuitry is on the order of 10 µA so as to provide a 5-year service life. The list of off-the-shelf integrated circuits which can operate in this restricted environment is limited and rarely useful. As a result, fully-custom analog integrated circuit design is essential. These circuits are referred to as ASICs (Application Specific Integrated Circuits). Design is done at the transistor level, with individual device currents on the order of 20 nA. What other industries would consider to be minor "leakage" currents are used to power whole ICD monitoring systems. These feats are assisted by the constant-temperature environment of the human body and the fact that all of the electronics are enclosed in a hermetically sealed titanium case with low humidity.

The sense amplifier must accurately count the rate of cardiac depolarizations. Because of the low amplitude of the electrogram signals, amplification is necessary. Due to the wide range in the amplitude of electrogram signals, fixed sensing thresholds typically used in pacemakers cannot be used. Automatic gain control (AGC) or automatic threshold control (ATC) techniques are required. The realization of these systems is constrained by tight physical size and power restrictions. Extensive testing during the design phase is essential to bring confidence in the detection system to a very high level. This usually involves playing recordings from multi-electrode catheters through the proposed analog circuitry while monitoring system response. In practice, perfect performance has not yet been demonstrated. Awareness of ICD sense amplifier limitations can enable physicians to better recognize and, in many cases, minimize the occurrence of various oversensing and undersensing problems.

ACKNOWLEDGMENTS

Thanks to Ben Pless (Ventritex) for his assistance. Fig. 14 is used by permission of the American Heart Journal.[44]

1. Gregorian R, et al. Analog MOS Integrated Circuits for Signal Processing. New York: John Wiley & Sons;1986.

2. Allen P, Holberg D. CMOS Analog Circuit Design. New York: Holt, Rinehart and Winston;1987.

3. Ott HW. Noise Reduction Techniques in Electronic Systems. New York: John Wiley & Sons;1975.

4. Strong P, et al. Biophysical Measurements, 1st ed. Beaverton, Oregon: Tektronix, Inc.;1973.

5. Bahill A. Bioengineering: Biomedical, Medical and Clinical Engineering, Englewood Cliffs:Prentice-Hall;1981.

6. Webster JG. Medical Instrumentation. Boston: Houghton Mifflin;1978.

7. Rosenqvist M, Norlander R, Andersson M, et al. Reduced incidence of myopotential pacemaker inhibition by abdominal generator implantation. PACE 1986;9 :417-421.

8. Hayes DL, Vlietstra RE. Pacemaker malfunction, Ann Intern Med 1993;119:828-835.

9. Erlebacher JA, Cahill PT, Pannizzo F, et al. Effect of magnetic resonance imaging on DDD pacemakers. Am J Cardiol 1986;57:437-440.

10. Lauck G, von Smekal A, Wolke S, et al. Effects of nuclear magnetic resonance imaging on cardiac pacemakers. PACE 1995;18:1549-1555.

11. Gimbel JR, Johnson D, Levine PA, et al. Safe performance of magnetic resonance imaging on five patients with permanent cardiac pacemakers. PACE 1996;19:913-919.

12. Abber JC, Langberg J, Mueller SC, et al. Cardiovascular pathology and extracorporeal shock wave lithotripsy. J Urol 1988;140:408-409.

13. Venditti FJ, Martin D, Long AL, et al. Renal extracorporeal shock wave lithotripsy performed in patient with implantable cardioverter defibrillator. PACE 1991;14:1323-1325.

14. Rasmussen MJ, Hayes DL, Vlietstra RE, et al. Can transcutaneous electrical nerve stimulation be safely used in patients with permanent cardiac pacemakers? Mayo Clinic Proc 1988;63:443-445.

15. Embil JM, Geddes JS, Foster D, et al. Return to arc welding after defibrillator implantation. PACE 1993;16:2313-2318.

16. Man KC, Davidson T, Langberg JJ, et al. Interference from a hand held radio frequency remote control causing discharge of an implantable defibrillator. PACE 1993;16:1756-1758.

17. Seifert T, Block M, Borggrefe M, et al. Erroneous discharge of an implantable cardioverter defibrillator caused by an electric razor. PACE 1995;18:1592-1594.

18. Dodinot B, Godenir JP, Costa AB, et al. Electronic article surveillance: a possible danger for pacemaker patients. PACE 1993;16:46-53.

19. McIvor ME. Environmental electromagnetic interference from electronic article surveillance devices: interactions with an ICD. PACE 1995;18:2229-2230.

20. Madrid AH, Moro C, Martin J, et al. Interferences of the implantable defibrillators caused by slot machines. PACE 1996;19:675. (abstract)

21. Barbaro V, Bartolini P, Donato A, et al. Do European GSM mobile cellular phones pose a potential risk to pacemaker patients? PACE 1995;18:1218-1224.

22. Naegeli B, Osswald S, Deola M, et al. Intermittent pacemaker dysfunction caused by digital mobile telephones. J Am Coll Cardiol 1996;27:1471-1477.

23. Fetter J, Ivan V, Benditt, DG, et al. Digital cellular telephones do not necessarily interfere with implantable cardioverter defibrillator (ICD) operation. PACE 1996;19:676. (abstract)

24 Stanton MS, Grice S, Trusty J, et al. Safety of various cellular phone technologies with implantable cardioverter defibrillators. PACE 1996;19:583. (abstract)

25. Madrid AH, Moro C, Chadli, et al. Interferences between automatic defibrillators and mobile phones. PACE 1996;19:676. (abstract)

26. Hofgärtner F, Müller Th, Sigel H. Können mobil-Telefone im C- und D-netz Herzschrittmacher Patienten gefärden? Dtsch Med Wschr 1996;121:646-652.

27. Singer I, Adams L, Austin E. Potential hazards of fixed gain sensing and arrhythmia reconfirmation for implantable cardioverter defibrillators. PACE 1993;16:1070-1079.

28. Ellenbogen KA, Wood MA, Stambler BS, et al. Measurement of ventricular electrogram amplitude during intraoperative induction of ventricular tachyarrhythmias. Am J Cardiol 1992;70:1017-1022.

29. Callans DJ, Hook BG, Marchlinski FE. Effect of rate and coupling interval on endocardial R-wave amplitude variability in permanent ventricular sensing lead systems. J Am Coll Cardiol 1993;22:746-750.

30. Perry GY, Kosar Em. Problems in managing patients with long QT syndrome and implantable cardioverter defibrillators: a report of two cases. PACE 1996;19:863-867.

31. Ellenbogen KA. Cardiac Pacing, Boston:Blackwell;1992. pp 86-89

32. Bardy GH, Ivey TD, Stewart R, et al. Failure of the automatic implantable defibrillator to detect ventricular fibrillation. Am J Cardiol 1986;58:1107-1108.

33. Brewer JE, Perttu JS, Brumwell DA, et al. Dual level sensing significantly improves automatic threshold control for R-wave detection in implantable defibrillators. PACE 1996; (in press Nov)

34. Mann DE, Kelly PA, Damle RS, et al. Sensing problems in a third generation implantable cardioverter defibrillator. PACE 1994;17:761. (abstract)

35. Wase A, Natale A, Dhala AA, et al. Sensing failure in a tiered therapy implantable cardioverter defibrillator: role of auto adjustable gain. PACE 1995;18:1327-1330.

36. Sperry RE, Ellenbogen KA, Wood MA, et al. Failure of a second and third generation implantable cardioverter defibrillator to sense ventricular tachycardia: implications for fixed-gain sensing devices. PACE 1992;15:749-755.

37. Saksena S, Poczobutt-Johans M, Castle LW, et al. Long-term multicenter experience with a second-generation implantable pacemaker-defibrillator in patients with malignant ventricular tachyarrhythmias. J Am Coll Cardiol 1992;19:490-499.

38. Callans DJ, Hook BG, Kleiman RB, et al. Unique sensing errors in third-generation implantable cardioverter-defibrillators. J Am Coll Cardiol 1993;22:1135-1140.

39. Kelly PA, Mann DE, Damle RS, et al. Oversensing during ventricular pacing in patients with a third-generation implantable cardioverter-defibrillator. J Am Coll Cardiol 1994;23:1531-1534.

40. Kelly PA, Mann DE, Damle RS, et al. Oversensing during ventricular pacing in patients with a third-generation implantable cardioverter-defibrillator. J Am Coll Cardiol 1994;23:1531-1534.

41. Rosenthal ME, Paskman C. Noise generation during bradycardia pacing with the Ventritex Cadence/CPI Endotak ICD system: incidence and clinical significance. PACE 1996;19:677. (abstract)

42. Spotnitz HM, Ott GY, Bigger JT, et al. Methods of implantable cardioverter-defibrillator-pacemaker insertion to avoid interactions. Ann Thor Surg 1992;53:253-257.

43. Haffajee C, Casavant D, Desai P, et al. Combined third generation implantable cardioverter-defibrillator with dual-chamber pacemakers: preliminary observations. PACE 1996;19:136-142.

44. Brooks R, Garan H, McGovern BA, et al. Implantation of transvenous nonthoracotomy cardioverter-defibrillator systems in patients with permanent

endocardial pacemakers. Am Heart J 1995;129:45-53.
45. Lampert RJ, McPherson CA, Lewis RJ, et al. Inappropriate sensing of atrial stimuli in patients with a third generation defibrillator and DDD pacemaker. J Am Coll Cardiol 1996;27:348A-349A. (abstract)
46. Glikson M, Hammill SC, Hayes DL, et al. The importance of noise reversion in pacemaker-ICD interactions. PACE 1996;19:737. (abstract)
47. Reiter MJ, Mann DE. Sensing and tachyarrhythmia detection problems in implantable cardioverter defibrillators. J Cardiovasc Electrophysiol 1996;7:542-558.
48. Jordaens L, Vertongen P, Provenier F, et al. A new transvenous internal cardioverter defibrillator: implantation technique, complications, and short-term follow-up. Am Heart J 1995;129:251-258.
49. Bardy GH, Ensuring automatic detection of ventricular fibrillation. Circulation 1992;86:1634-1635.
50. Lawrence JH, Fazio GP, DeBorde R, et al. Electrical but not mechanical stunning after endocardial defibrillation. Eur JCPE 1992;2:121 (abstract).
51. Jung W, Manz M, Moosdorf R, et al. Failure of an implantable cardioverter-defibrillator to redetect ventricular fibrillation in patients with a nonthoracotomy lead system. Circulation 1992;86:1217-1222.
52. Natale A, Sra J, Axtell K, et al. Undetected ventricular fibrillation in transvenous implantable cardioverter defibrillators: prospective comparison of different lead system-device combinations. Circulation 1996;93:91-98.
53. Berul CI, Callans DJ, Schwartzman DS, et al. Comparison of initial detection and redetection of ventricular fibrillation in a transvenous defibrillator system with automatic gain control. J Am Coll Cardiol 1995;25:431-436.
54. Ruetz LL, Bardy GH, Pearson AM, et al. Paired post-shock electrogram amplitudes for standard and integrated bipolar sensing. PACE 1994;17:743 (abstract).
55. Brady P, Friedman P Stanton M. Effect of failed defibrillation shocks on electrogram amplitude in a transvenous lead system. PACE 1994;17:785 (abstract).
56. Tchou PJ, Kroll MW. The Angemed Sentinel implantable antitachycardia pacer cardioverter defibrillator in Implantable Cardioverter - Defibrillators, Estes NAM, Manolis AS, Wang PJ (eds). Marcel Dekker Inc., New York 1994.
57. Jung W, Manz M, Moosdorf R, et al. Changes in the amplitude of endocardial electrograms following defibrillator discharge: comparison of two lead systems. PACE 1995;18:2163-2172.
58. Callans DJ, Swarna US, Schwartzman D, et al. Postshock sensing performance in transvenous defibrillation lead systems: analysis of detection and redetection of ventricular fibrillation. J Cardiovasc Electrophys 1995;6:604-612.
59. Smith JR, Kadish AH, Inbar S, et al. Local electrogram changes in response to a high-voltage intracardiac shock in humans. J Cardiovasc Electrophysiol 1996;7:387-397.
60. Mattioni T, O-Toole M, Riggio D, et al. Ineffective high energy shocks do not adversely effect subsequent fibrillation detection time in patients with a non-thoracotomy implantable defibrillator lead system. PACE 1994;17(II):850. (abstract)
61. Ellis JR, Martin DT, Venditti FJ. Appropriate sensing of ventricular fibrillation after failed shocks in a transvenous cardioverter-defibrillator system. Circulation 1994;90:1820-1825.
62. Lehmann MH. Hybrid nonthoracotomy systems: lessons from the brouhaha. PACE 1994;17:1802-1807.
63. Porterfield JG, Porterfield LM, Levine JH, et al. Compatibility of a nonthoracotomy lead system with a biphasic implantable cardioverter-defibrillator. Am J Cardiol 1996;77:586-590.
64. Gottlieb CD, Schwartzman DS, Callans DJ, et al. Effects of high and low shock energies on sinus electrograms recorded via integrated and true bipolar

nonthoracotomy lead systems. J Cardiovasc Electrophysiol 1996;7:189-196.

15

Tachyarrhythmia Detection

Stan M. Bach, Jr., BSEE, MD, Michael H. Lehmann, MD, and Mark W. Kroll, PhD

ETECTION of ventricular tachyarrhythmia in currently available ICDs relies primarily on an evaluation of the sequence of ventricular event timing intervals obtained from a rate sense amplifier and comparator circuitry. (Chap. 14) The term "sensing" is reserved for the noting of a depolarization (ventricular event); "detection" is the processing of these sensed depolarizations and noting the presence of an arrhythmia. These timing intervals (also called R-R intervals) are classified by comparing them to a programmable parameter known as a *rate zone limit (boundary)*. Depending upon an R-R interval's relationship to the programmed boundaries, algorithmic detection criteria such as duration (specified in time or number of events) may be applied to the sequence of depolarizations.

Each time a ventricular event is sensed, a timing period known as the *tachyarrhythmia sense refractory period* is started. If another ventricular event is sensed within this period, it is not counted. This prevents incorrect counting of device-filtered signals which typically have more waveform peaks than the original signal. Tachyarrhythmia sense refractory periods are shorter than those encountered with a pacemaker, and range over 70-200 ms depending upon the manufacturer and device operational mode. The sense refractory period may be programmable with a minimum value corresponding to a non-programmable "blanking period". In addition, the sense refractory period should not be longer than half the cycle length programmed for the boundary of the highest rate tachyarrhythmia sense zone. Otherwise, at certain tachyarrhythmia rates it would be possible for every other device-interpreted depolarization to fall inside the refractory period. As a result, alternate depolarizations would not be sensed, causing the rate to be counted at only half its true value. A suitably short sense refractory period, therefore, will ensure that even such an incorrectly measured rate is still faster than the programmed high rate boundary.

A *post-bradycardia pace/sense refractory period* may be separately programmable in order to reduce the incidence of counting the pacing-evoked repolarization response ("double counting"). In order to accomplish this, the value of the post-bradycardia pace/sense refractory period would have to be in a range which exceeds 200 ms. This feature should be used with caution, however, since a ventricular tachycardia (VT) which emerges during pacing may be temporarily masked by a lengthy refractory period (e.g. 400 ms) thereby delaying detection.

Ventricular fibrillation (VF) and VT are the rapid cardiac rhythm disturbances targeted for automatic treatment by ICDs. VF is relatively easy to detect because its rate is so much higher than the normal physiologic range (technically greater than 300 beats/min, but potentially slower with antiarrhythmic drugs). VF produces a chaotic appearance when viewed from large surface area electrodes, but may look transiently monomorphic with closely spaced bipolar electrodes. In contrast, VT often results in a monomorphic appearance on the surface ECG and on any internal cardiac electrograms. The hemodynamic effect of VT is highly variable, however, and its rate may overlap (be slower than) rhythms originating in the atria. The primary supraventricular tachycardias (SVTs) which may be misinterpreted as VT by an implantable device, because of rapid ventricular rate, are sinus tachycardia and atrial fibrillation. Sinus tachycardia represents a physiological response to exercise, stress, etc. whereas atrial fibrillation is a pathological condition in which the ventricular rate may be highly variable.

When the rates of ventricular and supraventricular rhythms overlap, additional algorithms known as rhythm onset and stability may be applied to the cycle length sequence. An *onset algorithm* attempts to prevent classification of sinus tachycardia as abnormal on the assumption that this physiological tachycardia begins more gradually than VT. A *stability algorithm* attempts to prevent classification of atrial fibrillation with a fast ventricular response as "abnormal" (i.e., ventricular in origin) on the assumption that its cycle length variability is greater than that of VT. These algorithms have limitations, however. An onset algorithm will not separate non-sinus SVT from VT, since non-sinus SVT begins abruptly and typically also results in a stable high ventricular rate. Furthermore, spontaneous VT may not always be promptly detected when using a stability algorithm, since VT may exhibit some cycle length variability.[1] An *electrogram morphology algorithm* may assist in further correct rhythm stratification, although widespread applicability of this approach remains to be demonstrated. Algorithms may be combined in logical fashion, e.g., onset *and* stability (meaning both must be met), in an attempt to improve specificity.

After therapy has been delivered, some devices apply a different algorithm to the ventricular interval sequence. Others provide the ability to combine algorithms in a different logical manner or to modify the programmable parameter settings of the initially selected algorithm.

This chapter is a synopsis of tachyarrhythmia detection algorithms currently employed in ICDs. Information about these algorithms has not been widely available, and the algorithms are undergoing change because they are new. The chapter should be regarded as an overview of various approaches to tachyarrhythmia detection. For further information about detection algorithms, individual device physician's manuals should be consulted. Company sponsored training courses are also a valuable source of information. Further complexities related to programming ICD detection algorithm parameters are discussed in Chap. 19.

Detection Zones

ICD arrhythmia detection is presently based on the detection zone concept. The range of ventricular rhythm cycle lengths is divided into a bradyarrhythmia, a normal, and one or more (in some cases up to four) tachyarrhythmia zones (Fig. 1). The boundary between the normal zone and the tachyarrhythmia (presumably monomorphic VT) zone may be called the TDI or tachycardia detection interval. Other designations are the TACH A cycle length, TACH-0 cycle length, or the primary rate limit (PRL), depending upon the manufacturer. If the tachycardia zone is subdivided, the next shorter cycle length zone has a lower boundary called the FTI (fast tachycardia interval), the TACH B cycle length, the TACH-1 cycle length, or the SRL (secondary rate limit). In the nomenclature of all device manufacturers, the highest rate zone (defined by the shortest cycle lengths) is called the "fibrillation" zone, although rapid monomorphic VT may frequently be classified here as well. Its cycle length limit may be called the fibrillation detection interval (FDI), and its corresponding rate is referred to as the fibrillation rate limit.

Each time a ventricular event is sensed, the value of a timer is saved. The difference between this timer value and the previous

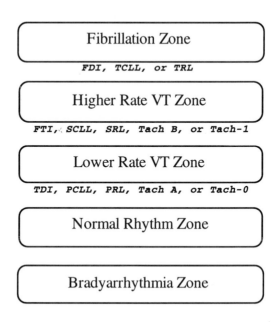

Figure 1. Therapy and detection zones. ICD arrhythmia detection algorithms have been designed to divide the range of possible ventricular rates into non-overlapping zones whose boundaries are specified by a variety of terms. Since devices directly measure time intervals between sensed depolarizations, most nomenclature refers to cycle length rather than rate. Abbreviations: FDI = Fibrillation Detection Interval; FTI = Fast Tachycardia Interval; TDI = Tachycardia Detection Interval; Tach A or Tach-0 = slower tachycardia limit; Tach B or Tach-1 = faster tachycardia limit; PCLL = Primary Cycle Length Limit; SCLL = Secondary Cycle Length Limit; TCLL = Tertiary Cycle Length Limit (more often called PRL, primary rate limit, SRL, secondary rate limit, and TRL or tertiary rate limit, respectively). FTI may be longer or shorter than FDI in one manufacturer's nomenclature and programmer.

event's value is computed. This gives the cycle length time within the precision of the device timer (about 1-10 ms, depending upon the device). In some cases, the timer may be reset to zero after it is read; this allows a direct read of the cycle length without a subtraction. These calculations can be done with great speed using a few microprocessor instructions or dedicated circuitry.

Every cycle length interval detected (it must be longer than the device tachyarrhythmia sense refractory period) resides somewhere in the cycle length (or rate) map range shown in Fig. 1. A detected interval residing within a tachycardia or fibrillation zone boundary increments a corresponding counter for the zone each time it occurs. The count may be incremented for that zone only, or for the zone of the current interval and all lower tachyarrhythmia rate zones. The advantage of the latter scheme is that rhythm cycle lengths residing in more than one zone will probably be detected and treated sooner. Without simultaneously incrementing lower rate zone counters or adding additional zone count summation criteria, it is possible for rhythms to go undetected if adjacent cycle lengths alternately reside in different zones (see next section). All of these cycle length ranges are physician programmable with certain logical restrictions, such as limitation of the bradycardia pacing zone boundary to a cycle length value greater than the lowest rate tachyarrhythmia cycle length zone boundary.

The detection ranges generally provide a direct linkage to level of therapy aggressiveness. For instance, a rhythm evaluated as having a cycle length in the lowest tachyarrhythmia rate zone, e.g. 500-350 ms, may be treated with antitachycardia pacing followed by shock. A second rhythm whose rate is in the next higher zone, e.g. 350-270 ms, may first be treated with low strength shock followed by a higher strength shock. A very fast rhythm of less than 270 ms cycle length may be treated by a maximum strength shock. Under the tactic of *monotonic therapy aggression,* the therapy provided by the ICD will not revert to lower energy levels (or back to antitachycardia pacing) during a single episode of VT even if the rate is reduced (say, by conversion to a slower VT) to place it in a lower zone. Thus, a shock could be provided in such a case even though antitachycardia pacing might normally be delivered as a first line therapy for a VT of the same rate (had it begun de novo).

Device interpreted rates of polymorphic (in contrast to monomorphic) rhythms are not very predictable from the corresponding electrogram recordings. Automatic gain control or threshold tracking circuitry can miss small fractionated depolarizations preceded by larger ones. (Chap. 14) These occasional signal "dropouts" result in cycle lengths falsely interpreted as long. If, however, this phenomenon occurs frequently during a tachyarrhythmia episode, however, detection in a lower zone, extended time to detect, or non-detection will result. This may be more of a problem when an unsuccessful shock for VF is delivered by a transvenous defibrillating lead with integrated sensing electrodes.[2-4] It is thus important that the highest rate zone boundary be carefully selected (and verified by testing) in order to ensure reliable detection of fibrillation. Other factors, such as a short coupling interval of premature beats can also cause amplitude variability.[5]

Duration Requirements for Detection

In order for a tachyarrhythmia to be recognized and assigned to a given rate zone, it must exhibit a minimum number of appropriate cycle lengths. This *duration criterion* for detection may be defined in various ways: the number of consecutive cycle lengths in a zone required for tachyarrhythmia detection; the total number of cycle lengths in a zone; X out of the last Y cycle lengths in a zone; elapsed time; average rate; or some combination of these. When consecutive cycle lengths within a zone are required for detection, a single cycle length residing in the normal zone resets the detection counter(s) to zero. This increases the specificity of the algorithm, but it also may prolong detection for those rhythms with cycle lengths near and intermittently longer than the TDI. If consecutive cycle lengths are required, the criterion is used only in zones intended for the detection of hemodynamically tolerated monomorphic VT. During monomorphic VT, the device circuitry will detect virtually all ventricular depolarizations. The criterion may be sensitive enough to detect if there is sufficient difference between the device TDI and the longest cycle length of the patient's observed VTs. This ensures that future variable rate monomorphic VTs will be unlikely to reset a device detection counter.

During polymorphic rhythms, most of the device interpreted cycle lengths are predominantly short, often highly variable, and occasionally "long" due to signal dropout. Because of these occasionally long interpreted cycle lengths, the *X out of Y criterion* may be used. This criterion requires a certain proportion of the preceding cycle lengths to be in a given zone for detection of VF or VT. The values of X and Y (where X < Y) may both be programmable, there may be a menu of choices, or the percentage may be fixed. These algorithms use a "sliding window." (Fig. 2) That is, if 8 out of 10 cycle lengths is the criterion, but only 7 out of the last 10 are shorter than the FDI, then the next time an event is detected, only the most recent 10 cycle lengths are analyzed; the most remote cycle length is discarded. Thus, the analysis window (10 R-R intervals) "slides" over the cycle length sequence. An algorithm may apply the X out of Y criterion to all zones, with independent X and Y values programmed for each zone.

In order to not prolong detection, a *safety-net duration timer* (commonly called the "extended high rate" or "sustained high rate" criterion) may be employed. Prolonged detection may occur when rhythm cycle lengths occur in more than one zone and a consecutive

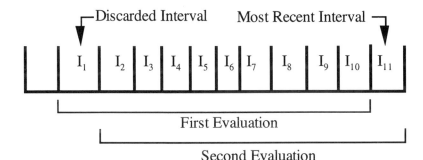

Figure 2. Sliding window for duration detection. Using this concept, only a certain number (in this case 10) of the most recent cycle lengths are evaluated. Within this window, if a certain number of tachycardia intervals occur (e.g. 8) detection may be declared ("X out of Y criterion" where X = 8 and Y = 10 in this example). Both the window width (number of most recent intervals evaluated, Y) and the number required for detection (X) may be programmable. Alternatively, the window may be utilized with a consecutive number requirement (in effect a "Y out of Y" criterion). In such a case, a single interval longer than the zone cycle length limit would reset the detection counter to zero.

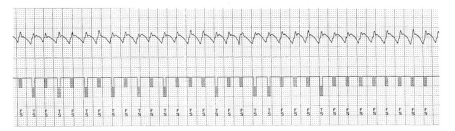

Figure 3. An induced arrhythmia whose rate wanders between the tachycardia zone and the fibrillation zone. *TS* refers to tachycardia sense and *FS* refers to fibrillation sense. This patient, with a PCD 7217B, had a delayed detection interval of 12 seconds. The VF rate cutoff and number of required intervals were then both lowered.

number of cycle lengths in one of the zones is required for detection. An example would be a rhythm whose cycle lengths wander between the tachycardia zone (consecutive criterion used) and the fibrillation zone (X out of Y criterion used).[6] (Fig. 3)

The safety-net duration timer begins when a potentially sustained tachyarrhythmia is initially declared; as long as the detection criteria have not been reset, i.e., normal rhythm has not been sensed, the timer continues to run. Once the timer expires, a tachyarrhythmia detection is declared.

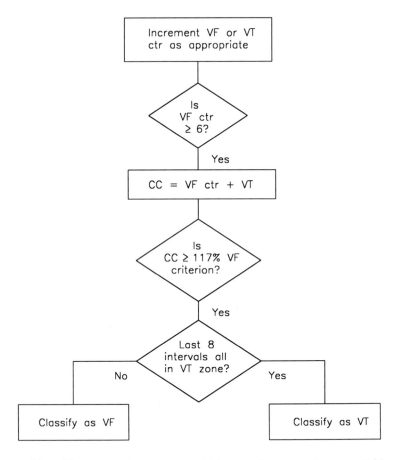

Figure 4. Use of the summation criterion which sums the counts in two neighboring tachycardia zones (VT and VF) after each sensed depolarization. This eliminates the problem of an arrhythmia evading detection by wandering between the two zones. CC is the combined counter; *VF criterion* is the number of intervals to detect VF (12 in example of Fig. 5); and *VF ctr* and *VT ctr* are the respective event counters. The 117% factor (actually equal to the fraction 7/6) for the summation was chosen to be low enough so that there is minimal detection delay yet must be greater than 1 so that it does not come into play before the satisfaction of normal VF criterion during a consistently high rate.

Another way of handling the zone boundary wandering problem is to use a *summation criterion* which adds the total tachyarrhythmia interval counts in the two neighboring zones. Usually shocks are delivered when the timer expires or a critical summation total is reached, since it is presumed the arrhythmia has continued too long. The approach of the Medtronic Jewel is shown in Fig. 4 (algorithm) and Fig. 5 (example).

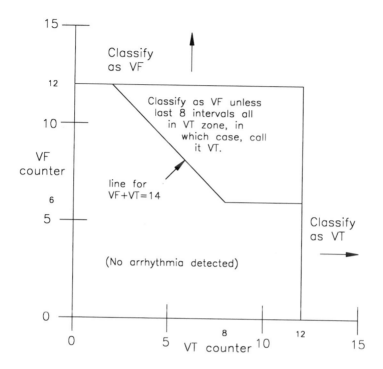

Figure 5. Example of summation (combined count) criterion used in the Jewel 7219 as described algorithmically in Fig. 4. In this case the VF and neighboring VT detection count criteria are both programmed to 12 intervals. The combined count criterion is then automatically calculated as 14 = 117% of 12 intervals. (Fig. 4) Note that the VF count must also be above 6 to satisfy the combined count criterion. This approach has the effect of lowering the VF count "threshold" below 12 for declaration of VF for VT counts of ≥ 3. (For either a VF or VT count criterion different from 12 these numbers will be changed.)

An *average of the cycle length intervals* may be used to direct therapy at the time of detection. An average cycle length may be an average of the last 4 detected intervals, or an exponential average. An exponential decaying average is calculated by multiplying a fraction ("weight" factor) times the previous average and adding this number to another fraction multiplied by the current interval. Typically, the previous average is weighted more heavily (e.g., 60%) than the current interval (e.g., 40%).

Some non-X out of Y algorithms require that a *total (not necessarily consecutive) count* of cycle lengths in a detection zone be accumulated to satisfy the detection duration criterion. In one algorithm, used in the original CPI PRx, total counts are not accumulated unless 3 consecutive tachycardia intervals are first detected.

Subsequently, if 2 consecutive cycle lengths in the normal zone are found, detection is reset and counting begins anew. Detection may also be reset if a fixed percentage (e.g., 30%) of the accumulated intervals reside in the normal zone. In this algorithm, counts are incremented in the zone of the interval and in all lower tachyarrhythmia zones. If the requisite total count for a zone has accumulated, but the last 4 intervals are not all in the same zone, the detection duration is extended until this criterion is met or until a maximum interval duration count has accumulated. At that point, the average of the last 4 intervals is used to place the arrhythmia within a detection zone.

Another non-X out of Y algorithm simply requires that the number of tachycardia intervals be greater than the programmed number for the zone. In this scheme, used in the Ventritex Contour and its predecessors, both the current interval and the average of this interval and the previous three intervals must be in a zone to increment its count. If the current interval and the average are in different zones, the count in the zone with the shorter cycle length is incremented. If either the average or the interval itself is in the normal zone, the interval is not counted. If both the interval and its average are in the normal zone, a sinus counter is incremented. An accumulated number of counts in the sinus counter causes a reset of the tachycardia detection counter; whereas the sinus counter is reset when a single tachycardia interval is declared.

Detection During and After Capacitor Charging

Because charging of the defibrillator high voltage capacitors creates significant noise within the pulse generator enclosure, some device algorithms do not attempt detection during this time. In others, if the rhythm spontaneously terminates during charging, and the algorithm recognizes this fact, capacitor charging is halted. If, after charging the high voltage capacitors, an algorithm recognizes that the arrhythmia has spontaneously terminated, the charge may not be delivered but, instead, simply held and permitted to slowly dissipate, or dumped to an internal load resistor. This is known as a "second look" detection capability.

After charging has begun, non-delivery of a charge to the patient, in response to a spontaneously terminating rhythm, is known as *noncommitted shock*. For instance, if VF is detected, *reconfirmation* (redetection of a tachycardia interval) is attempted after the high voltage capacitors are charged. Delivery of the shock after charging has begun, irrespective of the tachyarrhythmia condition, is known as *committed shock* Most algorithms employ noncommitted shock under some circumstances, but committed shock at other times.

Detection of a fibrillation interval results in a synchronous shock. If no event at all is found during a *time-out period* (typically 1 or 2 seconds), then the tachycardia is presumed to be ongoing with signal dropout; the shock will then be delivered asynchronously, particularly if the detection occurred in the highest or "fibrillation" zone. This is a form of committed shock. On the other hand, if intervals longer than TDI are detected during the synchronization time, the shock may not be delivered during further analysis of the rhythm. This is the noncommitted aspect of an algorithm. Noncommitted or committed shock may be a programmable option.

Onset Algorithms

Onset algorithms (summarized in Fig. 6 and explained in more detail below) identify a VT by examining a series of cycle lengths for an abrupt decrease in duration. These algorithms are intended to be used in the rate range where ventricular rates during sinus tachycardia (assumed gradual onset) overlap those of monomorphic VT (assumed abrupt onset), to avoid false positive detection. In some devices, an onset algorithm may be implemented by making continuous measurements of cycle length shortening independent of whether an interval shorter than that of the lower rate VT zone boundary has been measured. Other applications require a certain number of cycle lengths in the VT zone before a retrospective evaluation of the sequence is done. Onset algorithms are not used when cycle length intervals reside in the highest detection zone. Note that onset algorithms, by their design, may be unable to recognize the start of monomorphic VT during sinus tachycardia.

Onset algorithms have a *delta*, or change in cycle length, requirement which must be met before the rhythm can be declared as having an abrupt cycle length change. Meeting the requirement means that the device-computed delta exceeds the programmed parameter value. The delta may be programmable in milliseconds, in % of previous cycle length, or in % cycle length shortening. When described in % cycle length shortening, the selections are numbers like 10-50%. When the delta is described in % of previous cycle length, then numbers like 50-95% are encountered. The other method of specifying the delta is in time (ms), with programmable values in the range of 50-500 ms.

R-R Interval Sequence (I_n)

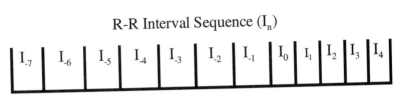

Alg. 1 $$\frac{I_n}{avg(I_{n-1},I_{n-2},I_{n-3},I_{n-4})} < \Delta(\%) \text{ and } either\ I_{n-2}\ or\ I_{n-3} > TDI$$

Alg. 2 $$\frac{avg(I_n,I_{n-1},I_{n-2},I_{n-3})}{avg(I_{n-4},I_{n-5},I_{n-6},I_{n-7})} < \Delta(\%)$$

Alg. 3   First, require 8 intervals < PRL cycle length   (These 8 are designated above as I_0 to I_7 although the depicted interval sequence only goes to interval I_4 for readability.) Find maximum interval-to-interval difference in previous intervals; the shorter of these two intervals (generating this difference) is called the "pivot interval" (I_0 above). Then require:

$$1-\frac{I_0}{I_{-1}} > \Delta(\%) \text{ and, in 3 out of the 4 intervals } \{I_0, I_1, I_2, I_3\},$$

$$1-\frac{I_k}{avg(I_{-3},I_{-4},I_{-5},I_{-6})} > \Delta(\%) \text{ where } k = 0,1,2,3$$

Alg. 4   First, require 2 consecutive intervals in zone TACH-0 (I_0 and I_1 above). Then require: $I_{-1} - I_0 > \Delta(ms)$ and *either* I_{-2} or $I_{-3} > I_0$ *or* $I_{-2}-I_0 > \Delta(ms)$

Alg. 5   Either $avg(I_{-1}, I_{-2}, ... I_{-m}) - I_0 > \Delta(ms)$ or $I_1 - I_0 > \Delta(ms)$; *and* all subsequent (Y) intervals $< avg(I_{-1}, I_{-2}, ... I_{-m}) - \Delta(ms)$; *and* X out of Y intervals < ODI

Figure 6. Onset algorithms, applied to a succession of tachycardia intervals which begin with I_0. Comparisons are done by subtraction or ratio. The result is then compared to a programmed designated onset delta (Δ). For example, if the two values (either interval averages or single intervals) are compared by subtraction, then the result, in ms, would have to be > Δ. If the two values are compared by ratio, then this fraction (as a percentage) would have to be less than (% of previous) or greater than (% change) the programmed delta (specified in %). Some algorithms use multiple logically connected comparison results, as shown above. Algorithms may operate continuously; others wait for one or more intervals and then examine the intervals retrospectively. I_n represents the R-R interval that has just been sensed and I_{n-1} is the one just previous, etc; *avg* is average; *ODI* is Onset Detection Interval (programmed independently of lower zone boundary). See text for further details and Fig. 1 for *PRL, TACH-0* and *TDI* definitions.

Onset algorithms necessarily use various actual or average reference cycle length(s) with which subsequent cycle lengths are compared. (Fig. 6) This reference may be the average of 4 consecutive cycle lengths (Algs. 1-3, Fig. 6). The 4 cycle length average reference may be continuously computed (using the "sliding window" concept) as the average of four intervals preceding the most recent four intervals (Alg. 2—Medtronic PCD 7217), or the average of the four intervals preceding the current interval (Alg. 1—Medtronic Jewel). Another implementation continuously computes the "sinus average" as the average of the intervals which precede those Y intervals used in the X out of Y algorithm (Alg. 5—Telectronics Sentry). Other algorithms (Algs. 3 and 4) defer computation of an average cycle length until intervals begin to reside in the tachycardia zone or above. The benefit of this approach is that battery energy is not continuously expended in making the calculation (assuming microprocessor code is used to implement the algorithm). One algorithm (Alg. 3—CPI Mini and predecessors) first identifies the most abruptly shortened interval (compared with the previous one). Then, skipping the 2 intervals preceding the shortened interval, the 4 previous intervals are used to compute the reference average cycle length.

Another algorithm (Alg. 4—Intermedics) does not compute an average interval for its reference, but instead applies criteria to each of the 3 intervals preceding the first 2 tachycardia intervals. After the previous average of intervals has been computed and the onset delta criterion met, algorithms may require additional criteria to be satisfied before the rhythm is declared as having rapid onset. In one algorithm (Alg. 5), all intervals after the first tachycardia interval must meet the delta requirement, when compared to the reference cycle length average. In addition, X out of Y intervals must be shorter than a separately programmable cycle length called the onset detection interval (ODI).

Most of the complexity in onset algorithms is designed to lessen the possibility of the onset algorithm being satisfied by premature beats, couplets, and their compensatory pauses in the presence of sinus tachycardia which progresses into the VT zone. As a consequence, VTs which begin with highly variable cycle lengths may not satisfy the criterion using the programmed parameter value. The overlap between the onset characteristics of SVTs and VTs means that a price must be paid for the use of this feature. One study showed that setting the onset level to its lowest level (minimum cycle length shortening of just 9%) would still result in the missing of 5-13% of VTs.[7]

Most, but not all, device algorithms back up the onset algorithm with a separate duration criterion in case the onset criterion is not fulfilled but the rate remains high for a programmable duration (measured in time or cycle lengths). This is done out of concern that a rapid VT might occur in the setting of exertion, which, in turn, may cause the onset algorithm to detect a smaller rate change than the programmed delta value, leading to non-detection of the arrhythmia.

In some algorithms, the cycle length criterion for the VT zone boundary may be separately programmable from that used during the onset evaluation. For instance, if VT begins during exercise, the onset criterion may not be met. If exercise testing reveals the patient's inability to sustain a heart rate above a certain level, then placing an "extended high rate" zone boundary within the lowest tachycardia zone would allow detection if the rhythm was fast enough *and* long enough. The assumption is that such a rhythm is probably VT. In this programming setup, a rhythm with a lower rate which satisfies the onset criterion would also be treated as VT. Fisher et al. demonstrated overlap of exercise rate changes in healthy people and VT onset rate changes in arrhythmia patients.[8] However, when the study was repeated with exercise in the VT population exclusively, there was no overlap.[9]

Stability Algorithms

Atrial fibrillation (AF) is characterized by an irregular ventricular response whereas monomorphic VT is typically more stable. Stability algorithms attempt to capitalize on this difference by using cycle length variability analysis.[10-12] The programmable stability parameter is usually specified in milliseconds with a range of 1-130 ms, depending upon the device. In one algorithm (Medtronic Jewel and PCD 7217), each tachycardia cycle length must not vary from any of its 3 predecessors by more than the programmable ms difference. If this variance is exceeded (i.e., presumed "AF"), the detection count is reset. In another algorithm (CPI PRx), the current cycle length is declared stable or unstable depending upon whether the difference between it and the most recent 4 interval running average remains less than or exceeds, respectively, a programmed value. (The running average of 4 consecutive intervals includes the current cycle length being evaluated.) If the unstable interval count exceeds a fixed proportion (e.g., 20%) of the total programmed duration, the rhythm is declared unstable (presumed "AF," i.e., not meriting therapy). In yet another algorithm (Intermedics Res-Q), the individual cycle length to previous cycle length differences must not vary by more than the programmed difference. A consecutive number of intervals, not variable by more than the programmed millisecond difference, is required for arrhythmia detection.

The overlap between stability values for VTs and SVTs can limit the value of this enhancement in particular patients. A setting which allows 100% sensitivity in detecting VTs will still typically admit some SVTs.[7] In a simulation study applying the PCD 7217B stability algorithm to induced VTs, a stability setting of 50-60 ms, combined with a number of intervals to detect criterion of 12-14, detected all regular VTs and 90% of irregular VTs (the latter comprising about 10% of the induced VTs); however, there were occasionally significant (>8 s) detection delays (especially at relatively slower VT rates, e.g., < 160 BPM) as well as inappropriate detection of AF in ≥ 10% of VTs.[12] Another study involved 16 patients with AF and 16 with monomorphic VT (rates < 220 beats/min) for whom a CPI PRx was implanted.[13] With stability settings spanning the entire range from 8-55 ms, 90-100% of some 30 AF episodes and 100% of 24 induced VTs were correctly classified; during a 292 patient-month followup in 24 patients programmed with stability settings of 24 or 31 ms with a duration of 10 intervals—and a sustained rate duration criterion of 30 seconds—there were no episodes (documented or suspected) of untreated VT. It should be emphasized that the VTs in this study were monomorphic and fairly regular. Near-fatal VT-underdetection, however, has been documented when a stability algorithm (Medtronic PCD 7217) was utilized in the setting of drug induced VT irregularity.[11]

Like the onset algorithm, the stability algorithm may be supported by an extended or sustained high rate criterion, ensuring therapy delivery after a preset time delay even if the tachycardia is classified as unstable.[13] This may avoid non-detection of a rapid, irregular ("AF" like) VT—at the expense, however, of permitting repetitive therapy delivery in the event of actual AF. Stability algorithms are usually available only in the lowest tachycardia rate zone. (See also Chap. 19.)

Combinational Detection Criteria

ICD systems permit individual activation of additional detection criteria. In the most simple combinational case, the criteria can be treated in a logical AND fashion. For example, if onset and stability are both activated, then in order to declare an arrhythmia, the duration criterion, the onset criterion, and the stability criterion must all be met. This improves the algorithm specificity (fewer "false positive" detections) at the expense of sensitivity (increased risk of missing VT or VF) and would, at the present time, only be occasionally employed. A somewhat less specific, but more sensitive combination, would be to select an OR option where either the onset or stability criteria and the duration criterion need to be satisfied before arrhythmia detection is declared. The extended (sustained) high rate criterion is employed in an OR logical fashion with the previous combinations. A continuous high heart rate for a sufficient duration and cycle length, results in arrhythmia detection. One device algorithm permits selection of one of ten logical combinations of detection algorithms. Most other device selections are relatively limited.

Post Therapy Detection

Detection algorithms are designed with the knowledge that rhythms arising after therapy delivery may have to be detected differently from those which arise from normal rhythm. For instance, an initial relatively high ventricular rate with rapidly progressive cycle length prolongation is not uncommon after defibrillation shocks. Initial detection criteria and/or parameters may not be suitable for this situation, since such post-shock accelerated ventricular rhythms are usually just transient phenomena. However, it is also recognized that an ineffective therapy means that cardiac function may deteriorate because of tachycardia-induced ischemia. Thus, it is desirable to have an algorithm which will recognize truly ineffective therapy and respond quickly.

Approaches to analyzing post-therapy rhythms include utilizing the initial detection algorithms with or without a different set of programmed parameters, invoking a different detection algorithm, or delaying detection for a fixed number of intervals until transient post-shock tachycardia subsides. The key question that needs to be answered is: When is an episode considered to have ended? If an episode is incorrectly declared to have ended, then the same initial (and ineffective) therapy may be applied as a result of a seemingly "new" detection. On the other hand, if recognition of tachyarrhythmia termination is erroneously delayed, then arrhythmias that were truly converted and arise once again will be treated with more aggressive therapy unnecessarily, since the algorithm incorrectly determined that conversion of the previous episode did not take place. Post-therapy detection consists of two algorithm components; a restored normal rhythm criterion (end of episode) and a redetection criterion.

In the most flexible implementations, programmable set-ups allow the device to be totally reconfigured post-therapy. That is, any parameter or set-up (AND vs. OR, for instance) may be changed for the post-therapy detection. Another example might be changing the device from a three zone configuration to a one zone configuration with a separately programmable cycle length limit after shock therapy. A delay period (in time or intervals) may first be provided to allow a transient rhythm, caused by therapy, to terminate. In one rapid detection implementation, it may take only four consecutive same zone intervals shorter than the tachycardia cycle length limit to result in redetection.

One device (CPI PRx) incorporates a "zone zero" that may impact on post-therapy responses. If the patient's heart rate is in zone 1 ("VT") but drops marginally to zone 0 ("sinus rhythm") following therapy, and then returns to zone 1 following further therapy, the software interprets this as an acceleration. A therapy shock may be delivered in this case, even though the programmed zone 1 antitachycardia pacing therapy may not have been completed. The specific details follow: If the last 4 intervals during redetection have an average interval lying in Zone 0 but 3 of the 4 intervals lie in Zone 1 then the tachycardia will be deemed to be continuing, but with a rate in Zone 0; Zone 1 therapy will be delivered. If, at the subsequent redetection, the last 4-interval average places the rhythm in Zone 1 this is then interpreted as an acceleration and monotonic therapy aggression is provided. Thus a shock can be delivered when antitachycardia pacing was expected for the "same-rate" tachycardia.

The declaration of the end of episode (return to normal rhythm) typically employs 1 of 3 criteria, depending upon the device: (1) Consecutive number of intervals longer than TDI (or FDI in the case of a single zone reconfiguration); this number of intervals may be fixed at 4 or 8. (2) X out of Y programmed intervals longer than TDI. (3) Expiration of a timer (e.g., 30 seconds) without redetection.

Morphology Detection

Morphology assessment of intracardiac electrograms has been incorporated into various ICD models. An early version, found in the CPI Ventak P, was called *Probability Density Function* or *PDF*. A later version, found in the PRx is known as *Turning Point Morphology*. The shocking lead electrogram is used for the algorithm's input signal. These algorithms assume that there is a loss of isoelectric time during ventricular tachyarrhythmias and no such loss during supraventricular rhythms. These algorithms lacked specificity, but have been employed with some success in certain clinical situations when the patient's normal shocking lead QRS signal is narrow. These algorithms have not been carried over into the later CPI Mini.

The Medtronic Jewel Plus 7218 measures the *width of the QRS complex* (far- and/or near-field electrograms)[14] to differentiate VTs from SVTs as another simple morphological discrimination. VT is detected when the QRS width (measured only in complexes with sufficiently high slew rates) increases for a programmed X out of Y intervals. The utility of this approach remains to be proven clinically, as the width can increase with high sinus rates[15] and chronically between followups.[16] Many patients lack sufficient high slew rate complexes to allow the width measurement.[17]

The future of electrogram morphology analysis is likely to include the development of an algorithm which "learns" the normal electrogram for the patient and then compares each unknown electrogram complex to this normal, to test if they are similar. The normal electrogram is first characterized by extracting a feature set, e.g. the sequence of slopes (signal derivatives) in the depolarization waveform.[18] Analysis of a sufficient number of complexes allows an average feature set to be obtained. This feature set or *template* is stored in the device memory. When a potential tachyarrhythmia (a series of cycle lengths less than the TDI) occurs, the algorithm begins extracting a feature set from each new complex and comparing it to the template. A sufficient number of "abnormal" declarations would result in a VT or VF diagnosis. For a discussion of this type of approach and other morphology algorithms see the review article by Jenkins et al.[19]

Increasing the specificity of a morphology analysis requires increased computing power of the implanted device. The task may be done in hardware, i.e., with dedicated transistor circuits, or it may be done with a general purpose microcomputer which is programmed. The latter approach is easier to develop because changes are done more quickly. However, dedicated circuitry can analyze signals quickly and at a lower battery current cost.

Clinical Caveats and Future Considerations

Detection algorithms utilized in ICDs are, currently, quite simplistic because of size and power consumption restrictions and because the tachyarrhythmia device industry itself is still relatively young. Enhancements to distinguish monomorphic VT from supraventricular rhythms generally were developed without testing with a large database of signals. Although clinical performance data are beginning to accumulate,[10-13] such algorithms should continue to be employed with caution and only when absolutely clinically necessary since underdetection of VT is a possibility.[11,12] Even the "simple" task of setting rate zone boundaries must be done with care to minimize risks of underdetection. (Chaps. 19, 21)

A likely addition to devices to improve discrimination of tachyarrhythmia is *atrial sensing*. An algorithm using atrial sensing would attribute a tachyarrhythmia to the fastest cardiac chamber.[20] In the case of a 1:1 atrial to ventricular activation ratio, the AV interval could be examined.[21] Addition of atrial sensing is not without cost, however, which includes increased opportunity for lead fractures, possibly increased device size, and over- and under-sensing problems. With advances in integrated circuits, signal processing techniques long employed in Holter monitors and elsewhere are likely to be incorporated into newer devices. These techniques will allow much better discrimination between normal and abnormal rhythms. Output from sensors now available for pacemakers (minute ventilation, temperature, etc.) are likely to be utilized in future discrimination algorithms.

All of this added sophistication in detection will come at the expense of increased programming difficulty unless care is taken by device manufacturers to provide complete information to physicians regarding how the device analyzes normal and abnormal patient rhythms. In the future, automated tools should be incorporated into device programmers. This would allow recording of the patient's tachyarrhythmias (either via electrograms or cycle length sequences); testing recognition of such stored rhythms utilizing various algorithm parameter settings could then be accomplished without repeatedly inducing VT, and/or exercising the patient.

ACKNOWLEDGMENT:

Fig. 3 is used with the permission of the Journal of Interventional Cardi-ology. Special thanks to Dan Huntwork (Angeion) and Walter Olson, PhD (Medtronic).

1. Geibel A, Zehender M, Brugada P. Changes in cycle length at the onset of sus-tained tachycardias—importance for antitachycardia pacing. Am Heart J 1988;115:588-592.
2. Jung W, Manz M, Moosdorf R, et al. Failure of an implantable cardioverter-defibrillator to redetect ventricular fibrillation in patients with a nonthoracotomy lead system. Circulation 1992;86:1217-1222.
3. Lawrence JH, Fazio GP, DeBorde R, et al. Electrical but not mechanical stunning after endocardial defibrillation. Eur JCPE 1992;2:121 (abstract).
4. Natale A, Sra J, Axtell K, et al. Undetected ventricular fibrillation in trans-venous implantable cardioverter defibrillators: prospective comparison of dif-ferent lead system-device combinations. Circulation 1996;93:91-98.
5. Callans DJ, Hook BG, Marchlinski FE. Effect of rate and coupling interval on endocardial R-wave amplitude variability in permanent ventricular sensing lead systems. J Am Coll Cardiol 1993;22:746-750.
6. Lindsay BD. Troubleshooting new ICD systems. J Interven Cardiol 1994;7:473-485.
7. Neuzner J, Pitschner HF, Schlepper M. Programmable VT detection enhance-ments in implantable cardioverter defibrillator therapy. PACE 1994;18:539-547.
8. Fisher JD, Goldstein M, Ostrow E, et al, Maximum rate of tachycardia develop-ment: sinus tachycardia with sudden exercise vs. spontaneous ventricular tachycardia. PACE 1983;6:221-223.
9. Mercando AD, Gableman G, Fisher JD, Comparison of the rate of tachycardia development in patients: pathologic vs. sinus tachycardias. PACE 1988;11:516. (abstract)
10. Swerdlow CD, Chen P, Kass, RM, et al. Discrimination of ventricular tachy-cardia from sinus tachycardia and atrial fibrillation in a tiered-therapy car-dioverter-defibrillator. J Am Coll Cardiol 1994;23:1342-1355.
11. Swerdlow CD, Ahern T, Chen P, et al. Underdetection of ventricular tachy-cardia by algorithms to enhance specificity in a tiered-therapy cardioverter-defibrillator. J Am Coll Cardiol 1994;24: 416-424.
12. Garcia-Alberola A, Yli-Mäyry S, Block M, et al. RR interval variability in irregular monomorphic ventricular tachycardia and atrial fibrillation. Circula-tion 1996;93:295-300.
13. Higgins SL, Lee RS, Kramer RL. Stability: an ICD detection criterion for dis-criminating atrial fibrillation from ventricular tachycardia. J Cardiovasc Elec-trophysiol 1995;6:1081-1088.
14. Gillberg JM, Olson WH, Bardy GH, et al. Electrogram width algorithm for dis-crimination of supraventricular rhythm from ventricular tachycardia. PACE 1994;17:866. (abstract)
15. Swerdlow CD, Mandel WJ, Ziccardi T. Effects of rate and procainamide on electrogram width measured by a tiered-therapy implantable cardioverter-defibrillator. PACE 1996;19:734. (abstract)
16. Brachmann J, Seidl K, Hauer B, et al. Intracardiac electrogram width measure-ment for improved tachycardia discrimination: initial results of a new implant-able cardioverter-defibrillator (ICD). J Am Coll Cardiol 1996;27:96A-97A. (abstract)
17. Ruetz LL, Bardy GH, Mitchell LB, et al. Clinical evaluation of electrogram width measurements for automatic detection of ventricular tachycardia. PACE

1996;19:582. (abstract)
18. Davies DW, Wainwright RJ, Tooley MA et al. Detection of pathological tachycardia by analysis of electrogram morphology. PACE 1986;9:200-208.
19. Jenkins JM, Caswell SA. Detection algorithms in implantable cardioverter defibrillators. Proc IEEE 1996;84:428-445.
20. Schuger CD, Jackson KJ, Steinman RT, et al. Atrial sensing to augment ventricular tachycardia detection by the automatic implantable cardioverter defibrillator: a utility study. PACE 1988;11:1456-1464.
21. LeCarpentier GL, Baga JJ, Yang H, et al. Differentiation of sinus tachycardia from ventricular-tachycardia with 1:1-ventriculoatrial conduction in dual-chamber implantable cardioverter-defibrillator—feasibility of a criterion based on the atrioventricular interval. PACE 1994;17:1818-1831.

16

Anti-Tachycardia Pacing and Cardioversion

Michael L. Hardage and Michael B. Sweeney

ALTHOUGH the primary focus of this text is on defibrillation issues, it is important to provide a discussion of therapies for ventricular tachycardias (VTs, that is, non-fibrillation tachyarrhythmias). In fact, tachycardia therapy is delivered much more frequently than ventricular fibrillation (VF) therapy in the general population of patients presenting with ventricular tachyarrhythmias in whom have implanted tiered therapy devices have been implanted. Patients who experience only primary ventricular fibrillation, exclusive of any tachycardia, are in the minority. The fibrillation-only patient typically experiences far fewer arrhythmia episodes than do patients with VT or supraventricular tachycardia (SVT). Although some patients present with fibrillation as the only documented or induced arrhythmia, many of these same patients had their VF episodes initiated by VT or have subsequent tachycardia episodes. About a third of the patients with ICDs implanted for cardiac arrest develop spontaneous monomorphic VTs and the vast majority are pace terminable.[1]

This chapter provides an overview of techniques and devices that have been employed to treat tachycardias. A historical perspective is presented, followed by the major issues confronting designers of these devices. The emphasis is more on engineering considerations, with some clinical observations from the authors' perspective.

The Ideal Anti-tachycardia Device

The ideal device for treating tachycardias would have several desirable characteristics, including the ability to detect hemodynamically compromising atrial or ventricular arrhythmias and immediately terminate them prior to onset of symptoms. A broad spectrum of therapies would be available, from sensor driven dual chamber bradycardia support pacing, intelligent "self-teaching" antitachycardia pacing algorithms, to a broad range of shock energies appropriate for various arrhythmias. It would not respond to sinus tachycardias nor atrial arrhythmias that produce rapid ventricular rates by delivering termination therapy to the ventricles. For example, atrial fibrillation producing rapid ventricular response would be treated by a low energy shock delivered to the atrium. It could apply appropriate therapy for each arrhythmia type in order to minimize patient discomfort. If a VT could be terminated by burst pacing it would do so as opposed to delivering high energy shocks. Its therapies would never accelerate slow monomorphic VT to faster VT or VF. It would offer extreme flexibility in its ability to be programmed for any type of patient or arrhythmia. It would also maintain a complete history of all arrhythmia episodes including an electrogram of the entire event, time and date the event occurred, the therapies delivered, and a status report of the device function at the time. It would periodically perform self diagnostic checks on its circuitry, the power source, and the integrity of the electrodes and their device connections. It would have the ability to inform the patient of any irregularities found from self-checks, and would have the capability of sending it's entire diagnostic history transtelephonically to the following physician's office or to a central computer for analysis by design engineers. The device would employ a small diameter single catheter containing all electrodes for detection of arrhythmias and therapy delivery. The pulse generator would be extremely small, such that it could be implanted by the electrophysiologist in the EP lab under local anesthesia. Finally, it would last several years and be low cost.

Unfortunately, technology and real world constraints at this time have not enabled this ideal device to be developed. The good news is that most of the features that have yet to be realized are being developed by researchers and manufacturers, and will become reality in the next few years. The limiting factors that separate the ideal device from current reality will be discussed in later sections.

History of Tachycardia Treating Devices

Some of the earliest attempts at terminating tachycardias (in the 1960's) came from employing simple demand bradycardia pacemakers in a magnet-induced asynchronous pacing mode. Otherwise known as underdrive pacing, the stimuli occur asynchronous to the tachycardia, randomly timed throughout diastole, and have a low probability of terminating the tachycardia. There were other variations of simple anti-tachycardia pacemakers, including rate doubling during magnet application and another system that would increase rate up to approximately 300 beats/min upon magnet activation. Other early magnet activated systems included units that would deliver single or double extrastimuli that were coupled to sensed intrinsic beats, with the coupling interval decreasing several ms after each beat. Another system consisted of a passive (no battery) implantable receiver and an external patient activated transmitter. The external unit would couple radio frequency energy into the implanted unit at rates adjustable from 50-400 beats/min. Although this system has not been implanted for several years, it did achieve some success in both atrial and ventricular applications. In fact there are still a few patients with units remaining implanted today, although most of these patients have by now received implanted tiered therapy defibrillators. Other systems included simultaneous atrioventricular (AV) pacing, dual demand pacing, and orthorhythmic pacing.

One feature common to the previously described early systems was the concept of patient activation. For the limited population of patients with well tolerated VT, who are "trainable" to activating their device and who remain calm during their arrhythmia the patient activated units could be effective. Many VT patients were, however, unable to perform the activation of their device due to hemodynamic intolerance of their arrhythmia caused by sudden onset of presyncopal symptoms. Also, it was necessary to always have the external control device (magnet or transmitter) in constant proximity to avoid prolonged arrhythmia duration. Many of these units also lacked backup bradycardia pacing if the patient's post-termination rhythm was asystole or sinus bradycardia.

The first widely available commercial system that automatically detected and treated VT/SVT was the CyberTach 60 (1980). This system was based on an available multiprogrammable bradycardia pacemaker. It responded to eight intervals shorter than the programmed detection interval by bursting for a programmable rate and duration. It was used primarily in the atrium to treat SVT in select patients who were screened against having rapid AV conduction due to accessory pathways and in whom atrial fibrillation did not produce rapid ventricular rates. There were a few implants for VT, although these patients were severely screened to ensure that burst pacing did not accelerate the VT into faster potentially lethal arrhythmias. Because implantable defibrillators were not available at the time the ventricular implants were particularly difficult to manage clinically. A later refinement of the CyberTach system came in the form of the InterTach/InterTach 2, which embodied multiple detection criteria and a wider variety of pacing regimens. As Intec and later CPI defibrillators became available throughout the 1980's, many VT patients received CyberTach/InterTach devices to burst pace terminate VT and a separate defibrillator (AID, AID B, Ventak) to protect against any accelerated rhythms resulting from burst pacing.[2]

In addition to burst pacing devices, other automatic systems included dual demand pacing and pacemakers capable of delivering single or dual extrastimuli which could iteratively scan diastole. The dual demand systems typically behaved as standard bradycardia pacemakers until the sensed rate exceeded the tachycardia detection rate, at which time they paced asynchronously in an attempt to underdrive pace terminate the tachycardia. One example of a dual chamber dual demand system was the Medtronic Symbios multiprogrammable DDD pacemaker, which could automatically respond to a supraventricular tachycardia either by burst atrial pacing or by activation to an underdrive pacing mode with near simultaneous atrial and ventricular pacing.

Automatic systems are now used almost exclusively, although only for control of atrial arrhythmias. With the advent of arrhythmia ablation techniques, even atrial application of antitachycardia-only devices has limited utility. The primary application for tachycardia terminating devices remains in the ventricle, although all devices implanted in the ventricle now are part of tiered therapy defibrillators. The possibility that antitachycardia pacing can accelerate what had been a relatively hemodynamically stable VT to rapid VT or VF necessitates backup defibrillation.[3]

During the late 1970's and early 1980's parallel development work was ongoing towards development of devices that could terminate tachycardias by using low energy cardioversion shocks of 0.5 mJ-2.5 J. Although a detailed discussion on cardioversion follows in a later section of this chapter, a few comments are appropriate on the historical perspective. It soon became obvious that the same types of limitations that were characteristic of antitachycardia pacemakers were also common to cardioversion devices. The probability of success and of accelerating a hemodynamically stable monomorphic VT to a potentially lethal VT or VF was found to be similar to that of pacing. But, the cardioversion units were larger and required larger, non-standard electrode systems. Also, patient discomfort from shocks was no small consideration.

Prevention of Tachycardias by Devices

Most cardiac arrhythmias require the presence of an electro-physiologic substrate and some initiating event to precipitate the arrhythmia. The primary techniques employed to prevent arrhythmias include pharmacologic agents, ablation or surgical resection. Various techniques have been studied in order to use pacing as a method of suppressing tachycardias, both atrial and ventricular. Pacing can alter the electrophysiologic substrate and/or suppress the initiating trigger mechanism of arrhythmias. Although there has not been widespread success in pacing suppression of tachycardias, a brief review of some of the techniques is presented.

There have been limited reports of standard bradycardia pacing in preventing tachycardias. The success is believed to arise from prevention of atrial and ventricular extrasystoles that trigger tachycardias. Some patients exhibit a narrow range of heart rate in which premature ventricular complexes (PVCs) are minimal. Theoretically if one could maintain the heart rate within that rate range then the extrasystoles and thus the arrhythmia would be suppressed.

Other techniques that have been attempted to prevent tachycardias included overdrive suppression, continuous high rate pacing, coupled stimulation, and train stimulation, all of which rely on suppression of extrasystoles or prevention of reentrant circuit formation. Dual chambered pacing was also investigated using short AV delays to suppress supraventricular tachycardia, although some negative effects were observed including poor hemodynamic response in some patients from short AV delays. Another approach to tachycardia prevention included a single pulse delivered after what would normally be an arrhythmia-inducing PVC. The single pulse was effective in preventing the R-on-T event from initiating arrhythmias in an animal model.

Other tachycardia prevention techniques are based on the observation that single subthreshold conditioning stimulus delivered during atrial or ventricular refractory period would prevent pacing capture of a subsequent pacing pulse delivered well outside the tissue refractory period. It would then seem that conditioning stimuli might be able to inhibit initiation of reentrant tachycardias.

While research is ongoing on tachycardia prevention methods, to date there has been limited success. Perhaps further investigations will lead to preventative features that can be incorporated into future generation devices.

Termination of Tachycardias by Pacing

The object of terminating tachycardias by pacing is to restore the patient to normal sinus rhythm as quickly as possible with little or no discomfort, to minimize the probability of degrading the arrhythmia to a more hemodynamically compromising one, and to minimize the energy consumption of the implanted antitachycardia device. Because of recent advances in supraventricular ablation techniques, antitachycardia pacing will probably be used most frequently in ventricular applications. However, any ventricular application will be concomitant with a tiered therapy defibrillator due to the need to have defibrillation backup in cases of paced acceleration of VT to rapid VT or VF. The advent of microprocessor controlled implanted devices has led to more intelligent antitachycardia devices, capable of treating a variety of VT rates and morphologies. Clinical acceptance of these devices has in the recent few years improved greatly

The probability of antitachycardia pacing (ATP) succeeding in terminating the VT is related to the ability of the pacing stimulation wavefront to arrive at the location of the reentrant circuit within the myocardium in such a manner that the circuit is modified or interrupted.[4] The factors influencing this process include the distance of the pacing electrode from the reentrant circuit, the pacing stimulus energy,[5] and the timing of the pacing stimuli[6] relative to the conduction velocities and refractory periods of the myocardium.

In simplified terms, the reentrant circuit can be thought of as a conduction wavefront propagating along a tissue mass of somewhat circular geometry. This circular conduction will consist of a portion of refractory tissue and a portion of excitable tissue. To terminate the circuit one needs to provide a pacing stimulus at the exact time and location when the tissue just comes out of refractoriness. If this occurs the paced stimulation wavefront proceeds toward the advancing wavefront of the circuit, colliding with the wavefront and interrupting the circuit. If the pacing stimulus arrives too soon it will be ineffective because the tissue will still be in refractoriness. If the stimulus arrives too late, it will generate wavefronts both towards the advancing wavefront and towards the "tail" of the circuit. Although one pacing generated wavefront will collide with the advancing wavefront of the reentrant circuit and

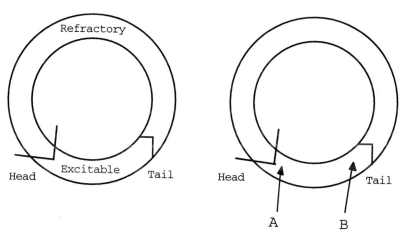

Figure 1. Simple reentry circuit model: Conduction proceeds around a circular tissue mass, with part of the tissue being refractory and an excitable gap of tissue. Introduction of an ATP impulse too early (arrow *A*) does not terminate the circulating wavefront since it will stimulate the excitable *Tail*, thereby sustaining the circuit. A critically timed pulse introduced just when the tissue comes out of refractoriness (arrow *B*) will fail to stimulate the *Tail*, and will collide with the *Head* (leading edge) of the wavefront, thereby interrupting the circuit.

will halt its progress, the latter pacing generated wavefront will act to sustain the reentrant circuit.[7] (Fig. 1)

ATP Techniques

There have been many techniques with concomitant terminology developed by clinicians and manufacturers to investigate effective ATP regimens. Although clinical trials have shown that there seem to be a few techniques that have the best termination properties, for the sake of completeness many of the ATP modalities will be presented here.

Underdrive pacing was one of the earliest ATP techniques, and relied on pacing at rates slower than the tachycardia to introduce randomly timed pacing pulses throughout diastole in an attempt to terminate. It didn't work well, and often required protracted time periods for success to be achieved. Critically timed extrastimuli delivered at various times during diastole worked much better. Because tachycardia episodes can vary in cycle length from one episode to the next, the need to alter the timing of the extrastimuli became apparent.

Programmed extrastimuli (PES) usually consists of 1 or at most a few pulses, and when the timing of their occurrence relative to the previous depolarization is changed for each successive attempt the PES are *scanned*. When a pulse is moved closer to the previous depolarization event then it is *decrementally scanned*. *Incremental scanning* moves the pulse further in time from the previous depolarization.

Quite different from PES is *train pacing*, in which ultra rapid pacing of up to a few thousand beats per minute is used to terminate reentrant tachycardias. The type of VT amenable to termination by this technique has its termination zone immediately after refractory period ends. Train pacing is started during the refractory period, and continues long enough only to produce a single capture.

The most common form of ATP is *burst pacing* which delivers multiple stimuli at a fixed cycle length between 50 and 100% of the tachycardia cycle length. Acceleration risk is minimized by keeping the number of pulses in a burst, the rate of the burst, and the number of bursts to the minimum required to terminate the VT. Most ATP regimens used by contemporary devices employ variations on this basic theme of burst pacing. Each *burst*, or attempt, consists typically of 2-20 pulses. The *number of bursts* used is typically 1-15. The rate of each burst can either be a fixed predetermined rate (*fixed burst*) or more frequently is a rate which is calculated based on the rate of the VT being treated (*adaptive burst*).[8]

The most frequently utilized burst rate is adaptive, varying from 70 to 90% of the average tachycardia cycle length. Although one can demonstrate excellent fixed rate burst pacing in the electrophysiology (EP) lab for a particular patient, when that patient experiences VT at home under a different autonomic nervous tone the VT may be different from that observed in the EP lab. Changes in posture or state of excitability can produce differing VT autonomic tone and thus different VT rates within the same patient over the same reentrant circuit. Adaptive burst pacing produces a rate proportional to the current VT, thereby attempting to place stimuli in the same relative position in diastole to terminate the reentrant circuit.

When a single burst is ineffective in terminating the VT, multiple bursts are utilized. Since the first burst was ineffective, it probably indicates that additional bursts delivered at the same rate will be no more effective. Therefore, scanning of the bursts is generally employed, typically decremental scanning. In this regimen, the first burst rate is calculated as a percentage of the average VT cycle length (adaptive). The second burst cycle length will then be either slightly faster (*decremental scanning*) or slower (*incremental scanning*) than the first burst. One can also produce alternating in-

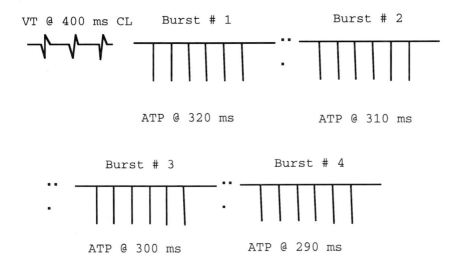

Figure 2. ATP example: Patient exhibits VT @ 400 ms cycle length. ATP device programmed to 80% adaptive burst pacing, 4 bursts of 6 pulses per burst. Decremental scanning is programmed on with a 10 ms step size. After initial detection, device bursts for 6 pulses @ 320 ms (400 ms x 0.8), then if the VT persists a second burst occurs at 310 ms (320 - 10 ms step size). A third and fourth burst will occur at 300 and 290 ms, respectively if VT sustains. Dashes (...) represent redetection of VT after unsuccessful burst.

cremental and decremental scanning bursts (*incremental/decremental scanning* or *centrifugal scanning*). Scanning bursts are also termed *concertina* or *accordion* bursts. Decremental scanning is typically preferred clinically, and the amount that each successive burst is made faster (*scanning step size*) is generally 5-20 ms.

As an example (Fig. 2), a clinical scenario might consist of a patient presenting with hemodynamically stable monomorphic VT of 400 ms cycle length. A typical ATP device regimen might include programming of adaptive burst pacing at 80% of the patient's VT cycle length, 4 bursts with 6 pulses per burst, and decremental scanning with a 10 ms step size. After detection of the VT the device would burst at 320 ms (400 VT cycle length x 0.8) for 6 pulses. If the VT was sustained, then the device would burst 6 more pulses at an interval of 310 ms (320 ms of first burst minus the 10 ms scanning step size). If the VT continues, then the third burst would be 6 pulses at 300 ms (310 - 10), then a fourth burst if necessary at 290 ms.

In a tiered therapy device, if all ATP bursts were unsuccessful then the next programmed VT therapy would be delivered. If any of the ATP bursts accelerated the VT to a faster VT or VF, then an appropriately more aggressive shock would be delivered. When an ATP burst is unsuccessful, the patient's rate is monitored to determine if VT is continuing. Redetection of the VT between bursts typically requires some programmable number of intervals. Some devices employ the number of intervals used to initially detect the VT as the number of intervals to redetect VT between bursts. If the initial number of intervals to detect VT is set to a large value to avoid treatment of nonsustained VT, prolonged redetection between bursts will occur.

A variation on fixed or adaptive burst pacing is *ramp pacing*, in which the cycle lengths of the pulses vary within each burst. An *incremental ramp* produces bursts that increase in cycle length progressively after the first interval, whereas a *decremental ramp* (or *autodecremental ramp*) has progressively decreasing intra-burst intervals. The amount of change from interval to interval within a ramp burst is termed the *intra-burst step size*.

Ramp bursts can be scanned in a similar fashion to scanning bursts previously explained. Thus an *incremental, decremental,* or *incremental/decremental scanning* ramp is produced.

Another clinical example (Fig. 3) of the patient with the 400 ms VT might include a device programmed to decremental scanning adaptive autodecremental pacing, with an adaptive rate of 80%, a scanning step size of 10 ms, an autodecremental step size of 5 ms, with 3 bursts of 4 pules per burst. Upon detection of the VT the initial interval of the initial burst would be at a cycle length of 320 ms (400 x .8), with the second and third intervals at 315 and 310 respectively. Note that there are only 3 intervals produced by 4 pulses. If the VT sustains then the first interval of the second burst is scanned decrementally, by 10 ms resulting in an interval of 310 ms (320 of first burst - 10) with second and third intervals of 305 and 300 ms, respectively. If needed, the third burst would have intervals of 300, 295 and 290 ms.

Decremental scanning and autodecremental bursts can produce very rapid pacing rates, especially if several bursts and pulses per burst are used to treat a rapid VT. The clinician may decide that there is some maximum rate beyond which bursting is undesirable either due to acceleration propensity or ineffectiveness of the pulses due to tissue refractoriness. Most devices support programming of a maximum burst pacing rate, or *minimum burst cycle length* (*minimum BCL*). If during the scanning process the cycle length of a burst attempts to become shorter than the minimum BCL, subsequent pulse intervals are delivered at the minimum BCL.

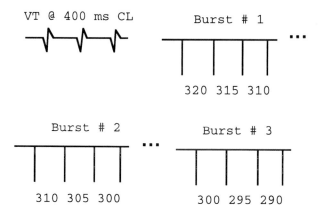

Figure 3. Scanning autodecremental example: Patient presents with VT @ 400 ms cycle length. ATP device programmed to scanning adaptive autodecremental bursts, with 80% adaptive interval, 3 bursts with 4 pulses per burst, scanning step size of 10 ms, and autodecremental step size of 5 ms. The first burst starts with 320 ms (400 ms x 0.8), the next interval in the first burst is 315 (320 - 5 ms autodec. step size), and the third interval is 310 ms (= 315 - 5). If VT persists, a second burst occurs with an initial interval of 310 ms (320 ms of initial burst first interval minus 10 ms scanning step size), followed by intervals of 305 and 300 ms. If a third burst is necessary, it starts with 300 ms (310 - 10), followed by 295 and 290 ms. Dashes (...) represent redetection of VT after unsuccessful burst.

The first pulse in a burst can be delivered synchronously with an R-wave to initiate timing of subsequent pulses, or can be delivered at some programmable coupling interval to the R-wave. The coupling interval between the R-wave and the first pulse in a burst can be scanned, producing *shifting burst* pacing.

Another variation on burst pacing is a method of adding 1 or more PES at the end of each burst, and scanning the PES coupling interval to the last pulse in the burst (*burst plus PES*). Another variation (*burst plus one*) includes adding an additional pulse with each subsequent burst in a regimen.

There are two commonly used approaches in calculating *adaptive burst rates during redetection of VT* following unsuccessful ATP bursts. One approach is to use the initially detected VT rate to calculate the burst rate and subsequent scanned burst steps following unsuccessful burst attempts. Another technique recalculates the adaptive burst rate between bursts. For example, if a 400 ms VT is accelerated to 350 ms cycle length by the first ATP burst, the first described technique continues to burst as though the VT cycle length was 400 ms. The second approach readjusts to the faster VT rate, and bursts faster than initially. This can produce acceleration of VT in some patients, while in others whose VT slows after a burst it may decrease the probability of acceleration.

Some devices (Telectronics Sentry 4310 and predecessors) incorporate a *memory* function that remembers what the cycle length of the previous successful scanned burst was for a VT with a similar cycle length. The subsequent VT episode is then treated with a burst that is the same rate as that previous successful one, thereby eliminating the time elapsed by attempting unsuccessful scanning burst rates.

An important parameter unrelated to timing of ATP pulses is the *pulse amplitude and width*. Because the pacing electrode may be physically distant to the reentrant circuit, it is important to pace with sufficient pulse energy to assure capture and thus propagation of the wavefronts to the reentrant circuit. Tiered therapy devices typically employ bradycardia support as well as ATP. It is important to have the ability to independently set the ATP pulse amplitude to a value different from that of the bradycardia function. Since the bradycardia pacing can sometimes occur 100% of the time, conservation of the battery energy is maximized when the bradycardia pulse energy is titrated to a sufficiently low but safe level. However, ATP occurs relatively infrequently and therefore setting the ATP pulse energy to a high level enhances effectiveness of VT termination with negligible degradation of the device battery longevity.

An additional consideration is that of the *pacing mode* during ATP bursting. Most devices burst in the asynchronous mode, but at least one device bursts in the demand pacing mode. In the presence of T-wave over-sensing, demand burst pacing can result in a burst rate at double the desired rate. This results in a loss of effectiveness in penetrating the reentrant circuit, and thus an overall reduced ability of ATP to terminate the tachycardia.

Clinical Effectiveness of ATP

Many investigators have reported varying levels of ATP effectiveness, both in the atrium and the ventricle. A thorough review of the literature is beyond the scope of this chapter, but a few comments regarding ATP effectiveness are provided. One recent review is provided by Rosenqvist.[9] There are several factors influencing ATP effectiveness, including patient selection, thorough EP workup to demonstrate ATP effectiveness, location of the pacing electrode relative to the reentrant circuit, ATP pulse energy, and delivering the proper number of critically time pulses. Thorough testing is a valuable approach to ensure ATP effectiveness. (But, see also later section on empiric approaches.)

Once it has been demonstrated that a patient is a candidate for an ATP device for treatment of VT, a tiered therapy device is implanted in the operating room. Although the patient may have never presented with VF nor ever had VT accelerate to VF during EP workup, there is a small but finite probability that acceleration will occur at some point in the future. Patients with ejection fractions under 0.3 have a much higher rate of acceleration.[10] If defibrillation backup is not available, the acceleration can quite likely be lethal. At the time of implant often very little effort is made to assess ATP effectiveness, since anesthesia can have profound effects on inducibility of the patient's clinical VT. Thus at implant the ability of the tiered therapy device to terminate VF is assessed. At the time of pre-hospital discharge, the patient is restudied in the EP lab, free from the effects of general anesthesia.

The ability of tiered therapy devices to support noninvasive programmable stimulation allows repeated EP studies without the requirement of temporary catheter insertion. The clinical VT is induced repeatedly in order to find an ATP programming regimen that works repeatedly with no acceleration of the arrhythmia. However, it must be born in mind that the reported failure rate of ATP for spontaneous VT is only *half* that of induced VT.[11] This may reflect selection bias as only those with good electrophysiology results tend to have the feature activated.[12] It may also reflect the slower rates of spontaneous VT or changes in ischemia or autonomic tone.

It is important to test the patient fully loaded on clinical doses of any cardioactive drugs that will be taken post discharge. If any changes in cardioactive medications occur subsequently, then retesting for ATP effectiveness is wise. Also, if the patient experiences spontaneous episodes in which the ATP is either ineffective (leading to cardioversion shocks) or accelerates the VT to VF (producing VF shocks) some titration of the ATP parameters during an EP restudy is required.

For VT patients who are appropriate candidates for ATP devices, excellent ATP effectiveness is available provided soundly designed tiered therapy devices are available. In a population of 338 patients implanted with a Ventritex Cadence, ATP was effective in terminating 94% (3982 episodes) of a total of 4242 episodes of spontaneous VT. Five percent (200 episodes) were unsuccessfully treated, requiring subsequent cardioversion shocks to

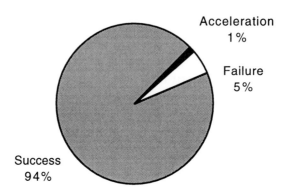

Figure 4. Clinical results of anti-tachycardia pacing with the Cadence ICD. The pie chart covers 1040 patients with 17,115 episodes of VT.

terminate the VT. The remaining 1% of the VT episodes (60) accelerated to either rapid VT or VF, requiring a high energy shock to terminate the episode. A later analysis of 1040 patients implanted with the same device ,for as long as 42 months indicated quite similar percentages of success, failure, and acceleration of VT from ATP. Of 17,115 episodes of spontaneous VT, 16,112 (94%) were treated successfully with ATP, 769 (5%) episodes were unsuccessfully treated, and 234 (1%) of the episodes were accelerated. Other studies have shown similar low rates of acceleration.[13] These data illustrate the potential advantages of treating VT with ATP as a primary therapy.[14] (Fig. 4)

Low Energy Cardioversion Shocks

In addition to pacing to terminate non-fibrillation arrhythmias, low energy cardioversion has received a great deal of attention from investigators. The concept of cardioversion differs from that of anti-tachycardia pacing in that cardioversion attempts to depolarize simultaneously (and thereby render refractory) a very large number of myocardial cells, especially those in the diastolic portion of the reentrant circuit, thus terminating the arrhythmia

This approach requires a different electrode system than the standard pacemaker leads employed by antitachycardia pacemakers. The typical pacing output pulse contains approximately 25 µJ = 5 V · 10 mA · 0.5 ms (Chap. 4) which is 1/100,000 of the energy of a 2.5 J cardioversion shock. Much larger surface area electrode systems are used in cardioversion to avoid excessive current densities that would otherwise exist if standard pacing electrodes were used. It has been shown that excessively high current density pulses can cause local tissue damage. The other necessity for using different electrode types arose from the need to distribute the electric field generated from the shock to as much ventricular mass as possible. This led to development of catheter electrode systems that utilized multiple fairly large surface area electrodes on the order of 1-2 cm^2.

While there are no clear conventions in cardioversion terminology, low and medium energy cardioversion is mentioned throughout the literature. It is useful to consider low energy cardioversion as shocks of energies up to approximately 0.5 J, and medium energy cardioversion energies ranging from 0.5 to approximately 10 J. The distinction between low and medium could refer to the perceived discomfort of the patient resulting from a shock. Although there are potentially many factors influencing perceived patient pain, such as electrode type and location, most patients begin to describe discomfort at approximately 0.5 J. At 0.1 J, little or no sensation is felt. Virtually all patients describe shocks of 1 J or greater as very uncomfortable.

The original speculation that low energy cardioversion would be more effective than ATP for terminating VT never materialized. Comparable success/failure/acceleration data occurred for cardioversion and for ATP. Each method has advantages and disadvantages. ATP requires little battery energy and is well tolerated by the patient. However, longer elapsed time is required to deliver scanned bursts compared to cardioversion. Cardioversion, on the other hand, requires special circuitry to generate the high voltage shock that is not well tolerated by patients for energy levels above approximately 0.5 J.

Tiered therapy devices support both ATP and low energy cardioversion therapies. Almost all slow monomorphic VT episodes are treated with ATP successfully, but there is the occasional patient for which ATP is unsuccessful yet low energy shocks are effective. Regardless of the method, backup defibrillation is mandatory to protect against accelerated rhythms.[15]

Empiric Approaches to ATP Programming

The fact that responses to ATP may be different for spontaneous versus laboratory-induced VTs, and be affected by various other factors, has led some investigators to adopt certain empiric ap-

Table 1. Example of empiric bifurcated approach to ATP programming.*

	Slow VT	Fast VT
Decision cutpoint	CL > 320 ms	260 < CL ≤ 320 ms
Method	burst or ramp	ramp
Number of pulses	3-5	7-11
Initial pulse cycle length	60-75% VT rate	91-97% VT rate
Minimum pulse cycle length	240 ms	240 ms unless very fast VT in which case: 200 ms
Decrementation interval	Ramp: 10 ms Burst: 30 ms	10 ms
Number of ATP attempts	1-4 (usually 2)	1-4 (usually 2)

* Courtesy of Gust Bardy, MD; CL = cycle length; VT = ventricular tachycardia.

Table 2. Example of empiric universal ATP programming.[16]

Phase	Therapy	Attempts	Pulses	Coupling Interval	Decrement
1	autodecremental ramp	≤7	5-11	91% of VT CL	10 ms between pulses
2	adaptive burst	≤6	7	84% of VT CL	10 ms between bursts
3	cardioversion shock				

CL = cycle length; VT = ventricular tachycardia.

proaches to programming at least the initial values of ATP parameters (with subsequent reprogramming over time, as needed). One such approach, shown in Table 1, bases the ATP schema on VT cycle length, using a 320 ms cutpoint.

Another approach, shown in Table 2, provides an even more general schema of progressive therapy culminating in cardioversion. Interestingly, the latter universal approach successfully terminated some 98.4% = 1315/1337 VT episodes with only a 1. % incidence of VT acceleration to VF requiring defibrillation in 162 patients; sudden death rate was < 1% per year.[16] More studies of the effectiveness of empiric approaches to ATP programming are needed.

Complications in Tachycardia Terminating Devices

The most frequent complication of ATP/cardioversion devices occurs when supraventricular tachycardias (sinus tachycardia or atrial fibrillation) produce rapid ventricular responses in excess of the patient's VT rate, also called *rate crossover*. A simple rate cutoff detection algorithm is fooled by such clinical scenarios, as previously described. The utilization of rate crossover detection algorithms such as sudden onset or rate stability, while occasionally effective, can often lead to failure to treat the patient's clinical VT. On rare occasions, inappropriate therapy delivery for detection of rapid rates due to atrial fibrillation or sinus tachycardia can lead to induction of VT. This inadvertently initiated VT is subsequently treated with ATP and/or cardioversion.

Another common clinical complication of ATP/cardioversion is acceleration of VT to VF, resulting in the requirement of delivery of a high energy defibrillation shock.[17] (See preceding discussion in "Clinical Effectiveness of ATP" section.) Thorough clinical workup can minimize such occurrences.   Occasionally, cardioversion shocks delivered synchronously with ventricular systole but asynchronously with atrial systole can produce atrial fibrillation, with resultant rapid ventricular response. This can, in turn, trigger inappropriate therapy delivery (i.e., for SVT mimicking VT).

ACKNOWLEDGMENT:
We thank Gust Bardy, MD for Table 1.

1.   Mitra RL, Hsia HH, Hook BG, et al. Efficacy of antitachycardia pacing in patients presenting with cardiac arrest. PACE 1995;18:2035-2040.
2.   Newman DM, Lee MA, Herre JM, et al. Permanent antitachycardia pacemaker therapy for ventricular tachycardia. PACE 1989;12:1387-1395.
3.   Hardage ML, Sweeney MB, Automatic Tachycardia Terminating Burst Pacemakers, The Third Decade of Cardiac Pacing. Mount Kisco, New York, Futura Publishing, 1982 pp 293-307.
4.   Abildskov JA, Lux RL. Mechanisms in the interruption of reentrant tachycardia by pacing. J Electrocard 1995;28:107-114.
5.   Waxman HL, Cain ME, Greenspan AM, et al. Termination of ventricular tachycardia with ventricular stimulation: salutary effect of increased current strength. Circulation 1982;65:800-804.
6.   Gardner MJ, Waxman HL, Buxton AE, et al. Termination of ventricular tachycardia. Evaluation of a new pacing method. Am J Cardiol 1982;50:1338-1345.
7.   Fisher JD, Kim SG, Waspe LE, et al. Mechanisms for the success and failure of pacing for termination of ventricular tachycardia: Clinical and hypothetical considerations. PACE 1983;6:1094-1105.
8.   Fisher JD, Johnston DR, Kim SG. Implantable pacers for tachycardia termination: stimulation techniques and long-term efficacy, PACE 1986;9:1325-1333.
9.   Rosenqvist M. Pacing techniques to terminate ventricular tachycardia. PACE 1995;18:592-598.
10. Heisel A, Neuzner J, Himmrich E, et al. Safety of antitachycardia pacing in patients with implantable cardioverter defibrillators and severely depressed left ventricular function. PACE 1995;18:137-141.
11. Porterfield JG, Porterfield LM, Smith BA, et al. Conversion rates of induced versus spontaneous ventricular tachycardia by a third generation cardioverter defibrillator. The Ventak PRx phase 1 investigators. PACE 1993;16:170-173.
12. Pinski SL, Fahy GJ. The proarrhythmic potential of implantable cardioverter-defibrillators. Circulation 1995;92:1651-1664.

13. Catanzariti D, Pennisi V, Pangallo A, et al. Efficacy and safety of antitachy-
    cardia pacing in ICD patients: analysis of two-years followup. Eur JCPE
    1995;5:248-252.
14. Pacifico A, Nasir N, Doyle T, et al. Safety and efficacy of antitachycardia pac-
    ing with a new third generation implantable cardioverter defibrillator, XV
    Congress of the European Society of Cardiology, 1993.
15. Jackman WM, Zipes DP. Low-energy synchronous cardioversion of ventricular
    tachycardia using a catheter electrode in a canine model of subacute myocardial
    infarction, Circulation 1982;66:187.
16. Connelly DT, Cardinal D, Foley L, et al. Is routine pre-discharge testing neces-
    sary for patients with implantable cardioverter-defibrillators? PACE
    1996;19:614. (abstract)
17. Hammill SC, Packer DL, Stanton MS, et al. Termination and acceleration of
    ventricular tachycardia with autodecremental pacing, burst pacing, and car-
    dioversion in patients with an implantable cardioverter defibrillator. PACE
    1995;18:3-10.

17

Implantation: Pre-operative Evaluation to Discharge

Wolfram Grimm, MD and Francis E. Marchlinski, MD

THOROUGH preimplant evaluation of the patient's physical condition and arrhythmias is crucial to successful ICD implantation and long-term clinical efficacy of the implanted device. The first approved devices in the United States used epicardial lead systems which have demonstrated long-term stability of the defibrillation threshold (DFT).[1,2] The less invasive nonthoracotomy lead system approach, however, appears to result in a significantly lower perioperative morbidity and mortality with an excellent short-term clinical efficacy.[3-5] Since nonthoracotomy lead systems can be implanted in virtually all patients when biphasic shock waveforms are being used[3] with similar low intraoperative DFTs as compared to what has been reported for conventional epicardial lead systems with monophasic shock waveforms, the nonthoracotomy approach has already become the primary method of ICD implantation.

For both the transvenous and the epi- or pericardial lead system approaches for ICD implantation, however, intraoperative defibrillation testing is mandatory in order to ensure that the energy required for defibrillation is always less than the energy that the device is able to deliver.[6] (Clinical variables are unable to predict the DFT even with simple modern unipolar systems.[7]) The awareness of potential surgical complications associated with ICD implantation[8] including infections of the ICD system is a prerequisite to avoiding their occurrence and, therefore, will also be briefly discussed in this chapter.

Table 1. Preimplantation assessment

Patient's physical condition and underlying heart disease

- ◆ Presenting arrhythmias: type, rate, frequency, and hemodynamic tolerance
- ◆ Heart failure, ischemia, previous cardiac surgery
- ◆ Serious systemic disorder
- ◆ Conditions predisposing for ICD infection, e.g., diabetes mellitus, preexisting skin infections
- ◆ Electrocardiogram
- ◆ Chest X-ray
- ◆ Routine hematology and blood chemistries (systemic disorder)
- ◆ Catheterization, ventriculography and coronary angiography (need for: revascularisation, aneurysmectomy or valve replacement), exercise testing or thallium scintigraphy (provocable ischemia, maximum achievable heart rate), echocardiography or radionuclide angiography (ventricular function)
- ◆ Exercise testing for maximum achievable heart rate (to assist rate cutoff programming)
- ◆ Holter or telemetry monitoring of rate, frequency and duration of spontaneous nonsustained VT, unsuspected bradyarrhythmias, and supraventricular tachyarrhythmias
- ◆ Need for psychological support

Electrophysiological testing

- ◆ Induction and termination of VT or VF, effectiveness of antitachycardia pacing
- ◆ Arrhythmia mechanism and location
- ◆ Response to antiarrhythmic drugs
- ◆ Future ablative therapy
- ◆ Arrhythmia prevention using electrical stimulation therapy
- ◆ Maximum rate of 1:1 AV conduction; below the rate cutoff for future device therapy?
- ◆ Inducibility of supraventricular tachyarrhythmias (particularly important in patients with a history of SVT
- ◆ AV conduction disturbances, e.g., HV interval > 100 ms
- ◆ Prolonged bradyarrhythmias or asystole after electrical cardioversion or defibrillation

---

AV = atrioventricular conduction, SVT = supraventricular tachycardia, VF = ventricular fibrillation, VT = ventricular tachycardia.

Preimplant Evaluation

All ICD candidates should undergo preoperative assessment of their physical condition, kind and severity of the underlying heart disease, and unsuspected systemic conditions, as summarized in Table 1. Reversible causes of the presenting arrhythmia such as severe electrolyte disturbances, acute ischemia, or proarrhythmic drug effects need to be excluded as far as possible. Exercise testing is important for estimating maximum achievable physiological heart rate which should be well below the future programmed rate cutoff for device therapy.

In addition, prophylactic treatment with beta blockers or calcium channel blockers (which depress atrioventricular [AV] nodal conduction) should be considered for patients prone to atrial fibrillation with a rapid ventricular response, since the majority of unnecessary ICD shocks during followup are triggered by atrial fibrillation with a rapid ventricular response in our experience,[9] and treatment with digitalis alone is usually not sufficient to control the ventricular rate during exercise in many patients with atrial fibrillation.

In order to select the appropriate device, mode of implantation, and device programming for the individual patient, a thorough preoperative electrophysiologic evaluation is essential. The information obtained by the preimplant electrophysiologic study (Table 1) includes maximum rate of 1:1 AV conduction, potential for bradyarrhythmias, particularly post-cardioversion/ defibrillation, and the characteristics of any inducible supraventricular or ventricular tachycardia. In patients with inducible sustained monomorphic VT, the effectiveness of antitachycardia pacing for VT termination should be assessed. For survivors of out-of-hospital VF, with no history of monomorphic VT, it may be possible to bypass the electrophysiologic study but this approach is not widely accepted.[10]

Finally, electrophysiologic testing may be useful to determine "best" antiarrhythmic drug therapy in patients presenting with frequent episodes of sustained ventricular tachyarrhythmias, symptomatic nonsustained VT, or additional supraventricular tachyarrhythmias. In patients without frequent episodes of sustained ventricular tachyarrhythmias, symptomatic nonsustained VT, or additional supraventricular tachyarrhythmias, no antiarrhythmic drug therapy is probably the "best" antiarrhythmic drug therapy prior to ICD implantation, since antiarrhythmic drug therapy is unlikely to improve clinical device efficacy, may exert proarrhythmic and negative inotropic effects, and may alter the defibrillation threshold in an unpredictable way in the individual patient.

Implantation Using Nonthoracotomy Lead Systems

Due to a decrease in morbidity and mortality associated with implantation of nonthoracotomy lead systems as compared to epicardial lead systems, (Chap. 22) the nonthoracotomy lead system approach has already become the method of choice for ICD. For a complete discussion of various electrode designs, possible single, two, or multiple electrode pathways for defibrillation and the importance of shock waveforms using nonthoracotomy lead systems the reader is referred to Chaps. 6, 7, and 9, respectively.

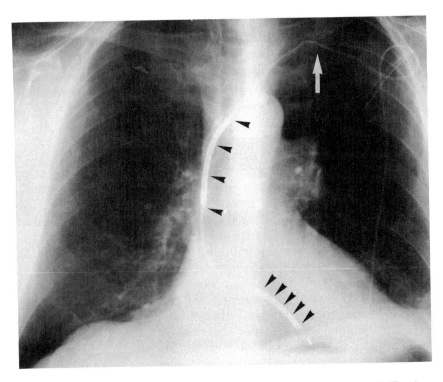

Figure 1. Chest X-ray of a completely transvenous lead system using a 12 F tripolar catheter (Endotak C lead). Insertion of the lead was performed via puncture of the left subclavian vein (white arrow). The shocking cathode, (distal electrode in the right ventricular apex), and the shocking anode, (proximal electrode between the superior vena cava and the right atrium) are marked with black arrows.

For implantation of nonthoracotomy lead systems, one or more electrode catheters are inserted under fluoroscopic control usually via the left cephalic or subclavian vein so that the distal tip of the rate sensing electrode is located in the right ventricular apex. In addition to the rate sensing and pacing electrode, a distal and a proximal spring electrode may also be located on a single endocardial lead system for morphology sensing as well as cardioversion and defibrillation. (Fig. 1)

Another nonthoracotomy lead system consists of a right ventricular apical lead with bipolar sensing and pacing electrodes and a defibrillating coil electrode in conjunction with a second defibrillation lead placed in the coronary sinus or superior vena cava Fig. 2. Any transvenous lead system may be combined with a subcutaneous patch electrode or a subcutaneous array electrode as an

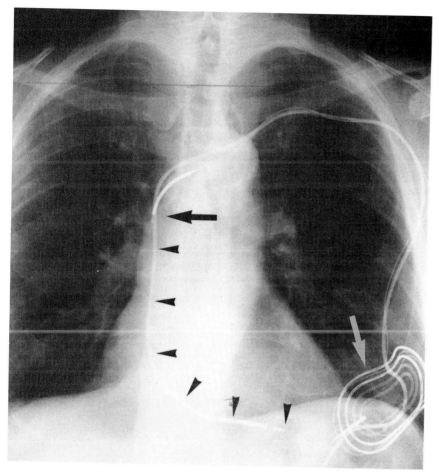

Figure 2. Chest X-ray showing a nonthoracotomy lead system with a three electrode configuration for dual pathway defibrillation. The right ventricular lead
(small black arrows) was used as rate sensing and pacing electrode as well as
common shocking cathode. The second transvenous lead which was positioned in
the superior vena cava (large black arrow) served as first shocking anode and the
subcutaneous chest patch electrode (white arrow) as second shocking anode.

additional shocking electrode which is usually implanted subcutaneously or submuscularly over the cardiac apex. (Fig. 2)

In our experience, implantation of subcutaneous *patch electrodes* or *array electrodes* was almost always required (in addition to
endocardial defibrillation leads) when the device implanted was
only capable of delivering monophasic shock waveforms. *Subcutaneous array electrodes* consisting of three 20.5 cm long coils covering
an area of about 150 cm^2 may be superior to standard subcutaneous patch electrodes with respect to intraoperative DFTs, bleeding
complications, and patient discomfort.[11] While the array electrodes

may be inserted through the same incision utilized for a pectoral implantation,[11] the electrodes' benefit may not be fully realized in patients with high DFTs until inserted through a lower antero-lateral chest incision to permit placement of the coils posteriorly at an infrascapular location.

Multiple lead configurations can be tested in order to determine the configuration which provides the lowest DFT by changing shock pathways, polarity, or lead position. Biphasic waveforms currently enable endocardial lead systems to achieve acceptable DFTs in most cases without the need for subcutaneous patch or array leads.[3] (Fig. 1)

The pectoral implant approach has achieved rapid acceptance. This is typically used with a Hot Can system with a unipolar defibrillation lead system. The ICD is either implanted subcutaneously or subpectorally, typically through a left intraclavicular incision. The subcutaneous location reduces patient pain and facilitates device replacement. The subpectoral location may lower the infection risk (due to increased circulation) and obviates cosmetic issues. When necessary (e.g., because of preexisting transvenous hardware on the left side) a right-sided infraclavicular venous-access approach may be utilized,[12] although higher DFTs can be expected.[13]

Implantation Using Epicardial Lead Systems

Epicardial lead implantations are now the exception rather than the norm. However, due to the occasional patient with an extremely high DFT, this option must be available. Various procedures may be used to implant epicardial lead systems (Fig. 3): median sternotomy, left anterior thoracotomy, as well as subxyphoid and subcostal.[14-18] Each particular approach has certain advantages and disadvantages. The left anterior approach, for example, causes postoperative pain and is associated with a higher pulmonary complication rate than that associated with a median sternotomy. Both subxyphoid and subcostal approaches have the least pulmonary complications but provide less visualization of the heart and are therefore less practical in patients with prior thoracic surgery or in those undergoing concomitant coronary artery surgery. Epicardial patch lead implantations have even been performed via thoracoscopy.[19]

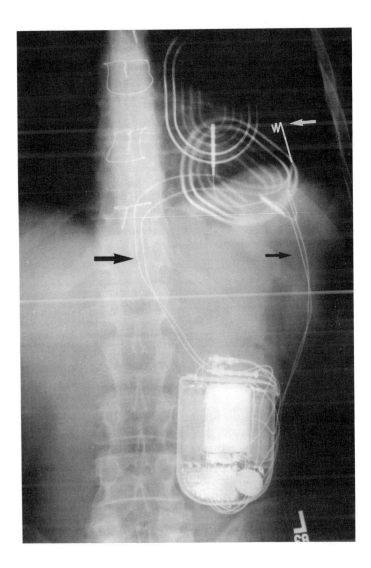

Figure 3. Chest X-ray showing an epicardial lead system consisting of two patch electrodes for defibrillation and two screw-in leads for sensing and pacing (white arrow). The generator is implanted subcutaneously in the left paraumbilical region. The patch leads (small black arrow) and the screw-in leads (large black arrow) are tunneled subcutaneously into the generator pocket.

If *concomitant thoracic surgery* is performed, obviously a median sternotomy should be used. Alternatively, and more simply, a nonthoracotomy lead system (using biphasic waveforms) may be implanted in a second procedure a few days after cardiothoracic surgery which may decrease mortality and morbidity in some of these patients.

With either one of the surgical approaches described above, 2 defibrillation patch electrodes are usually placed epi- or pericardially. The sensing electrograms may be obtained from 2 epicardial screw-in leads (Fig. 3) or a single transvenous lead with the tip positioned in the right ventricular apex.

Assessment of sensing and pacing lead function and DFT testing are described below. At the end of the procedure, the pulse generator is ordinarily placed in the left upper quadrant or paraumbilical region of the abdomen. (Fig. 3) New smaller devices are often implanted in the subclavicular region.

Assessment of Sensing and Pacing Lead Function

Following insertion of sensing, pacing and defibrillation electrodes, using either one of the described nonthoracotomy or thoracotomy approaches, sensing and pacing lead function are assessed as outlined in Table 2. If inadequate values for sensing or pacing thresholds are obtained, the leads need to be repositioned until satisfactory values can be measured. Signal amplitude from the sensing leads should be measured during sinus rhythm as well as during ventricular pacing and induced VT/VF before permanent implantation in order to ensure that undersensing will not be a problem under any condition. In addition, T-wave oversensing at maximum sensitivity of the ICD should be excluded in order to avoid inappropriate ICD shocks resulting from double counting (i.e., sensing of both QRS complexes and T-waves). (Chap. 14)

Avoidance of ICD-Pacemaker Interactions

All currently available pacemakers may potentially interfere with appropriate ICD function.[20] (See Chap. 14, "Sensing Limitations" for a theoretical treatment.) Concomitant unipolar pacemaker therapy is contraindicated in ICD patients since the pacemaker may fail to sense VF and continue to pulse. As a consequence, the ICD may sense only the larger amplitude unipolar pacing spikes during

VF and not the arrhythmia. (Preliminary observations suggest that this problem may be ameliorated with ICD lead systems utilizing "true bipolar" ventricular sensing,[21] but more extensive confirmatory data are needed regarding this issue.)

In addition, double sensing of unipolar (and even bipolar) pacing spikes and the QRS complex may result in inappropriate triggering of ICD shocks. Therefore, pacemaker leads should be placed at a maximum distance from the ICD's rate sensing leads, and the pacemaker generator should be programmed to the lowest amplitude and maximum sensitivity for normal pacemaker function. This will usually minimize the likelihood of any pacemaker-ICD interaction. Implant-related considerations and testing for device-device interactions in patients with preexisting pacemakers (or arising when dual-chamber devices are implanted in the setting of a preexisting ICD) are discussed further in Chaps. 14 and 23.

Defibrillation Threshold Assessment

Importantly, all patients - regardless of the presenting arrhythmia - require intraoperative induction of VF (using programmed stimulation, shock delivered during the T-wave, or AC current) in order to demonstrate the ability of the ICD system to reliably terminate VF, since device therapy for a hemodynamically tolerated VT always has the potential to accelerate the arrhythmia to VF; and inappropriate device therapy for a supraventricular rhythm may initiate rapid VT or VF de novo.

In addition, any patient without VF as a presenting arrhythmia has the potential for developing VF in the future; indeed this terminal arrhythmia has been documented in association with sudden death in some ICD patients, in whom DFT testing had not been performed due to a belief that DFT testing was not necessary for patients presenting with sustained VT.[22] In order to shorten the implant procedure, and thus potentially decrease the risk of ICD infection, we usually perform testing of cardioversion thresholds and antitachycardia pacing for VT at the time of predischarge electrophysiologic study and not intraoperatively.

Traditionally, DFT testing was performed using an external cardioverter defibrillator (ECD) hooked up to the lead system. Recently, device based testing has been introduced. With this approach there is no ECD and the ICD, under programmer control, performs the VF induction and delivers all defibrillation shocks. This has the advantage of eliminating the ECD and the temporary connections.

Table 2. Parameters to assess for adequate ICD sensing and pacing lead function.

- Amplitude of rate sensing leads (> 5 mV) during sinus rhythm, VT/VF, and ventricular pacing (if concomitant pacemaker present)
- Duration of rate sensing electrograms (< refractory period of the device to avoid double counting, usually < 100 ms)
- Lead impedance; slew rate > 0.5 V/s (if available)
- Morphology sensing signals (should differentiate between supraventricular rhythms and VT to allow for analysis of treated events in devices with electrogram storage capability)
- Location of leads for rate sensing when concomitant pacing systems are being used (stimulus amplitude < 0.5 mV on rate sensing electrogram with maximum pacing output); VOO -pacing with maximum output of concomitant pacemaker during induced VT/VF in order to ensure adequate sensing and therapy delivery by the device; exclusion of double counting of stimulus artifact and QRS in paced beats immediately after shock delivery
- Pacing threshold < 1.5 V at 0.5 ms pulse width (possible cycle length dependent changes of the pacing threshold particularly if future antitachycardia pacing is considered)

However, it uses up shock energy from the ICD and, occasionally, requires the use of a transthoracic rescue shock. For Hot Can implants device based testing is especially attractive. Without it one must use a "dummy can" placed in the pectoral pocket and connected to the ECD. The dummy can is then sterilized while its connection lead is discarded.

Before VF induction and DFT testing, a low-energy test shock (e.g. 1-5 J) is routinely delivered during sinus rhythm to assess voltage, lead impedance and integrity of all electrical connections between the leads and the ECD. In addition, effectiveness of bradycardia backup pacing should be tested prior to VF induction and DFT testing to ensure that backup pacing can immediately be applied if prolonged bradycardia or asystole should occur after cardioversion or defibrillation.

The goal of DFT testing is to ensure that the energy required for defibrillation is always less than the energy that the device is able to deliver. Guidelines for DFT testing are shown in Table 3. It is important to realize two limitations that apply to the concept of DFT testing: First, both stored and delivered energy are simple parameters to describe discharges and waveform efficiency is critically dependent on pulse duration, capacitance, and electrode. (Chap. 4) Second, the term DFT reflects a certain probability of successful defibrillation rather than some "absolute" amount of energy required to defibrillate the heart. (Chap. 5) To define the sigmoidal curve describing the probability of a successful defibrillation for any given energy delivered (Fig. 1, Chap. 5), multiple VF inductions with attempted defibrillation at several energy levels would be required.

Table 3. DFT testing guidelines.*

Goal

- ◆ Energy output of device exceeds (by 50 % or more) the energy uniformly successful in terminating VF on 3 trials; e.g. 20 J with 30 J output device

  or

- ◆ Energy output of the device exceeds (by 100 % or more) the energy uniformly successful in terminating VF on 2 consecutive trials without prior failures ; e.g. 15 J with 30 J output device

Safety precautions

- ◆ Close hemodynamic monitoring (arterial line in all patients, pulmonary artery catheter in high-risk patients)
- ◆ Application of a synchronized, low energy test shock (e.g. 1 J) during sinus rhythm before DFT testing to assess integrity of all electrical connections
- ◆ Immediate transthoracic rescue shock by a precharged external defibrillator if the first shock (and backup shock) fails to terminate VF (preapplied, self-adhesive patches recommended)
- ◆ Post shock bradycardia backup pacing immediately available if required
- ◆ ≥ 3 minute pause between inductions (monitor arterial pressure and ST-segment elevations)
- ◆ Capability of responding to all emergencies such as myocardial perforation with cardiac tamponade, prolonged ventricular fibrillation requiring open chest cardiac massage,[25] electromechanical dissociation, coronary artery (or bypass) erosion by epicardial patches including the need for heart-lung bypass

* Assumes delivery of test shock within 10 -15 seconds after VF induction; the longer the duration of VF, the higher the energy required for termination.[24]

Safety considerations preclude such exhaustive testing in man. *For clinical purposes, therefore, DFT may be defined as the lowest energy value at or above which VF can reproducibly be terminated.*[6,23]

In our early experience with epicardial shocking lead systems we found that a safety margin of at least 10 J for termination of VF should be sought intraoperatively in order to ensure successful defibrillation postoperatively.[6] A similar safety margin is desirable for nonthoracotomy lead systems with biphasic waveforms.

Of note, no prospective studies are available to determine the best method for DFT testing in humans.[25,26] In order to induce VF, ultra-rapid burst pacing, or delivery of T-wave shock, (or application of 4-6 s of AC current) will usually suffice in the majority of patients. The first shock should be delivered 10-15 s after VF induction (Table 3), and at least 3 minutes should be allowed between consecutive VF inductions for hemodynamic recovery.

Since presently available devices have a maximum output of 30-40 J, we usually begin DFT testing with the external cardioverter defibrillator set to deliver 15-20 J, as shown schematically in Fig. 4; the test shock energy is then decreased in 5 J steps until the delivered energy fails to terminate induced VF, necessitating a backup

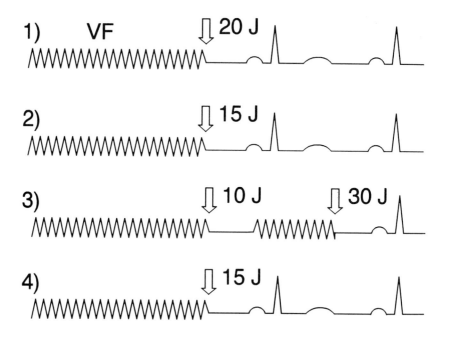

Figure 4. Example of intraoperative DFT testing in a hemodynamically stable patient with an external defibrillator attached to the previously implanted leads. Confirmation of VF termination with 15 J (example #4) may be performed after the ICD is already attached to the leads obviating the need for an extra VF induction to show proper ICD function.

shock with higher energy (e.g. 30 J). If the first backup shock also fails to terminate the arrhythmia, a high energy shock is immediately delivered through cutaneous self-adhesive patch electrodes (e.g. R2-pads) by a pre-charged external defibrillator (200-360 J). By using this approach, the time to successful termination of induced VF episodes rarely exceeds 20 s in duration.

If more than 20 J (biphasic waveform) are required for termination of VF, an attempt should always be made to decrease the DFT by: (1) changing the polarity of the delivered shock, (2) altering the position of the transvenous defibrillation leads, (3) adding another defibrillation lead, or (4) using a device with higher shock energy or a better biphasic waveform.

Because of patient safety concerns, some investigators have advocated that DFT testing be as restrictive as possible.[27] In our experience including more than 400 primary ICD implants at 2 centers as well as in the experience of other centers, multiple shocks to optimize the defibrillation threshold in hemodynamically stable pa-

Table 4. Sequential approach to high DFTs.*

♦ Assess integrity of all electrical connections manually and by delivering a low energy test shock during sinus rhythm.

♦ Exclude possibility, in epicardial system implantations, that energy is being shunted from the heart, e.g.: patches are too close or touching (lead impedance may be low), exclude patch crinkling, and air or fluid under the patches (lead impedance may be high).

♦ Change lead location (across septum/right atrium in cases with epicardial patches).

♦ Change lead polarity.

♦ Use larger lead (for epicardial implantations), or additional (e.g., subcutaneous patch or array) leads allowing for two or multiple pathways.

♦ Use a device with a high energy shock capability (e.g. 40 J).

♦ Repeat DFT testing off antiarrhythmic drugs (particularly class IB and IC agents, and amiodarone, if possible).

♦ If acceptable DFTs cannot be obtained with any of the described methods, consider cardiac transplantation in patients at high risk for sudden cardiac death.

* Use of biphasic shock waveform assumed

tients did not result in an increase in intraoperative morbidity or mortality.[28] Also, except in patients with severely depressed left ventricular function, DFT testing does not appear to impair cardiac output.[29] Particularly in patients with high DFTs vigorous testing with altered lead positions and polarity etc. (Table 4) should be performed to enhance the margin of safety for effective defibrillation, since patients with high DFTs still have a considerable arrhythmia-related death rate during followup.[30,31]

An alternative method to assess DFTs is to determine the upper limit of vulnerability (ULV). With this method, high energy shock is delivered into the T-wave during pacing, and the energy is reduced until fibrillation is induced. The highest level at which VF is induced is defined as the ULV. There is a good correlation between the DFT and the ULV.[32-34] The ULV value depends on the exact placement of the shock in the T-wave.[35] Thus the correlation between the DFT and ULV is dependent on the T-wave shocks being delivered with the proper timing.[36,37] (See Chap. 5, "Upper Limit of Vulnerability" for more detail.) Theoretically, a DFT could be estimated with only one fibrillation episode. Importantly, the ULV (*plus* 3 J) is a good estimator of the 100% successful energy for defibrillation.[38] A larger experience with this approach is needed, however, prior to its general adoption.

Intraoperative ICD Testing and Programming

(*This and the following paragraph are not relevant for device-based testing and apply only to ECD testing of the DFT.*) Once a satisfactory DFT has been demonstrated using the ECD, the ICD is attached to the implanted leads and VF is induced once more in order to ensure that VF is appropriately sensed and terminated by the implanted ICD system before the generator pocket is closed by the surgeon. In addition, we routinely ensure appropriate position of transvenous leads after DFT testing by fluoroscopy in all patients with nonthoracotomy lead systems in order to correct any lead displacements that may have occurred during DFT testing or during final fixation and subcutaneous tunneling of the leads to the generator pocket.

It is strongly advised that ICD system testing be performed with the generator placed in the skin pocket. For one thing, this will help to ascertain adequacy of communication with the programmer replicating real world condition of wand placement over the generator pocket; this will also serve as a check against the device being inadvertently flipped over (and rendered incommunicable) when placed inside the pocket. VF testing with device inside the generator pocket also allows for detection of *electrical shunting* at the ICD-lead interface connector interface, which might not be apparent if testing occurs without the device being in contact with subcutaneous tissue and fluids. Although uncommon, such shunting could occur as a result of either (a) micro-separation between the epoxy header and titanium can (perhaps as a result of prior heat/cold exposure) thereby exposing the feedthrus or (b) loose cap screw permitting the setscrew to come into contact with body fluids. (See Chap. 9, "Potential Complications.") With the generator placed in the pocket, electrical shunting may manifest as failed defibrillation during VF testing, and "new" appearance of noise on the intracardiac electrogram with a possible drop in pacing lead impedance. If such shunting is detected, retesting with a new generator is required.

At the end of the implant procedure, we routinely program the device to active mode. Immediate postoperative device activation ensures prompt therapy if rapid VT or VF, occurs, avoiding any time delays to external cardioversion or defibrillation (also, the latter may have a decreased efficacy in patients with patch leads due to an insulation effect of the patches.) In patients with epicardial implants, several studies have shown an increased incidence of sustained VT and VF in the early postoperative period in.[39-41] The occurrence of perioperative sudden death in that earlier era was sometimes associated with deactivated ICDs.[22,26]

Predischarge Testing

Before discharge from the hospital, we routinely perform an electrophysiologic study to reassess appropriate detection and termination of VF (and VT, when relevant) by the implanted device. Importantly, a chest X-ray should be obtained prior to (and fluoroscopic inspection is advised at the time of) predischarge testing in order to document appropriate lead position. In addition, evaluation of pacing thresholds and sensing parameters including electrogram amplitude and morphology of rate sensing electrodes and morphology sensing electrodes should be evaluated prior to VF induction and device testing, where available.

In patients with uniform VT, we vigorously test antitachycardia pacing and/or low energy cardioversion at predischarge testing, since we do not test antitachycardia pacing or cardioversion thresholds intraoperatively in order to reduce the duration of the implant procedure. Some investigators, however, simply prescribe antitachycardia pacing therapies in a generic fashion based on the notion that spontaneous VT cycle lengths and responses to pacing maneuvers may differ considerably from those VTs induced in the somewhat artificial predischarge electrophysiology laboratory setting. (See Chap. 15, "Empiric Approaches to ATP Programming.")

In a large clinical experience with routine ICD testing (373 prehospital discharge and 293 within 1-6 months after implantation), failure of the ICD to terminate VF was observed in only 0.6% of tests.[42] On the other hand, operative revision or significant programming revisions were required in 5-10% of 49 patients undergoing routine predischarge and 1-month testing following ICD implantation.[43] Although the necessity for performing a postoperative electrophysiologic study in all patients remains controversial, predischarge testing is mandatory when any of the following apply:

1. Adequate intraoperative defibrillation testing could not be performed, e.g. in a hemodynamically unstable patient following concomitant myocardial revascularization.
2. The intraoperative DFT was within 10 J of the maximum device output.[6]
3. A change in the antiarrhythmic drug treatment is made, which may alter rates and/or cardioversion/defibrillation thresholds of the arrhythmia.[44]

Table 5: Surgical complications associated with ICD implantation.

Complication	Examples	Incidence
Perioperative mortality*[†]	(thoracotomy in 230 of 241 study patients)	3 %
Respiratory complications[†]	adult respiratory distress syndrome, pneumonia, pneumothorax, large pleural effusion	11 %
Postoperative bleeding	generator pocket, duodenal ulcer, cardiac compression syndrome	2 %
Thromboembolic events[†]	pulmonary emboli, cerebral stroke, subclavian vein thrombosis, arterial embolization	3 %
ICD infection[†]	requiring removal of the device	5 %
Lead related complications[‡]	lead migration, lead or adapter break, insulation defect, loose setscrew, patch crinkling	8 %
Other surgical complications	perforation of the right ventricle or septum, erosion of the generator pocket, generator migration, wound dehiscence, superficial wound infection, large seromas of the generator pocket[§]	10 %

*   Within 30 days after implant or before hospital discharge
†   Lower incidence reported for nonthoracotomy ICD systems[Error! Bookmark not defined.,8,16,17]
‡   The incidence of lead displacements may be higher in complete nonthoracotomy lead systems vs. epicardial lead systems[5,14,17]
§   Usually benign and spontaneously resolving, puncture should not be performed in the absence of major discomfort to avoid infection

Surgical Complications of ICD Implantation

Our experience[8] with surgical complications in the first 241 patients with ICD implantation, using almost exclusively the thoracotomy approach for placement of the defibrillation leads, is summarized in Table 5. Of note, despite vigorous intraoperative testing of the DFT in all hemodynamically stable patients we did not see any adverse consequences of our efforts to optimize DFTs and no intraoperative deaths occurred in our ICD patients. The use of endocardial nonthoracotomy defibrillation leads appears to result in significantly lower perioperative mortality ($\leq 1\%$ versus 3-5%), and morbidity in most series. However, postoperative displacement of transvenous leads may occur in up to 10% of patients during short-term follow up and remains a source of concern.[5]

ICD infections requiring the removal of the device occurred in 13 of 241 patients in our series including 112 ICD generator replacements (5% per patient, 4% per implanted device). Blood cultures and generator pocket cultures were negative in only 1 of these 13 patients (after 2 weeks of antibiotic treatment). However, blood cultures and/or generator pocket cultures were positive for *Staphylococcus aureus* in 8 (65%), *Staphylococcus epidermidis* in 2 patients, *Pseudomonas* in 1, and *Serratia* and *Escherichia coli* in 1. ICD infections usually occurred within 3 months after initial ICD implantation (9 patients) or generator replacement (2 patients). Only 2 patients had an ICD infection more than 3 months after ICD implant or generator replacement respectively.

In order to decrease the incidence of ICD infections we routinely:

1. treat predisposing factors such as diabetes mellitus, immunosuppression, preexisting sources of infections, especially skin infections close to the implantation site,
2. perform careful skin preparation,
3. administer prophylactic perioperative antibiotic treatment including agents against staphylococci (e.g. vancomycin), although this approach is not validated by any prospective controlled studies,
4. keep the implant procedure as short as possible, and
5. monitor the patient closely for early signs of infection such as tenderness of the wound, swelling, redness, drainage, or fever.

For detailed discussion of infection control see Chap.18. Erosion can usually be treated with local surgical intervention and device replacement is rarely warranted.[45]

Implantation in the Electrophysiology Lab

There are many reports of successful nonthoracotomy ICD system implantation in the electrophysiology laboratory. Some institutions use general anesthesia[46,47] while some use local anesthesia and intravenous sedation.[48,49] Average implantation times reported run from 1 to 2 hours[48] unless a subcutaneous patch is required.[50] Complication rates are low. One report of 27 patients described 1 minor abdominal pocket hematoma and an incision site cellulitis.[48] A report of 62 patients found no infections and 1 hematoma.[46] Another group of 78 patients implanted under general anesthesia had 2 cases of congestive heart failure, a moderate-sized pocket hematoma, a small pneumothorax, and a benign lead dislodgment.[50] There were no complications found with a study of 37 patients.[48] In a larger series of 105 patients, there was 1 intraoperative rupture of the subclavian vein and 1 late infection.[47]

Including all minor complications the overall experience reported above gives a complication rate of only 10/309 = 3.2%. From these early reports it appears that nonthoracotomy ICD systems can be implanted successfully in the electrophysiology laboratory with few complications. We expect that this trend will continue and that the operating room will be reserved for the occasional patient with extremely high DFTs or (less likely) receiving concomitant open chest surgery.

Generator Replacement

Many of the principles guiding ICD implantation are equally applicable at the time of generator replacement: assessment of preexisting ICD leads for acceptability of position (chest x-ray) and pacing and sensing functions (Table 2); documentation of appropriate sensing and conversion of induced VF by the ICD; and close adherence to operative practices that serve to minimize the risk of infection. DFT testing via the preexisting defibrillator leads to document a ≥10J energy margin is certainly desirable. Such an assessment, however, carries with it the implication of replacing or revising the preexisting leads in the event that a very narrow energy margin is found. DFT testing of preexisting leads becomes more critical in patients with known high DFTs or with suspected impairment of ICD defibrillation capability based on possible lead problems (e.g., mild lead dislodgment, etc). The importance of thorough pacing, sensing and defibrillation testing has recently been emphasized in regard to patients with preexisting epicardial leads, some 16% of whom may require lead revision or replacement procedures due to asymptomatic malfunction detected at the time of generator replacement.[51]

ACKNOWLEDGMENTS:

This chapter writing was supported in part by the Sidney Kimmel Research Center-Philadelphia Heart Institute. Table 5 is adapted from Grimm et al.[8]

1. Frame R, Brodman R, Furman S, et al. Long-term stability of defibrillation thresholds with intrapericardial defibrillator patches. PACE 1993;16(II):208-212.
2. Wetherbee JN, Chapman PD, Troup PJ, et al. Long-term internal cardiac defibrillation threshold stability. PACE 1989;12:443-450.
3. Block M, Hammel D, Böcker D, et al. A prospective randomized cross-over comparison of mono- and biphasic defibrillation using nonthoracotomy lead configurations in humans. J Cardiovasc Electrophysiol 1994;5:581-590.
4. Saksena S, and the PCD Investigators. Defibrillation thresholds and perioperative mortality associated with endocardial and epicardial defibrillation lead systems. PACE 1993;16:202-207.
5. Bardy GH, Hofer B, Johnson G, et al. Implantable transvenous cardioverter defibrillators. Circulation 1993;87:1152-1168.
6. Marchlinski FE, Flores BF, Miller JM, et al. Relation of the intraoperative defi-

brillation threshold to successful postoperative defibrillation with an automatic implantable cardioverter defibrillator. Am J Cardiol 1988;62:393-398.

7. Raitt MH, Johnson G, Dolack GL, et al. Clinical predictors of the defibrillation threshold with the unipolar implantable defibrillator system. J Am Coll Cardiol 1995;25:1576-1583.

8. Grimm W, Flores BF, Marchlinski FE. Complications of implantable cardioverter defibrillator therapy: followup of 241 patients. PACE 1993;16: 218-222.

9. Grimm W, Flores BF, Marchlinski FE. Electrocardiographically documented unnecessary, spontaneous shocks in 241 patients with implantable cardioverter defibrillators. PACE 1992;15:1667-1672.

10. Dolack GL, Poole JE, Kudenchuk PJ, et al. Management of ventricular fibrillation with transvenous defibrillators without baseline electrophysiologic testing or antiarrhythmic drugs. J Cardiovasc Electrophysiol 1996;7:197-202.

11. Kall JG, Kopp D, Lonchyna V, et al. Implantation of a subcutaneous lead array in combination with a transvenous defibrillation electrode via a single infraclavicular incision. PACE 1995;18:482-485.

12. Schofield IJ, Rankin I, Bennett DH. Right sided pectoral implantation of an "active can" transvenous implantable cardioverter-defibrillator with single right ventricular lead. Br Heart J 1995;74:204.

13. Epstein AE, Kay GN, Plumb VJ, et al. Elevated defibrillation threshold when right-sided venous access is used for nonthoracotomy implantable defibrillator lead implantation. The Endotak investigators. J Cardiovasc Electrophysiol 1995;6:979-986.

14. Watkins L, Taylor E. The surgical aspects of automatic implantable cardioverter defibrillator implantation. PACE 1991;14:953-960.

15. Watkins L, Mirowski M, Mower MM, et al. Implantation of the automatic defibrillator: the subxyphoid approach. Ann Thorac Surg 1982;34:515-520.

16. Brodman R, Fisher JD, Furman S, et al. Implantation of the automatic cardioverter defibrillators via median sternotomy. PACE 1984;7:1363-1369.

17. Lawrie G, Griffin JC, Wyndham CRC. Epicardial implantation of the automatic implantable defibrillator by left subcostal thoracotomy. PACE 1984;7:1370-1374.

18. Cannom DS, Winkle RA. Implantation of the automatic cardioverter defibrillator (AICD). practical aspects. PACE 1986;9:793-809.

19. Frumin H, Goodman GR, Pleatman M. ICD implantation via thoracoscopy without the need for sternotomy or thoracotomy. PACE 1993;16:257-260.

20. Epstein AE, Kay GN, Plumb VJ, et al. Combined automatic implantable cardioverter-defibrillator and pacemaker systems: implantation techniques and followup. J Am Coll Cardiol 1989;13:121-131.

21. Haffajee C, Casavant D, Desai P, et al. Combined third generation implantable cardioverter-defibrillator with dual-chamber pacemakers: preliminary observations. PACE 1996;19:136-142.

22. Lehmann MH, Thomas A, Nabih M, et al. Sudden death in recipients of first-generation implantable cardioverter defibrillators: analysis of terminal events. J Interven Cardiol 1994;7:487-503.

23. Lehmann MH, Saksena S. Implantable cardioverter defibrillators in cardiovascular practice: Report of the Policy Conference of the North American Society of Pacing and Electrophysiology. PACE 1991;14:969-979.

24. Winkle RA, Mead RH, Ruder MA, et al. Effect of duration of ventricular fibrillation on defibrillation efficacy in humans. Circulation 1990;81:1477-1481.

25. Marchlinski FE. Nonthoracotomy defibrillator lead systems - a welcomed addition but still a lot to learn. Circulation 1993;87:1410-1411.

26. Lehmann MH, Steinman RT, Schuger CD, et al. Defibrillation threshold testing and other practices related to AICD implantation: do all roads lead to Rome? PACE 1989;12:1530-1537.

27. Meesmann M. Factors associated with implantation related complications. PACE 1992;15:649-653.
28. Frame R, Brodman, R, Furman S, et al. Clinical evaluation of the safety of repetitive intraoperative defibrillation threshold testing. PACE 1992;15:870-877.
29. Meyer J, Möllhoff, Seifert T, et al. Cardiac output is not affected during intraoperative testing of the automatic implantable cardioverter defibrillator. J Cardiovasc Electrophysiol 1996;7:211-216.
30. Pinski SL, Vanerio G, Castle LW, et al. Patients with a high defibrillation threshold: clinical characteristics, management and outcome. Am Heart J 1991;122:89-95.
31. Epstein AE, Ellenbogen KA, Kirk KA, et al. Clinical characteristics and outcome of patients with high defibrillation thresholds - a multicenter study. Circulation 1992;86:1206-1216.
32. Chen P-S, Shibata N, Dixon EG, et al. Comparison of defibrillation threshold and the upper limit of ventricular vulnerability. Circulation 1986;73:1022-1028.
33. Kavanaugh KM, Harrison JH, Dixon EG, et al. Correlation of the probability of success curves for defibrillation and for the upper limit of vulnerability. PACE 1990;13:536. (abstract)
34. Chen P-S, Feld GK, Mower MM, et al. The effects of pacing rate and timing of defibrillation shock on the relationship between the defibrillation threshold and the upper limit of vulnerability in open chest dogs. J Am Coll Cardiol 1991;18:1555-1563.
35. Fabritz CL, Kirchhof PF, Behrens S, et al. Myocardial vulnerability to T wave shocks: relation to shock strength, shock coupling interval, and dispersal of ventricular repolarization. J Cardiovasc Electrophysiol 1996;7;231-242.
36. Chen P-S, Feld GK, Kriett JM, et al. Relation between upper limit of vulnerability and defibrillation threshold in humans. Circulation 1993;88:186-192.
37. Hwang C, Swerdlow CD, Kass RM, et al. Upper limit of vulnerability reliably predicts the defibrillation threshold in humans. Circulation 1994;90:2308-2314.
38. Swerdlow CD, Ahern T, Kass RM, et al. Upper limit of vulnerability is a good estimator of shock strength associated with 90% probability of successful defibrillation in humans with transvenous implantable cardioverter defibrillators. J Am Coll Cardiol 1996;27:1112-1118.
39. Hii JTY, Gillis AM, Wyse DG, et al. Risks of developing supraventricular and ventricular tachyarrhythmias after implantation of a cardioverter-defibrillator, and timing the activation of arrhythmia termination therapies. Am J Cardiol 1993;71:565-568.
40. Kim SG, Fischer JD, Furman S, et al. Exacerbation of ventricular arrhythmias during the postoperative period after implantation of an automatic defibrillator. J Am Coll Cardiol 1991;18:1200-1206.
41. Kelly PA, Cannom DS, Garan H, et al. The automatic implantable cardioverter-defibrillator: efficacy, complications and survival in patients with malignant ventricular arrhythmias. J Am Coll Cardiol 1988;11:1278-1286.
42. Brunn J, Block M, Weber M, et al. Routinely performed tests of the defibrillation function of ICDs are not mandatory. NASPE 1996;19:605. (abstract)
43. Goldberger J, Inbar S, Burke J, et al. Utility of one month transvenous implantable defibrillator tests. PACE 1996;19:676. (abstract)
44. Gottlieb CD, Horowitz LN. Potential interactions between antiarrhythmic medication and the automatic implantable cardioverter defibrillator. PACE 1991;14:898-904.
45. Har-Shai Y, Amikam S, Bolous M, et al. The management of soft tissue complications related to pacemaker implantations. J Cardiovasc Surg 1995;35:211-217.
46. Strickberger SA, Niebauer M, Man KC, et al. Comparison of implantation of nonthoracotomy defibrillators in the operating room versus the electrophysiology laboratory. Am J Cardiol 1995;75:255-257.

47. Trappe HJ, Pfitzner P, Heintze J, et al. Cardioverter-defibrillator implantation in the catheterization laboratory: observations in 105 patients. Zeit fur Kardiol 1995;84:385-393.
48. Stix G, Anvari A, Grabenwöger, et al. Implantation of a unipolar cardioverter/defibrillator system under local anaesthesia. Eur Heart J 1996;17:764-768.
49. Tung RT, Bajaj AK. Safety of implantation of cardioverter-defibrillator without general anesthesia in an electrophysiology laboratory. Am J Cardiol 1995;75:908-912.
50. McCowan RJ, Slayyeh Y, Cook F, et al. Transvenous implantation of cardioverter defibrillators in the electrophysiology laboratory at CAMC. W Virg Med J 1995;267-269.
51. Janosik D, Bjerregaard P, Quattromani A, et al. Asymptomatic malfunction of chronic epicardial lead systems detected during cardioverter defibrillator replacement. PACE 1996;19:677. (abstract)

18

ICD Infection Avoidance: Science, Art, Discipline

Richard B. Shepard, MD and Andrew E. Epstein, MD

IN THE PAST complications of various kinds have been reported in 53% of ICD patients followed 24 ± 20 months.[1] These on the whole have been non-severe (e.g., postoperative atalectasis or inappropriate shocks[1]) compared to the problems for which the ICD systems were implanted. ICD system infection, however, represents a very serious complication. It occurs in up to 7-8% of patients[2] and nearly always requires ICD removal.[3] Multiple additional operations may be required. The cost of prolonged hospitalization, to monitor these high risk patients while they remain unprotected (owing to ICD explantation) during treatment aimed at eradication of their infection, is obviously substantial.[4]

To prevent a cascade of problems, all persons involved in ICD operations should work toward obtaining a zero infection rate. This goal can be approached[2] if not completely reached. That is the hypothesis advanced and supported here.

The purpose of this chapter is to describe in practical terms how one surgeon and one electrophysiologist have avoided defibrillator hardware infections. We know that not only our methods, but also patient status, co-workers, institutional factors and unknowns (usually described as chance) determine the incidence of infection. The methods presented have been successful in our hospital.

Lessons From the Pacemaker Experience

Pacemakers and infection
Pacing systems have been widely implanted since 1961 and to a lesser extent since 1958. Clinical experience with them has involved more patients and much longer time periods than the experience with implantable defibrillators. Transvenous pacemaker lead infections have become prevalent enough to prompt development of

special lead extraction equipment and skills.[5-8] The overall pacemaker patient experience of more than 33 years provides anticomplication information applicable to the current transvenous and pectoral era. That experience includes the observations that infection is the "bane of implantable device therapy", and that *any seemingly localized infection of an implanted device may be much more ubiquitous than is at first apparent.*[3]

Reported infection incidence after pacemaker implantation varies from 0–19%.[8] Some institutions have very infrequent infection occurrence. Frame and associates reported their rate, calculated on the basis of 91 infections in 8,508 pulse generator implantations, as only 1.06%[7] [0.87–1.32%].[a]

Frame and associates also reviewed the literature and concluded that when an infected pacemaker lead is retained, the risk of death (up to 25%) due to sepsis exceeds the risks associated with lead removal.[8] Removal risks are not trivial, though. They include arrhythmias, rupture of the tricuspid valve, rupture of the right atrial or ventricular wall, cardiac tamponade, rupture of the chordae, tearing of the cephalic or subclavian veins, embolization of the lead or a portion of it, septic thrombus formation, impairment of venous return, and direct spread of infection.[8]

Transvenous *ICD* leads, particularly those with integrated sensing and defibrillator functions, have larger diameters and greater lengths than pacemaker leads. Defibrillator patients also have a high incidence of left ventricular dysfunction. Removal of infected transvenous ICD leads, therefore, is highly likely to be more dangerous than is removal of infected pacemaker leads.[9] Even so, when a defibrillator becomes infected the balance of risks favors removal. There are some limited reports of successful management of ICD infection with very aggressive debridement and continuous irrigation of the pocket.[10] In general, however, *not removing* an infected ICD system should be considered radical management.[3,11]

The methods we use to minimize the occurrence of infections associated with defibrillators evolved first with pacemaker and then with defibrillator experience. The evolving changes have been in details, such as in using submuscular initial placement of ICD pulse generators in certain patients.

---

a. The *95% confidence intervals* have been, in some cases, calculated by the authors of this chapter and are enclosed in *square brackets* [ ].

Table 1. UAB pacemaker infection summary 1971–1993 using authors' protocol for 2347 PGs.

	Patients	Infections	Rate	Conf. Limits
Infection within 2 months				
CPBP history	952	2	0.21%	[0.04–0.84%]
CPBP history	468	2	0.43%	[0.07–1.71%]
Infection 2 months – 1 year	1420	0	0.00%	[0.00–0.34%]
Total within 1 year	1420	4	0.28%	[0.09–0.77%]
Total for 1971–93 followup	1420	7	0.49%	[0.22–1.06%]

CPBP is cardiopulmonary bypass. Infections occurring after procedures done elsewhere are excluded. One year infection rate per operation is 4/2347 = 0.17% [0.05–0.47%].

The UAB pacemaker experience

The University of Alabama at Birmingham (UAB) Department of Surgery has maintained a computer database of pacemaker patient information since 1972.[12] For the 273 pacemaker patients managed between 1961 and 1972 before the database began, retrospective information was collected and entered in the 1970's. The amount of information about each patient increased as computers became smaller and cheaper.[13] During the 9.5 year period from June 1961 through 1970, 172 patients (103 with transvenous electrodes) had 338 pacemaker procedures not associated with a cardiopulmonary bypass operation.[14] Seven infections occurred, 3 within 30 days. One of these was superficial and was related to skin sutures not being removed at the patient's home location; another occurred after a physician did an emergency cutdown on the pulse generator outside an operating room. Of the 4 late infections, 2 followed trauma to the pulse generator at 6 and 8 months, and 2 followed non-pacemaker infections more than a year post-implantation. The total short- and long-term incidence of infection in this 1961–1970 period was 7 in 172 patients which is 4.1%, [1.8–8.5%], or 7 in 338 operations which is 2.1%, [0.9–4.4%].

During the 23 year period from January 1, 1971 through December 31, 1993, 2112 UAB patients had their first pacing system and 2989 pacemaker pulse generators implanted. The number of these patients with early or late pacemaker associated infections (wounds, hardware, or bacteremia) has been 28/2112 = 1.33% [0.90–1.94%]. Of these 28 infections, 15 (53.6%) occurred among the 627 patients (29.7% of the 2112) who also at any time had a cardiopulmonary bypass (CPBP) operation. *Among the 2112 patients are 1420 (67%) whose pacemaker procedures were done by the senior author, or were directly (hands-on) supervised by him, and were managed by our methods.* Through 1993 these 1420 patients had 2347 pulse generators, and 468 (33%) had a cardiopulmonary bypass operation at any time.

Table 2. UAB pacemaker infections, 1971–1993.

Timing	Description	Action taken	Result
< 2 weeks (1987)	A portion of the PG pouch incision line was superficially infected.	PG pouch wound excision and reclosure.	Healed. No pacing system infection.
< 2 weeks (1984*)	Sternal wound infection after repair of truncus arteriosus and aortic valve replacement.	Old pacing system removal; new system implanted later.	Healed without further infection.
2 – 8 weeks (1985*)	Sternal wound infection after surgical enlargement of VSD (diagnosis: tricuspid atresia and transposition of the great vessels, with pacemaker).	Old system removed new system implanted later with thoracotomy.	Healed without further infection.
2 – 8 weeks (1991)	Drainage from lateral end of PG pouch wound. Infection was superficial.	PG pouch wound excision and reclosure.	Healed. No pacing system infection.
> 1 year (1986)	Persistent staphylococcal bacteremia following hospitalization for stroke. Myasthenia gravis patient; prednisone.	Removal of transvenous pacing system in toto.	Cure of infection; no new implant. Tachybrady syndrome.
> 1 year (1986)	Transvenous lead infection 5 years after implantation. Source of bacteria was abcess in jaw.	Removal of transvenous pacing system in toto.	Infection cured; no new implant.
> 1 year (1987)	Child with automobile accident trauma to PG pouch. Already scheduled for ERI replacement.	Excision of necrotic tissue and new PG. Infection superficial; pouch contents sterile.	Cure.

* Mixed CPBP and pacer protocols. PG is pulse generator. VSD is ventricular septal defect.

Only 7 of 1420 patients have had infections = 0.49% [0.22–1.06%]. Of the infections, 4/1420 = 0.28% [0.09–0.77%] occurred within 2 months of a UAB operation. Two of these were *superficial* infections of a short segment of the pulse generator pouch skin suture line; they were recognized early, and were treated by wound excision and reclosure, without hardware removal and without recurrence in long-term followup.

The other two infections within 2 months of pacemaker implantation occurred after congenital heart disease cardiopulmonary bypass operations done by surgeons with management protocols optimized for the bypass procedures. These 2 infections involved the sternum and infected the pacemaker leads. Complete removal of the 2 pacing systems was necessary.

The remaining 3 of the 7 infections occurred more than a year after the pacemaker operation and were related to a jaw abcess, to trauma, and to bacteremia following intravenous fluid and drug treatment of a cerebrovascular problem in an immunosuppressed patient. Table 1 is a summary of infection rates in these

1420 patients. Table 2 gives the details of those infections. The inference from these data is that pacemakers may become infected early or late from non-pacemaker operations, from trauma, from other infections, and from transient bacteremia associated with intravenous lines. The overall results are comparable to the most recent and best results for surgical implantation.[15]

The anti-infection protocol developed for these 1971–1993 pacemaker patients has been applied to the 1984–1993 defibrillator patients with only minor modifications. It is described later in this chapter.

The ICD and Infection

Published Results From Other Centers

Hammel and associates have reported data from 205 non-thoracotomy ICD implantations in 200 patients.[16] Early infection occurred in 2 patients. Late infection appeared in 5 during followup of 20 ± 10 months. The combined early and late infection rate was 7 in 200 patients, or 3.5% [1.5–7.4%]. Their earlier data concerning 50 patients from the 1989–1991 time period, with a shorter mean followup time of 13 ± 5 months, showed an infection rate of 2.0% [0.1–12.0%].[17] These 50 patients consisted of 43 with successful non-thoracotomy implantation plus 7 requiring epicardial patch electrodes.

In a multicenter series of 439 patients for whom non-thoracotomy ICD implantation data (CPI Endotak 60 series) were submitted in 1993 to a FDA evaluation panel, the incidence of pulse generator pocket was 3.2% [1.8–5.6%], with an infection rate of 2.0% [0.9–4.0%], skin erosion rate 0.5% [0.1–2.0%], seroma rate 0.2% and hematoma rate 0.5%. In a different multicenter set of 757 patients with another non-thoracotomy defibrillator (Medtronic Transvene), the data submitted to the evaluation panel showed a similar complication rate of 5.5% [4.1–7.5%], including an infection rate of 3.2% [2.1–4.8%] skin erosion rate of 0.7% [0.2–1.6%], seroma rate 0.8%, and hematoma rate 0.8%.

Table 3 shows data compiled from 11 studies published during 1989–1995 which had at least partial use of thoracotomy implant techniques. The total number of ICD patients is 1663. Infection occurred in 58. The infection rate for all of the patients combined into one group with both epicardial and transvenous leads was 3.5% [2.7–4.5%]. If 50,000 ICD's had been implanted worldwide by January 1995, and if the data in Table 3 are a repre-

Table 3. Infection data from 11 studies with thoracotomy and mixed implant approaches.

Paper	Pts.	Inf.	Rate	Comments
Hammel[17]	50	1	2.0% [0.10–12.0%]	Subcutaneous patch pocket infection; only the patch was removed.
Mitchell[18]	40	0	0 % [0 –10.9%]	Extrapericardial patches.
Grimm,[1]	241	13	5.4% [3.0–9.3%]	Infections required removal of the ICD in 13 patients. There were 353 implants counting replacements.
Bardy[19]	84	1	1.2% [0.06–7.6%]	Pulse generator pocket infection.
Saggau[20]	107	3	2.8% [0.73–8.6%]	
Pfeiffer[21]	140	11	7.9% [4.2-14.0%]	Pocket infection alone (10), lead and pocket (1). *Staphylococcus* (7), *E. coli* (2), unidentified (2). All but one unit replaced.
Zaim[22]	110	3	2.7% [0.7-8.4%]	Pocket infection alone in all 3. Count does not include 2 infections of mediastinal incision site.
Trappe[23]	335	13	3.9% [2.2-6.7%]	Initial implant (5) with replacement (8); all infected devices were removed.
Wunderly[24]	207	8	3.9% [1.8–7.7%]	4 infections after initial implantation and 4 after changes.
Winkle[25]	270	7	2.6% [1.1–5.5%]	*Serratia* (1), *Staphylococcus* (6); System removed (5), ICD only (1), death from sepsis (1).
Pinski[26]	79	5	6.3% [2.4–14.8%]	CABG patients: 34 received ICDs then and 25 later.
Totals	1663	65	3.9 % [3.1 - 5.0%]	

CABG = coronary artery bypass graft operation; Inf. = infections. No attempt is made to correct for followup time or the incidence of replacement implants. As is the case throughout this chapter, square brackets [ ] denote 95% confidence intervals.

sentative sample of worldwide experience, then more than 1500 defibrillator infections had occurred by that time.

Table 4 shows entirely *non-thoracotomy* implantation data. There were 21 infections (2.1%) in 984 patients [1.4–3.3%]. These 95% confidence limits just overlap those for the 65 infections in the 1663 mixed-approach patients described in Table 3. This would suggest that the infection rate for nonthoracotomy implants has been reduced from that of the thoracotomy implants; the rate is still significantly higher than the 0.5% rate which we would expect with pacemakers.

Table 4. Infection data from 6 studies with purely non-thoracotomy implant approaches.

Paper	Pts.	Inf.	Rate	Comments
Carlson[28] (Endotak)	207	5	2.4% [0.9–5.9%]	Followup period was 4.7 ± 2.9 months.
Hammel[16]	200	5	2.5% [0.9-6.1%]	Infections arose from device pocket (2), patch pocket (2), and skin incision site (1).
Jones[29] (Transvene)	148	2	1.4% [0.2–5.3%]	Both infections were in the pocket and the devices were reimplanted on the right side.
Nunain[30]	154	1	0.6% [0.0-4.1%]	System removed for infection after revision of the lead.
Schwartzman[31]	170	7	4.1% [1.8-8.6%]	All 7 devices removed.
Trappe[32]	105	1	1.0% [0.0-6.0%]	All implants performed in catheterization laboratory.
Totals	984	21	2.1 % [1.4–3.3%]	

No attempt is made to correct for followup time or the incidence of replacement implants. As is the case throughout this chapter, square brackets [ ] denote 95% confidence intervals.

The findings of Saksena and the Medtronic PCD Investigator Group, who compared complications in 1221 endocardial and epicardial ICD system implantation patients, had an opposite trend.[27] *Infection that required system revision* developed in 3.6% = 22/605 of endocardial implantation [2.34–5.54%] and in 1.6% = 10/616, [0.83–3.07%] of epicardial implantations (p < .03). This difference was attributed to the multiple surgical fields or incisions and lead tunneling procedures associated with nonthoracotomy implantation of the monophasic PCD.

The Authors' Experience
Infection

By January, 1994, the total number of ICD operations of all types done by the surgeon and cardiologist author-pair of this chapter was 251 in 180 patients. The median patient followup time was 26.8 months, the mean 34.3 months, and the maximum 118 months. Among these 251 procedures, 139 were for the original implantation (34 transvenous), and 112 were for pulse generator implantation or replacement, lead repair or new lead implantation. *No* pulse generators or leads became infected, i.e., 0% infection rate [0.0–1.88%]. The dates of implantation ranged from 1984 through 1993. None of these 251 procedures were done concomitantly with a cardiopulmonary bypass operation.

The upper 95% confidence limit (CL) of 1.88% for the infection rate at our institution is below the lower 95% CL (3.1%) for the pooled data of Table 3. Thus one could, with 95% confidence, say that the authors' experience is better than the average reported rate in the literature (for such mixed implant approaches) to both a statistical and clinical level of significance.

Pulse Generator Pouch Wound Revision
Five pulse generator pouch wounds were revised prophylactically because of localized incision skin-edge ischemic spots. If allowed to remain, the latter could result in infection of the underlying subcutaneous tissue. Abnormal post-operative appearances of these incision lines were recognizable as potential problems within about 3 days of ICD implantation. In those 5 patients for whom we judged that skin-edge ischemic sites would not resolve within a few additional days, *the object of wound revision was to prevent short and narrow segments of newly necrotic skin, which either had or would become infected, from producing an extension of infection into the subcutaneous tissue overlying the pouch.* Wound revision would prevent infection spread into the deep subcutaneous and peri-pouch tissue. In each instance one could look at the pouch skin incision and see 2 or 3 mm wide segments of discolored skin edges. These progressed to narrow bands of dry and beginning moist necrosis. Points of surgical judgment were *whether tiny sites of dry necrosis at the skin edge would heal over, and if or when the wound should be revised.*

These patients were obese and had protruding abdomens. In contrast to many obese patients, each had relatively thin abdominal-wall subcutaneous tissue. *None of the pulse generators in these 5 patients had been implanted in the subrectus position as they now would be in similar patients.* Tension on the skin suture line was especially tight when each patient stood up. Collateral arterial blood supply and venous drainage around the incision sites had, in high probability, been diminished by division of nearby perforating vessels during pouch construction. Surgical revision consisted of excision of the skin edges and immediately adjacent subcutaneous tissue, and then creation of skin, or rectus muscle and skin, flaps. These maneuvers allowed skin closure with less tension and with adequate blood supply. Antibiotics were used for only a few days after operation. No infection has become manifest in followup.

Such operations are *anti-pouch-infection, preventive re-operations.* Here, this preventive re-operation rate was 5 in 180 patients or 2.8% [1.0–6.7%]. Viewed as a percentage of *operations* rather than of patients, the wound revision rate was 6 (the 1 patient mentioned above had 2 procedures) among 251, or 2.4% [0.98–5.4%]. No implanted device infection or hardware removal for infection has occurred in any of these patients (mean followup time 13.7 months; minimum 6.5 months).

When ICD pulse generators are to be implanted in the *pectoral* position, similar considerations regarding wound blood supply, preservation of perforating vessels, minimization of skin tension, and possible submuscular location will apply. Additionally, the implanter must recognize and abort skin ischemia early. Coverage of the subcutaneous tissue with well perfused skin is a necessity.

Mechanisms for ICD Infection.

Defibrillators may become infected by contamination in the operating room or catheterization laboratory, by intravenous line contamination or other external sources, and by within-body sources such as urine or gums. In addition, internal or external pressure on tissue can produce ischemia, erosion, and infection. Unless special care is taken during implantation, post-implantation reduction in blood supply to pouch skin is more likely when the pouch has to be made large, for an ICD pulse generator, than when it can be small for a pacemaker. If ischemia occurs, necrosis and infection may follow.

The Concept Of Biofilm

Bacteria which grow on medical devices can form an organic matrix, a biofilm which to a large extent protects the organisms from bactericidal agents.[33] The biofilm for coagulase negative staphylococci is a mixture of about 80% teichoic acid and 20% protein into which the bacteria are embedded.[34] In a study of *Pseudomonas aeruginosa* infected implants in rabbits, microcolonies of gylcocalyx-coated bacteria were in the biofilm. The bulk of the biofilm was host generated and typically contained phagocytes trapped within a thick mesh of fibrin. The embedded bacterial microcolonies are thus shielded from body defenses.[35] In an intensive care unit study of 68 transcutaneous vascular catheters placed in patients for 1–14 days, 81% were found colonized by bacteria growing in biofilm.[36] Biofilm constitutes the resilient plaque on teeth and on cardiac pacemakers.[36,37] Biofilm is highly resistant to sterilization by antibiotics and at present makes hardware removal necessary for eradication of infection. Khoury has reported that the killing of biofilm bacteria by antibiotics can be dramatically enhanced by relatively weak electric fields of 1.5 V/cm.[33]

With indolent bacteria, the time from contamination to clinical manifestation may be greater than a few weeks, and the source and time of contamination uncertain.

Ischemia Of The Wound Without Infection

As described in the authors' experience above, wound edge ischemia, if recognized and managed, need not lead to infection of the device. A willingness to spend enough time in the operating room to obtain just the right wound closure, and early approach to wound revision if ischemia or early erosion occur will avoid the much bigger problem of device infection.

ICD Pouch Skin Discoloration Without Infection

ICD pouch skin can become mildly discolored when blood flow patterns change without infection. We have in a moderate number of instances seen an almost distinctive, subtle change in appearance of the skin over ICD pulse generator pouches when no infection was present then or subsequently. The appearance was, we believe, that of dermal mild hyperemia. Skin blood flow pattern changes were brought on by the large defibrillator-pouch construction when the process divided perforating vessels. These vessels pass through the muscle and fascia into the subcutaneous tissue. They supply and drain blood to and from the skin. When they are divided, arterial supply and venous drainage routes are altered. We tell patients before operation that for their safety our decision regarding orientation of the pulse generator in the abdominal wall will be made during the implantation procedure. The decision will be based on positioning the pulse generator so that division of the larger perforating vessels can be minimized.

Fluid In Pouch Without Infection

In the immediate post-implantation period a small amount of fluid may become palpable in an abdominal or chest wall pouch. The palpable fluid can be blood from micro-vessel oozing that continued for a short time after the operation. The amount is minimal when hemostasis has been excellent. Another source of fluid, when patch electrodes have been implanted by thoracotomy, is pericardial fluid that reached the pouch by following the path of the wires from the patch electrodes. A third source is the body wall, when subcutaneous patches or pulse generators rub on subcutaneous tissue. When patients are anticoagulated, intra-pouch rubbing may result in accumulation of blood rather than seroma fluid. During the time of healing, patients should minimize motions that produce rubbing of the implanted hardware on the surrounding tissue, and they *should avoid excessive bouts of such motion in the future.* Just as a shoe can produce an external blister, a hard pulse generator in the body wall can produce local tissue injury even years later.

We have observed only small amounts of fluid in pulse generator pouches, and do not remove it. A pouch containing sterile fluid and defibrillator hardware could easily become contaminated during the removal process. *For defibrillator patients, and for pacemaker patients since 1970, we have successfully followed this no-tap policy.*

Difference Between Erosion And Infection

Erosion can lead to infection, and infection can lead to erosion. Excess mechanical pressure on adjacent tissue from a *sterile* implanted defibrillator lead or pulse generator can erode the tissue. Erosion is more apt to occur if the local blood supply has already been compromised. When sterile erosion begins, early surgical intervention is necessary to avoid infection. If erosion is a result of infection within the pouch, or if infection has occurred as a result of erosion, the ICD must be removed.

Sterile erosion of ICD pouch tissue can nearly always be prevented by anticipatory surgical technique. Such technique preserves blood supply, avoids pressure points and minimizes tension on suture lines. Subrectus placement of the defibrillator pulse generator (or subpectoral placement of small ICD pulse generators) will nearly abolish the hazard of erosion due to pressure on the skin from within. Submuscular positioning does lengthen the surgical portion of replacement operations. Conceivably subrectus placement can produce problems (we have seen none) such as ICD erosion into the peritoneal cavity or temporary masking of an infection. A retroperitoneal repositioning can be used.[38]

Infection of the ICD hardware

The sequence of events when defibrillator infection actually occurs will depend on the organism, local blood supply and other factors. *Almost no ICD system infection will be identifiable as such until 5 or more days after implantation.* Fever before this time is nearly always due to a problem with lungs, urine, drug reaction or some other systemic cause. If an infection of the defibrillator hardware does occur, inflammation and secondary erosion plus eventually intravascular infection with all of its very serious consequences will take place. If infection begins with the leads instead of with the pulse generator, this sequence may be altered in time or order but will be no less serious. It will virtually always progress, despite antibiotic therapy, unless the device is removed.[8] Almost never can the leads be left in place if the pulse generator must be removed.[11] (In some very rare circumstances the patient and physician may judge it better for the patient to live as long as possible with recurrent symptoms and recurrent antibiotic administration rather than undergo an extensive operation for lead removal.[39] Extensive debridement and continuous antibiotic infusion may also be an option.[10])

Late Infections
A urinary tract or other infection, even years after operation, may result in infection of an implanted device. *We advise all ICD patients to see their physician if they get a superficial infection (as from a thorn), if they develop infected teeth or gums, or if they acquire an organ system infection.*
    In the 1960's we saw several pacemaker infections which occurred years after operation. We then began to recommend that pacemaker patients planning dental work or other procedures follow the prophylactic antibiotic regimen recommended by the American Heart Association for prosthetic heart valve patients. This same regimen has been applied to all of our defibrillator patients.

Pre-Operative Anti-Infection Management

Lungs, urine, skin, and the rest of the body should be as infection free as possible before defibrillator implantation. In addition, the following special considerations apply.

Use Of Antibacterial Soap Baths
Numerous studies have shown that antibacterial agents such as povidone-iodine and chlorhexidine gluconate can reduce the skin bacterial count. We routinely in the past used povidone-iodine baths (showers) the day before operation, and now for several years have used a chlorhexidine preparation. Study results comparing these and other agents are not entirely consistent,[40-42] perhaps in part related to which organisms were being studied. The use of chlorhexidine in pre-operative showers produced a significant decrease in skin staphylococcal colony counts when the showers were both *evening and morning*, and chlorhexidine was more effective than povidone iodine in diminishing skin colonization in patients before operation.[40] Multiple showers were more effective than single

showers. We request that patients shower 3 times the day before an early morning implantation procedure.

Some cardiopulmonary bypass patients also have received during the bypass operation implantable defibrillator electrodes for possible later use. Because these patients in the postoperative period have mediastinal drainage tubes and temporary transcutaneous epicardial pacing wires, they face (for ICD pulse generator implantation) the additional infection hazard of bacterial growth at the skin exit sites of the tubes and temporary wires. These sites should be kept as bacteriologically clean as is possible. In addition, *tape should be kept away from potential defibrillator incision sites* because it sometimes abrades the skin.

Patients with urinary tract infections, pulmonary infections, or teeth and gum problems of severe nature should have these abolished or controlled before defibrillator implantation. In some patients with peridontal infections we have thought it clinically prudent to go ahead with defibrillator implantation, and later to proceed with dental work under antibiotic coverage.

A rare patient will have a chronic mild infection which may not be curable but is controllable. An example is a man with a 20 year old, occasionally draining sinus tract from an old osteomyelitis of the tibia. Should this man who by standard criteria badly needs an ICD have one implanted? We have done one such patient without a consequent problem so far.

Anticoagulation Management

The pre-operative anticoagulation state is important in avoiding post-operative hematomas. When heparin as been used, we stop it at or before midnight the evening before operation.

For most patients receiving coumadin, we prefer to reduce the dose rather than stop coumadin entirely. Our object is to have the prothrombin INR in the 1.5–2.0 range on the day of ICD implantation. One or 2 days later, the coumadin dose is switched back to the original dose and the prothrombin time is allowed to increase slowly. When the INR 1.5–2.0 regimen has been used, we have not observed episodes of arterial, venous, or prosthetic valvular thrombosis associated with the temporary reduction in coumadin dose.

Protection For Anticipated Incision Sites

Some services protect against pulmonary emboli by using *prophylactic subcutaneous heparin* in most patients. If the patient is to have an ICD implanted, the responsible physicians must make sure that the heparin is not repeatedly injected in the abdominal wall at the anticipated pulse generator pouch site. The physician also should be sure that *ECG monitor electrodes* are not applied to an anticipated pectoral or abdominal wall incision site. If the monitor electrodes stay on the skin long enough, they will cause skin surface irritation and increase the odds that infection will occur.

Maintenance Of Systemic And Local Ability To Kill Bacteria
Occasionally patients are poorly nourished and/or immunologically incompetent or compromised for various reasons. These patients provoke special thought regarding the ratio of benefit to risk. Decisions regarding implantation timing or even no implantation may be necessary.

Patients with autoimmune disease may receive prednisone, azathioprine or other immunosuppressants. We have implanted defibrillators without complications in patients receiving azathioprine and prednisone.

During the perioperative period we do not try to keep the blood glucose level lower than high normal, and do follow the wounds for infection or healing problems more closely in diabetic patients than in others. In one vascular surgery study, diabetes was identified as a risk factor when cefamandole was given preoperatively and for 8 hours thereafter, but in contrast was not a risk factor when the antibiotic was given every 6 hours for 48 hours after operation.[43]

For ICD patients, prophylactic antibiotics used intravenously are vancomycin 10 mg/kg every 8 hours (with the dose and/or dosing interval reduced if the creatinine level is greater than 1.5 mg/dl), and ceftazidime 1 gram every eight hours. *These are begun intravenously about 2 hours before operation and are continued for 24 hours after operation.* Except for duration this regimen is the same as that used for cardiopulmonary bypass procedures at UAB; broad spectrum bacterial antibiotic susceptibility has been continually monitored for institutional effectiveness. *If for some reason an intravenous line must be kept in longer than 24 hours, the intravenous antibiotics are also continued.* After intravenous line removal, we have given an oral cephalosporin for 24–48 hours. Variations in duration of cephalosporin administration have been related to intravenous line entrance site appearances after line removal.

What is the *optimal duration* of antibiotic administration after defibrillator operations? Regarding surgical wound infections in 561 multicenter patients after vascular surgical operations, Richet et al[43] reported univariate and multivariate analyses of risk factors. The multivariate analysis showed that when lower extremity surgery was associated with delayed operation, previous vascular surgery, or insulin dependent diabetes, patients who received cefamandole just before operation and for 48 hours after operation had an infection rate less than that in patients who received the antibiotic for only 8 hours after operation.[43] The surgical wound infection rates were not statistically significantly different among the 4 hospitals in the study, although the range was 1.9–5.8%. These vascular surgery data imply that it may be wise to continue prophylactic antibiotics after defibrillator implantation for 48 hours.

The Operation

Location, Incision, and Tunneling
When an *old incision site* is present, one must plan the pulse generator replacement incision so that blood supply to both sides will be adequate for healing. Best exposure for safe dissection of scar tissue around leads at the pulse generator, necessary for delivery of the pulse generator onto the body wall, is obtained by an incision directly over the entrance site of the leads into the pulse generator. If this is not the original incision site, the new incision blood supply may be compromised by the original incision scar. *To avoid the problem, the implanter usually can, with forethought at the time of original ICD implantation, position the pulse generator so that the leads enter it near the original incision, not several centimeters away.*

If a non-defibrillator abdominal operation has been done in the past, the desired site for the ICD pouch may have fascia or fascia and peritoneum fused to the skin, or an unrecognized hernia may be present. *Avoidance* of such a site is wise. When a colostomy has been on the left, we have placed the pulse generator on the right. Pathways for the leads being implanted are kept well away from the colostomy region. Extra thought and care in draping are also necessary.

When the implanting physician is making a subcutaneous tunnel from the pectoral region to a pulse generator pouch in the abdominal wall, in an obese person with a protruding abdomen, it would be easily possible with the tunneling instrument to penetrate muscle and peritoneum. Thinking about this will result in one being very sure that the tunnel is being made in the correct tissue plane.

Operating Room Factors Influencing Infection Rate
All incisions expose tissues to bacteria. Other things being equal, short operations with less tissue exposure time and less anesthesia

time should result in fewer infections than would occur in longer operations. One review of postoperative posterior spinal wound infections found *surgery duration greater than 5 hours, high volume of personnel moving through the operating room* and *instrumentation* as risk factors for infection. Risk increased with the complexity of the procedure.[44] Another study of post-sternotomy mediastinitis in cardiac surgery patients found that *diabetes, obesity, length of surgical intervention, total time spent in the operating room,* and the *duration of endotracheal intubation* were risk factors associated with the infection.[45]

Literature review concerning prosthesis-related infections in orthopedic practice was carried out by Wymenga and associates.[46] They concluded that such infections were initiated by *contamination with bacteria-carrying particles from the air, as a result of dispersion of skin scales from individuals in the operating room.* The authors stated that a small number of infections were caused by hematogenous seeding of bacteria, that glycocalyx (biofilm) plays an important role in the pathogenesis of prosthesis-related infections; and further that clean-air systems in combination with perioperative systemic antibiotics reduced prosthesis-related infections from 3–4% to a few per thousand. Similar findings have been reported by others.[47]

Planners of new electrophysiology laboratories to be used for ICD implantation might wish to set up air filtering facilities comparable to those used for operating rooms.

Reducing Bacterial Contamination

Even in the most bacteriologically safe device implantation room, airborne and skinborne bacteria enter surgical wounds. The actions described below help to reduce the number of live bacteria in the wound to as near zero as is possible in the practical sense.

Distraction can result in wound contamination. Planning and discipline will minimize distraction. Everyone is asked to speak up if anyone sees an accidental or unconscious break in sterile technique.

Sterility protocols regarding intravenous line management should be strictly followed by all personnel at all times. Contamination opportunities occur frequently both in the implantation room and in the patients' rooms.

Draping should be done not only to set up the sterile field, but also to minimize odds of accidental contamination occurring later. *Wounds and hardware to be implanted are kept covered when not in use.* If drape contamination should occur, appropriate re-draping must be carried out.

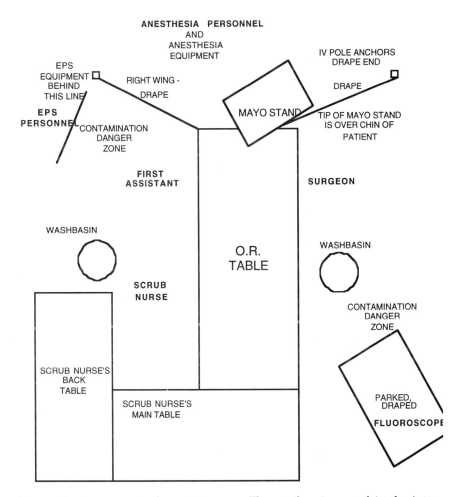

Figure 1. Arrangement of operating room. The sterile wires used in the intra-operative electrophysiologic study are carried laterally to the patient's right by being held in folds of the right wing-drape at operating table level or higher. The external rescue defibrillator (with sterile external paddles), is located behind the right wing. The paddles are adjacent to the Mayo stand in a pouch on the sterile side of this drape. (See Shepard[53] and text below for more information.)

Fig. 1 shows the layout of a UAB operating room. The room is arranged so that during ICD implantation sterility maintenance is made as easy as possible. Fluid-impervious sterile drapes are placed so that the lower neck, the entire antero left-lateral chest wall and the anterior abdominal wall are within the sterile field.

Both pectoral regions are within the sterile field so that either left or right subclavian vein can be used. Sterile drapes cover the remainder of the operating table and the Mayo stand. The electrophysiologist's external cardioverter defibrillator (ECD), used for threshold testing, is in the EPS equipment location.

Portions of the sterile field not actually in use are kept covered to avoid gloves or instruments coming into contact with skin. A *no-touch-the skin technique* is used even though the skin has been thoroughly prepared in the usual surgical sense. Even very thorough skin preparation only temporarily reduces bacterial activity in the skin. Sterile towels should cover any exposed skin within the sterile field of operation. The pulse generator and leads are not allowed to rub on the skin. Similar procedures and precautions apply in the catheterization laboratory.

Unneeded people are kept out of the implantation room. The more people in the room, the greater is the chance of airborne or direct contamination of the wound or instruments from a person.

Glove perforation during surgical procedures is frequent. Wong and associates in one study of 48 adult patients undergoing open heart operations found 185 occult punctures in 162 gloves, among 514 gloves tested.[48] Only 20 punctures were recognized at the time or before the end of the operation. They found that 61% of gloves worn by scrub nurses and 23% of those worn by surgeons had one or more punctures. *The data imply that members of the operating team should wear 2 gloves and/or change gloves several times during ICD operations.*

During *fluoroscopy*, we use *outer gloves of the leaded rubber type* and lead-containing eyeglasses. (Even though roentgenogram exposure during any one ICD procedure is low for the implanter, the electrophysiologist should keep in mind that he or she will be exposing hands and eyes many times over many years, and should by practical precautions minimize exposure during each procedure.)

Although extremely useful in bringing about hemostasis within a reasonable time period, the radio frequency coagulator can contribute to occurrence of infection. It kills tissue by exploding cells with local heat produced by the modulated radiofrequency current. The operator has the choice of leaving a great deal or only a little necrotic tissue in the wound, based on how thoughtfully he or she uses the device. Thoughtful dissection and little use are better.

The radio frequency coagulator can also trigger ICD sensing circuits and can change pacemaker programming. Not so well known is its ability to cause ventricular fibrillation under some circumstances not associated with pacemakers or defibrillators.[49] Also not well known is its ability to induce RF currents in nearby pacemaker wires[50] or by capacitive coupling to produce laparo-scopic-instrument burns of tissue.[51,52]

Once the ICD leads have been inserted, we avoid further use of the radio frequency coagulator and instead then use a *sterile hot-wire, fountain-pen-size, disposable cautery* (commercially available). The hot spot on the tissue is frustratingly small; however, the smallness is an advantage from the infection prevention point of view. No excess tissue damage occurs.

Drains provide a path for bacterial entry into wounds. Even closed drainage systems are potential sources of wound con-tamination. Entry of bacteria occurs along the periphery of the tube or drain. *We do not leave drains in wounds containing pacemaker or ICD hardware.* Abbreviating the surgical drying-up process will save time. It will also increase the risk of hematoma development and the degree of need for a drain.

Subcutaneous Tissue and Skin Closure

Because wound problems can be much more serious when ICD hardware is present than when not, usually the *person with the most experience* in device implantation should close the incisions. Assis-tants must be taught the special requirements and techniques of im-plantable device wound closure and management. When they have been properly trained by the most experienced person, then this rule may be relaxed.

Redundant leads within the pulse generator pouch should be placed posterior to the pulse generator. At replacement time it is then not in the way when the incision into the pouch is being made.

When the pulse generator is in the *subrectus or subpectoral position* the replacement operation may be more difficult than if the device were in the subcutaneous position. Scar over fascia and muscle may hide the old incision line in the fascia. To make identifi-cation of that exact site easier, use of synthetic, monofilament, *col-ored* sutures in closing the muscle and fascia during the initial im-plantation procedure will sometimes help the person opening the wound years later. That will save time, prevent excess dissection, and thereby is an anti-infection measure.

In the *subcutaneous tissue*, interrupted sutures are likely to necrose less fat than are continuous sutures. In the *skin*, knots at the ends of a continuous subcuticular suture line should be buried more deeply than the subcuticular level to avoid erosion of the knots through the skin and subsequent possible infection.

Local Antibiotic Use

Because a few bacteria must inevitably get in any wound, pectoral or abdominal wall, no matter how great the precautions, *local antibiotic irrigation* (500 mg of polymixin B and 1 g of methicillin in 1 L of normal saline) of the pouch and incisions, and of the defibrillator hardware in the subcutaneous tissue has been the authors' practice.[53] Irrigation also serves to flush out small globules of loose, fatty tissue.

When the pouch is opened for *pulse generator replacement* years after the original ICD implantation procedure, one sees in about a third of the patients loose material which has the consistency of not quite hard-boiled egg white. The fact that this material is sterile is an impressive illustration of the point that the wound must be sterile at the close of the first operation. The finding of the material at pulse generator replacement time is one reason we irrigate the ICD pulse generator pouch and the lead tunnels with antibiotic solution.

The chemical properties of some antibiotics applied locally make them irritating and might cause micro-scarring at endocardium or myocardium. We avoid contact of antibiotic irrigation solution with electrodes which touch endocardium or myocardium, but not with patch electrodes which are to be placed on pericardium or in the chest wall. During thoracotomy ICD implantation operations we do not place antibiotic solution on the myocardial surface, lungs or pleura.

Care After the Operation

On the morning after implantation, removal of intravenous lines, heparin locks, and catheters will reduce the chance of an infection occurring from these potential bacterial-entry sites.

To prevent hematoma formation related to the pulse generator rubbing on raw surfaces, patients who are anticoagulated and have leads or a pulse generator in the pectoral region should be advised to limit motion of the humerus during the wound healing time. For the same reason, when the pulse generator is in the abdominal wall, patients should limit the amount of body bending during the healing period.

When a patient with a large abdomen and little subcutaneous tissue stands, tension on an abdominal pulse generator pouch suture line increases. Both the incision and the rest of the pouch skin should be examined when such a patient, or a very thin patient, is standing. If tension or pressure is excessive, and/or skin necrosis is beginning, wound revision may be necessary.

Patients should not wear clothes or belts which put pressure on the pulse generator pouch. In *amputees*, leg prosthesis fastenings of some types push on the most inferior aspect of an abdominal pouch. Pressure points may change when patients go from supine to erect positions. Pressure points must be eliminated.

Patients and nurses should be asked to keep ICD incision regions dry. Following thoracotomy, women with large overhanging breasts sometimes perspire repeatedly in the space between breast and chest wall. Keeping the overhanging breast skin separated by clean, dry gauze from the incision line will prevent skin maceration.

Final Thoughts

With many ICDs now small enough for routine implantation in the pectoral region, the procedure will be done in many more locations than in the past. An increasing number of implants will be performed in the catheterization laboratory.[32] Only small amounts of tissue will be cut or dissected. *The apparent surgical simplicity of ICD implantation can be an infection—and erosion—producing trap.* Even though the mean reported infection rate for nonthoracotomy implants (about 2.1 %) is about half that of the thoracotomy implants (3.9%), it is still about 4 times that which we would expect for pacemaker implants based on our experience and other reports. Thus greater diligence is required.

Persons not involved with long-term ICD patient management may be unaware of the special hazards of device infection. They may, without realizing they are doing so, become lax in sterile technique when in a hurry or tired. These persons need supervision and training.

Persons in an expert group may become lax in maintaining routines because success seems constant and easy. Unless the leaders prevent relaxation of implantation-room discipline, the complication rate will eventually increase. *Think infection-prevention at all times* is a phrase which can, by the leaders' actions, be brought to life in device implantation operations.

Most surgical wound infections are acquired in the operating room and hospital, either from the patient's own microbial flora or from the staff.[54] This chapter has described one set of methods to minimize the incidence of infection. Much effort is required for small improvement. Such actions as being extra careful in skin preparation and draping, avoiding intraoperative contact with the skin, changing gloves, irrigating the wounds and the device with antibiotics, maintaining surgical discipline, and keeping lifelong antiinfection precautions for ICD patients in effect may take extra time (and expense) and be frustrating in some ways. Yet, the reason for doing these things and for continuing to evaluate protocols is to reduce the ICD infection rate to as near zero level as possible.

Thereby, we carry out the physicians' charge: *primum non nocere.*

1. Grimm W, Flores BF, Marchlinski FE. Complications of implantable cardioverter defibrillator therapy: followup of 241 patients. PACE 1993;16:218–222.
2. Shahian DM, Williamson WA, Martin D, et al. Infection of implantable cardioverter defibrillator systems: a preventable complication? PACE 1993;16:1956–1960.
3. Furman S. Implantable cardioverter defibrillator infection (Editorial). PACE 1990 13:1351.
4. Ferguson TB, Ferguson CL, Crites K, et al. The additional hospital costs generated in the management of complications of pacemaker and defibrillator implantations. J Thorac Cardiovasc Surg 1996;111:742-752.
5. Sloman G, Strathmore N. Permanent pacemaker lead extraction. PACE 1993;16:2331–2332.
6. Colavita PG, Zimmern SH, Gallagher JJ, et al. Intravascular extraction of chronic pacemaker leads: efficacy and followup. PACE 1993;16:2333–2336.
7. Espinosa RE, Hayes DL, Vlietstra RE, et al. The Dotter retriever and pigtail catheter: efficacy in extraction of chronic transvenous pacemaker leads. PACE 1993;16:2337–2342.
8. Frame R, Brodman RF, Furman S, et al. Surgical removal of infected transvenous pacemaker leads. PACE 1993;16:2343–2348.
9. Frame R, Brodman RF, Furman S. Infections of nonthoracotomy ICD leads: a note of caution (Editorial). PACE 1993;16:2215–2216.
10. Lee JH, Geha AS, Rattehalli NM, et al. Salvage of infected ICDs: management without removal. PACE 1996;19:437-442.
11. Mull DH, Wait MA, Page RL, et al. Importance of complete system removal of infected cardioverter-defibrillators. Ann Thorac Surg 1995;60:704-706.
12. Shepard RB, Robinson PR, Russo AG, et al. Use of a programmable desk calculator for pacemaker patient data handling. Proceedings of VIth World Symposium on Cardiac Pacing, Montreal, Canada. Claude Meere (ed), Montreal Heart Institute and University of Montreal, Montreal, Laplante-plus, Langeoin, Inc., Quebec, 1979;Chapter 25–11.
13. Shepard RB, Blum RI, The Computer Applications Committee of The American College of Cardiology: Cardiology office computer use: primer, pointers, pitfalls. J Am Col Cardiol 1986;8:933–940.
14. Shepard, RB, with assistance of Vaughn E, and Redmond S. Cardiac pacemaker experience:1961–1970. Amer Surg 1971;37:691–699.
15. Ferguson TB, Lindsay BD, Boineau JP. Should surgeons still be implanting pacemakers? Ann Thorac Surg 1994;57:588-597.
16. Hammel D, Scheld HH, Block M, et al. Nonthoracotomy defibrillator implantation: a single-center experience with 200 patients. Ann Thorac Surg 1994;58:321–327.
17. Hammel D, Block M, Konertz W, et al. Surgical experience with defibrillator implantation using nonthoracotomy leads. Ann Thorac Surg 1993;55:685–693.
18. Mitchell JD, Lee R, Garan H, et al. Experience with an implantable tiered ther-

apy device incorporating antitachycardia pacing and cardioverter/defibrilla-tor therapy. J Thorac Cardiovasc Surg 1993;105:453–462; Discussion 462–463.

19. Bardy GH, Hofer B, Johnson G, et al. Implantable transvenous cardioverter-defibrillators. Circulation 1993;87:1152–1168.

20. Saggau W, Sack FU, Lange R, et al. Superiority of endocardial versus epi-cardial implantation of the implantable cardioverter defibrillator (ICD). Eur J Cardiothorac Surg 1992; 6:195–200.

21. Pfeiffer D, Jung W, Fehske W, et al. Complications of pacemaker-defibrillator devices: diagnosis and management. Am Heart J 1994;127:1073-1080.

22. Zaim S, Connolly M, Roman-Gonzalez J, et al. Perioperative complications of cardioverter defibrillator implantation: the Emory experience. Am J Med Sci 1994;307:185-189.

23. Trappe HJ, Pfitzner P, Klein H, et al. Infections after cardioverter defibrillator implantation: observations in 335 patients over 10 years. Br heart J 1995;73:20-24.

24. Wunderly D, Maloney J, Edel T, et al. Infections in implantable cardioverter defibrillator patients. PACE 1990;13:1360–1364.

25. Winkle RA, Mead RH, Ruder MA, et al. Long-term outcome with the automatic implantable cardioverter-defibrillator. J Am Coll Cardiol 1989;13:1353–1361.

26. Pinski SL, Mick MJ, Arnold AZ, et al. Retrospective analysis of patients under-going one- or two-stage strategies for myocardial revascularization and im-plantable cardioverter defibrillator implantation. PACE 1991;14:1138–1147.

27. Saksena S for The PCD Investigator Group. Clinical outcome of patients with malignant ventricular tachyarrhythmias and a multiprogrammable implantable cardioverter-defibrillator implanted with or without thoracotomy: an interna-tional multicenter study. J Am Coll Cardiol 1994; 23:1521–1530.

28. Carlson MD, Biblo LA, US P2/Endotak Investigators. Initial experience with a transvenous implantable cardioverter defibrillator system using a biphasic shock. J Am Coll Cardiol 1994;23:112A. (abstract).

29. Jones GK, Dolack GL, Kudenchuk PJ, et al. Complications following implanta-tion of non-thoracotomy lead system cardioverter-defibrillators. J Am Coll Cardiol 1994;1A-484A:111A. (abstract)

30. Nunain SO, Roelke M, Trouton T, et al. Limitations and late complications of third-generation automatic cardioverter defibrillators. Circulation 1995;91:2204-2213.

31. Schwartzman D, Nallamothu N, Callans DJ, et al. Postoperative lead-related complications in patients with nonthoracotomy defibrillation lead systems. J Am Coll Cardiol 1995;26:776-786.

32. Trappe HJ, Pfitzner P, Heintze J, et al. Cardioverter-defibrillator implantation in the catheterization laboratory: observations in 105 patients. Zeit fur Kar-diol 1995;84:385-393.

33. Khoury AE, Lam K, Ellis B, et al. Prevention and control of bacterial infections associated with medical devices. ASAIO 1992;38:M174–M178.

34. Hussain M, Wilcox MH, White PJ. The slime of coagulase-negative staphylo-cocci: Biochemistry and relations to adherence (Review). FEMS Microbiol Rev 1993;104:191–207.

35. Buret A, Ward KH, Olson ME, et al. An in vivo model to study the pathobiology of infectious biofilms on biomaterial surfaces. J Biomed Mater Res 1991;25:865–874.

36. Passerini L, Lam K, Costerton JW, et al. Biofilms on indwelling vascular cathe-ters. Critical Care Medicine 1992;20:665–673.

37. Marrie TJ, Costerton JW. Morphology of bacterial attachment to cardiac pace-maker leads and power packs. J Clin Microbiol 1984;19:911–914.

38. DeFilippi VJ, Gottlieb L, Bump T, et al. Retroperitoneal placement of an ICD generator: a solution to a difficult problem. PACE 1996;19:130-131.

39. Thomas O, Leenhardt A, Masquet C, et al. Constriction péricardique due aux patchs épicardiques des défibrillateurs automatiques implantables. Arch Mal Coeur 1994;87:931-935.

40. Kaiser AB, Kernodle DS, Barg NL, et al. Influence of preoperative showers on staphylococcal skin colonization: a comparative trial of antiseptic skin cleansers. Ann Thorac Surg 1988;45:35-38.

41. Aly R, Maibach HI. Comparative antibacterial efficacy of a 2-minute surgical scrub with chlorhexidine gluconate, povidone-iodine, and chloroxylenol sponge-brushes. Am J Infect Control 1988;16:173-177.

42. Dineen P. Hand-washing degerming: a comparison of povidone-iodine and chlorhexidine. Clin Pharmacol Ther 1978;23:63-67.

43. Richet HM, Chidiac C, Prat A, et al. Analysis of risk factors for surgical wound infections following vascular surgery. Am J Med 1991;91:170s-172s.

44. Massie JB, Heller JG, Abitbol JJ, et al. Postoperative posterior spinal wound infections (Review). Clinical Orthopaedics & Related Research 1992;284:99-108.

45. Semper O, Leclerc Y, Cartier R, et al. Post-sternotomy mediastinitis: strategy of treatment. Annales de Chirurgie 1991;45:770-773.

46. Wymenga AB, Van Dijke BJ, Van Horn JR, et al. Prosthesis-related infection. Etiology, prophylaxis and diagnosis (Review). Acta Orthopaedica Belgica 1990;56:463-475.

47. Kwasny O, Scharf W, Schemper M. Prevention of infection in implantation of femur head prosthesis. Lagenbecks Archiv fur Chirurgie 1989;374:227-231.

48. Wong PS, Young VK, Youhana A, et al. Surgical glove puncture during cardiac operations. Ann Thorac Surg 1993;56:108-110.

49. Hungerbuhler RF, Swope JP, Reves JG. Ventricular fibrillation associated with use of electrocautery. JAMA 1974;230:432-435.

50. Shepard RB, Russo AG, Breland VC. Radiofrequency electrocoagulator hemostasis, and chronically elevated pacing thresholds, in cardiopulmonary bypass procedure patients. Proceedings of VIth World Symposium on Cardiac Pacing, Montreal, Canada. Claude Meere (ed), Montreal Heart Institute and University of Montreal, Montreal, Laplante-plus, Langeoin, Inc., Quebec, 1979;Chapter 35-2.

51. Tucker RD, Voyles CR, Silvis SE. Capacitive coupled stray currents during laparoscopic and endoscopic electrosurgical procedures. Biomed Instrum Technol 1992;26:303-311.

52. Voyles CR, Tucker RD. Education and engineering solutions for potential problems with laparoscopic monopolar electrosurgery. Am J Surg 1992;164:57-62.

53. Shepard RB, Goldin MD, Lawrie GM, et al. Automatic implantable cardioverter defibrillator: surgical approaches for implantation. J Cardiac Surg 1992;7:208-224.

54. Ayliffe GA. Role of the environment of the operating suite in surgical wound infection (Review). Reviews of Infectious Diseases 1991;13:S800-S880.

19

Safety Margins for Sensing and Detection: Programming Tradeoffs

Walter Olson, PhD

FOR DEFIBRILLATION energy, at least a 10 J safety margin between the estimate of the defibrillation threshold for a patient and the programmed shock energy is a widely accepted requirement for proper ICD function. Safety margins for sensing and for rate detection are also critical requirements but they are not as widely considered and evaluated during implant testing and followup. *Sensing* of an event occurs at the instant in time when the processed electrogram signal exceeds a reference threshold. *Detection* classifies each sensed event and analyzes the recent series of events with algorithms to initiate therapy. A *sensing safety margin* is needed to compensate for variability in electrogram amplitudes, whereas a *detection safety margin* is required to compensate for cycle length variability during an episode or between episodes. This chapter describes these sensing and detection safety margins; offers practical methods for their estimation; and discusses implications for programming ICD sensing and detection parameters.

Normal Sensing and Detection of Fibrillation

Bipolar electrograms from 2 ventricular electrodes are applied to adaptive circuitry that senses each ventricular depolarization. Current ICDs use the time between successive sensed R-waves to classify each R-R interval. These recent classified R-R intervals are counted to determine when and what type of therapy is to be delivered. This reliance on the ventricular rate to detect and discriminate between ventricular tachycardia (VT), fast ventricular tachycardia (FVT) and ventricular fibrillation (VF) is very sensitive but lacks specificity for excluding supraventricular tachycardias. Single chamber ICDs use either automatic gain control or automatic

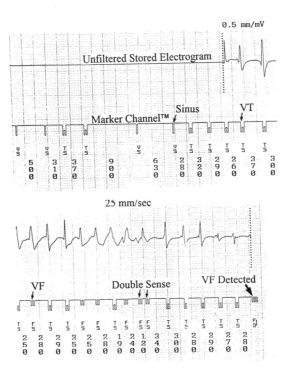

Figure 1. Spontaneous VF episode record with the unfiltered stored electrogram (upper trace) and the Marker Channel™ (lower trace) that shows the time intervals (in ms) between successive sensed ventricular depolarizations (left edge of each marker symbol). Abbreviations: VS = "sinus" interval sensed (single large pulse), TS = tachycardia interval sensed (pair of large pulses), FS = fibrillation interval sensed (pair of small pulses), FD = fibrillation detected (three small pulses). Medtronic Jewel™ Model 7219.

threshold control and ventricular cycle length classifiers with a variety of counting algorithms for detection.[1,2] (Chaps. 14, 15). The type of rhythm detected should be appropriate for the automatic programmed therapy even if the electrophysiologic classification of the rhythm is not strictly correct. For example, very fast VTs with cycle lengths < 240 ms should probably be treated with the same shocks used for VF.

Fig. 1 shows an example of initial detection of spontaneous VF by the Medtronic Jewel 7219. The unfiltered stored electrogram displays large variations in morphology and rate. The Marker Channel indicates when each event during this rhythm was sensed (left edge of each symbol), together with its cycle length from the preceding sensed event classified as VF (short double marker), VT (larger double marker) or sinus (single larger marker). Note that one

R-wave was double sensed and that 21 VT and VF events were sufficient to meet the combined count for detection of VF that was marked by the short triple marker at the end of the strip. Capacitor charging for a shock then began (not shown).

After initial detection, the tachyarrhythmia may be confirmed during or after capacitor charging. The shock is synchronized to the R-wave and should avoid T-waves. Algorithms for post-therapy redetection of VT and VF and detection of episode termination operate simultaneously after therapy delivery of. All of these processes are dependent on reliable sensing of R-waves in the electrogram during any possible rhythm. Undersensing or oversensing during each part of an episode can have different consequences. Current algorithms detect only sustained high ventricular rates without considering atrial depolarizations or hemodynamic information that may be available in future ICDs.

Undersensing of Ventricular Fibrillation

All current ICDs use filtering and adaptive sensing to automatically achieve very high sensitivity for low amplitude VF electrograms while avoiding inappropriate sensing of T-waves. Some devices use automatic gain control while others use automatic threshold control. These two methods of sensing can be equivalent if the gain, filtering and the dynamics of the adaptation are comparable.[1] (Chap. 14) Both techniques are susceptible to undersensing during VF when large variations in R-wave amplitude occur with successive R-waves.

Electrogram waveforms with a simultaneous marker channel, that shows sensing of R-waves, are both needed to evaluate sensing performance. Fig. 2 shows these two simultaneous recordings during a problematic episode of induced VF. Sinus rhythm electrogram amplitude for this lead position was less than 2 mV which is below the minimum of 5 mV that is generally recommended. During implantation the Jewel system is normally tested at 1.2 mV programmed sensitivity to provide a 4:1 sensing safety margin for the routinely programmed 0.3 mV adaptive sensitivity thereby requiring a 4-fold larger minimum R-wave amplitude to be sensed during testing. The upper strip (Fig. 2) shows that after VF induction with the T-shock, VF was initially undersensed during two long intervals; then 10 R-waves were reliably sensed; the VF electrogram amplitude then decreased and was not sensed, so a bradycardia

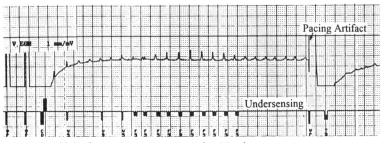

1.2 mV Sensitivity for Testing 4:1 Sensing Safety Margin

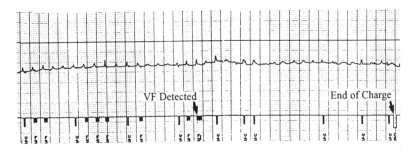

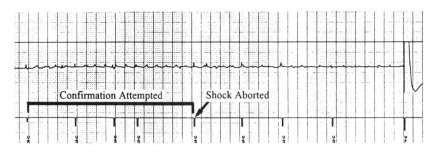

Figure 2. Undersensing of induced VF for an electrogram that was less than 2 mV in sinus rhythm. Sensitivity was programmed to 1.2 mV (4 x 0.3 mV to provide a safety margin). The marker channel shows that VF was detected in the middle strip, but confirmation did not occur on the lower strips, so the shock was inappropriately aborted. A rescue shock (not shown) restored sinus rhythm. Jewel Model 7219.

pacing pulse eventually occurred which briefly saturated the telemetered electrogram.

This amplifier's automatic threshold control does not increase after a pacing pulse. Undersensing continued and VF was eventually detected, as shown near the end of the upper strip when 18 of the last 24 events were classified as VF. Then, on the lower strip after capacitor charging was completed, the shock was inap-

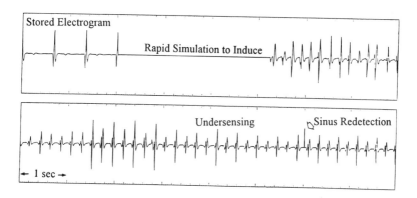

Figure 3. The stored filtered electrogram for induced VT shows variable amplitude electrograms with 240 ms cycle lengths that were undersensed and classified as sinus rhythm for at least 5 intervals prior to the open arrow that shows a "sinus" redetection marker.[3] Apparently the smaller electrograms during alternate beats were not sensed. The rhythm was externally cardioverted after 38 s. Ventritex Cadence Model V-100.

propriately aborted because undersensing of VF resulted in classification of 4 consecutive intervals as sinus during the confirmation process. A manual rescue shock (not shown) was needed to restore sinus rhythm.

If the safety margin had been eliminated by programming the sensitivity from 1.2 mV to 0.3 mV, VF might have been detected without incident, but the inadequate safety margin would not have been exposed. In this patient the lead was repositioned to obtain at least a 5 mV sinus rhythm electrogram, and reliable VF sensing with a 4:1 safety margin was demonstrated. For the PCD and Jewel, the nominal 0.3 mV sensitivity is programmed in nearly all patients. For a few patients with very large electrograms, T-wave oversensing has been avoided by using 0.6 mV sensitivity and a large VF sensing safety margin was maintained. The Jewel has 0.15 mV maximum adaptive sensitivity that has been useful to avoid lead repositioning in selected patients with small electrograms.

Two similar episodes of VF undersensing that led to failure to reconfirm VF and no shock for up to 38 seconds were reported for the Ventritex Cadence V-110 ICD.[3] The stored electrogram shown in Fig. 3 has large R-wave amplitude variability prior to the sinus redetect marker during VF. With no marker channel, the authors presume that the automatic gain control caused VF undersensing severe enough to cause the 5 consecutive non-tachyarrhythmic intervals needed to redetect "sinus" rhythm (arrow). The sinus redetection criterion was reprogrammed from "nominal" (5 beats) to "slow" (7 beats) to reduce inappropriate "sinus" redetection. A subsequent induced VF was promptly detected and treated. Undersensing for highly variable VF electrogram amplitudes in some patients, also has been observed for CPI/Guidant Ventak devices.[4]

Undersensing during supraventricular rhythms is much less of a concern; however, it is not benign in ICD patients. Electrogram amplitudes can vary substantially (up to 24%) in sinus rhythm, and even larger changes can occur for premature beats.[5] Callans et al reported five patients with episodes in which the Cadence ICD undersensed smaller sinus electrograms after premature beats or short runs of VT which caused inappropriate bradycardia pacing that initiated sustained VTs.[6] This ICD proarrhythmia was detected and terminated by device therapy. Increasing the programmed bradycardia pacing rate may reduce long escape intervals, and diminish the likelihood of inducing VT if sinus undersensing occurs; however, this will increase the number of paced beats which might increase the risk of inducing VT and which also reduces ICD longevity. The undersensing of sinus electrograms occurred because the automatic gain control in the Cadence ICD adapts by averaging electrogram amplitude for several beats. This type of device proarrhythmia probably also can occur when premature ventricular beats with low amplitude bipolar electrograms are undersensed, inappropriately triggering bradycardia pacing that could induce VT. Fig. 4 illustrates how the Jewel with automatic threshold control avoided such an occurrence by correctly sensing two ectopic beats that had very small electrogram amplitudes compared to the preceding sinus beats. The limited increase in the threshold (less than 10 times programmed sensitivity) and the decaying threshold with time permitted rapid adaptation to this large change in amplitude. Thus, rapid automatic adjustment of the adaptive sensing function, be it automatic gain or automatic threshold control , is important to avoid undersensing that may cause proarrhythmic pacing.

Since little or no programmability of sensing is available in many ICDs, the lead position is critical for reliable sensing of VF. At the time of implant, the electrogram and marker channel (when available) should be recorded and examined to evaluate the quality of sensing. Poor correlation of sinus and VF electrogram amplitudes[7,8] and practical experience has led to the recommendation of 5 mV as the minimum acceptable sinus rhythm electrogram amplitude for all manufacturers. It is important to inspect VF electrograms looking for large abrupt changes in R-wave amplitude (Fig. 3)

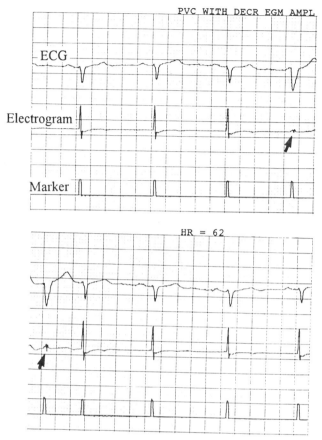

Figure 4. Holter recording of surface ECG, telemetered bipolar electrogram and telemetered marker channel showing that automatic threshold control can sense electrograms that are very small (arrows) compared to the sinus rhythm R-waves. This avoids inappropriate bradycardia pacing that may be proarrhythmic. Jewel Model 7219.

or very fractionated electrograms that may indicate the sensing electrode tip is located on or near an infarct. *Smaller but consistent R-waves during VF are preferred to large but variable amplitudes.*

The electrogram signal quality should be evaluated during the implant procedure when lead repositioning is most feasible. Sometimes sensing lead repositioning or replacement may be required to correct sensing problems.

Oversensing of T-waves, Myopotentials, and Noise

ICD sense amplifiers are about 10 times more sensitive than pacemaker sense amplifiers, and the blanking period after each sensed event must be short enough to allow sensing of another R-wave at

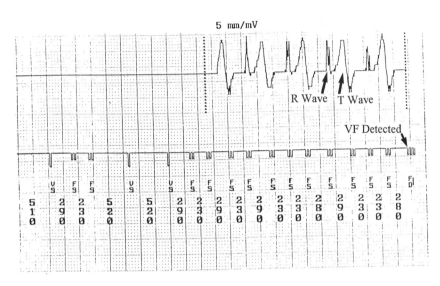

Figure 5. Stored episode record for an inappropriate VF detection due to T-wave oversensing when R-wave amplitude was only 2 mV whereas T-waves during sinus tachycardia were large with high slew rates. Jewel Model 7219.

the very short cycle lengths typical of VF. Post-sense blanking periods ranging from 70 to 165 ms have been used in various ICDs to turn off the sensing long enough to avoid double counting of a single ventricular depolarization. These blanking periods are too short, however, to prevent T-wave oversensing. The long refractory periods used to ignore T-waves in bradycardia pacemakers cannot be used. The T-wave amplitude is reduced by the bandpass filter and rejected by the adaptive sensing which relies on the filtered R-wave being larger than the filtered T-wave. (Chap. 14) If the R-wave decreases due to problems at the electrode-tissue interface or the T-wave increases due to drugs, electrolyte imbalances, or congenital long QT syndrome[9] then T-wave oversensing and double counting of the rhythm may cause inappropriate detection and therapy. This has been observed in rare cases, as shown on the stored electrogram in Fig. 5. The unfiltered stored electrogram shows that the R-wave in sinus rhythm is only about 2 mV and the unfiltered T-wave is over 3 mV in amplitude. Both the R-waves and the T-waves were being sensed during sinus tachycardia and VF was inappropriately detected.

Since a surface ECG is not available, conceivable alternative interpretations of the stored electrogram in Fig. 5 are fast bigeminy or VT with alternating cycle lengths and morphology. These interpretations are unlikely because of the short coupling intervals that would be implied. If we assume the recordings in Fig. 5 truly indicate T-wave oversensing, then the real problem is that the filtered R-waves amplitudes have become comparable to the T-wave amplitudes and adaptive sensing, with either automatic gain control or automatic threshold control, cannot distinguish between the two types of electrical events that are seen. Correction of this problem will require that either the T-waves be reduced or the R-waves increased to the recommended minimum value of 5 mV in sinus rhythm. Repositioning or replacement of the sensing lead may be the only remedy.

The very high sensitivity of ICD amplifiers and the consequences of serious oversensing restricts sensing electrode configurations to bipolar only. Two closely spaced sensing electrodes on an endocardial lead or two epicardial electrodes (rather than unipolar sensing) are essential to avoid inappropriate sensing of myopotentials, environmental noise and P waves. Integrated bipolar sensing of the voltage between a transvenous right ventricular tip electrode and a right ventricular shocking coil electrode is possibly more susceptible to noise than sensing between two closely spaced small tip and ring electrodes because the long right ventricular coil can pick up more noise signals.

Oversensing of T-waves after paced beats is common because ICD sensing systems make the post-pace sensitivity high to assure adequate sensing during VF. However, this post-pace T-wave oversensing cannot cause inappropriate detection because at least every other cycle length is long.[10] (While T-wave oversensing post-pacing should not lead to "false" VT/VF detection, increased amplifier gain during ventricular pacing in some ICD systems has been reported occasionally to result in sensing of spurious noise or respiratory artifact that could either mimic tachyarrhythmia or act to inhibit the ICD pacing function.[11,12])

Isolated incidents of inappropriate detection and shocks due to environmental electrical noise have been reported for radio controlled toys[13] and electromagnetic theft surveillance devices.[14] (Chap. 14) One case of myopotential oversensing was reported for a Res-Q ICD with a unipolar endocardial electrode.[15] Loose setscrews, faulty adapters and lead fractures have caused oversensing and inappropriate therapy.[16-18] Stored electrograms, marker channels and Holter recorders can be used to diagnose these problems. (Chap. 21)

Programming Detection Zone Boundaries

Patient-specific programming of the fibrillation detection interval (FDI) below which VF is detected by the ICD and the tachycardia detection interval (TDI) below which VT is detected by the ICD are important programmable detection parameters. (Chap. 15) These ICD zone boundaries are programmed as cycle lengths (ms) by some manufacturers or as heart rate (beats/min) by others. Such opposite conventions can cause human errors if rates and intervals are confused, particularly when needing to "increase" or "decrease" them if the direction of the change is opposite what was intended. The possibility of error is compounded by the fact that the interval and rate have equal numerical values at 245 ms or 245 bpm which is close to the values typical for VF cycle lengths. Most cardiac electrophysiologists prefer to use intervals, but the rate is often preferred when hemodynamic consequences are considered. Consistency in stating the units utilized for a particular device will help to avoid misinterpretations of the programmed detection zone boundaries.

Both the variability of tachyarrhythmia cycle lengths and the uncertainty of the exact time of sensing each depolarization wavefront must be considered in selecting the detection safety margin. The variability of spontaneous ventricular tachyarrhythmias is illustrated in Fig. 6, which shows stored electrograms and marker channels for a cluster of 4 episodes that occurred during a 30 minute tachyarrhythmia "storm". All 4 episodes were detected as VF and each episode was terminated by the first shock. Note that the unfiltered stored electrogram morphologies were quite different for each episode and the actual cycle lengths varied from 270 to 330 ms. The FDI for the VF zone was programmed to 320 ms (nominal). The VT zone extended from the programmed TDI of 400 ms (nominal) to the FDI.

The monomorphic rhythm in panel A of Fig. 6 was sensed well, although the 360 ms interval classified as VT was sensed much later in the local electrogram as evident from the timing of the beginning of the marker symbols show. The rising edge of the local electrogram that was classified as VT (arrow) had a smaller slope that was not sensed. Note that the next interval was only 220 ms, which makes up the difference. This sensing "jitter" can increase the cycle length variability.

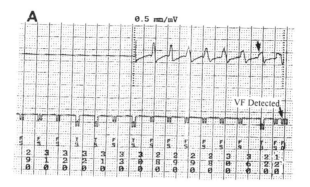

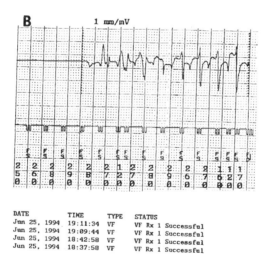

DATE	TIME	TYPE	STATUS
Jun 25, 1994	19:11:34	VF	VF Rx 1 Successful
Jun 25, 1994	19:09:44	VF	VF Rx 1 Successful
Jun 25, 1994	18:42:58	VF	VF Rx 1 Successful
Jun 25, 1994	18:37:58	VF	VF Rx 1 Successful

Figure 6. Four stored episodes of spontaneous VF recorded during a 30 minute tachyarrhythmia "storm". The 4 episodes occurred in the order *A, B, (above) and C, D (next page)*. Large variability of electrogram morphology is evident but no under-sensing occurred. Jewel Model 7219. See text for details.

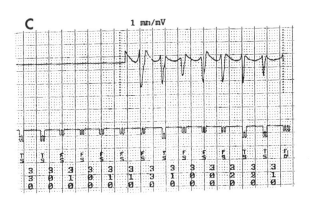

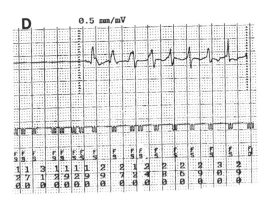

Figure 6. (*continued*)

In panel B, the electrogram morphology is variable, so inter-mittent oversensed events with 120 ms intervals are acceptable for this complex waveform though the actual cycle lengths were 260-290 ms. Oversensing during true VF is actually desirable because detection and therapy will occur sooner. In panel C, the times of sensing on the waveforms are quite consistent but small differences in cycle lengths affect the classification of events as either VT

("*TS*") or VF ("*FS*"). The Jewel detection algorithm may use the sum of the VT and VF counts to avoid delaying detection for rhythms with events that occur in two zones. (Chap. 15) Panel D again shows oversensing of VF for very wide local R-waves.

The inter-episode variability for sensed cycle lengths during induced VT and VF for individual patients is shown in Fig. 7. In panel A, the cycle length data for 30 induced episodes are shown for 1 year of intensive defibrillation threshold testing followup in 1 patient. Each horizontal row shows 20 cycle lengths for one induced episode where each tick mark indicates an individual cycle length. The bold letter that is positioned at the median cycle length for each episode codes the surface ECG rhythm diagnosis. The rows for all episodes are rank ordered by the median cycle length on the graph. For panel A, the VF cycle lengths were variable but the median was less than 240 ms and there is a gap from 240 ms to 260 ms between the VFs and the VTs. Two groups of VTs based on cycle lengths are apparent. With all this information, an FDI of 260 ms and a TDI of 340 ms would appear adequate. In panel B, for another patient, 41 episodes are displayed with the same format. Note that the separation of VF and VT based on cycle length alone is less clear. The VT intervals are more variable than in panel A, yet the VF intervals are less variable than in panel A. A similar value of 260 ms for FDI is reasonable, but the TDI may need to be as high as 380 ms to assure VT detection.

Unlike Fig. 7, where many episodes are shown for each patient, in routine clinical practice only a few induced episodes are available to guide the programming of the detection zone boundaries for a given ICD. Therefore, a larger rate detection safety margin may be needed because of uncertainty about the variability in tachyarrhythmia cycle lengths.

Detection Zone Boundaries and Algorithms

The names, nominal values and ranges for the three rate detection zones for three widely used ICDs are shown in Fig. 8. Each device can be programmed for 1 zone i.e., VF only; a 2-zone VF and VT configuration; or the full VF, FVT, and VT 3-zone setup. Different methods of counting the intervals that fall in the various detection zones for these 3 ICDs have been described and compared.[2] (Chap. 15)

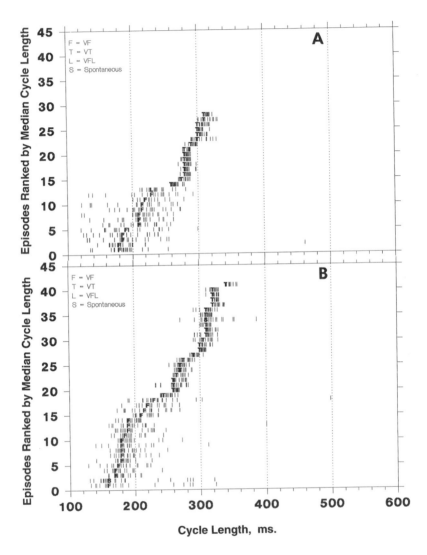

Figure 7. Inter-episode variability of induced VT and VF sensed cycle lengths during 1 year of intensive followup for 2 patients (panels A and B). The individual cycle lengths of each detected rhythm are plotted as a horizontal row of ticks with the median cycle length labeled (in bold) with the rhythm type determined from the surface ECG. Rows for each tachyarrhythmia episode are rank ordered by the median cycle length values.

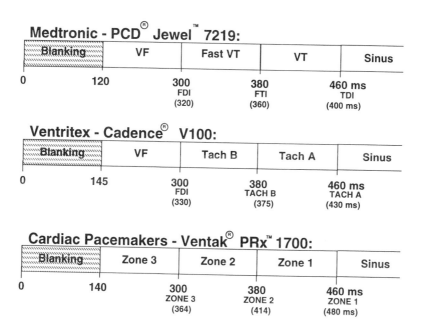

Figure 8. Ventricular rate detection zone and boundary names, nominal values, and programmable zone boundary ranges are shown for three widely used ICDs. The detection algorithms for counting beats classified into the zones are quite different for the three devices.[2]

For the Jewel programmed for Fast VT via the VT zone, VF detection uses an X of Y counter (VFCNT) for cycle lengths in the VF zone and a single consecutive counter (VTCNT) for both the FastVT and the SlowVT zones. (Chap. 15) These two counters are independent and the VT counter is reset to zero by a single "sinus" interval. If the VT counter reaches its limit, SlowVT (VT) is detected if all of the last 8 events are in the SlowVT zone. If any of the last 8 events are in the FastVT zone, then FastVT via VT (FVT) is detected. A combined counter that uses the sum of these two counters (VFCNT + VTCNT) may detect VF, or if all of the last 8 cycle lengths are in the VT zone, then VT or FVT may be detected.

For the Ventritex Contour (and its predecessors), the 3 tachyarrhythmia zones have separate independent Tach counters for VF (VFCNT), Tach B (BCNT), and Tach A (ACNT). The average of the 4 latest cycle lengths (CLAVE) is compared to the latest cycle length and if both are less than or equal to Tach A, the one in the shorter detection interval zone determines which counter increases. If either the latest cycle length or CLAVE is greater than Tach A, then no counter increases. If both the latest cycle length and

CLAVE are greater than Tach A, then the "sinus" rhythm counter increases. All three Tach counters are reset to zero when the "sinus" rhythm counter reaches 5 and the "sinus" rhythm counter is reset to zero when any Tach counter increases. The first counter to reach the detection limit determines the detected zone.

For the CPI/ Guidant Mini (and its predecessors), the 3 tachyarrhythmia zones, (designated 3, 2, 1) have 3 counters (3CNT, 2CNT, and 1CNT, respectively) that are not independent. The latest cycle length increments its zone counter as well as all lower rate tachyarrhythmia zones. A zone count is reset to zero if 4 consecutive cycle lengths are classified in slower rate zones. A single "sinus" cycle length increments all non-zero tachy counters to compensate for possible VF undersensing, but 2 consecutive "sinus" cycle lengths reset all tachyarrhythmia zone counters. Tachyarrhythmia zone counts due to "sinus" cycle lengths must be less than 30% of the count limits, otherwise single "sinus" cycle lengths do not count for tachyarrhythmias. When any counter reaches its limit, detection occurs when either: all of the last 4 cycle lengths are in the same zone; the limit for a shorter zone is also met; or a maximum duration limit counter is reached. (Chap. 15) Detection is completed only when both at least 1 counter reaches its limit and one of these 3 conditions is met whereupon, the CLAVE for the last 4 cycle lengths determines the detected zone.

Consistency Plots for Three Detection Algorithms

The detection algorithms for classifying and counting cycle lengths in the Jewel, Cadence, and PRx were tested and compared by applying large numbers of simulated rhythms with a broad range of cycle lengths and also a broad range of standard deviations of cycle length. The purpose of this testing was to determine how consistently the algorithms detect an arrhythmia when the latter's cycle lengths are close to a zone boundary, particularly as the cycle length variability (standard deviation) increases. These simulated rhythms only test the performance for possible rhythms that are uniformly (normally) distributed and do not represent the distribution of clinical tachyarrhythmias.

Rhythm variability was simulated with strings of 50 cycle lengths that were generated with Gaussian statistics specifying cycle length means in 5 ms steps and standard deviations in 3 ms steps over the ranges shown in Fig. 9.

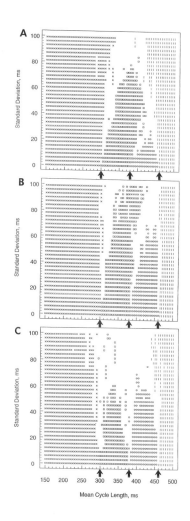

Figure 9. Consistency (9 of 10 times) of simulated detection is shown as a function of the mean (horizontal axis) and standard deviation (vertical axis) of the Gaussian cycle length strings applied to each simulated detection algorithm. These "consistency plots" were generated for the Jewel (Panel A), for the Cadence (Panel B) and for the PRx (Panel C). When 90% consistency did not occur, no symbol was plotted resulting in the white space near the zone boundaries. The symbol "X" denotes consistent detection of VF or Zone 3; "□" is FVT, Tach B, or Zone 2; "O" is VT, Tach A, or Zone 1; and "|" is no detection during the series of 50 cycle lengths. The programmable ICD detection zone boundaries were 300 ms, 380 ms and 460 ms (heavy black arrows). See text for further details.

   At each of the 2,414 points on these "detection consistency"
graphs, 10 rhythms with different random number generator seeds,
but with the same statistics (i.e., an identical mean and standard
deviation values for all 10 cycle length strings), were applied to a
computer emulation of each ICD's tachyarrhythmia detection algorithm. If at least 9 of the 10 results at each point were the same,
then a "consistent detection symbol" was plotted showing the type
of detection that consistently occurred. When 90% consistency was
not attained, no symbol was plotted resulting in the white space
near the boundaries. The programmable detection zone boundaries
were 300 ms (VF or Zone 3), 380 ms (FVT, Tach B, or Zone 2) and
460 ms (VT, Tach A, or Zone 1) as shown by bold arrows on each
cycle length axis.
   Fig. 9 shows these "detection consistency" plots for the Jewel
(Panel A), for the Cadence (Panel B) and for the PRx (Panel C).[2]
For algorithms A and B, VF was consistently detected for mean cycle lengths less than 300 ms even for high standard deviation, while
for algorithm C there were rhythms with high standard deviation
that had mean cycle lengths that were 10 to 20 ms below 300 ms,
yet they were not consistently detected as VF. For the middle
tachyarrhythmia zone, algorithm B consistently detected the most
variable rhythms; algorithm A was less consistent; and algorithm C
was least consistent for very large rhythm variability. For the slow-
est VT zone, algorithm A consistently allowed only about 30 ms of
variability, while algorithms B and C allowed up to 60 ms of variability. Human VT cycle length variability has been shown to decrease with time to less than 30 ms after the first few cycle lengths.[21]
For algorithm A, many of the high variability slow VTs were detected consistently in the middle FastVT zone. (This would result in
more aggressive therapy, i.e., shock being delivered, which might be
desirable since use of antitachycardia pacing in a case of highly
variable VT might be more likely to accelerate the rhythm to VF.)
The data in Fig. 9 imply that high variability rhythms in the slow
VT zone, typical of atrial fibrillation are unlikely to be detected as
tachyarrhythmias by these ICD algorithms. Note that algorithm A is
best at not detecting in this region, followed by algorithm C, and
finally, algorithm B which is most likely to detect highly variable
rhythms in the zone boundary between slow VT and no detection.
Overall, algorithm B had 83% consistency, algorithm A was 82%
consistent, and algorithm C had 71% consistency for the ranges of
axes chosen for Fig. 9 and the selected programmable zone boundaries. Consistency of detection for rhythms that are close to zone

boundaries is a desirable property for a detection algorithm. All 3 algorithms perform well for low variability rhythms.

Zone -Boundary Programming Tradeoffs

For a sudden-death survivor with no inducible VT, the *single zone* detection for VF requires only the selection of the FDI. To assure VF detection even for VF slowed by various antiarrhythmic drugs, the FDI should be programmed in the 320-340 ms range. Sinus tachycardia in adults will usually not approach this range; however, atrial fibrillation may result in rapid conduction to the ventricle that can cause false positive VF detection. If atrial fibrillation causes inappropriate shocks and the VF cycle lengths are typically 200-240 ms in the drug free state, then of course the FDI can be shortened. While FDIs in the 320-340 ms range will not compensate for VF undersensing that doubles the sensed intervals, they will tolerate considerable jitter of the sensed cycle length as described for Fig. 6. Thus, the safety margin between the VF cycle lengths and the programmed FDI can often be 80-120 ms or more.

For the patient with VT as well as VF, or at least the risk of VT degenerating into VF, a *two zone* detection system is needed that requires programming the FDI and the TDI. The same considerations described above for VF alone apply, except that now the cycle length of the VT also must be considered. If the VT is slow, in the range of 340-600 ms, then the FDI should remain in the 320-340 ms range and the TDI should be *at least* 40 ms greater than the VT cycle length to allow for some VT variability. The selection of the TDI would also depend on the minimum achievable sinus tachycardia cycle length (which can be assessed by treadmill testing or Holter monitor). The ventricular rate during atrial fibrillation may occur in either the VT or the VF zone. Compared to atrial fibrillation, however, VT is commonly faster, in the range of 260-340 ms. If these fast VTs can be pace terminated, then programming the FDI in the 240-300 ms range has the advantage of avoiding shock delivery for many of these VTs. However, such short FDI values also create some risk of underdetecting VF as VT and thereby delivering ineffective therapy, if the VF cycle length prolongs due to changes in drugs, electrolytes, autonomic tone, or unknown factors.

Alternatively, fast VTs in the 240-300 ms range can be detected as FVT using VF-type counting with the Jewel programmed for 2 zones: VF and FVT via VF. These 2 zones share the sensitive X of Y type counter and when the counter threshold is reached, FVT is detected only if all of the last 8 beats are in the FVT zone. Any other combination of VF and FVT beats will result in VF detection. This reduces the risk of inappropriately detecting true VF as VT and delivering ineffective ATP or low energy cardioversion.[19]

When patients have both slow VT and fast VT that requires more aggressive therapy, as well as VF that requires shocks, then a full *three zone* detection system may be used. The FDI must be chosen to assure detection of VF; the Fast Tachy Interval (FTI), or Tach B interval, or Zone 2 interval may be programmed to separate well-tolerated VT from poorly-tolerated VT; and the TDI should be programmed to detect slow VT while rejecting sinus tachycardia and atrial fibrillation. The Jewel FTI may be programmed either above the FDI (FVT via VT) or below the FDI (VT via VF) to select the type of counting used in the FVT zone.

VT and VF Detection in an ICD Trial

The programmed values of FDI and TDI for 2 zone detection used during the PCD 7217 clinical study are shown in the "flower" plot in Fig. 10 for 387 patients. In this figure the number of patients programmed with each combination of FDI and TDI is displayed by the number of "petals" on the "flower" at each coordinate. The range of TDI values used is considerably greater than the range of FDI values used. The width of the VT zone for each flower is equal to the time difference on the ordinate (Y-axis) from the flower down to the diagonal line of identity. There are only a few patients with less than the recommended minimum 40 ms separation between the FDI and the TDI.

During the same PCD clinical study, there were 269 patients with 1454 episodes of induced VT and VF where the physician's rhythm diagnosis and the device's rhythm classification could be compared. There was agreement on 575 episodes of induced VF and agreement on 723 episodes of induced VT. While there were 151 VT episodes overdetected as VF by the ICD, there were only 5 episodes of VF (0.86%) that were underdetected as VT. The ECGs for these 5 rhythms were highly organized ventricular flutters. These data suggest that the PCD was appropriately programmed, as described in Fig. 10, to minimize undertreatment of life-threatening rhythms.

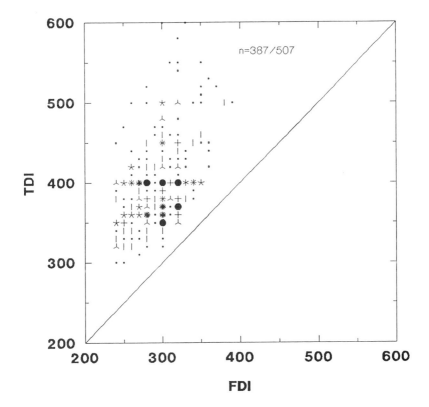

Figure 10. Physician-programmed values for the Tachycardia Detection Interval (TDI) and the Fibrillation Detection Interval (FDI) for 2 zone VT and VF detection are shown for 387 PCD patients. The number of patients with each combination of values is shown as the number of line segments or "petals" radiating from each coordinate pair in this "flower plot". Dots represent single patients and the large black discs represent many patients. The line of identity is shown.

VF Detection Safety Margins

Histograms of the median cycle lengths for induced arrhythmias detected by the PCD as VF (1,731 episodes) or detected as VT (1,560) are shown in Fig. 11. Note that the distributions overlap because the FDIs vary from 240 to 400 ms. The peak of the VF distribution occurs at about 220 ms and for VT at about 350 ms.

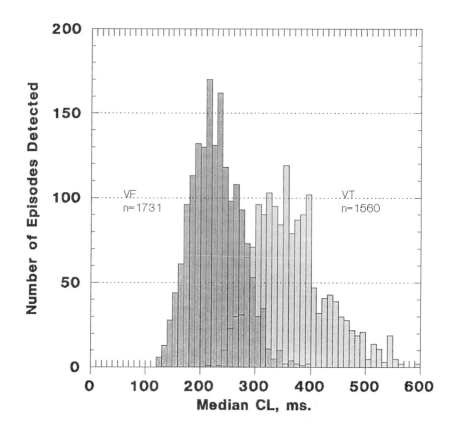

Figure 11. Histograms showing the distribution of induced VT and VF median cycle length for the programmed detection TDIs and FDIs shown in Figure 10. There were 1,731 induced VF episodes and 1,560 induced VT episodes. PCD Model 7217.

     The VF detection safety margins for these same episodes are shown in Fig. 12. The VF detection uses an X of Y counter that is nominally 18 of 24 intervals, which is 75%. Thus, for this VF detection algorithm, the difference between the programmed FDI and the 75th percentile of the cycle lengths used for detection determines the safety margin for detection. This means that if the FDI were programmed to only 10 ms more than the 75th percentile of the intervals used for detection, then VF would just barely be detected. It can be appreciated from the figure that in the great majority of patients, the safety margin for VF detection was ≥ 40 ms.

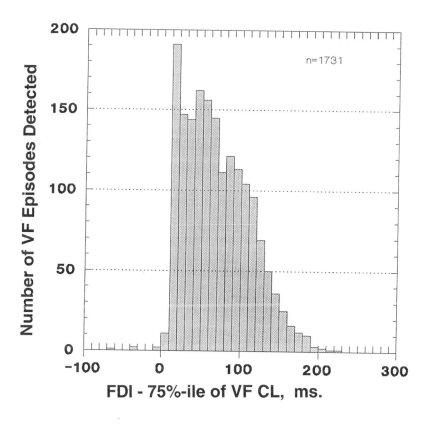

Figure 12. The distribution of safety margins for VF detection for the 1,731 induced VF episodes with the median cycle lengths shown in Figure 11 and the programmed values of FDI shown in Figure 10. The VF safety margin is the FDI minus the 75th percentile of the sensed intervals stored in the ICD memory. This ICD uses an X of Y type VF detection algorithm so, typically, 18 of the last 24 intervals must be less than the FDI. The 75th percentile of the intervals sensed represents the value of the FDI at which detection of that particular episode would have just failed. Hence, FDI minus the 75th percentile is the VF detection safety margin. PCD Model 7217.

In Fig. 12, the large number of detected VF episodes with very low safety margins is not cause for alarm, however, because the ECG analysis for this study (as discussed above) showed that most of these rhythms were really VTs that were overtreated. The inter-episode variability described above contributes to the wide range of VF safety margins.

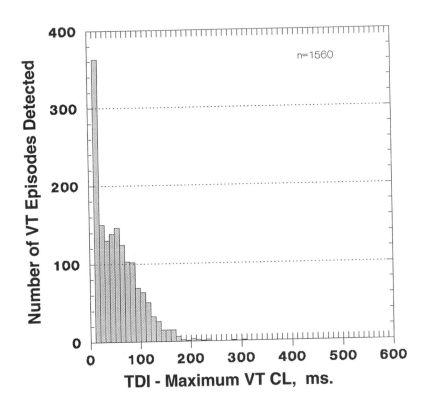

Figure 13. The distribution of safety margins for VT detection for the 1,560 induced VT episodes with median cycle lengths shown in Figure 11 and the programmed values of TDI and FDI shown in Figure 10. The VT safety margin is the TDI minus the maximum VT cycle length (CL) of the intervals used for detection. The consecutive VT counter used in this ICD has this VT safety margin. The large spike in the histogram near zero is caused by tachyarrhythmias that gradually cross the TDI. Most represent sinus tachycardia. PCD Model 7217.

VT Detection Safety Margins

The safety margins for detection of many VT episodes compiled from PCD memory interval data are shown in Fig. 13. For this ICD, the VT detection safety margin is defined as the programmed TDI minus the maximum VT cycle length of the intervals used for detection. (The safety margin for detection, however, is always algorithm specific.) In the figure, it is evident that in most patients, the safety margin for VT detection was ≥ 40 ms.

The large bin for the smallest safety margins in the histogram of Fig. 13 was investigated further by comparing the intervals before and after therapy. The post-therapy cycle lengths did not change for many of those episodes, indicating most likely that supraventricular tachycardias (especially sinus tachycardia) may have been inappropriately detected. An alternative, less likely explanation is that VTs slowly accelerated across the TDI and were not terminated. Almost 10% of the rhythms detected as VT were of this type.

Programming Time to Detection and Redetection

Tradeoffs to consider when programming the number of intervals to detection (NID) or the time to detection include the duration of nonsustained ventricular tachyarrhythmias, the need to reject inappropriate sensing due to lead problems or noise, the time for the patient to become syncopal, and the likely time for ischemia to develop. For all counting algorithms, the NID or time for detection of a sustained tachyarrhythmia has some effect on the sensitivity of detection.

Consecutive counting algorithms reset the VT counter when a single sinus interval occurs. While such algorithms are excellent for rejecting atrial fibrillation, they become increasingly susceptible to undersensing that could delay detection of VT when the NID is programmed to large values.

An X of Y counter that is used for VF detection can ignore some long intervals. Nonetheless, finding 12 of 16 VF intervals in a rhythm is easier (more sensitive) than finding 18 of 24 VF intervals even though both have a 75% proportion, because the minimum proportion of VF intervals must be sustained for a longer total time period (i.e. 18 vs. 12 intervals). Algorithms that use averaging are susceptible to underdetection when undersensing causes large variability in the running average cycle lengths.[2]

Most ICDs allow programming of shorter redetection times following therapies within an episode to reduce the duration of episodes requiring multiple therapies. The disadvantage of a short redetection time, however, is that many post-therapy arrhythmias are nonsustained and convert to sinus rhythm soon after the therapy is completed. Redetection times that are too short to allow this termination to occur may commence another pacing therapy that interferes with termination of the arrhythmia or reinitiates VT. Shorter redetection times may be used to increase sensitivity of VF redetection for leads that are susceptible to post-shock undersensing.

Programming Optional Stability Algorithms

Optional cycle length stability algorithms are used to improve rejection of AF for the VT detection zone and are available with the PCD, Jewel, PRx, Mini, and Res-Q. The stability algorithms reject tachyarrhythmias occurring in the VT zone if the cycle length variability exceeds a programmed value. (Chap. 15) Swerdlow found that PCD stability programmed to 40 ms reduced inappropriate detection of induced atrial fibrillation by 95% in 20 patients, reduced inappropriate detection of paroxysmal atrial fibrillation by 95% in 6 patients, and reduced inappropriate detection of chronic atrial fibrillation by 99% in 9 patients while maintaining appropriate detection of all induced VT (339 episodes) and spontaneous VT (877 episodes).[20]

The tradeoff in using the stability criterion is that the variability of atrial fibrillation must consistently exceed the variability of the VT to be detected. Several studies have shown that monomorphic VT cycle length variability rarely exceeds 30 ms.[21-23] Polymorphic VT with larger cycle length variability usually self-terminates (nonsustained VT), becomes monomorphic, or spontaneously accelerates to VF. The first 5-7 beats of spontaneous VTs are often polymorphic before becoming monomorphic. When stability is used to reject the more variable atrial fibrillation, some risk of underdetecting variable VT is unavoidable. Underdetection due to use of the stability criterion occurred in 0.2% of induced VT and 0.4% of spontaneous VT.[20] For slower VTs that are well tolerated, the benefit may outweigh the risk. Swerdlow[20] recommends using PCD stability of 40 ms when *all* of the following apply:

1. Patients have a history of chronic or paroxysmal atrial fibrillation with cycle lengths likely to be shorter than the TDI.
2. The VT is monomorphic and hemodynamically stable.
3. The VT is slow enough that inappropriate detection of atrial fibrillation is likely without use of the stability criterion.
4. Hemodynamically unstable (usually more rapid) VTs are detected and treated as though they were VF.
5. Variability in spontaneous monomorphic VT cycle length does not exceed 40 ms except at the onset of VT.

6. Induced monomorphic VT is detected with a stability criterion of 40 ms.
7. The programmable number of intervals for detection is 16 or less.

Many physicians elect to wait until atrial fibrillation causes inappropriate detection before turning on stability because then there is a real patient specific benefit to balance the risk of underdetecting VT. Stability was used in about 20% of PCD patients during the clinical study in Europe, Canada and the USA. (See Chap. 15 for clinical experience with use of stability algorithms.)

Programming Optional Onset Algorithms

Optional onset detection algorithms discriminate between the sudden change in ventricular rate at the start of spontaneous VT and the gradual acceleration of sinus tachycardia when the rates of these two rhythms overlap. The Medtronic PCD and Jewel, CPI/Guidant Mini (and its predecessors), Ventritex Contour (and its predecessors), Telectronics Sentry 4310 (and its predecessors), and the Intermedics Res-Q have optional onset algorithms. The onset may be programmed as a percentage change (PCD and Jewel) or as an absolute change in milliseconds (Mini, Contour). (Chap. 15). Sustained high rate criteria are used to limit the duration of the high rate in the VT zone. Swerdlow studied the PCD onset programmed at an 87% value and found 98% rejection of sinus tachycardia, but also 4 episodes (0.5%) of symptomatic hemodynamically stable sustained VT were not detected. In one of these episodes the VT cycle length was documented to gradually cross the TDI without satisfying the onset criteria. There were also instances in which premature beats during sinus tachycardia satisfied the onset criteria and detection ensued. The onset algorithm was improved for the Jewel but no clinical data are available.

Swerdlow recommends use of the PCD onset when the benefit outweighs the risk of underdetecting 0.5% of hemodynamically stable VTs. This benefit may arise when inappropriate detection of sinus tachycardia has occurred and is likely to recur due to the TDI needed to detect slow VT in a patient in whom beta blockers (for blunting the rate of sinus tachycardia) are not tolerated or are contraindicated. The PCD onset algorithm has been used sparingly (only 3.3% of patients) for very slow VTs during clinical studies.

Programming Optional Morphology Algorithms

In earlier CPI/Guidant devices, an electrogram morphology algorithm can be programmed ON to add specificity to the rate detection. The probability density function (PDF) measures the proportion of time that the signal deviates from the isoelectric line throughout the entire cardiac cycle. (Chap. 2) During VF there is relatively little isoelectric signal, so that PDF is satisfied. When the PDF option is utilized, both the rate and the PDF criteria must be met to detect the tachyarrhythmia.[24] Fast ventricular tachycardia and ventricular flutter that need to be shocked may not satisfy PDF. In these instances use of the PDF has been reported to delay detection, particularly if the duration of the EGM depolarization is less than 100 ms.[25] The turning point morphology (TPM) uses a similar measurement, but when satisfied, it accelerates the therapy that is delivered.

In the Jewel Plus 7218 ICD, the width of R-waves in electrograms are measured and compared to a threshold to discriminate VT from supraventricular rhythms with normal conduction.[26] The time of bipolar sensing is used to center a 200 ms measurement window in which the beginning and ending points of the far-field R-wave are determined with programmable slew rate criteria to measure the R-wave width. At least 6 of the last 8 beats of the detected rhythm based on rate alone must be wider than the programmable width threshold to detect VT. This algorithm has a passive mode that permits complete testing and documentation of the criterion for spontaneous episodes to determine if it is helpful and safe before enabling it. (See Chap. 15 for further discussion of morphology.)

Confirmation and Synchronization

Spontaneous termination of ventricular tachyarrhythmias during charging was the most common cause of inappropriate shocks for committed ICDs.[27] Tachyarrhythmia confirmation is useful to avoid inappropriate shocks. Aborting shock therapy, however, wastes considerable battery energy. The disadvantage of confirmation was shown in Fig. 2 where undersensing during VF for 4 consecutive beats inappropriately aborted the shock. For nonsustained tachyarrhythmias, increasing the time for detection via the number of intervals for detection or the pre-therapy delay is preferred unless the patient becomes syncopal during this period. Memory data can be used to determine when the number of aborted shocks becomes excessive. Rarely, ICDs have required replacement because repetitive inappropriate high voltage capacitor charging has depleted the battery.

Shocks are synchronized to the local bipolar sensed electrogram so that they are delivered into an R-wave, and to avoid oversensed T-waves, in case the rhythm may actually be supraventricular. Undersensing can also cause synchronization problems. For example, a case was reported[28] in which the second blanking period following a single double-sensed R-wave caused undersensing of the next R-wave, that inappropriately aborted a VT cardioversion shock; subsequent redetection with automatic delivery of a successful shock occurred within 6 seconds. Sensing malfunctions during confirmation and synchronization should be considered during troubleshooting of ICDs.

Episode Termination

If detection of episode termination in ICDs is too specific, then several actually separate episodes in a tachyarrhythmia "storm" may be treated as one "episode" by the ICD until all programmed therapies are inappropriately exhausted. If, however, detection of episode termination is too sensitive, then undersensing following unsuccessful shocks may cause the ICD to inappropriately detect episode termination, subsequently detect another "episode" and repeatedly apply the same ineffective therapy during what is actually only one episode. This inappropriate detection of episode termination has been caused by severe post-shock undersensing for some integrated bipolar endocardial leads, particularly for short tip-to-RV coil electrode spacing.[29] Recovery of the post-shock electrogram amplitude up to 1-2 minutes after the shocks may result in delayed redetection of the VF, either with or without episode termination, and recycling of ineffective therapy.

The limited number of shocks for one episode is designed to avoid incessant shocking when some type of oversensing continuously satisfies the detection algorithm. In rare cases, this safety feature has been thwarted when T-wave oversensing in sinus rhythm caused shocks that, in turn, created a transient rhythm, such as an idioventricular rhythm, which did not exhibit T-wave oversensing; this lack of T-wave oversensing then continued for a period long enough to satisfy episode termination (as short as 3 beats in some ICDs) followed by a return to sinus rhythm with the T-wave oversensing that again caused inappropriate detection of a new "episode". Unfortunately this type of inappropriate therapy that causes a transient rhythm change may occur repeatedly without any limit to the number of "episodes". It is difficult to design algorithms to prevent such phenomena because actual ventricular tachyarrhythmia "storms" often contain clusters of valid episodes.

Summary and Conclusions

Adequate safety margins for both sensing and detection are needed for reliable clinical application of ICD technology. Sensing of R-waves in bipolar electrograms during low amplitude VF and rejection of T-waves in other rhythms require adaptive amplification or adaptive thresholds. Temporary reduction of programmed sensitivity during induced episodes of VF can be used to evaluate a sensing safety margin. Total variability of ICD sensed R-R intervals is the sum of actual tachyarrhythmia cycle length variability and the sensing jitter due to R-wave shape variability. Safety margins for ICD detection algorithms that classify each R-R interval depend on the type of counting algorithm used. Tradeoffs for programming zone boundaries require consideration of both the ventricular tachyarrhythmias to be detected and the supraventricular tachyarrhythmias to be rejected. Optional algorithms that add detection specificity should be used only when the need to avoid inappropriate detection outweighs the slight risk of VT underdetection. The great flexibility provided to reprogram ICD parameters to solve patient specific problems can also cause trouble if accidental, inadvertent, or misconceived programming occurs. Future improvements in detection will use atrial sensing to perform dual chamber rhythm analysis, new methods for analyzing ventricular electrogram morphology, and sensors to monitor heart failure and control the therapy.

ACKNOWLEDGMENT:
Special thanks to Charles Swerdlow, MD for his review and insights.

1. Olson WH: Tachyarrhythmia sensing and detection. In: Implantable Cardioverter-Defibrillator, I Singer (ed). Armonk, NY: Futura Publishing Co., Inc. 1994, Chapter 4, pp 71-107.
2. Olson WH, Gunderson BD, Fang-Yen MC, et al. Properties and performance of rate detection algorithms for three implantable cardioverter-defibrillators. Computers in Cardiology 1994. IEEE Computer Society Press, 1995:65-68.
3. Mann DE, Kelly PA, Damle RS, et al. Undersensing during ventricular tachyarrhythmias in a third-generation implantable cardioverter defibrillator. PACE

1994;17:1525-1530.
4. Bardy GH, Ivey TD, Stewart R, et al. Failure of the automatic cardioverter defibrillator to detect ventricular fibrillation. Am J Cardiol 1986;58:1107-1108.
5. Callans DJ, Hook BG, Marchlinski FE. Effect of rate and coupling interval on endocardial R-wave amplitude in permanent ventricular sensing lead systems. J Am Coll Cardiol 1993;22:746-750.
6. Callans DJ, Hook BG, Kleiman RB, et al. Unique sensing errors in third-generation implantable cardioverter-defibrillators. J Am Coll Cardiol 1993;22:1135-1140.
7. Ellenbogen KA, Wood MA, Stambler BS, et al. Measurement of ventricular electrogram amplitude during intraoperative induction of ventricular tachyarrhythmias. Am J Cardiol 1992;70:1017-1022.
8. Leitch JW, Yee R, Klein GJ, et al. Correlation between the ventricular electrogram amplitude in sinus rhythm and in ventricular fibrillation. PACE 1990;13:1105-1109.
9. Perry GY, Kosar Em. Problems in managing patients with long QT syndrome and implantable cardioverter defibrillators: a report of two cases. PACE 1996;19:863-867.
10. Frazier DW, Stanton MS. Pseudo-oversensing of the T-wave by an implantable cardioverter defibrillator: a nonclinical problem. PACE 1994;17:1311-1315.
11. Kelly PA, Mann DE, Damle RS, et al. Oversensing during ventricular pacing in patients with a third-generation implantable cardioverter-defibrillator. J Am Coll Cardiol 1994;23:1531-1534.
12. Rosenthal ME, Paskman C. Noise generation during bradycardia pacing with the Ventritex Cadence/CPI Endotak ICD system: incidence and clinical significance. PACE 1996;19:677. (abstract)
13. Man KC, Davidson T, Langberg JJ, et al. Interference from a hand held radiofrequency remote control causing discharge of an implantable defibrillator. PACE 1993;16:1756-1758. (also letter: PACE 1994 17:685)
14. Mathew P, Lewis C, Neglia J, et al. Interaction between electronic surveillance systems and implantable defibrillators: insights from a fourth generation ICD. Submitted to PACE.
15. Sandler MJ, Kutalek SP. Inappropriate discharge by an implantable cardioverter defibrillator: recognition of myopotential sensing using telemetered intracardiac electrograms. PACE 1994;17:665-671.
16. Almeida HF, Buckingham TA. Inappropriate implantable cardioverter defibrillator shocks secondary to sensing lead failure: utility of stored electrograms. PACE 1993;16:407-411.
17. Epstein AE, Shepard RB. Failure of one conductor in a nonthoracotomy implantable defibrillator lead causing inappropriate sensing and potentially ineffective shock delivery. PACE 1993;16:796-800.
18. Daoud EG, Kirsh MM, Bolling SF, et al. Incidence, presentation, diagnosis, and management of malfunctioning implantable cardioverter-defibrillator rate-sensing leads. Am Heart J 1994;128:892-895.
19. Olson WH, Peterson DK, Ruetz LL, et al. Discrimination of fast ventricular tachycardia from ventricular fibrillation and slow ventricular tachycardia for an implantable pacer-cardioverter-defibrillator. Computers in Cardiology 1993. IEEE Computer Society Press, 1993:835-838.
20. Swerdlow CD, Chen PS, Kass RM, et al. Discrimination of ventricular tachycardia from sinus tachycardia and atrial fibrillation in a tiered-therapy cardioverter-defibrillator. J Am Coll Cardiol 1994;23:1342-1355.
21. Geibel A, Zehender M, Brugada P, et al. Changes in cycle length at the onset of sustained tachyarrhythmias - importance for antitachycardia pacing. Am Heart J 1988;115:588-592.
22. Volosin KJ, Beauregard LM, Fabiszewski R, et al. Spontaneous changes in ventricular tachycardia cycle length. J Am Coll Cardiol 1991;17:409-414.

23. Olson WH, Bardy GH: Cycle length and morphology patterns at onset of spontaneous ventricular tachycardia and fibrillation. PACE 1986;9:284. (abstract)
24. Langer A, Heilman MS, Mower MM, et al. Considerations in the development of the automatic implantable defibrillator. Med Instrum 1976;10:163-167.
25. Routh AG, Larnard DJ. The probability density function as an arrhythmia discriminator in cardiac electrogram analysis. Miami Technicon International Conference, 1987;IEE TH0206:19-22.
26 Gillberg JM, Olson WH, Bardy GH, et al. Electrogram width algorithm for discrimination of supraventricular rhythm from ventricular tachycardia. PACE 1994;17:866. (abstract)
27. Maloney J, Masterson M, Khoury D, et al. Clinical performance of the implantable cardioverter defibrillator: electrocardiographic documentation of 101 spontaneous discharges. PACE 1991;14:280-285.
28. Swerdlow CD, Ahern T, Chen PS, et al. Underdetection of ventricular tachycardia by algorithms to enhance specificity in a tiered-therapy cardioverter-defibrillator. J Am Coll Cardiol 1994;24:416-424.
29. Jung W, Manz M, Moosdorf R, et al. Failure of an implantable cardioverter-defibrillator to redetect ventricular fibrillation in patients with a nonthoracotomy lead system. Circulation 1992;86:1217-1222.

20

Patient Followup Systems

Ted P. Adams

THE NEED for patient followup systems for pacemakers evolved out of the unpredictability of component failure, mechanical breakdown, and battery end of life associated with the early devices of the 60's and 70's. As reliability and predictability of the devices improved, the character of patient followup changed to involve patient diagnostic data as well as device monitoring. The genesis of ICD/patient followup has followed the same path but in a time span of only 5 years versus 15 years for pacemakers. The device reliability has improved such that the current generations of ICD followup systems are already more concerned with providing data regarding the condition of the patient than of the device.

Typically, there are 4 parts to the recommended followup procedures. These are: system evaluation, capacitor forming, device history and patient evaluation, and reprogramming. In some cases, the followup may also include re-induction of the patient's arrhythmia to test the device response. Clinical aspects of ICD followup are covered in more detail in Chap. 21 (Troubleshooting).

System Evaluation

Battery Condition

The most fundamental form of device evaluation is measurement of the battery condition to determine the remaining monitoring life and the remaining shock capacity. (In most devices these parameters are interrelated.) Every manufacturer specifies an "elective replacement indicator" (ERI) which is based upon the remaining battery capacity. Determination of the presence or absence of the ERI is a necessary part of the followup procedure.

The early Intec, Inc. devices (AID B, AID C, Ventak C) used a lithium vanadium pentoxide (LiV$_2$O$_5$) battery which had a relatively constant voltage throughout its lifetime when under low current loads. This made evaluation of the battery condition by measurement of battery voltage virtually impossible. The only way to evaluate the battery condition was to test it under load and this was done by measuring time required to charge the capacitors. The variable leakage exhibited by the "unformed" output capacitors and a surface charge effect giving an "unused" battery a shorter than normal charge time necessitated a two-step process to determine the remaining capacity. Thus, a capacitor forming charge cycle was required, followed by a measurement charge cycle. Determination of ERI in these devices was both cumbersome and wasteful of battery energy.

Most current ICD devices use lithium silver vanadium oxide chemistry (SVO) in the battery. With this battery, the open circuit voltage (synonyms are: unloaded voltage, monitoring voltage) is a reasonable indicator of the remaining capacity. Interrogation of the implanted device via telemetry yields both a direct measurement of the battery voltage and/or a message indicating whether ERI has been reached. The Angeion Sentinel and Pacesetter Aegis use SVO cells for the defibrillation shock delivery but use a lithium iodide cell for the monitoring current. The Res-Q I device uses a lithium carbon monofluoride chemistry whose open circuit voltage is not indicative of the remaining capacity. With this device, a charge time measurement and post-charge battery voltage measurement is recommended after capacitor forming to determine remaining capacity. It uses 3 cells, one of which is partially discharged during manufacturing, so that a clear voltage drop (of about one third) occurs when this first cell is discharged.

The ERI voltage varies with manufacturers even though they may use the same type of power source. (Table 1) The differences in recommended ERI voltages are a function of the particular cell's power delivery capacity, the overhead monitoring current (See Chap. 10), and the maximum capacitor storage energy. Thus, it is important to know the recommended ERI voltage for the particular manufacturer and model being evaluated. In general, the voltage measurement should not be made within a half hour after a charge sequence (including capacitor reforming) as the reading may be erroneous and usually pessimistic.

An (assumed) rule of thumb is that there is a 3 month safety margin of time after the ERI before the device will malfunction. Unfortunately, this cannot be relied on for several reasons. First, the manufacturers will not specify a "grace period" as they are concerned that physicians and patients would be tempted to abuse it.

Table 1. Elective Replacement Indicator (ERI) for various ICDs.

Model	Cells	ERI
Angeion Sentinel	3*	5.15 V
CPI PRx	2	4.75 V
CPI Mini	1	Combination of voltage and charge time
Intermedics Res-Q	3	8.15 V
Medtronic Jewel	2	4.91 V or charge time ≥ 14.5 s
Medtronic PCD 7217	2	4.97 V
Pacesetter Aegis	3*	5.15 V
Telectronics Guardian 4215	1	2.52
Telectronics Sentry 4310	1	Combination of last "valid" voltage, total charging since the valid voltage, and battery rundown characteristic. Typical ERI is at 2.52 V.
Ventritex Cadence	2	5.10 V
Ventritex Cadet	1	2.55 V
Ventritex Contour	1	2.55 V

All voltages are measured before charging.
* One of the three cells is a LiI monitoring cell which is not used in the ERI measurement.

Secondly, the time available after an ERI is significantly reduced by shock delivery and, to a lesser extent, continuous bradycardia pacing. (See Appendix of Chap. 12 and "Performance in Devices" section of Chap. 10.) Thirdly, the ERI is set at different estimated reserves. Finally, high dosage X-rays can remove battery capacity.[1]

A second voltage parameter is sometimes specified, the so-called end of life (EOL) voltage. By definition, if this voltage is reached, the device may no longer be capable of functioning within specification or may be incapable of any useful function. The EOL voltage is usually specified as a *loaded voltage*. In general, the loaded voltage is the voltage of a cell (battery) while under a significant load. This is equal to the open circuit voltage less the voltage lost across the internal series resistance. Specifically for the ICD, the most severe load is seen during capacitor charging and hence "charging voltage" is synonymous with loaded voltage. Thus the EOL voltage is measured during charging. The device should be replaced before the EOL voltage is reached. If EOL is indicated during followup, immediate replacement should be considered. The EOL indication seen at followup gives no acute information; it means that sometime, in the past, the battery voltage was excessively low during the charging of the capacitors which, in turn, happened with defibrillation, noncommitted shock charging, or capacitor reforming.

Lead Integrity

The next important system check is an assessment of lead integrity. Implantable defibrillators have 2 lead/electrode systems, 1 for pacing/sensing and 1 for delivering the high current shock. The devices which include bradycardia pacing also have the capability for directly measuring the lead impedance on the sensing lead or have a method of accessing pacing threshold margin. The integrity of the pacing lead can be inferred from these tests. Each type of pacing lead has a characteristic impedance. A measured impedance more than twice or less than half the nominal value may indicate a broken wire or broken insulation, respectively. (See also Chap. 9, "Clinical Surveillence of Lead Function and Integrity.")

In order to measure lead impedance, it is necessary to pass current through the heart. In the case of the pacing/sensing leads, this is relatively innocuous as it is only necessary to measure the voltage and current in a pacing pulse. The device can then calculate the lead impedance (typically between 300 and 1000 Ω).

With the defibrillation leads, the assessment is more difficult since pacing pulses are not delivered to the defibrillating electrodes. The impedance measurement can only be made when a shock is delivered. Thus, if the device has not generated any shocks, an assessment of the shocking leads cannot be made electrically. If a lead problem is suspected, the alternative is to cause the device to generate a shock or to look for lead anomalies under fluoroscopy.

The Ventak PRx, Jewel, and Sentinel devices have outputs whose pulse widths vary with lead impedance. These values are stored in memory and are converted to impedance values when the device is interrogated. The Guardian measures the voltage and current of a shock and can telemeter the calculated impedance when interrogated. Neither the PCD 7217, nor the Res-Q I devices have provisions for noninvasively measuring lead impedance. The lead impedance in the latter devices could be ascertained by using an oscilloscope to measure the tilt during a provoked output pulse (and then calculating the impedance), but this method is not recommended by any of the manufacturers. All newer models include the capability of measuring impedance on the shocking leads during or following a discharge.

Typical impedances for defibrillation leads are on the order of 30-80 Ω. The large sizes of the electrodes and higher voltages used account for the lower impedance than seen with pacing leads. The impedance will vary from patient to patient depending on the size of the electrodes, the number of electrodes, the location of the electrodes and the physiology of the patient.

All modern devices a have a real-time continuous electrogram telemetry capability that can be used at followup to help evaluate the quality of the intracardiac electrogram used for detection. This function can also be used as an indirect indicator of lead function. A broken lead wire, for example, may be indicated by a very low amplitude, intermittent, or non-existent electrogram. The presence of spike artifacts in the electrogram may also be an indicator of lead problems (e.g., fracture, or extracardiac/external noise).

Capacitor Reforming

A special characteristic of implantable defibrillators, as distinct from pacemakers, is the need for periodic forming of the output capacitors. This process is a consequence of the need for defibrillator designers to use electrolytic capacitors to store the energy prior to a shock. Electrolytic capacitors are the only currently available type of capacitor with sufficient energy density to physically fit into the small space available in an implanted device. This type of capacitor has an inherent characteristic of having relatively high leakage currents if they have not been recently charged. Charging the capacitor causes a healing effect which reduces leakage to acceptable levels. Over time the leaks reappear, and, unless healed ("reformed"), the implanted device could have an excessively long charge time when next charged.

The reforming is generally recommended to be done in 2-4 month intervals depending on the capacitor type, inverter (DC-DC converter) circuit design, battery power, and last occurrence of a shock. The recommended forming schedule for various manufacturer's devices is shown in Table 2.

The consequence of failing to form capacitors on schedule is not catastrophic for the device; its functionality and reliability are not compromised. The effect on the *patient*, however, could be catastrophic in extreme cases. To protect the device and patient from certain component failures, most defibrillators are designed to abort a shock if the capacitor cannot be charged within a specified time. An unformed capacitor will take longer to charge. When the battery is near end of life and the capacitor is unformed, a shock could be aborted due to excessive charge time; in contrast, a formed capacitor may have been capable of reaching a full charge before an excessive charge time is registered. One unpublished animal study found an implanted device which had not had a shock or reforming for 3 years. The device required 45 seconds to charge the capacitor.

Table 2. Reforming intervals for various ICDs.

Model	Manual / Automatic	Reforming Interval (months)*
Angeion Sentinel	Automatic	4
CPI Ventak P, early PRx	Manual	(2)
CPI PRx II, III, P2	Automatic	2
CPI later PRx	Automatic	2 then 1[†]
CPI Mini	Either[§]	3 then 1[†]
Intermedics Res-Q	Manual	(4)
Intermedics Res-Q II	Automatic	2, 3, or 4
Medtronic PCD 7217	Manual	(3)
Medtronic Jewel	Either	1, 2, (3), 4, 5, or 6
Pacesetter Aegis	Automatic	4
Telectronics Guardian 4210	Automatic	2
Telectronics Guardian 4215	Automatic[§]	100 days
Telectronics Sentry 4310	Automatic[§]	100 days
Ventritex Cadence	Automatic	3, 6, 9, or 12
Ventritex Cadet	Automatic	3 or 6
Ventritex Contour	Automatic	3 or 6

* Reforming intervals shown in parentheses are those recommended by the manufacturer.
† The device switches to monthly reforming near the end of life.
§ Counts a full energy therapy charge as a reform — referred to as "smart" reforming.

If a longer than recommended interval between forming should occur, there is no permanent damage done to the device and the normal forming procedure should be followed. Conversely, there is no harm done to the device by forming more often than recommended. The only harm in doing too frequent forming is a decrease in the remaining shock capacity. While all manufacturers either require reforming or provide it automatically, it is not clear that all capacitors require this process; perhaps the battery benefits the most. See discussions in Chaps. 10 and 11.

Device History Evaluation

All of the devices have an internal memory which can provide data on the functional history of the defibrillator. In the earliest generation defibrillators, "memory" was essentially a simple shock counter which alerted the physician that a shock had occurred, and served as a secondary indicator of ERI. These early devices were "hardwired" (i.e., not under software control), wherein a large space and current drain premium had to be paid for memory. Current devices are all microprocessor controlled with a still noticeable but substantially lower impact on size and current drain.

It is now possible for the devices to record large amounts of virtually any kind of discrete information. The only serious limitation is the amount of continuous cardiac analog data that can be stored. Currently, only short segments of electrogram data can be stored, usually totaling about one minute. With a given amount of memory, engineers can trade off precision, resolution, and duration to reach the final compromise in the design of the analog data storage. The number of data bits in each sample of analog data impact its precision, and the number of samples taken each second determine the resolution. The maximum duration of stored electrogram data, then, is determined by the size of the memory divided by the word length (used by the analog to digital converter) and the number of samples required per second. As technology improves the density of digital memories, one can expect longer and more accurate analog data storage and the addition of analog data from other physiologic sensors, as well, in future devices.

Getting the data from the implanted device is deceptively simple for the user, but very complex in its engineering. All the data must be digitized and stored in a binary number format (ones and zeros) in the implanted device memory. The stored information is typically encoded and transmitted out by switching a carrier frequency on and off in a timing sequence that can be decoded by the receiver (programmer) into ones and zeros. These data strings are then reassembled into alphanumeric form (words and numbers) or into analog format (electrogram) before being displayed to the user. Because of the need to conserve power in the implanted device, the carrier frequency is chosen as a compromise between it's transmissibility through the metal can and the body (wherein low frequencies work best) and the need for relatively short data transmission times (wherein high frequencies work best). Since the carrier signal emerging from the implanted device has limited power, the receiving antenna could be made sensitive enough to allow detection several inches away. However, increasing sensitivity to the signal also increases sensitivity to noise. This can make the signal unintelligible. The solution is to put the programming head as close to the transmitting antenna as possible to maximize the signal-to-noise ratio.

Before interrogation of the device to retrieve the stored data, it is necessary to properly position the programming head over the device. If the programmer has a "correct position" indicator, a trial and error approach to finding the proper location is possible, but referring to the manual for position diagrams is preferred.

Diagnostics Report   **Ventritex, Inc.**

Model: V-115   Serial #: 0000
Print Report Date/Time: 01-Jan-1996 / 12:00

Episodal Diagnostics

Episode 2 of 2 (Most Recent) : 31-Dec-1995 20:11 (EGM 1)		
Initial Diag.: Fib (CL 170 ms)		Diag. Time: 2.00 sec
Therapy	Result	Additional Episode Information
Defib 550V	Below Rate Detection (CL 740 ms)	None

Episode Duration: 15 sec

Last H.V. Charge Time:	6.4 sec
Last H.V. Lead Impedance:	40 ohms
Last H.V. Delivered Energy:	16.4 J

Episode 1 of 2 (Least Recent) : 29-Dec-1995 09:32 (EGM 2)		
Initial Diag.: Tach (CL 360 ms)		Diag. Time: 3.00 sec
Therapy	Result	Additional Episode Information
ATP x 1	Below Rate Detection (CL 740 ms)	None

Episode Duration: 10 sec

Successful BCL: 306 ms
Burst 1:306, 296, 286, 276, 266, 256, 246 ms

Lifetime Diagnostics

Device Charging History

50 - 100 V:	0
150 - 200 V:	0
250 - 300 V:	3
350 - 400 V:	1
450 - 500 V:	0
550 - 600 V:	12
650 - 700 V:	4
750 V:	4

Bradycardia Pacing

Percent Brady Paced: 11.0 %

Figure 1. Cadet telemetry example. This page gives the history of the most recent therapies delivered. In the above case there has been a successful use of antitachy-cardia pacing and later, defibrillation. CL = cycle length; H.V. = high voltage (therapy); BCL = burst cycle length.

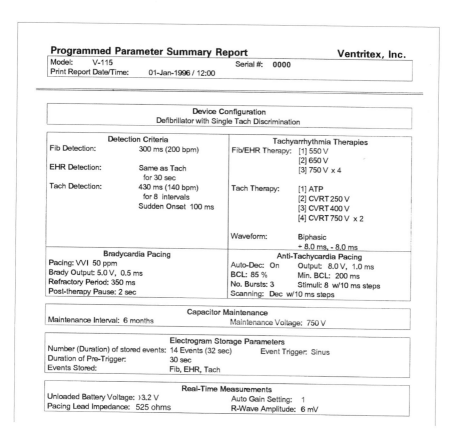

Figure 1. Cadet telemetry example (continued). This page gives the device configuration as programmed. Note that the capacitor reforming interval is 6 months; the unloaded battery voltage is > 3.2 V. An electrogram output page from the same device is shown as Fig. 14 in Chap. 14. EHR = extended high rate; CVRT = cardioversion shock therapy; BCL = burst cycle length.

Modern ICDs generally provide such data as programmed settings, patient related data such as implant date and lead type serial numbers, etc., event detection history, therapy delivery history, and limited R-R (i.e., beat to beat) interval data or electrogram storage. The large amount of stored data presents another problem for the device designer in developing a low power, error free, yet high speed telemetry system for recovery of the data. These goals are somewhat mutually exclusive and provide a design challenge.

The requirement for backward compatibility with existing telemetry systems designed for pacemakers has added to the problem for some manufacturers. That tradeoff can make reception of the telemetered data take considerably longer than with conventional pacemakers. This, in turn, necessitates that the programmer head be held in place in the receiving position for up to a full minute or even more. During the data transmission it is important that the programming head not be moved so as not to introduce any telemetry errors.

Recovery of the device history data is a valuable tool in determining whether the device's programmed settings are suitable for proper detection and therapy delivery. This information can also be valuable in determining the effectiveness of a particular drug regimen or in analyzing a potential device anomaly.

The particular data recorded and format of the printed data varies substantially among manufacturers. In addition, since there are no standards covering the telemetry scheme, every manufacturer has optimized the data telemetry for their particular needs, leading to total incompatibility of implanted devices and programmers among manufacturers. Thus it is necessary to have the proper interrogation device (programmer) available at followup and owing to the complexity of these devices, advance study of the manual of the device involved in the followup is recommended.

An example of telemetered patient data from a modern device is shown in Fig. 1. See Chaps. 14, 19, and 21 for examples of stored intracardiac electrograms.

Noninvasive Programmed Stimulation

Upon review of the telemetered data, the physician may discern that certain arrhythmias are not easily terminated by the programmed cardioversion or antitachycardia pacing regimen.

Present ICD's have noninvasive programmed stimulation (NIPS) which causes the implanted device to generate pacing pulses upon command from the programmer. The programmer is set up to transmit such commands when it receives a trigger input from another source. The usual source is an electrophysiology stimulator. This setup provides the capability for provoking tachycardias and then testing various antitachycardia pacing regimens. In using this setup, it is important to understand that there are certain unavoidable delays between the output of the electrophysiology stimulator and the output pulse of the implanted device. When the programmer receives an input trigger signal, it must set up the correct telemetry codes and then transmit the data. At the receiving end, the ICD must interpret the code and then deliver the pacing pulse. All of this takes time, on the order of 10-30 ms, depending on such parameters as microprocessor speed, telemetry data length, and telemetry data rate. For any given system, however, this delay is fairly constant. It is important to know the actual delay time so that it can be taken into consideration when pulses are synchronized with or triggered from the surface ECG.

Reprogramming

After evaluation of the device history data and/or further evaluation and testing of the patient, reprogramming of the device parameters is often warranted. Even if tachyarrhythmia detection criteria and therapy specifications are not altered after a particular followup interrogation it is common practice to at least reprogram (by resetting to 0) the tachyarrhythmia event counters thereby creating a new reference date for tabulation of events.

Reprogramming requires that the proper programmer and software be used for compatibility with the implanted device. As with receiving telemetry, attention must be paid to positioning of the programming head in the correct location over the device. Unless the programmer has a head position indicator, it will be necessary to refer to the manual for diagrams of proper positioning as each manufacturer's device is unique. Programming requires significantly less time to transmit data than interrogation and can usually be completed in a couple seconds at most.

Followup Safety Considerations

Followup procedures can cause complications. The two most common are loss of pacing function during capacitor reforming and device turn-off due to magnet resetting.

The Medtronic PCD 7217 turns off bradycardia pacing during capacitor reforming. This device behavior can lead to syncope in patients that are pacemaker dependent.[2] Since alternate applications of the magnet can make the CPI PRx (or Mini if so programmed) either active or inactive, it is possible to accidentally deactivate the device during removal of the programming wand.

Remote Followup

Unlike pacemaker patients, most ICD patients do not have an in-home method of checking the battery condition or functionality of the implanted device available to them. This makes periodic visits to the following physician a mandatory requirement for assessment of the device as well as the patient.

The only remote followup available today are arrhythmia monitoring services which offer various kinds of Holter or transient arrhythmia recording, some with transtelephonic ECG transmission capability. If the device has functioned while the recording is in progress, the recordings can yield information on the performance of the device, but this information still does not address battery condition.

In general, patients do not have any control over the operation of the device. However, with some devices currently available, it is possible to inhibit operation of the device by placing a magnet over the device. (See Appendix) This can be important with patients who experience frequent false shocks (i.e., for sensed events other than tachyarrhythmias) provided they are capable of handling the task of placing the magnet properly. This problem is more difficult than with pacemakers, as various types of magnets are recommended (bar, donut, etc.) for various ICDs and each device has a specific location where the magnet is effective. Therefore, it is critical to know the type of implanted device and its peculiarities with respect to magnet operation before attempting to modify its operation with application of a magnet.

The Future

The information relative to specific devices will certainly become outdated as the devices are replaced by newer models, but the general principles of patient followup and the need for close attention to the details of each device will persist. As the sophistication of the devices grows with time and more experience with the behavior of both the devices and patients is gained, one can predict that future devices will provide even more data. The challenge is to make that data relevant to the physician's needs for management of the patient without compromising utility, reliability, or longevity.

ACKNOWLEDGMENTS:
The magnet table was prepared with the help of Regina Jarandilla, RN.

Appendix: Magnet Function Table

Device	Suspends Tachycardia Detection & Therapy	Suspends Brady-cardia Therapy	Suspends Noninvasive Programmed Stimulation	Audible Tone or Tones	Comments
Angeion Sentinel 2000	Yes[†]	No	No	None	
CPI Ventak 1550-1600	Yes[*]	N/A	N/A	Yes	R-wave synchronous tones indicate device is Active; continuous tones indicate device is Inactive.
CPI PRx 1700, 1705	Yes[*]	No	No	Yes	If Tachy Status is disabled, magnet has *no* effect - even if magnet function is enabled. If Tachy Status is enabled, each new application for ≥ 30 s will toggle the device between Monitor only (Inactive with continuous tone) and Monitor and Therapy (Active with R-wave synchronous tone).
CPI Ventak P2 1620, 1625; PRx II 1715; PRx III 1720-1725,	Yes[*]	No	Yes, Fib mode; No, Burst Pacing Mode	Yes	Enable/Disable Magnet function is programmable. If Magnet function is disabled, application of a magnet will have no effect on device status between Active (R-wave synchronous tones) and Inactive (continuous tones).
CPI Mini 1740, 1741, 1745, 1746	Yes[*]	No	Yes	Yes	When programmed, magnet application of ≥ 30 s cycles operation from Off to Monitor Only to Normal and back to Off.
Intermedics Res-Q	Yes[†]	No	No	None	
Medtronic PCD 7217, Jewel 7219-7221	Yes[†]	No	No	None	Using the Cancel Magnet and/or the Resume Detection function on the programmer will restore detection capabilities while the magnet programming head (or a stand-alone magnet) is applied.
Pacesetter Aegis 2600	Yes[†]	No	No	None	
Telectronics 4202, 4203	Yes[†]	Yes	No	None	
Telectronics 4210, 4211, 4215, 4310	Yes[†]	No	No	None	Magnet application will abort programming and Emergency Function in Progress.
Ventritex Cadence V100-V112; Cadet V115; Contour 135,145	Yes[†]	No	No	None	

† Therapy will be only *temporarily* inhibited for as long as magnet is applied.
* Magnet will inactivate device when applied for ≥ 30 seconds, if previously Active; application of magnet for < 30 s will only temporarily inhibit tachycardia detection and therapy. Once the device is in the Inactive mode, a new magnet application of ≥ 30 s is required to convert to Active mode.
N/A is not applicable

1. Rodriguez F, Filimonov A, Henning A, et al. Radiation-induced effects in multi-programmable pacemakers and implantable defibrillators. PACE 1991;14:2143–2153.
2. Lehmann MH, Personal communication.

21

Troubleshooting Suspected ICD Malfunction

Mark E. Rosenthal, MD, J. Todd Alderfer, MD, and Francis E. Marchlinski, MD

THE ICD has made a dramatic impact on the management of patients with ventricular tachycardia (VT) and fibrillation (VF), markedly reducing the risk of sudden cardiac death in this high-risk group. In addition, the ICD has evolved from a relatively simple, non-programmable device to a complex unit with multiple options for tachycardia detection and therapy. As ICD technology has developed, a variety of clinical scenarios have arisen which force the electrophysiologist to differentiate appropriate from inappropriate device function. This chapter seeks to outline essentials of routine ICD clinical followup and then identify the most common types of clinical problems, other than infection, encountered during ICD followup. (Table 1) The differential diagnosis and plan for management of these problems will be discussed.

Table 1. Common clinical problems encountered during ICD followup

ICD therapy in the asymptomatic or minimally symptomatic patient

Delayed ICD therapy in patients with documented VT/VF

Failure of ICD therapy in patients with documented VT/VF

Lack of detectable ICD therapy in patients with symptoms suggesting arrhythmia occurrence.

VT = ventricular tachycardia; VF = ventricular fibrillation.

Essentials of ICD Followup

During the early years of ICD therapy, routine followup was relatively simple. The first Ventak series of ICD produced by Cardiac Pacemakers, Inc. (CPI) had limited programmability, and device followup consisted primarily of evaluating the status of the generator's battery, accomplished by reforming the capacitors and then checking the time required to charge the capacitors. With aging of the generator, the charge time increases until a device-specific charge time is reached which indicates the elective replacement time. This procedure is still part of routine followup with the earlier generation CPI Ventak units (1550, 1555, and 1600). In addition, these models keep track of total device discharges as their only means of tracking delivered therapy. It is recommended that patients with the Ventak ICD be seen every two months for the first two years of followup, and monthly thereafter to reform the capacitors and check the charge time. Application of a magnet over the Ventak ICD causes the emission of an audible tone synchronous with the sensed ventricular electrogram, and should be done periodically during followup to confirm appropriate sensing.[1,2] (See Appendix of Chap. 20 for a table of magnet functions in various ICDs.)

The newer ICDs (e.g., Medtronic Jewel; Ventritex Cadence, Cadet, and Contour; CPI PRx III, Ventak P2, and Mini; Intermedics Res-Q; and Telectronics Guardian and Sentry 4130; Angeion Sentinel; and Pacesetter Aegis) require more detailed followup due to their sophisticated functions. At each followup visit, full device interrogation should include:

1. Review of all programmed detection criteria and therapies.
2. Real time measurements of remaining battery voltage, lead impedance, and sensed ventricular electrogram amplitude and morphology (if available).
3. Review of detected arrhythmias and therapy delivered (plus high voltage lead impedance [if available] in the case of shocks).
4. Retrieval of stored electrograms (if available) recorded from detected tachyarrhythmia events.
5. Determination of pacing threshold especially in devices programmed to deliver antitachycardia pacing.
6. In appropriate cases, determination of potential oversensing of T-waves or noncardiac signals through use of marker channels or real time electrogram recording.
7. Creation of a final printout of programmed ICD settings to assure that no unintended permanent changes were made during diagnostic testing.

These devices are also generally followed every 2-3 months with outpatient evaluations during the first two years after implantation and monthly thereafter. The elective replacement indicator is typically a predetermined battery voltage as opposed to a charge time. (See Chaps. 10 [Battery] and 20 [Followup].)

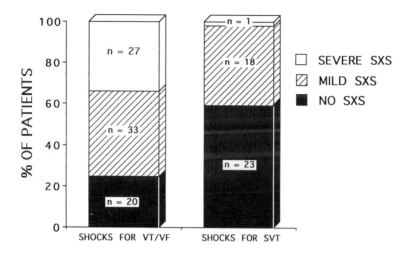

Figure 1. Symptoms severity prior to shock with ECG documented VT/VF and SVT. Mild symptoms included palpitations and mild presyncope. Severe symptoms included severe presyncope and frank syncope and occurred almost exclusively in patients experiencing VT/VF. However, no or mild symptoms were common before shock in patients having ventricular (67%) or supraventricular (98%) arrhythmias.

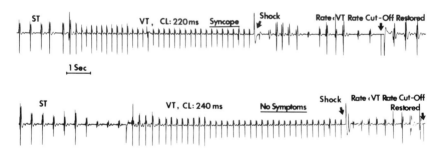

Figure 2. Stored electrograms from Cadence device showing rhythm leading to shock in two patients (top and bottom panels respectively). The change in morphology with the onset of the tachycardia is consistent with the diagnosis of VT. The symptoms preceding shock (first arrow in each panel) are indicated above recordings. Despite the very short cycle length, the VT shown in the bottom panel was not associated with any symptoms. The diagnosis of VT was confirmed despite the absence of symptoms from the rate and morphology of the electrogram. The change in amplitude of the electrogram during VT is due to the automatic gain control. ST = sinus tachycardia.

As nonthoracotomy systems are now standard, determination of stable endocardial lead position and stable subcutaneous

Table 2. Causes of ICD discharges in the asymptomatic or minimally symptomatic patient

Clinically appropriate
- ♦ Hemodynamically tolerated, uniform sustained VT
- ♦ Very rapidly detected and terminated VF or VT

Clinically inappropriate
- ♦ Supraventricular tachycardia
- ♦ Nonsustained VT or SVT (committed ICD device)
- ♦ Oversensing of internal non-QRS signals i.e., cardiac vs. other (non-cardiac) inside the body
    - T-wave or P-wave sensing
    - Lead or adapter fracture ("make-break potentials")
    - Lead or adapter insulation failure
    - Loose generator or adapter setscrew connections
    - Sensing of pacemaker stimuli
    - Automatic gain control-mediated oversensing[8]
- ♦ Other external signal source—e.g., electrocautery

SVT = supraventricular tachycardia

patch position and contour becomes even more crucial. As a result, a chest X-ray should be obtained within the first month of outpatient followup and then on an annual basis or as clinically indicated. (See Chap. 20 for more details on followup.)

ICD Therapy in the Absence of Severe Symptoms

Differential Diagnosis

High energy discharges may frequently be delivered by the ICD in conscious patients. Only a minority (10-20%) of patients develop frank syncope prior to the ICD discharge.[3,4] Approximately 30-40% of patients with an ICD will be totally asymptomatic at the time of high energy shock delivery.[5-7] (Figs. 1, 2)

When an ICD discharges in a conscious patient, the major question facing the electrophysiologist is whether the shock was "appropriate." (Table 2) This is especially relevant in light of the reported 20-30% incidence of unnecessary ICD shocks.[9-13] (Fig. 3) For a discussion of detection problems see Reiter and Mann.[14]

The major appropriate cause of ICD discharge in the conscious patient is tolerated, sustained uniform VT. Less commonly, very rapid VT/VF may be sensed so quickly that ICD discharge may occur prior to loss of consciousness with minor prodromal symptoms. As seen in Fig. 4, delivery of shocks may also result from limitations of the ICD or its programming (e.g., imperfect

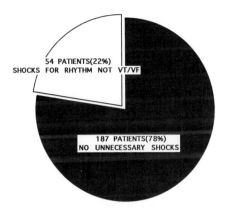

Figure 3. Incidence of ECG documented unnecessary ICD shock in 241 patients followed for 24 ± 20 mos. Fortuitous surface ECG was available in 184 patients while 57 had a stored electrogram device. Only 54 patients (22%) experienced a shock for a ECG documented rhythm other than VT /VF; of these 30 had 80 shocks for AF.

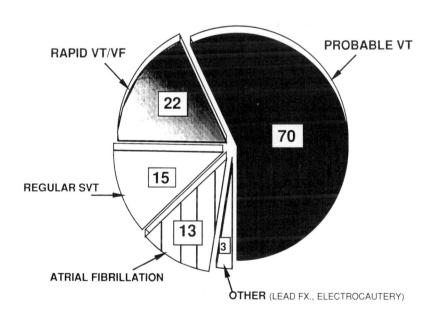

Figure 4. Rhythm leading to ICD shock based on analysis of stored electrograms in 32 patients experiencing 123 shocks. The diagnosis of VT was based on a change in electrogram morphology coincident with the onset vs. ECG documented sinus rhythm. The diagnosis of a regular SVT and AF was based on the absence of change in morphology with the onset of the tachycardia and the rhythm regularity. About 25% of shocks were delivered during suspected AF, regular SVT (such as sinus tachycardia and atrial flutter) or an external signal mimicking a rapid VT.

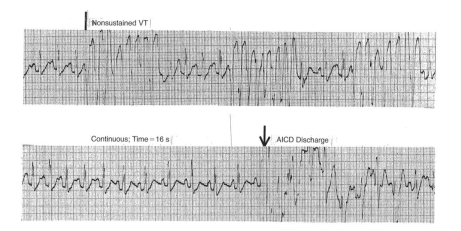

Figure 5. Repeated bursts of nonsustained VT leading to ICD shock (arrow) from a Ventak 1400 series committed device.

tachycardia discrimination) rather than an absolute device malfunction but still may be clinically inappropriate. The differential diagnosis of such shock delivery in the conscious patient includes:

1. Nonsustained VT (Fig. 5, 6) satisfying initial detection criteria but terminating during device charging in "committed" ICD units (e.g. Ventak 1550, 1555, 1600; PCD 7217). Even in some noncommitted ICDs, termination of nonsustained VT may not be recognized owing to lenient tachycardia confirmation criteria.

2. SVT which satisfies detection criteria for VT/VF. The most common example with early devices was AF;[5,12-16] (Fig. 7) although in low rate cutoff VT zones of tiered therapy ICDs, sinus tachycardia may be a more common cause of "false" detection of VT.

3. Detection of non-QRS cardiac signals such as P-waves or T-waves resulting in double counting and satisfaction of rate criteria (Fig. 8)

4. Detection of noncardiac signals which mimic VT/VF, resulting from sensing lead fracture[17] or insulation failure,[18-20] (Fig. 9) loose lead connections at the header or adapters, myopotentials,[21] and electromagnetic interference. (Fig. 10, Table 3, Chap. 14)

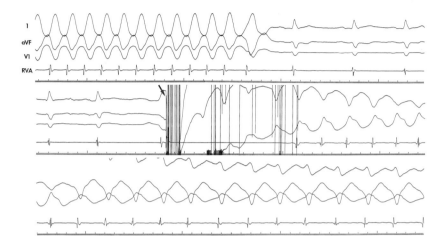

Figure 6. Nonsustained VT induced during electrophysiologic testing leading to an shock from a committed device (Ventak 1500 series). The shock (arrow) initiates a sustained VT. The three panels are continuous with surface ECG and RVA signal.

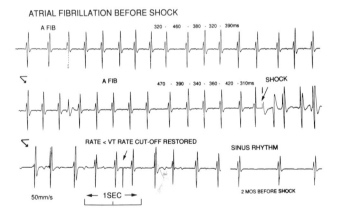

ATRIAL FIBRILLATION BEFORE SHOCK

A FIB   320 - 460 - 380 - 320 - 390ms

A FIB   470 - 390 - 340 - 360 - 420 - 310ms   SHOCK

RATE < VT RATE CUT-OFF RESTORED   SINUS RHYTHM

50mm/s   ◄— 1SEC —►   2 MOS BEFORE SHOCK

Figure 7. Electrograms from a Cadence ICD showing AF leading to shock occurring without symptoms. The panels are continuous except for the lower right which was NSR one month previously. At the beginning of the top panel a rapid irregularly irregular rate is observed. The morphology is identical to that of NSR, consistent with AF. The cycle length of the mean ventricular response during AF falls below the cutoff for shock delivery. The shock is followed by a slower ventricular response.

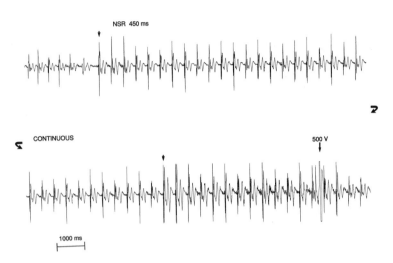

Figure 8. Stored electrograms from a Cadence ICD demonstrating oversensing of the T-wave during sinus tachycardia (*NSR*) at a cycle length of 450 ms leading to inappropriate shock (500 V—large arrow). The large T-waves were counted as R-waves (double counting). Small amplitude R-waves recorded during sinus rhythm resulted in gain increases from the automatic gain control (small arrows) which enhanced T-wave amplitude. Management would include decreasing the sensitivity (if programmable) and verifying sensing of induced VF at that sensitivity. Repositioning of the sensing lead to achieve lower amplitude R-waves would also help.

Table 3. Sources of electromagnetic interference which could possibly affect ICD function

Medical
  ♦ Electrosurgical equipment
  ♦ Magnetic resonance imaging devices*
  ♦ Therapeutic diathermy
  ♦ Pacemaker programming[22]
  ♦ Lithotripsy
Non-Medical
  ♦ Arc welding equipment and robotic jacks
  ♦ Industrial transformers and motors
  ♦ Electrical smelting furnaces
  ♦ Large radiofrequency transmitters such as radar
  ♦ Large stereo speakers* [23]
  ♦ Radiofrequency remote control devices[24]
  ♦ Slot machines[25]
  ♦ Cellular phones,[26] probably at most a problem for pacemakers and not ICDs[27-30]
  ♦ Store security systems[31]
  ♦ Magnetic wands such as those used in bingo[32]

* Effects on ICD primarily limited to device activation/inactivation due to effect of magnetic field on reed switch.

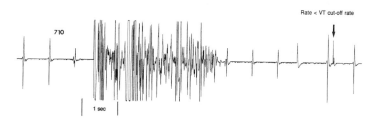

Figure 9. Burst of electrical noise leading to an aborted ICD shock documented on stored electrograms caused by an interruption of the insulation of the rate-sensing lead. The lead impedance was normal and not significantly changed from baseline.

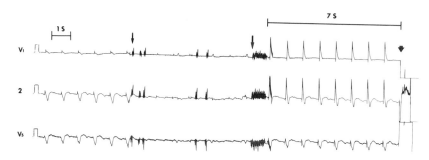

Figure 10. ICD discharge during threshold testing of a bradycardia pacing device. Radio frequency transmissions (narrow arrows) from the programmer (Cordis Programmer III, model #255A, Cordis Corp.) for the bradycardia pacemaker (Cordis Multicom II) triggered discharge (broad arrow) from a committed ICD (AID-BR, CPI).

Kelly et al recently described noise generated by the Cadence during ventricular pacing which was not related to lead malfunction, but probably related to the automatic gain control.[8] Such noise during ventricular pacing by the ICD was found to be related to breathing or Valsalva maneuver in some patients with a hybrid Cadence/Endotak integrated lead ICD system, and was also able temporarily to inhibit the ICD pacing.[33]

5. Interaction with permanent pacemakers: Sensed pacing artifacts (usually unipolar) may lead to double counting, typically during dual chamber pacing (Fig. 11), but occasionally during ventricular pacing if there is a long duration between the pacing stimulus and the paced QRS.[34,35] Asynchronous pacing can occur after ICD discharge due to undersensing of ventricular endo-

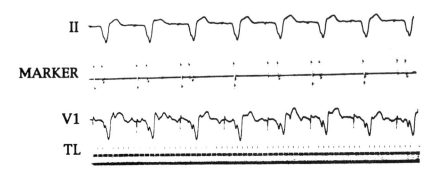

Figure 11. Oversensing of atrial pacing stimulus indicated on marker channel for sensed real time events. Surface ECG leads II and V1, along with marker channel are displayed through programmer of Ventak PRx. A-V sequential bipolar pacing from pacing system is evident on the surface ECG. Marker channel demonstrates intermittent sensed event coincident with atrial pacing stimulus as well as sensed QRS complex. Inappropriate triggering of the ICD device can be prevented by documenting a small amplitude bipolar pacing stimulus which is < 1 mV at the time of pacemaker placement. Programming of pacing amplitude output for chronic pacing should be kept at a minimum safe value.

cardial signals with subsequent sensing of pacing spikes and native QRS complexes which may also lead to satisfaction of rate criteria for VT/VF detection and subsequent therapy delivery.[35] Some pacemakers may be reprogrammed by an ICD shock from bipolar to unipolar pacing setting the stage for possible double counting (especially with dual chamber systems). These and other adverse device-device interactions can usually be avoided by appropriate ICD and pacemaker testing upon implantation of these devices. (Chaps. 17 and 23)

Two special circumstances possible only with tiered therapy ICD units, warrant mention. In these uncommon situations, inappropriate device function may lead to ICD-induced VT which may, in turn, precipitate subsequent device discharge with or without preceding arrhythmia symptoms.

Inability of the automatic gain control (Chap. 14) to allow for sensing of the sinus rhythm ventricular electrogram after frequent premature ventricular complexes or nonsustained VT associated with large amplitude electrograms may result in asynchronous bradycardia pacing with VT induction.[36,37] (Figs. 12, 13) Alternatively, oversensing of noncardiac "noise" or detection of supraventricular rhythms satisfying rate criteria for VT may trigger antitachycardia pacing which can induce a more rapid VT and subsequent high energy discharge.[38] (Figs. 14-16)

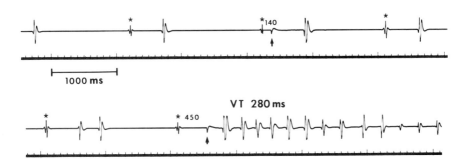

Figure 12. Stored electrograms from a continuous recording showing an episode of VT induced by bradycardia pacing after a nonsensed sinus beat. The morphology of the electrograms consistent with that recorded during surface ECG documented normal sinus rhythm are marked by asterisk (*). The arrow in each panel indicates an artifact that signals the end of the post pacing blanking period, which follows the pacing stimulus by 120 ms. After a series of larger amplitude PVCs, the gain in the automatic gain control adjusts and a low amplitude sinus complex is seen. This complex is not sensed and a pacing stimulus is introduced at the bradycardia pacing interval. The pacing stimulus (not shown) falls 330 ms = 450 - 120 after the nonsensed complex and probably initiated VT. Decreasing the bradycardia pacing interval prevented recurrence.

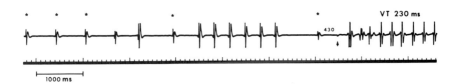

Figure 13. Stored electrograms of continuous recording showing an episode of VT induced by bradycardia pacing similar to Fig.12. Recordings are obtained from a Cadence ICD. The morphology of electrograms consistent with normal sinus rhythm are marked by asterisk (*). The arrow indicates an artifact that signals the end of the post pacing blanking period, which follows the stimulus by 120 ms. After nonsustained VT with larger amplitude signals, there is an automatic gain adjustment and a reduced amplitude sinus complex. This complex is not sensed and a pacing stimulus is introduced at the pacing interval. The presumed pacing stimulus (not shown) falls 310 ms = 430 - 120 after the complex and probably initiated the VT. Decreasing the bradycardia pacing interval prevented recurrence.

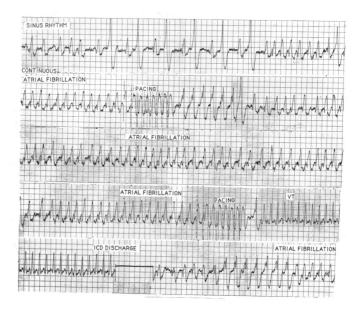

Figure 14. Continuous surface ECG rhythm strip demonstrating onset of AF with a rapid ventricular response (end of panel 1) which triggers bursts of antitachycardia pacing from the Cadence ICD (panels 2 & 4) with the initiation of VT (nonsustained in panel 2). The rapid VT seen in the panel 4 triggers a shock (panel 5) with termination of the VT but not of the AF. Drug therapy was then directed at preventing AF and slowing the ventricular response. Using rate stability criteria (in devices with this feature) and increasing the number of intervals required for arrhythmia recognition may also help.

Assessment

Prior to hospital discharge, all patients should be instructed to alert the followup physician should their device deliver a shock. Conscious patients with multiple ICD discharges should be admitted for immediate in-hospital monitoring. Multiple discharges in the absence of arrhythmia symptoms have been associated with atrial fibrillation or a lead disruption.[13] If single ICD shocks have occurred, prompt evaluation may be required, but this can usually be done in the outpatient setting.

    Complete ICD interrogation is essential. Full advantage should be taken of sophisticated telemetry functions which can reveal: (1) the rate of the detected rhythm, (2) the R-R intervals before and after the shock, and (3) electrogram recordings before and after the shock. (Table 4)

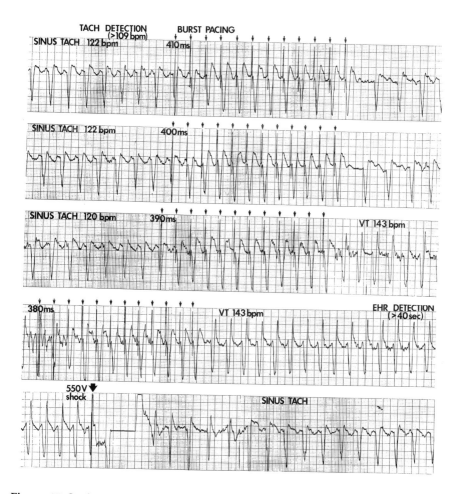

Figure 15. Surface ECG demonstrating sinus tachycardia with a rapid rate which falls above the cutoff for VT detection. This was not associated with any symptoms. The sinus tachycardia at a rate of 122 bpm triggers bursts of antitachycardia pacing from the Cadence ICD at progressively faster rates (panels 1,2, & 3) with the initiation of VT (panel 3). The VT at a rate of 143 bpm also triggers antitachycardia pacing seen in panel 4. Because of the extended period above the rate cutoff for VT detection without arrhythmia termination (EHR—extended high rate), the device defaults to deliver a defibrillation shock which terminates VT. In this patient the sinus tachycardia coupled with the pacing therapy resulted in VT initiation and a subsequent shock in the absence of severe arrhythmia symptoms. Activating the sudden onset criteria for arrhythmia detection may preclude device therapy for the gradually accelerated rate associated with sinus tachycardia.

Table 4. Criteria for rhythm classification using stored telemetry data.[41]

	Electrogram morphology vs. baseline	Mean cycle length	Cycle length variability >60 ms for 3 of 10 consecutive intervals
Probable VT	Different *	> 260 ms	No
Rapid VT/VF	Different *	≤ 260 ms	No / Yes
Probable Regular SVT	Same †	> 260 ms	No
Atrial Fibrillation	Same †	> 260 ms	Yes

* About 5-10% of VTs will have an electrogram morphology matching sinus rhythm.

† Aberrant conduction may cause a change in electrogram morphology if the recording leads are located ipsilateral to the location of bundle branch block.

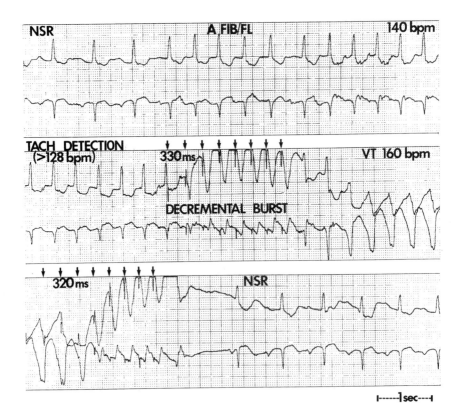

Figure 16A. Surface ECG recording demonstrating onset of atrial fibrillation/flutter with a rapid ventricular response (panel 1) which triggers bursts of antitachycardia pacing from the Cadence ICD (panel 2) with initiation of VT. The VT triggers additional antitachycardia pacing from the ICD (panel 3) with termination of the VT.

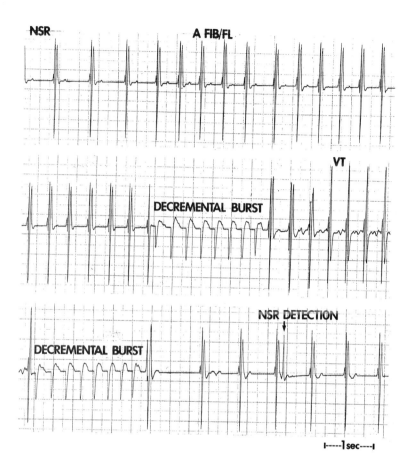

Figure 16B. Stored electrograms from an arrhythmia episode shown in Fig. 16A. The onset of atrial fibrillation/flutter is marked by the development of an increase in rate and only minimal R-R interval variability. The electrogram morphology matches that of sinus (NSR) shown at the beginning of the recording. The absence of a change in the electrogram morphology is consistent with the diagnosis of an SVT. Following the first burst of pacing (panel 2) the electrogram morphology changes and the rate increases modestly consistent with the diagnosis of VT. Following the second burst of pacing (panel 3), a stable supraventricular rhythm is restored and the electrogram returns to the baseline morphology.

Comparison of electrogram morphology during the patient's usual supraventricular rhythm and the detected tachycardia can be quite useful in determining the etiology of tachycardia. There is usually a distinct difference between VT/VF and an SVT, with the morphology of the latter resembling normal rhythm electrogram characteristics.[11,12,39-41] The stability of the R-R intervals prior to de-

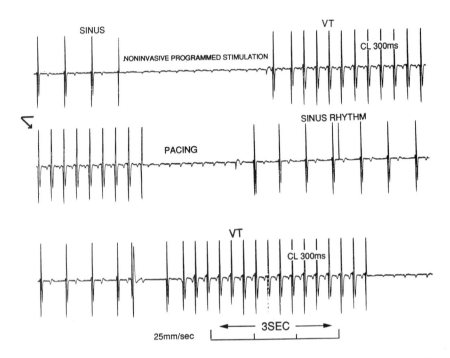

Figure 17. Intracardiac electrogram during VT mimicking that of sinus rhythm. Top two panels show an example of stored electrograms recorded from the Cadence ICD at the time of induced VT in the electrophysiology laboratory. The morphology during the induced VT is similar to that recorded during the sinus rhythm at the beginning of the tracing. An electrogram morphology during VT which is similar to that recorded during ECG documented sinus rhythm is noted in less than 10% of VT episodes.[40] Bottom panel shows stored electrogram recordings obtained at the time of spontaneous tachycardia leading to ICD therapy. The electrogram morphology also matches that recorded during sinus rhythm. Information obtained at the time of postoperative electrophysiologic testing related to the induced VT electrogram morphology and rate permitted accurate ECG diagnosis of the spontaneous arrhythmia as VT.

vice discharge may be used to differentiate VT from atrial fibrillation.

Unfortunately, diagnosis using morphology is limited by the fact that VT and SVTs may share identical ventricular electrogram morphology on occasion,[39-41] (Fig. 17) particularly with closely spaced bipolar electrodes which do not pick up far signals; and that sustained uniform VT may be quite irregular at times,[42,43] especially at onset.[44] In these latter instances, a careful review of the morphology during all induced arrhythmias, a knowledge of the maximum rate at which 1:1 A-V conduction occurs, and an assess-

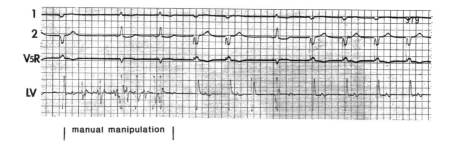

| manual manipulation |

Figure 18. Electrical artifact consistent with make-break potentials and intermittent lead disruption evident on real time electrogram recordings (LV) from ICD device (Cadence V100) with manual manipulation of the generator pocket.

ment of the clinical arrhythmia rate and previously documented electrogram characteristics will frequently permit the correct diagnosis. (Fig. 18)

Oversensing may be evaluated in a number of ways. The Ventak emits a beeping tone synchronously with sensed signals when a magnet is placed over the device. Evaluation of this audible tone with simultaneous ECG monitoring can aid in the detection of non-QRS signals being sensed by the device.[1,2] (Fig. 19) This maneuver should also be done with the patient performing a number of positional changes (e.g. twisting or bending) and with manipulation of the ICD generator in the pocket in order to detect myopotential sensing or lead fracture with "make-break" potentials. Deep breathing or Valsalva maneuvers may also be utilized in an attempt to bring out noise that may be amplified during ICD-mediated bradycardia pacing.[33]

In ICD units with *marker channels* (which indicate how the device "labels" successive sensed events or intervals), similar maneuvers may show device sensing at a time when there is no QRS. Extremely short R-R intervals (<160 ms) coupled with longer intervals registered just preceding ICD discharge are findings consistent with intermittent "make-break" potentials. In ICD units with real time electrogram recordings, similar maneuvers may show electrical artifact consistent with make-break potentials (Fig. 18). Devices capable of real time telemetry should be fully interrogated to determine impedance characteristics of the rate sensing leads as a clue to lead fracture (high impedance) or lead insulation failure (low impedance), either of which can cause oversensing of non-cardiac signals.

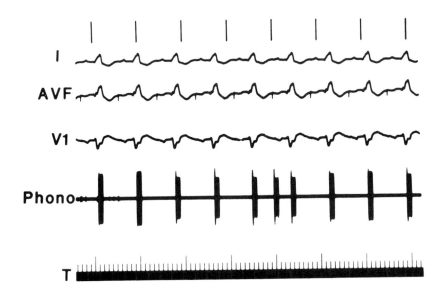

Figure 19. "Beepogram" recorded during paced rhythm by placing a magnet over Ventak 1550 or 1600 ICD device. Beeping tone is emitted for every sensed signal. Evidence of intermittent detection of atrial pacing stimulus as sensed ventricular event in patient who experienced ICD discharge in the absence of any arrhythmia symptoms. Surface ECG leads I, AVF, and V1 along with phonogram recordings of beeping which indicates the timing of sensed electrical events.

Nonthoracotomy lead systems incorporating sensing and shocking functions in a single endocardial lead system (Chap. 9) may also be the source of oversensing and inappropriate shocks. The original investigational CPI Endotak series of integrated transvenous leads was plagued by lead fractures; however, design modifications largely eliminated this problem. Epstein et al[20] reported malfunction in an Endotak-C series 60 lead in which there was documented oversensing with inappropriate shocking as well as ineffective shock delivery associated with oversensing. This lead uses the distal spring electrode as the anode for "integrated bipolar" sensing and the cathode for shock delivery; the combination of clinical findings suggested the distal spring electrode lead element as the common source of malfunction. Intraoperative testing was required to show high impedance with unipolar and bipolar pacing.

Dislodgement of transvenous ICD sensing leads partially to the right atrium may present with inappropriate shocks triggered by P-wave oversensing. Early recognition of this problem, readily accomplished by fluoroscopic or chest X-ray examination, followed by prompt lead revision is important to avert the catastrophic failure if the dislodged lead is of the integrated type.

Management

If the patient's history or device interrogation suggest an occasional appropriate discharge for VT, often no intervention is required. If frequent but appropriate shocks have been delivered, an alteration in ICD programming or therapy prescription may be desired for patient comfort and the preservation of generator longevity. The addition of an antiarrhythmic agent or catheter ablative therapy may decrease the incidence of spontaneous sustained or nonsustained VT.[45] However, if a change in antiarrhythmic therapy is made, reassessment of the rate (and, when relevant, interval stability) of induced VT, as well as the defibrillation threshold, should be performed due to the ability of some agents to significantly alter these important electrophysiologic parameters.[46] (Chap. 5, Table 2)

Sustained, hemodynamically tolerated VT can also frequently be treated with antitachycardia pacing or low energy cardioversion with avoidance of high energy discharges. In patients with a tiered therapy device, these options should be utilized when appropriate (Fig. 20A, 20B).

Due to the discomfort associated with even low energy shocks, antitachycardia pacing may be the better option. In patients with ICDs incapable of antitachycardia pacing, it may be necessary to upgrade the generator to a tiered therapy device. Occasionally, an antiarrhythmic drug may be required to slow the patient's spontaneous VT to facilitate antitachycardia pacing.

Nonsustained VT may require ICD reprogramming, e.g. increase in number of intervals for tachycardia detection, or device upgrade to a more sophisticated system (with noncommitted shock feature, for example) to prevent high energy discharges for this arrhythmia. This is especially a problem in committed devices which stop sensing once capacitor charging begins. In the Ventak series, some units allow for lengthening the interval from tachycardia detection to capacitor charging (first shock delay) to allow for self-terminating episodes of nonsustained VT. It may occasionally be necessary to upgrade the generator to a noncommitted ICD which senses during capacitor charging and takes a "second look" prior to delivery of a high energy shock and allows for the shock to be aborted. Hurwitz et al showed that this capability prevented high energy shocks from being delivered in 37% of patients studied with a Ventritex Cadence system.[47](Figs. 21, 22)

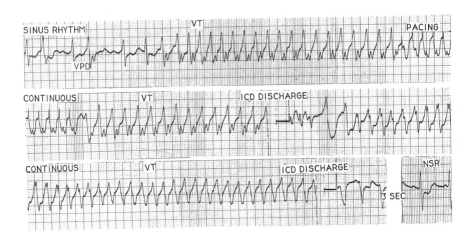

Figure 20A. Surface ECG recordings from a patient with recurrent episodes of hemodynamically tolerated VT. An ICD with antitachycardia pacing capabilities was substituted for a "shock box." A single burst (proven effective during testing) failed to terminate a spontaneous VT. A low energy shock (middle panel) accelerated this to a more rapid VT which was terminated by a higher energy shock.

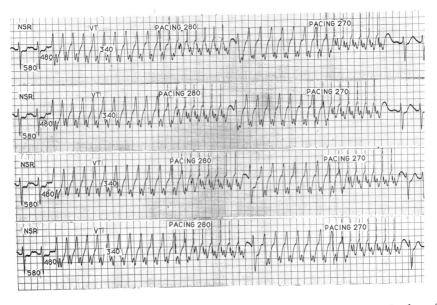

Figure 20B. Surface ECG recordings from a patient with recurrent episodes of hemodynamically tolerated VT. Repeated spontaneous episodes of VT are terminated with two bursts of antitachycardia pacing after reprogramming the antitachycardia algorithm to use a second burst at a shorter paced cycle length.

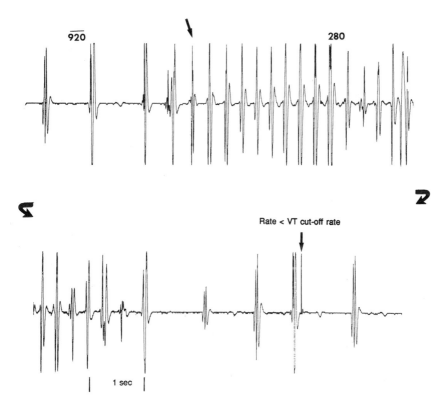

Figure 21. Nonsustained VT documented with stored electrograms. The Cadence ICD aborted the shock after initiation of charging because arrhythmia termination was recognized. The diagnosis of nonsustained VT was made on the basis of the rapid rate and the change in the electrogram morphology with the onset of the tachycardia. The stored electrogram information was helpful in determining the etiology of recurrent dizziness which occurred at the time of the repeated aborted ICD shocks.

It should be mentioned that the PCD 7217/19 system, although a committed unit with respect to detection of "VF" zone tachyarrhythmias, allows for programming of a specific number of intervals for tachycardia detection which may also permit the device to ignore nonsustained VT. Analogous flexibility for avoiding unnecessary treatment of nonsustained VT was achieved in earlier generation committed CPI Ventak devices (e.g., 1500 and 1550) through the availability of a programmable delay period prior to VT declaration.

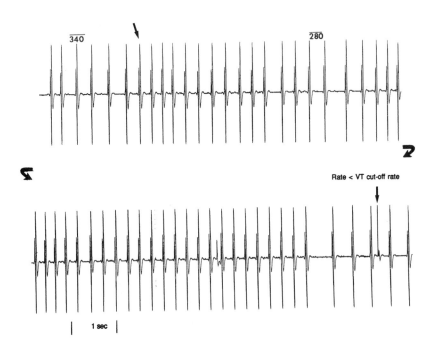

Figure 22. AF with a rapid ventricular rate and aborted ICD shock. The Cadence ICD aborted the shock after initiation of charging because slowing of the ventricular rate was recognized. The diagnosis of AF was made because of the variable ventricular rate and the absence of a change in the electrogram morphology with the tachycardia when compared to ECG documented sinus rhythm (not shown). The stored electrogram information was helpful in determining the etiology of recurrent palpitations which occurred at the time of the repeated aborted ICD shocks.

An ICD high energy discharge for SVTs satisfying the rate criteria for VT/VF may be approached in a number of ways. Radiofrequency ablation can be used to eliminate recurrent SVTs (atrial, atrioventricular [AV] reentrant, or nodal reentrant) or to interrupt AV conduction in cases of atrial fibrillation with rapid ventricular rates. Suppression of SVT with antiarrhythmic agents is an alternative approach. Reassessment of the rate of induced VT, pacing thresholds, and defibrillation efficacy is then necessary. If the rate of induced VT is significantly higher than that of the clinically observed SVT, the programmable rate cutoff of the ICD can be raised above the rate of the SVT, always providing an appropriate safety margin to ensure that VT detection is not adversely affected.

Newer ICD systems possess more sophisticated options for detection (Chap. 15) which can be used to prevent recognition of

ONSET OF ATRIAL FIBRILLATION WITH AVERAGE RR INTERVAL 350 MS
ICD PROGRAMMED WITH TACHYCARDIA DETECTION INTERVAL 400 MSEC, RATE STABILITY REQUIREMENT 60 MSEC

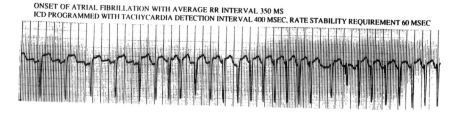

ONE BURST OF ANTITACHYCARDIA PACING DELIVERED DURING ATRIAL FIBRILLATION

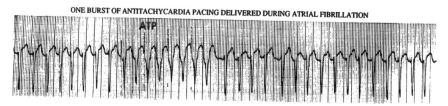

Figure 23. Rate stability criteria for preventing ICD therapy during atrial fibrillation. Regulation of the ventricular response during atrial fibrillation resulted in a burst of antitachycardia pacing during atrial fibrillation (bottom panel) despite the activation of a 60 ms rate stability criteria in the PCD 7217. Increasing the number of beats required to satisfy VT detection will enhance the benefit of rate stability criteria in eliminating ICD therapy for atrial fibrillation. A long detection time and rate stability should be activated only for the range of rates which do not produce any hemodynamic sequelae during VT.

atrial fibrillation as VT (rate stability criteria) or sinus tachycardia as VT (sudden onset criteria). However, these options are not foolproof. (Fig. 23) The ventricular response to atrial fibrillation may transiently regularize and satisfy criteria for rate stability, especially at very fast ventricular rates, thereby falsely prompting "VT" detection. On the other hand, sinus rate acceleration may precipitate VT of similar or only a slightly faster rate, which may fail to be recognized by the ICD if a sudden onset criterion is used. In addition, some VTs may also be associated with marked rate variability which may not satisfy rate stability criteria.[42,48] Therefore, careful selection of detection criteria is required to ensure appropriate therapy for VT in all patients.

If oversensing of non-QRS signals is determined to be the cause of a discharge, the specific etiology will need to be addressed. Depending on the type of ICD, T-wave sensing during ventricular pacing can be eliminated by prolonging the ventricular refractory period of the ICD (e.g., Contour and Jewel). A similar corrective measure might be helpful when oversensed breathing-related noise is sensed during bradycardia pacing by the ICD.[33] Another approach to reducing autogain-mediated oversensitivity during ventricular pacing by the ICD, at least with Ventritex device is programming a faster VVI pacing rate.[49]

T-wave sensing during supraventricular rhythms may also be prevented by changing a programmable sensitivity setting to a less sensitive value (e.g. Jewel). Care must then be taken, however, to avoid an inappropriately high sensitivity setting by documenting the reproducible sensing of VF at the new programmed sensitivity settings.

Lead problems, adapter breaks, and loose connections need surgical intervention for resolution. Malfunctioning endocardial leads should be explanted. However, fibrosis at the tip of the lead may prevent safe extraction, forcing abandonment of the lead. In integrated endocardial lead systems incorporating both sensing and shocking capabilities, identification of the lead site causing malfunction is crucial for therapy guidance. For example, since the distal spring electrode in the transvenous Endotak-C lead is involved in both sensing and shocking in lead-alone systems, failure of this electrode will require implantation of new sensing and shocking leads. Malfunction of the tip sensing electrode alone could be managed with only a new endocardial sensing lead; however, no consensus currently exists regarding the preferred management approach. Although it might be argued instead that replacement of the *entire* integrated lead is advisable given uncertainty regarding the possibility of progression of the fracture (e.g. with further mechanical stress) to involve additional lead elements, total lead replacement may expose the patient to other serious risks (associated with the extraction process itself or consequent to further reduction in vein lumen secondary to the additional integrated lead if the fractured one is abandoned).

Interaction with an implanted unipolar pacemaker will usually require revision of the pacemaker to a bipolar unit. Due to the remote possibility of pacemaker reprogramming after a high energy shock, selection of a "committed" bipolar generator as opposed to one with programmable polarity is desirable. In pacemakers with programmable polarity it is important to establish that bipolar pacing is maintained during ICD testing, without post-shock reset of the pacemaker to unipolar pacing.

Finally, the possibility of "ghost" shocks must be considered. These false perceptions are easily diagnosed with device interrogation, and treated with reassurance.[50]

Table 5. Causes of absent or delayed effective ICD therapy with documented VT/VF

Inactivated ICD
Undersensing of ventricular electrogram
♦ Diminution of sensed ventricular electrogram amplitude at lead-tissue interface
♦ Low amplitude ventricular electrogram after a failed high-energy discharge
♦ Marked fluctuation in electrogram amplitude in ICD with automatic gain control
♦ Lead malfunction or displacement
♦ Generator malfunction
Underdetection
♦ Inappropriately high rate cutoff selection
♦ Failure to satisfy multiple detection criteria
♦ Tachycardia rates at or near VT/VF detection interval in ICDs with multiple programmable tachycardia detection zones
Ineffective antitachycardia pacing algorithms or overly low energy shocks with VT
Delayed VF or VT detection in patients with permanent pacing systems due to sensing of large amplitude pacing stimuli or noise reversion[51]

Absent or Delayed Therapy in Patients with VT/VF

Differential Diagnosis

Occasionally, patients with documented VT/VF will have either no appropriate therapy delivered or a delayed therapy. (Table 5) The three most common causes for this phenomenon are: ICD sensing malfunction, inappropriate selection of tachycardia detection criteria (Fig. 24), and inappropriate selection of ICD therapy (which can prolong the time for termination of VT/VF despite normal sensing). The possibility of prior, inadvertent ICD inactivation should always be considered as well.

Undersensing by the ICD

Undersensing by the ICD may be due to ICD failure or deterioration of the sensed signal at the interface of the rate sensing electrode and tissue. All of the current ICD systems require a certain number (or proportion) of tracked of R-R intervals to be sensed which are shorter than the programmed detection interval for ICD therapy to be delivered. If the sequence of consecutive intervals is interrupted by transiently unsensed signals (resulting in erroneously long R-R intervals), the detection sequence may be reinitiated depending on the type of detection algorithm employed. (Chap. 15)

    In "noncommitted" ICD units, which sense during charging or prior to therapy delivery, this opportunity for resetting the detection process comes into play both during initial tachycardia detection and attempted reconfirmation. Resetting of the detection algorithm can lead to a delay in appropriate ICD therapy.

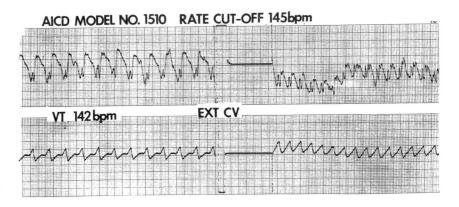

Figure 24. Sustained VT falling below the rate cutoff for VT detection two months following the initiation of oral amiodarone therapy. The VT induced one week after a loading dose of amiodarone was above the rate cutoff. Underdetection of VT occurred and external cardioversion was required. The administration of antiarrhythmic drugs with resultant VT rate below the rate cutoff is the most common cause for failure to detect VT. Detailed testing after all antiarrhythmic drug therapy is necessary to encourage optimum drug/device therapy. The VT rate cutoff should be programmed below the rate that results in hemodynamic compromise even if slow VT is not inducible.

Lead fracture or insulation breakdown may result in sensing failure in both endocardial and epicardial systems.[52] The history of a subclavian puncture technique used for implantation of an endocardial sensing lead should raise the possibility of lead disruption whenever appropriate sensing is delayed. There is an association of this implantation technique with "crush" injury to the lead if it is compressed between the clavicle and first rib.[53]

Poor electrogram sensing at the tissue-lead interface may occur for a number of reasons. Acute inflammation after initial lead placement may result in marked increases in pacing thresholds and decreases in sensing ability which may resolve over a number of weeks or persist chronically. Gradual deterioration of the sensed ventricular electrogram may also occur with time.

All current ICD systems utilize automatic gain control (or automatic threshold control—see Chap. 14) to increase the relative size of low amplitude signals during VT/VF to prevent undersensing. This does not always guarantee prompt tachycardia detection.[54] Some ICD systems can fail to redetect VF after an unsuccessful shock.[55-57] This uncommon phenomenon has been shown to be due to the inability of the automatic gain control to account for the

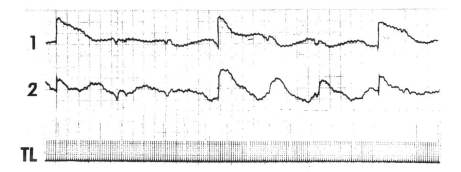

Figure 25. Large amplitude unipolar pacing spikes during VF precludes its detection. Committed bipolar pacing is preferred. Documentation of effective VF recognition with the pacemaker set in the fixed rate mode using the maximum voltage output is required whenever a concomitant bradycardia pacing system is employed. The pacing stimulus amplitude recorded by the ICD sensing system should be < 1 mV. After testing, the pacing unit should be programmed to the maximum sensitivity and minimum pacing amplitude.

marked decrease in electrogram amplitude, a problem possibly compounded by post-shock diminution of R-wave amplitude with certain transvenous leads, such as the Endotak C.[55]

Post-shock failure to detect VF was reported with the Ventritex Cadence ICD using a standard bipolar endocardial rate sensing lead (involving 2 of 98 patients)[56] and also using the integrated CPI tripolar Endotak-C 60 series lead (4 of 22 patients).[57] The Cadence (as well as the Cadet and Contour) have a programmable sinus redetection time of "nominal" (5 beats) and "slow" (7 beats); both reports suggest that programming to the "slow" redetection time may prevent this problem with VF redetection. Although a report by Ellis et al involving the Endotak C lead and the Ventak P generator reported no difference between initial VF detection time and redetection time after a failed shock, redetection times > 10 s were noted in 7.8% of VF episodes and > 12 s in 3.5%.[58]

Interactions with a permanent pacemaker can cause nondetection of VF by the ICD with subsequent failure of the device to deliver any therapy. (See also Chaps. 14 [Amplifier], 17 [Implantation], and 23 [Sudden Death Despite ICD Therapy]. In units with automatic gain control, the presence of asynchronous pacing artifacts (due to undersensing of VF by the pacemaker) can cause the ICD to ignore low amplitude ventricular electrograms during VF.[23,59,60] (Fig. 25) This problem appears to be limited pri-

marily to unipolar pacing systems, but can be seen with large amplitude bipolar pacing stimuli. "Noise reversion" to VOO pacing
(unipolar) during ventricular tachyarrhythmias may occur with
some bipolar pacemakers, potentially interfering with VT/VF detection.[51] Such an adverse pacemaker-ICD interaction might be
minimized by use of minimal noise-sampling periods and dual
chamber rather than VVI mode for the pacemaker.[51]

Underdetection By The ICD
Delay in ICD therapy can also be caused by tachycardia underdetection in devices which require multiple detection criteria for
VT/VF to be satisfied. A number of tiered therapy devices utilize
additional detection criteria besides rate; these include: rate stability, and sudden onset. Again, these additional programmable criteria are designed to improve specificity of VT/VF detection, but the
use of one or more of these may increase the time for detection criteria to be satisfied. Using a definition of underdetection as a delay
of ≥ 5 s for detection of VT/VF, Swerdlow et al noted that the incidence of this phenomenon in the PCD 7217 was 1.9% of total induced ventricular tachyarrhythmia episodes involving 9.6% of the
patients studied.[48] During clinical followup, underdetection occurred in 10% of patients with a total failure to detect 2 episodes of
polymorphic VT in 1 patient who required external cardioversion.
With respect to specific criteria for VT detection, the inability to
satisfy the sudden onset criteria or the rate stability criteria led to a
similar incidence of VT underdetection during clinical followup
(0.4%). Of note, in an earlier study,[61] Swerdlow et al demonstrated
1 reset of VT detection due to failure to satisfy the stability criteria
in 64% of VT episodes induced post implant in the electrophysiology laboratory, although the delays in the detection were ≤ 3.6 s.
(See also Chaps. 15 and 19)
    Tiered therapy ICD units permit the physician to program
multiple detection zones which allow for different therapies to be
delivered based on the rate of the detected tachycardia. In all devices, VT detection can be reset with a minimal number of intervals
falling above the interval required for VT detection. In the PCD
7217, for example, this occurs with a single interval longer than the
VT detection interval. Swerdlow et al noted such a reset phenomenon, with resultant detection delays of > 5 s, in 0.4% of VT episodes during long-term followup of patients with the PCD.[48] Consecutive VT intervals straying above and below the preset VT
detection interval can readily lead to delays in VT therapy. For VF
detection, generally a *cumulative* number of intervals rather than a

consecutive number of intervals less than the VF detection interval are required to initiate VF therapy. As a result, VF detection may also be delayed if the tachycardia rate is oscillating above and below the preset VF detection interval. This was noted in 0.4% of VT episodes induced in the electrophysiology laboratory and in 0.1% of VT episodes during long-term followup in Swerdlow's series.[48] Such a zone boundary wandering problem can be overcome with detection algorithms that use combined (VT and VF) counters. (Chap. 15) VT and VF detection criteria vary, and may be quite complex, in different ICD units; it is essential, therefore, to be familiar with the detection criteria in each device.

Errors in Programming of ICD Therapy Options

Inappropriate programming of ICD therapy delivery may also delay successful conversion of VT/VF despite prompt tachycardia detection. Antitachycardia pacing should be restricted primarily to use for relatively slow and hemodynamically tolerated VT where efficacy has been demonstrated during laboratory testing. If antitachycardia pacing is programmed as initial therapy for rapid, syncopal VT, it is less likely to be efficacious, and may delay life-saving high energy cardioversion until long after the patient has lost consciousness; in the interim, significant myocardial ischemia and acidosis may develop which may affect subsequent efficacy of delivered shocks. Selection of adequate shock energy amplitude is also required to avoid a prolonged delay in conversion of rapid VT/VF secondary to ineffective lower energy shocks.

Assessment And Management

The initial approach to the patient in whom there appears to be a delay in the delivery of appropriate therapy is thorough interrogation of the device. Real time measurements of sensed electrogram amplitude and rate sensing lead impedance may provide clues to sensing malfunction at the tissue-lead interface or in the lead itself. Evidence of overly high lead impedance (suggesting lead fracture), low lead impedance (suggesting insulation failure) or poor R-wave sensing suggests the need for implantation of a new rate sensing lead. Tachycardia detection criteria should be reviewed to ensure that there is an appropriate safety margin between all induced and clinical VT rates and the programmed rate cutoff. This is especially important if antiarrhythmic drug therapy has been added since implant. (Fig. 24) Detection criteria utilizing a combination of rate, stability, and sudden onset may have to be simplified with the elimination of all but rate criteria in order to avoid delayed tachycardia detection.

Programmable therapy should be reviewed to avoid delivery of antitachycardia pacing or low energy shock therapy during rapid hemodynamically unstable VT. When antitachycardia pacing is used for rapid VT, every effort should be made to document its efficacy at the time of device testing prior to discharge. (See appendix to Chap. 16) When utilized in this setting, the number of burst attempts should be minimized to avoid any delay in high energy shocks if required. A desire to avoid patient discomfort from a shock should never compromise the delivery of effective therapy for hemodynamically unstable ventricular tachyarrhythmias.

The strategy for assessing and correcting tachycardia undersensing depends on the ICD unit's telemetry features and sensing mechanism. The assessment of appropriate sensing may require induction of VT or VF or both in the electrophysiology laboratory. In the Ventak series of ICDs, Beepograms during VT/VF may allow for assessment of appropriate sensing.[5] (Fig. 19) With the limited programmability of this device, correction of undersensing may require implantation of a new rate-sensing lead unless a reversible cause such as drug therapy is present. In ICD units with marker channels, these markers can also be utilized during induced VT/VF to document undersensing (indicated by an observed deficit in number of "marked" ventricular events). If undersensing is noted, and an automatic gain control is not utilized, the sensitivity setting can be increased. In devices with automatic gain control with delay or failure to redetect VT/VF after an initial high energy discharge, the time to redetect sinus rhythm should be programmed to its maximum value to ensure appropriate VT/VF redetection. Berul et al suggest consideration of a pre-discharge ICD evaluation which includes programming an initial subthreshold shock to be delivered during induced VF to ensure appropriate VT/VF redetection.[57]

In patients with permanent pacemakers, failed ICD therapy should prompt a search for pacemaker-induced nondetection of VF. If a unipolar system was left in place at ICD implant, it should be replaced with a committed bipolar system. If a bipolar system was in place, VF should be induced under general anesthesia with the pacing amplitude and pulse width maximized, to ensure proper ICD function. The risk of nondetection of VF secondary to sensed pacing artifacts should be minimized by programming the pacemaker to the lowest pacing output that will allow for reliable capture. The pacemaker should also be programmed to its greatest sensitivity setting in order to maximize detection of small amplitude

Table 6. Causes of failed ICD therapy in patients with documented VT/VF

Battery Depletion
High Defibrillation Threshold
  ♦ Dislodgement of transvenous defibrillator leads
  ♦ Alteration of the contour of epicardial defibrillating patches
  ♦ Drug induced
  ♦ Spontaneous change in defibrillation threshold with time
Ineffective antitachycardia pacing algorithms or overly low energy shocks with VT
ICD component failure resulting in absent or inadequate pacing or shocking therapy

signals and, thereby, avoid pacing during VF. (Following these various maneuvers, the ICD should always be interrogated to ensure that any temporary programmed features, such as suspension of VT/VF detection, are replaced by the intended permanent programmed configuration.)

Failure of ICD Therapy With Documented VT/VF

Differential Diagnosis
Potentially, the most serious problem encountered during ICD followup is failure of the device to successfully terminate VT/VF, leading to either patient demise or the need for conventional resuscitation. (Table 6)

In a multicenter experience, Lehmann et al[62] analyzed terminal events in 51 ICD (first generation device) patients who died suddenly; 30 deaths were monitored. Two thirds of monitored episodes demonstrated VT/VF as the initial rhythm. Of the patients with documented or presumed tachyarrhythmic death (based on witnessed shocks), 41% had active, nondepleted devices with defibrillation thresholds ≤ 20 J (monophasic pulse), although possible contributory factors were noted in over half of these patients. Of note, battery depletion was present in 15% of the patients with documented or presumed tachyarrhythmic death, confirming the importance of routine followup of indicators of ICD battery reserve.

ICD therapy which had previously been found to be effective may lose its efficacy during long-term followup. Antitachycardia pacing may become ineffective due to increases in pacing threshold in the chronic setting[63] or lead fracture. Migration, crinkling, or folding of patch defibrillating leads may significantly increase the defibrillation threshold. (Fig. 26)

Epicardial or extra-pericardial patches which come in contact with each other may cause current to be shunted away from the myocardium, leading to ineffective high energy discharges. Dis-

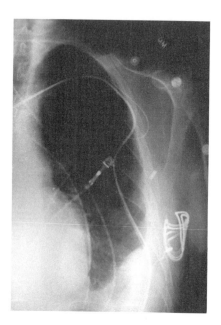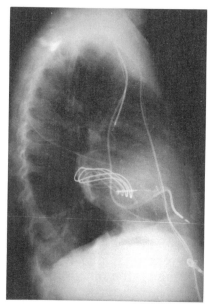

Figure 26. Marked folding of defibrillator subcutaneous patch lead (Medtronic Inc.) shown on PA (left) and lateral (right) chest films. The folding of the patch lead developed postoperatively. A marked increase in defibrillation threshold and failure to terminate induced VF were documented in this patient. Defibrillation lead impedance was increased. The patch lead was replaced but not repositioned, and effective defibrillation with a low threshold value was documented. Marked crinkling or folding of defibrillator patch lead associated with an increase in shocking lead impedance warrants retesting of ICD function to document efficacy even if failure to terminate spontaneous VT/VF has not yet been observed.

lodgement or migration of transvenous defibrillating electrodes may also lead to ineffective defibrillation. (Fig. 27, 28) With both epicardial and transvenous systems, defibrillating lead fracture can lead to failure to cardiovert or defibrillate.[64]

Occasionally, antiarrhythmic drugs may make VT incessant, resulting in only transient termination of VT with antitachycardia pacing. Although defibrillation thresholds in epicardial systems have a tendency to remain stable,[65] defibrillation thresholds may rise during followup in transvenous systems;[66] this is not usually clinically significant, however, especially with the use of biphasic waveforms.

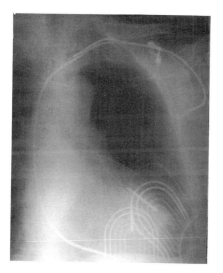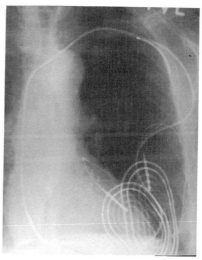

Figure 27. Migration of endocardial shocking lead (Medtronic) from left sub-clavian (left) to subcutaneous position (right) preventing defibrillation of induced VF. Marked changes in any shocking or sensing lead location warrants retesting of ICD function even if therapy failure has not previously been seen.

Antiarrhythmic medications such as amiodarone and Type IA and IC agents may also raise the defibrillation thresholds to un-acceptable values.[36,67-69] (Chap. 5, Table 2) Failure of initially effec-tive programmed values for high energy shocks to treat VF may also occur in patients with low safety margins.[70,71] (Chap. 5) The pres-ence of concomitant conditions such as myocardial infarction or ischemia, drug-induced torsade de pointes, or electrolyte abnor-malities, may produce ventricular arrhythmias refractory to previ-ously documented efficacious therapy. A more detailed discussion of failure of ICD therapy is provided in Chap. 23.

Assessment And Management

As in all instances of suspected ICD malfunction, patients who survive failed therapy require full interrogation of the device. Using whatever real time measurements are available, attention should be paid to the status of the rate-sensing lead, shocking leads, and gen-erator status. In units which can store events and subsequent deliv-ered therapy, this information should be reviewed to determine whether appropriate tachycardia detection occurred as well as the ICD's therapeutic response. In settings where antitachycardia pac-ing failed, the pacing threshold should be rechecked.

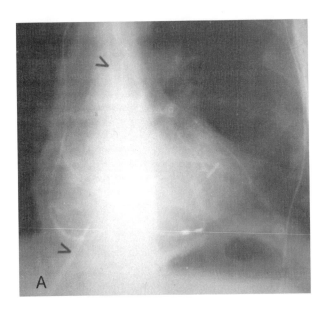

Figure 28. Migration of shocking lead to the inferior vena cava (arrow) and the proximal aspect of the rate sensing lead to the right ventricular outflow tract (arrow) and pulmonary artery. The change in position of the leads (CPI) was associate with ineffective defibrillation of induced VF. Lead repositioning was required.

Threshold measurements should be performed at or near the desired pacing rates to avoid missing rate-dependent increases in pacing threshold, particularly when class IC agents are being used. Antitachycardia pacing amplitude and pulse width should usually be set at maximal values. An inappropriately high pacing threshold will either force abandonment of antitachycardia pacing as a treatment option or require repositioning or replacement of the pace/sense lead. In some transvenous pacing lead systems, repositioning of the right ventricular lead may be possible if dislodgement is noted as the cause of high pacing thresholds prior to fixation of the lead.

Patients with documented failure of high energy shocks to terminate VT/VF will require re-evaluation of ICD function if battery depletion is not found to be the problem. The shocking lead impedance registered at the time of the last shock should be carefully checked.[72] Any increase in impedance should raise questions as to the integrity and position of the lead systems. A chest ro-entgenogram should be obtained to assess lead position and con-tour of epicardial patches. VT and VF should be induced in the electrophysiology laboratory under general anesthesia and the defi-brillation threshold determined. Impedance during shocks should be checked and compared to prior measurements including implant values.

If the defibrillation threshold is high, medications known to raise the threshold should be discontinued if possible. In non-thoracotomy systems, evaluation for lead dislodgement or migra-tion should be made, as even small changes in position may affect defibrillation efficacy. Occasionally, patients with marginal defi-brillation thresholds using an ICD system capable of delivering a single, unidirectional monophasic shock may benefit from the use of a biphasic shock or the addition of another current pathway. This would involve not only changing the ICD generator, but in some in-stances adding additional leads such as a left thoracic subcutane-ous patch lead or a superior vena cava lead.

Symptoms of VT/VF Without Noticed Shock

Differential Diagnosis
Patients with known VT or VF may develop symptoms (e.g. palpi-tations, near-syncope, or syncope) suggestive of arrhythmia, but without shock delivery. (Table 7) In most instances, this does not represent ICD malfunction. Such a phenomenon may result from supraventricular or ventricular arrhythmias with either too slow a rate or too short a duration to satisfy detection criteria. These oc-currences are more likely with use of a long first shock delay in the Ventak ICD or in noncommitted devices capable of a second look during ICD charging. Hemodynamically tolerated VT may initiate antitachycardia pacing and tachycardia termination with only a minimum of symptoms. Similarly, a brief trial of antitachycardia pacing may be successful in terminating VT associated with syn-cope without obvious ICD function (i.e. high energy shock delivery) being evident to the patient or witnesses. Inappropriate antitachy-cardia pacing (say, for some SVT) also might mimic symptoms of a spontaneous tachyarrhythmia.

Table 7. Causes of symptoms suggesting VT/VF without noticed shock.

Nonsustained VT or SVT not satisfying detection criteria

Hemodynamically tolerated VT terminating with antitachycardia pacing

Undersensing of VT

Oversensing of non-QRS signals or supraventricular tachyarrhythmias triggering symptomatic antitachycardia pacing

In patients who are dependent upon bradycardia pacing by the ICD, symptoms may develop if this is interrupted. Of note is that the PCD 7217 "turns off" bradycardia pacing during normal capacitor reforming which can lead to transient symptomatic bradyarrhythmias (possibly mistaken for symptomatic VT, if not monitored) at that time.

ICD malfunction may also be considered in this setting. As previously discussed, undersensing or underdetection of VT may result in the device ignoring a tachyarrhythmia that should have been detected and treated prior to spontaneous termination. ICD failure due to battery depletion or component failure could cause the same phenomenon. Oversensing of non-QRS signals or sinus tachycardia could cause the unique situation where pacing is initiated during normal rhythm with subsequent palpitations in the absence of a tachyarrhythmia.

Assessment And Management

In ICD units without the ability to store events and subsequent therapy history, the ability to determine the cause of symptoms suggesting arrhythmia, as well as the ICD response is limited. Although these devices can store the number of high energy discharges delivered, any correlation with clinical events would require prolonged continuous ambulatory ECG monitoring or the use of a patient-activated event recorder.

In patients with ICDs which store episode-related information, it is possible to review, by telemetry, the occurrence of tachyarrhythmias which satisfied detection criteria as well as any therapy delivered, and correlate these events with clinical symptoms. This can be helpful in determining the occurrence of nonsustained arrhythmias with aborted therapy as well as sustained arrhythmias eliciting few symptoms with termination by antitachycardia pacing. As mentioned above, stored electrograms can be helpful in differentiating supraventricular and ventricular tachyarrhythmias which may cause symptoms without high energy ICD discharge.[11,12,39-41] The use of a patient-activated event recorder may be necessary even in patients with these sophisticated ICD units if

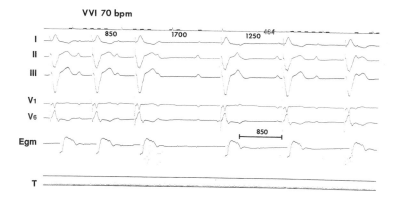

Figure 29. Intermittent T-wave oversensing during ventricular pacing through ICD system leading to marked symptomatic bradycardia. The bradycardia was prevented by increasing the post pacing refractory period and increasing the bradycardia pacing rate. The increase in pacing rate shortened the QT interval and decreased the likelihood of T-wave oversensing for any given post pacing refractory period. A backup approach would be to revise the sensing lead location or to implanting a separate bradycardia pacemaker and lead.

one suspects a symptomatic arrhythmia that does not satisfy programmed detection criteria.

The management of frequent episodes of symptomatic nonsustained tachyarrhythmias or sustained VT triggering antitachycardia pacing will often necessitate the administration of antiarrhythmic drugs or consideration of catheter ablation.[45] If the nonsustained episodes are causing only mild symptoms, drug therapy is counterindicated to avoid other interactions with device function. If frequent episodes of tachycardia cause significant patient symptoms or repeated therapy delivery, drug therapy should be started with the recognition that complete reassessment of ICD function will be required once steady-state drug levels are attained.

The inability to detect a tachyarrhythmia as the cause of near-syncope or syncope should trigger a search for an alternative cause, with appropriate therapy based on the etiology. If a bradycardia is found to be the cause of syncope or near-syncope, a bipolar—not unipolar- pacing unit should be utilized to avoid problems with double counting due to oversensing of pacing artifacts or nondetection of VF.[16,59] In ICDs capable of bradycardia pacing, appropriate sensing and pacing thresholds as well as normal lead impedance should be confirmed to exclude the possibility of an untreated bradycardia due to pacing system malfunction.[73] (Fig. 29)

Table 8. Approach to the ICD patient with possible device malfunction

Chest X-ray
   ♦ Evaluate lead position and possibility of fracture
Device Interrogation
   ♦ Real time measurements (battery status, pacing lead impedance, EGM amplitude)
   ♦ Review of programmed detection criteria for VT and VF
   ♦ Review of programmed therapy for VT and VF
   ♦ Review of diagnostic data (events, delivered therapy, shocking lead impedance)
   ♦ Review of R-R interval and stored electrogram data (comparison of EGM morphology
     during tachycardia with NSR) for tachycardia episodes
When sensing or detection malfunction is suspected which may lead to inappropriate therapy or de-
lay/failure in delivery of effective therapy
   ♦ Beepogram/marker channels/real time electrogram recordings
   ♦ Assessment of T-wave or pacing stimulus sensing
   ♦ Assessment during device manipulation
   ♦ Reassessment of sensing function after VT/VF induction
   ♦ Reassessment of programmed detection criteria for VT
   ♦ Assessment of possible device-device interactions in patients with pacemakers
   ♦ Assessment of VT/VF redetection after a failed high energy shock for VF
When primary failure of delivered therapy is suspected
   ♦ Reassessment of pacing threshold when ATP utilized
   ♦ Reassessment of DFT and ATP efficacy during induced VT/VF
   ♦ Review of contributing clinical factors such as concomitant antiarrhythmic therapy or
     change in myocardial substrate

ATP = antitachycardia pacing, DFT = defibrillation threshold, EGM = electrogram, NSR = normal sinus rhythm

Final Note

As ICD capabilities have expanded, the different problems encountered during clinical followup have multiplied as well. A full knowledge of device function and capabilities allows for formulation of
an appropriate differential diagnosis and plan of assessment and
therapy. (Table 8) It will be essential that device-specific phenomena be well known to the electrophysiologist to differentiate ICD
malfunction from proper function. Future advances in ICD technology should improve the ability of the clinical cardiac electrophysiologist to troubleshoot potential device complications and
hopefully decrease the overall incidence of these problems.

Acknowledgments
The authors would like to acknowledge the expert technical assistance of
Tessa David and Kathy Freeman in the production of this chapter and
the critical review by Charles Swerdlow, MD. Figs. 1 and 2 are adapted
with permission from the American Journal of Cardiology.[5] Fig. 3 is

adapted with permission from PACE.[12] Fig. 5 is adapted with permission from Annals of Internal Medicine.[6] Figs. 8 and 29 are adapted with permission from Journal of the American College of Cardiology.[37] Fig. 9 is adapted with permission from Journal of the American College of Cardiology.[47] Fig. 10 is adapted with permission from PACE.[46] Figs. 12 and 13 are adapted with permission from PACE.[36] Figs. 15, 16A, and 16B are adapted with permission from Journal of the American College of Cardiology.[38] Fig. 18 is adapted with permission from Grune and Stratton Inc.[74] Fig. 20 is adapted with permission from Futura Publishing Inc.[75] Fig. 21 and 22 is adapted with permission from Journal of the American College of Cardiology.[47] Figs. 25 and 28 are adapted with permission from Grune and Stratton Inc.[74]

1. Corbelli R, McAllister H, Rashidi R, et al. Initial Beep-o-gram experience: Assessment of automatic implantable cardioverter-defibrillator sensing function. PACE 1986;12:665A. (abstract)
2. Chapman, PD, Troup P. The automatic implantable cardioverter-defibrillator: Evaluating suspected inappropriate shocks. J Am Coll Cardiol 1986;7:1075-1081.
3. Axtell KA, Akhtar M. Incidence of syncope prior to implantable cardioverter-defibrillator discharges. Circulation 1990;82:211A. (abstract)
4. Kou WH, Calkins HG, Lewis RR, et al. Incidence of loss of consciousness during automatic implantable cardioverter-defibrillator shocks. Ann Int Med 1991;115:942-945.
5. Grimm W, Flores BT, Marchlinski FE. Symptoms and electrocardiographically documented rhythm preceding spontaneous shocks in patients with implantable cardioverter-defibrillators. Am J Cardiol 1993;71:1415-1418.
6. Marchlinski FE, Flores BT, Buxton AB, et al. The automatic implantable cardioverter-defibrillator: Efficacy, complications and device failures. Ann Int Med 1986;104:481-488.
7. Maloney J, Masterson M, Khoury D, et al. Clinical performance of the implantable cardioverter-defibrillator: electrocardiographic documentation of 101 spontaneous discharges. PACE 1991;14:280-285.
8. Kelly PA, Mann DE, Damle RS, et al. Oversensing during ventricular pacing in patients with a third generation implantable cardioverter-defibrillator. J Am Coll Cardiol 1994;23:1531-1534.
9. Newman D, Dorian P, Downar E, et al. Use of telemetry functions in the assessment of implanted antitachycardia device efficacy. Am J Cardiol 1992;70:606-621.
10. Grimm W, Flores BF, Marchlinski FE. Complications of implantable cardioverter-defibrillator therapy: Followup of 241 patients. PACE 1993;16:218-222.
11. Grimm W, Flores BT, Marchlinski FE. Shock occurrence and survival in 241 patients with implantable cardioverter-defibrillator therapy. Circulation 1993;87:1880-1888.
12. Grimm W, Flores BT, Marchlinski FE. Electrocardiographically documented unnecessary, spontaneous shocks in 241 patients with implantable cardioverter-defibrillators. PACE 1992;15:1667-1673.
13. Fogoros RN, Elson JJ, Bonnet CA. Actuarial incidence and pattern of occurrence of shocks following implantation of the automatic implantable cardioverter-defibrillator. PACE 1989;12:1465-1473.
14. Reiter MJ, Mann DE. Sensing and tachyarrhythmia detection problems in implantable cardioverter defibrillators. J Cardiovasc Electrophysiol 1996;7:542-

558.

15. Hook BG, Callans DJ, Kleinman RB, et al. Implantable cardioverter-defibrillator therapy in the absence of significant symptoms: Rhythm diagnosis and management aided by stored electrograms. Circulation 1993;87:1897-1906.
16. Edel TB, Maloney JD, Moore S, et al. Six-year clinical experience with the automatic implantable cardioverter-defibrillator. PACE 1991;14:1850-1854.
17. Horton RP, Canby RC, Roman CA, et al. Diagnosis of ICD lead failure using continuous event marker recording. PACE 1995;18:1331-1334.
18. Almeida HF, Buckingham TA. Inappropriate implantable cardioverter defibrillator shocks secondary to sensing lead failure: utility of stored electrograms. PACE 1993;16:407-411.
19. Almassi GH, Olinger GN, Wetherbee JN, et al. Long term complications of implantable cardioverter defibrillator lead systems. Ann Thorac Surg 1993;55:888-892.
20. Epstein AE, Shepard RB. Failure of one conduction in a nonthoracotomy implantable defibrillator lead causing inappropriate sensing and potentially ineffective shock delivery. PACE 1993;16:796-800.
21. Bardy GH, Troutman C, Poole VE, et al. Clinical experience with a tiered therapy multiprogrammable antiarrhythmia device. Circulation 1992;85:1689-1698.
22. Gottlieb C, Miller JM, Rosenthal ME, et al. Automatic implantable defibrillator discharge resulting from routine pacemaker programming. PACE 1988;11:336-338.
23. Karson T, Grace K, Denes P. Stereo speaker silences automatic implantable cardioverter-defibrillator. Letters to Editor. N Engl J Med 1989;320:1628-1629.
24. Man KC, Davidson T, Langberg JT, et al. Interference from a hand held radiofrequency remote control causing discharge of an implantable defibrillator. PACE 1993;16:1756-1758.
25. Madrid AH, Moro C, Martin J, et al. Interference of the implantable cardioverter defibrillator caused by slot machines. PACE 1996;19:675. (abstract)
26. Barbaro V, Bartolini P, Donato A, et al. Do European GSM mobile cellular phones pose a potential risk to pacemaker patients? PACE 1995;18:1218-1224.
27. Naegeli B, Osswald S, Deola M, et al. Intermittent pacemaker dysfunction caused by digital mobile telephones. J Am Coll Cardiol 1996;27:1471-1477.
28. Fetter J, Ivan V, Benditt, DG, et al. Digital cellular telephones do not necessarily interfere with implantable cardioverter defibrillator (ICD) operation. PACE 1996;19:676. (abstract)
29 Stanton MS, Grice S, Trusty J, et al. Safety of various cellular phone technologies with implantable cardioverter defibrillators. PACE 1996;19:583. (abstract)
30. Madrid AH, Moro C, Chadli, et al. Interferences between the automatic defibrillators and mobile phones. PACE 1996;19:676. (abstract)
31. McIvor ME. Environmental electromagnetic interference from electronic article surveillance devices; interactions with an ICD. PACE 1995;18:2229-2230.
32. Ferrick KJ, Johnston D, Kim SG. Inadvertent AICD inactivation while playing bingo. Am Heart J 1991;121:206-207.
33. Rosenthal ME, Paskman C. Noise generation during bradycardia pacing with the Ventritex Cadence/CPI Endotak ICD system: incidence and clinical significance. PACE 1996;19:677. (abstract)
34. Calkins H, Brinker J, Veltri EP, et al. Clinical interactions between pacemakers and automatic implantable cardioverter-defibrillators. J Am Coll Cardiol 1990;16:666-673.
35. Kim SG, Furman S, Matos JA, et al. Automatic implantable cardioverter-defibrillator: Inadvertent discharges during permanent pacemaker magnet tests. PACE 1987;10:579-582.
36. Callans DJ, Hook BG, Marchlinski FE. Paced beats following single nonsensed complexes in a "codependent" cardioverter defibrillator and bradycardia pacing system: Potential for VT induction. PACE 1991;14:1281-1287.

37. Callans DJ, Hook BG, Kleinman RB, et al. Unique sensing errors in third generation implantable cardioverter-defibrillators. J Am Coll Cardiol 1993;, 22:1135-1140.
38. Johnson NJ, Marchlinski FE. Arrhythmias induced by device antitachycardia therapy due to diagnostic specificity. J Am Coll Cardiology 1991;18:1418-1425.
39. Hook BG, Marchlinski FE. Value of ventricular electrogram recordings in the diagnosis of arrhythmias precipitating electrical device shock therapy. J Am Coll Cardiol 1991;17:985-990.
40. Callans DJ, Hook BG, Marchlinski FE. Use of bipolar recordings from patch-patch and rate sensing leads to distinguish ventricular tachycardia from supraventricular rhythms in patients with implantable cardioverter-defibrillators. PACE 1991;14:1917;-1922;.
41. Marchlinski FE, Gottlieb CD, Sarter B, et al. ICD data storage—value in arrhythmia management. PACE 1993;16:527-534.
42. Brachman J, Sterns LD, Hilbel T, et al. Regularity of spontaneously occurring VT and its influence on stability criteria for detection. Circulation 1993;88:1353. (abstract)
43. Volosin KJ, Beauregard MA, Fabiszewski R. Spontaneous changes in ventricular tachycardia cycle length. J Am Coll Cardiol 1991;17:409-414.
44. Geibel A, Zehender M, Brugada P. Changes in cycle length at the onset of sustained tachyarrhythmias—importance for antitachycardia pacing. Am Heart J 1988;115:588-592.
45. Willems S, Borggrefe M, Shenasa M, et al. Radiofrequency catheter ablation of VT following implantation of an automatic cardioverter defibrillator. PACE 1993;16:1684-1692.
46. Gottlieb CD, Horowitz LN. Potential interactions between antiarrhythmic medication and the automatic implantable cardioverter-defibrillator. PACE 1991;14:898-904.
47. Hurwitz JL, Hook BG, Flores BT, et al. Importance of abortive shock capability with electrogram storage in cardioverter-defibrillator devices. J Am Coll Cardiol 1993;21:895-900.
48. Swerdlow CD, Ahern T, Chen P, et al. Underdetection of VT by algorithms to enhance specificity in a tiered-therapy cardioverter-defibrillator. J Am Coll Cardiol 1994;24:416-424.
49. Reiter Michael J, Div. Cardiology, Univ. of Colorado Health Sciences Center, Denver, CO 80262. Phone: 303-270-5173. Personal communication.
50. Miller JM, Hsia HH. Management of the patient with frequent discharges from implantable cardioverter devices. J Cardiovasc Electrophysiol 1996;7:278-285.
51. Glikson M, Hammill SC, Hayes DL, et al. The importance of noise reversion in pacemaker-ICD interactions. PACE 1996;19:737. (abstract)
52. Stambler BS, Wood MA, Damiano RJ, et al. Sensing/pacing lead complications with a newer generation implantable cardioverter-defibrillator: Worldwide experience from the Guardian ATP 4210 clinical trial. J Am Coll Cardiol 1994;23:123-132.
53. Magney JE, Flynn DM, Parsons JA, et al. Anatomical mechanisms explaining damage to pacemaker leads, defibrillator leads, and failure of central venous catheters adjacent to the sternoclavicular joint. PACE 1993;16:445-457.
54. Bardy GH, Ivey TD, Stewart R, et al. Failure of the automatic implantable defibrillator to detect ventricular fibrillation. Am J Cardiol 1986;58:1107-1108.
55. Jung W, Manz M, Moosdorf R, et al. Failure of an implantable cardioverter-defibrillator to redetect ventricular fibrillation in patients with a nonthoracotomy lead system. Circulation 1992;86:1217-1222.
56. Mann DE, Kelly PA, Damle RS, et al. Undersensing during ventricular tachyarrhythmias in a third generation implantable cardioverter-defibrillator. Diagnosis using stored electrograms and correction with programming. PACE 1994;17:1525-1530.

57. Berul CI, Callans DJ, Schwartzman DS, et al. Comparison of initial detection and redetection of ventricular fibrillation in a transvenous defibrillator system with automatic gain control. J Am Coll Cardiol 1995;25:431-436.
58. Ellis JR, Martin DT, Venditti FJ. Appropriate sensing of ventricular fibrillation after failed shocks in a transvenous cardioverter-defibrillator system. Circulation 1994;90:1820-1825.
59. Singer I, Guarneri T, Kupersmith J. Implanted automatic defibrillators: Effects of drugs and pacemakers. PACE 1988;11:2250-2262.
60. Kim SG, Furman S, Waspe LE, et al. Unipolar pacer artifacts induced failure of an automatic implantable cardioverter/defibrillator to detect ventricular fibrillation. Am J Cardiol 1986;57:880-889.
61. Swerdlow CD, Chen PS, Kass RM, et al. Discrimination of ventricular tachycardia from sinus tachycardia and atrial fibrillation in a tiered therapy cardioverter-defibrillator. J Am Coll Cardiol 1994;23:1342-1355.
62. Lehmann MH, Thomas A, Nabih M, et al. Sudden death in recipients of first-generation implantable cardioverter-defibrillators: analysis of terminal events. J Interventional Cardiol 1994;7:487-503.
63. Saksena S, Polzobutt-Johanos M, Castle LW, et al. Long-term multicenter experience with a second generation implantable pacemaker-defibrillator in patients with malignant ventricular arrhythmias. J Am Coll Cardiol 1992;19:490-499.
64. Jones GK, Bardy GH, Kudenchuk PJ, et al. Mechanical complications following implantation of multiple lead nonthoracotomy defibrillator systems: implications for management and future system design. Am Heart J 1995;10:327-333.
65. Frame R, Brodman R, Furman S, et al. Long-term stability of defibrillation thresholds with intrapericardial defibrillator patches. PACE 1993;16:208-212.
66. Venditti FJ, Martin DT, Vassolas G, et al. Rise in chronic defibrillation thresholds in nonthoracotomy implantable defibrillator. Circulation 1994;89:216-223.
67. Guarneri T, Levine JH, Veltri EP, et al. Success of chronic defibrillation and the role of antiarrhythmic drugs with the automatic implantable cardioverter defibrillator. Am J Cardiol 1987;60:1061-1064.
68. Haberman RJ, Veltri EP, Mower MM. The effect of amiodarone on defibrillation threshold. J Electrophysiol 1988;5:415-423.
69. Marinchak RA, Friehling T, Kline RA, et al. Effect of antiarrhythmic drugs on defibrillation threshold: Case report of an adverse effect of mexiletine and review of the literature. PACE 1988;11:7-12.
70. Pinski SL, Vanerio G, Castle LW, et al. Patients with a high defibrillation threshold: Clinical characteristics, management and outcome. Am Heart J 1991;122:89-95.
71. Epstein AE, Ellenbogen KA, Kirk KA, et al. Clinical characteristics and outcome of patients with high defibrillation thresholds: a multicenter study. Circulation 1992;86:1200-1216.
72. Haddad L, Padula LE, Moreau M, et al. Troubleshooting implantable cardioverter defibrillator system malfunctions: the role of impedance measurements. PACE 1994;17:1456-1461.
73. Hayes DL, Vlietstra RE. Pacemaker malfunction. Ann Int Med 1993;119:828-835.
74. Marchlinski FE, Buxton AE, Flores B. Automatic Implantable Cardioverter Defibrillator: Followup and complications. In: Samet and El-Sheriff (eds:) Cardiac Pacing and Electrophysiology, 3rd Ed., Grune and Stratton 1990; Chapter 45, pp 743-758.
75. Marchlinski FE, Kleiman RB, Hook BG, et al. Advances in implantable cardioverter defibrillator therapy. In: Josephson ME, Wellens HJJ (eds): Tachycardias: Mechanisms and Management, Mt. Kisco, NY, Futura Publishing Co., Inc., 1993: pp405-420.

22

Clinical Results

Richard N. Fogoros, MD

URING the first 15 years of its clinical use, over 75,000 patients have received the implantable cardioverter defibrillator (ICD). While the concept of an ICD was initially regarded by much of the medical community with great skepticism, the ICD is now seen as one of the most important tools available for preventing death from ventricular tachyarrhythmias. The drastic change in how the ICD is perceived has come directly from the clinical results that have been seen with this device.

As impressive as the ICD has been in the clinical arena, however, over 300,000 Americans continue to die suddenly each year from ventricular arrhythmias. Implanting the ICD at a rate of over 20,000 patients per year (1995) including replacements, then, clearly has not yet made a measurable impact on the overall problem of sudden cardiac death. If the ICD is ever to make such an impact, its usage will have to be vastly increased.

Increasing the usage of the ICD will depend on several factors, including educating the public and the general medical community on the prevention of sudden death; availability of a device which can be implanted easily, safely and cheaply; and most importantly, conducting clinical trials using the ICD in patients who have not yet experienced sustained ventricular arrhythmias.

While much work remains to be done in defining the ultimate role of the ICD in preventing sudden cardiac death, that work is being driven by the promising clinical results which have been obtained to date with the device. The purpose of this chapter is to review those clinical results, and to discuss the strengths and weaknesses of the available data.

Efficacy of the ICD in Preventing Sudden Death

Since the introduction of the ICD in the early 1980's, implantation of this device was limited primarily to patients presenting with sustained, drug-resistant ventricular tachyarrhythmias which had caused a full-blown cardiac arrest, syncope, presyncope, or some other evidence of severe hemodynamic compromise.

Without the ICD, the expected outcome of such patients is dismal. Up to 40% will experience recurrent life-threatening arrhythmias within a year or two of their presenting arrhythmias.[1] Even the use of invasive electrophysiologic testing to select antiarrhythmic drug therapy has not improved the outcome for many of these patients, since approximately 60% will have inducible arrhythmias which cannot be suppressed by drug therapy during serial electrophysiologic testing.[2,3] The risk of recurrent events for patients whose arrhythmias are not suppressible is greater than 50% within a few years (Fig. 1); and if their left ventricular ejection fractions (EFs) are depressed to under .35 or .40, the risk is even higher.[2,4]

Even patients who leave the electrophysiology laboratory in the noninducible state (i.e., either their arrhythmias are not inducible during baseline testing, or the arrhythmias are rendered noninducible during drug testing) have an appreciable risk of recurrent arrhythmias over long-term followup, as shown in Fig. 1. Unfortunately, recurrent arrhythmias are usually devastating. For patients who have lost consciousness with their presenting arrhythmias, there is approximately an 80% probability that they will die suddenly with their next recurrence.[3,5]

It was the frustration of being unable to prevent the sudden death of a respected colleague, even after exhaustive efforts were made to control his arrhythmia medically, that led Mirowski to begin his efforts to develop an ICD.[6] During the time of Mirowski's pioneering work, many leaders in the field of cardiology were opposed to the very concept of an ICD.[7] Fortunately, however, the first clinical trials with the ICD occurred at a time when the use of electrophysiologic testing to direct therapy for ventricular arrhythmias was coming into its own, so there existed a relatively small but aggressive cadre of physicians who were receptive to new ideas for treating these lethal arrhythmias. When the earliest trials with the ICD in human subjects documented beyond any doubt that the ICD could indeed efficiently and reliably abort fatal ventricular tachyarrhythmias, this new therapy had a receptive audience.

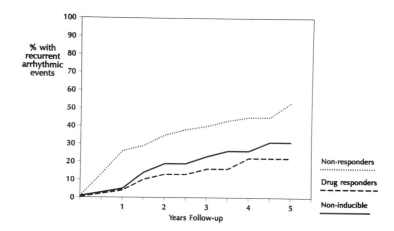

Figure 1. Actuarial incidence of recurrent sustained ventricular tachycardia or ventricular fibrillation among 217 cardiac arrest survivors, grouped according to their response to electrophysiologic testing. Nonresponders were patients with inducible ventricular tachyarrhythmias which could not be suppressed during serial drug testing. Drug responders were patients whose inducible arrhythmias were successfully suppressed during serial drug testing. Cardiac arrest survivors whose arrhythmias were noninducible comprised the third group. The incidence of recurrent events was significantly higher (p < .01) in nonresponders than in the other two groups. In this study, 77% of patients without ICDs who had recurrent events died suddenly.

In 1983, Mirowski et al published their experience with the first 52 patients to receive an ICD.[8] This series included only patients who had survived at least 2 episodes of arrhythmic cardiac arrest, and whose arrhythmias had proven refractory to pharmacologic therapy. During a mean followup period of 14 months, 62 episodes of symptomatic recurrent arrhythmias in 17 patients were automatically terminated by the ICD, and the estimated reduction in mortality due to the device was 52% at 1 year. These results were quite impressive, especially considering the primitive nature of the ICD used in this study, and the fact that the patient population was probably "sicker" than in later series (the requirement for surviving 2 cardiac arrests was dropped after this first series of patients). Electrophysiologists quickly became enthusiastic about the ICD. Over the years, numerous centers performed clinical studies with the ICD, and one finding has remained constant—all studies confirmed a very low incidence of sudden death in recipients of the ICD.

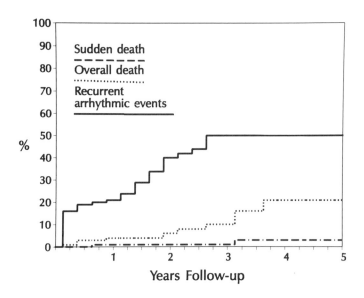

Figure 2. The actuarial incidence of recurrent arrhythmic events (sustained VT or VF), overall death, and sudden death in 70 survivors of cardiac arrest who received the ICD as primary therapy.

Beyond just surviving sudden death, the overall survival of ICD recipients also seemed generally favorable. Manolis et al[9] reported survival from sudden death to be 100% at 1 and 2 years in 77 recipients of an ICD, and overall survival to be 94% at 1 and 2 years. In the author's center,[3] for 70 survivors of sudden death who received an ICD, the actuarial sudden death survival rate was 99% at 1 year and 97% at 5 years (despite an incidence of recurrent arrhythmic events of 20% at 1 year and 50% at 5 years—Fig. 2); and the overall survival rate was 96% at 1 year and 79% at 5 years.

In the earliest large published single center trial, Winkle et al[10] reported the actuarial sudden death survival rate among 270 ICD recipients of the to be 99% at 1 year and 96% at 5 years, and overall survival to be 92% at 1 year and 74% at 5 years. Data from the registry maintained by Cardiac Pacemakers, Inc. showed that the first 3610 recipients of the ICD had a sudden death survival rate of 98% at 1 year, and 94% at 5 years; and an overall survival of 90% at 1 year and 70% at 5 years.[11] The Billitch registry reported similar overall survival among 1737 patients in 13 centers who received ICDs—survival was 90% at 1 year and 70% at 5 years.[12]

Table 1. Estimated 2-year cumulative rate of sudden death and total mortality in high-risk patients receiving various antiarrhythmic therapies, from published studies.[14]

Therapy	Sudden Death	Total Mortality
ICD	3.5%	16.6%
PVC-directed therapy	17%	≥ 25%
Empirical amiodarone	12%	34%
EP-directed therapy	14%	≥ 24%
Arrhythmia surgery	3.7%	37%

In a report from our center, we further assessed the efficacy of the ICD in preventing sudden death by comparing the actuarial incidence of sudden death in similar patients who did and who did not receive an ICD.[5] This study included 50 patients who had presented with ventricular tachyarrhythmias which produced loss of consciousness, which was inducible during electrophysiologic testing, and which could not be suppressed with antiarrhythmic drugs. Twenty one patients received an ICD, and 29 patients (who had either refused an ICD or who presented at a time when an ICD was not available) did not undergo device implantation but they received amiodarone instead. Among the 21 patients who received an ICD, there were no sudden deaths, although 13 patients had apparent recurrences of their arrhythmias which were treated successfully by their ICDs. The 29 who did not receive an ICD, however, had an actuarial incidence of sudden death of 31% at 1 and 2 years (p < .003 for sudden death with vs. without ICD).

Thus, by the late 1980's, it was well established that the ICD was extraordinarily successful in doing exactly what it was designed to do, that is, to prevent sudden cardiac death in patients who were at high risk for this event. Lehmann et al[13,14] compared the results of therapy with the first-generation ICDs to the results of other treatment modalities in similar groups of high-risk patients. As seen in Table 1, the outcome of patients treated with an ICD was substantially better than for patients receiving other therapies. The authors were sufficiently moved by the available evidence to suggest that the ICD, instead of being considered a treatment of last resort, should be considered the "gold standard" for the prevention of sudden cardiac death in survivors of cardiac arrest.

Indeed, low sudden death mortality rates with ICD therapy have been confirmed in several large recent series of cardiac arrest survivors, having a variety of different clinical substrates and at high risk for recurrent tachyarrhythmic arrests.[15-18] It should also be noted that the excellent sudden-death free survival with epicardial lead systems in patients with sustained ventricular tachyarrhythmias has been replicated by nonthoracotomy lead, tiered-therapy device systems.[19-21]

Effect of the ICD on Overall Survival

In the late 1980's, a relatively small but vocal group of physicians began to take issue with the published data on the efficacy of the ICD.[22,23] These physicians agreed with the finding that the ICD reliably prevents sudden cardiac death, but they asked, in effect, "What is the benefit (and what is the cost) of preventing sudden death with the ICD?" Essentially, they challenged the original assumption that the benefit of preventing sudden death was self-evident.

One of the major reasons the critics of the ICD were able to mount this challenge was the fact that there had never been a randomized, controlled trial with the ICD. While early investigators of the ICD have been criticized in retrospect for not conducting a randomized trial, there were compelling reasons why they could not have done so. First, these investigators were under intense pressure (given the negative atmosphere at the time toward the idea of an ICD), to demonstrate quickly whether the ICD could successfully terminate lethal arrhythmias. The cumbersome process of conducting a randomized trial was simply not a viable way to achieve this end. Second, at the time of the early clinical implantations, there were simply too many unknowns to allow a randomized study — these unknowns included the optimal lead design, lead configurations and lead size; the best methods of arrhythmia detection; optimal surgical approaches; and how to test defibrillation thresholds at the time of implantation. Since all these issues underwent significant evolution during the first clinical trials, at that time a meaningful randomized study would simply not have been feasible.

Despite all of the unknowns during the initial trials, and despite the relatively primitive nature of the early ICD system, the ability of the ICD to prevent sudden death was, in fact, quickly documented. And, once documented, the effective prevention of sudden death immediately rendered a randomized study with the ICD (in the type of high-risk patient who received the device in those early years) extremely difficult, if not unethical. Thus, the original decision not to undertake a randomized study of ICD therapy in patients with known sustained ventricular tachyarrhythmias has proved to be difficult to reverse until recently.

The previous lack of any randomized prospective study with the ICD left the door wide open for critics of the device. These critics advanced several arguments as to why the available data on the efficacy of the ICD are insufficient. These arguments can be grouped into four general categories.

The most serious of these arguments is simply that the lack of a randomized study rendered all the available data on the survival of patients with ICDs flawed.

Second, some have noted that only a minority of patients who had received ICDs in published reports had ever received shocks from their devices. If this were true, it would mean that the impressive survival statistics reported for the ICD have been "diluted" by the inclusion of patients who have never used their devices. Further, it would mean that even during a time when implantation of an ICD was reserved for only high-risk patients, many more of these expensive devices were being implanted than were actually needed. This argument carries obvious implications at a time when expansion of the usage of the ICD to lower-risk patients is being considered.

Third, it was argued that the patients who were the most likely to use their ICDs were those with the most severe underlying cardiac disease (since arrhythmias are more frequent in such patients). These patients may not receive much overall benefit from their devices, since they are likely to die relatively quickly from their underlying cardiac disease, and their overall survival may not be significantly prolonged even if they are rescued by an ICD. Implied in this argument is the notion that patients whose potential for long-term survival was relatively good (i.e., patients with less severe cardiac disease), are relatively unlikely to use their ICDs, since recurrent arrhythmias are less likely in these patients. Thus, the overall benefit of therapy with ICDs in these patients is also unclear.

Fourth, while the ICD does prevent sudden death, it creates a new set of complications and problems (including operative mortality) which cancel out at least some of the benefits of the device.

These arguments were raised toward the end of the era of the first generation ICDs, prior to the initiation of a variety of randomized clinical trials currently in progress. Nonetheless, responses to such criticisms remain relevant for proper interpretation and appreciation of the large body of observational data accumulated with regard to outcome with ICD therapy.

Argument 1: The lack of a randomized study in patients with sustained ventricular tachyarrhythmias negates the usefulness of any available data. This argument is no longer strictly correct and it is also impractical. If we limited medical therapy to only those treatments which have been proven in randomized prospective trials to be beneficial, physicians would have very little to do indeed. When an initial therapy has significant obvious benefit it becomes difficult to justify a broad randomized trial of the therapy. Would anyone today propose a randomized trial of antibiotics for bacterial infections?[24] Further, in the case of the ICD, there are in fact several lines of evidence which strongly suggest that the ICD has significantly prolonged the overall survival of its recipients during the first decade of its clinical use. It is not proper to simply dismiss these studies out of hand while awaiting the results of randomized trials.

One piece of evidence that the ICD has resulted in prolonged overall survival is that the use of the ICD has reduced the mortality of "high-risk" patients to equal the mortality of "low-risk" patients. In one study,[3] the selected use of the ICD in cardiac arrest survivors who were at highest risk for recurrent arrhythmic events (i.e., patients whose arrhythmias were inducible during serial drug testing and are not suppressible during serial drug testing) resulted in those patients having the same long-term survival as cardiac arrest survivors who were in lower risk categories (i.e., patients who did not have inducible arrhythmias or in whom inducible arrhythmias were rendered noninducible during drug testing). This result was found despite the fact that the high-risk cardiac arrest survivors had significantly more recurrent arrhythmic events than the low-risk patients. Thus, the ICD seems to have eliminated the excess mortality that would have been predicted on the basis of recurrent arrhythmic events.

Further, the actuarial survival of patients with ICDs who have received appropriate shocks from their defibrillators appears to be the same as the survival of patients who have never received appropriate shocks.[16,25,26] Again, this finding can only mean that the ICD eliminated the excess mortality associated with recurrent arrhythmias.

Several studies have used recipients of an ICD as their own "controls", constructing projected survival curves based on the incidence of appropriate shocks, to estimate what survival would have been without an ICD.[10,27,28] All such studies have concluded that survival was significantly improved by the ICD. (Two of these studies will be discussed in more detail below.)

Similar results have been found with specific patient sub-groups such as those with idiopathic dilated cardiomyopathy;[17,29] patients who are asymptomatic but at high risk;[30] and children with sustained ventricular tachyarrhythmias.[31]

Newman et al[32] conducted a case control study in which the survival of 60 consecutive recipients of an ICD was compared to 120 matched control patients treated without an ICD. The survival of the patients who received an ICD was significantly higher than that of the control patients.

The only randomized clinical trial published to date (involving patients with sustained ventricular tachyarrhythmias) was undertaken in the Netherlands by Wever, et al.[33] In that study, 60 consecutive survivors of cardiac arrest due to ventricular fibrillation (VF; 85%) or sustained ventricular tachycardia (VT; 15%), in the setting of prior myocardial infarction, were randomized to early ICD implantation or conventional therapy. Over a median follow-up of 24 months, 52% of the 31 patients initially assigned to conventional therapy ended up receiving an ICD. The cumulative incidence of combined primary endpoints (death, recurrent cardiac arrest and cardiac transplantation) was significantly reduced in the patients assigned to early ICD implantation (risk ratio 0.27, 95% CI .09-.85; p = .02). Although total mortality was clearly lower in the early ICD implantation group (13% vs. 35% with conventional therapy), the difference was not statistically significant—likely reflecting the study's small sample size.

Thus, several careful analyses of available data consistently suggest that the ICD prolongs the overall survival of its recipients. The data are strong enough that clinicians should certainly consider ICD implantation as an important (and, possibly preferred) therapeutic option in patients with symptomatic sustained ventricular tachyarrhythmias, especially when the latter are also inducible and not suppressible during electrophysiologic testing.

Argument 2: Only a minority of patients with ICDs require shocks. Numerous reports have now been published which show that ICDs have not, in fact, been overutilized. While some early studies seemed to show that only a minority of recipients of an ICD received shocks, this impression proved to be incorrect. Some early studies simply reported the proportion of ICD recipients who had received shocks at the time of data analysis. The incidence of appropriate shocks, however, is a longitudinal statistic (like the incidence of death), and is meaningful only when described with actuarial statistics. Studies employing actuarial methods have now shown that the cumulative risk of requiring at least 1 shock after implantation of an ICD increases most rapidly during the first 6 to 12 months after implantation, but continues to gradually and steadily increase for at least 5 years after implantation; and that by 2 to 4 years after implantation a majority of patients will have required a shock.

In our series of 209 patients with an ICD, there was a cumulative incidence of appropriate shocks of 34% at 1 year, 49% at 2 years, 59% at 3 years, 63% at 4 years, and 69% at 5 years.[25] Myerburg et al[34] reported an incidence of 67% at 16 months. Veltri et al[35] reported an incidence of > 50% at 20 months. Grimm et al[29] showed that the majority of patients with severely depressed left ventricular function (EF ≤ .30) had an appropriate shock by 3 years; for an EF > .30 this required 5 years. In a series of 300 ICD recipients with a history of VF in the setting of chronic coronary artery disease, by 5 years the cumulative incidence of an appropriate shock was about 55%; and for a shock of any type, 90%.[16] Using appropriate statistical methods, then, at least when the ICD is reserved for patients presenting with symptomatic, sustained ventricular tachyarrhythmias (often which have not responded to antiarrhythmic therapy), the majority of implantees eventually are rescued by their device at least once. Thus, the application of therapy with the ICD, at least during the first decade of its use, seems to have been appropriate.

The finding of high cumulative device utilization rates has held up in the more recent experience with third generation/transvenous lead ICD systems. For example, a study of 2834 patients implanted with the Medtronic PCD device (nonthoracotomy systems in 48%) found that 57% received tachyarrhythmia therapy (successful 98% of the time) from their ICD.[36] It should also be noted that the fact that the cumulative incidence of appropriate device discharges continues to rise over time carries important implications regarding the need for generator replacement; even if a patient with prior sustained VT or VF has not yet received an appropriate shock by the time the ICD battery has run down, generator replacement is warranted because a moderate proportion of these patients will subsequently receive a needed shock (for the first time) from their replacement device.[37]

Argument 3: Patients with severe underlying cardiac disease may not significantly benefit from the ICD, since they are likely to die of their underlying disease even if sudden death is prevented. Patients with less severe underlying disease may not benefit since they are less likely to require shocks. While mortality in ICD patients (as with all patients) is influenced by EF[38] the "appropriate shock" surrogate analysis suggests that survival is improved with the ICD regardless of the EF.

Tchou et al[27] analyzed results of therapy in 70 consecutive patients who received an ICD for sustained ventricular tachyarrhythmias which could not be controlled with medication. Twenty five patients had left ventricular EFs < .30. During followup, only 1 of the 25 had sudden death. The 2 year overall survival of these patients with severe underlying heart disease was 87%, compared to a projected survival without the ICD (based on the incidence of appropriate shocks) of 57% (p = .025). Patients treated with an ICD whose left ventricular EFs were > .30 had an overall 2 year survival of 100%, compared to a projected survival of 60% (p < .0015). This series was later updated by Akhtar et al[39] after 300 patients had received an ICD. The overall survival remained significantly higher than projected survival, whether the left ventricular EF was higher or lower than .30, for up to 8 years of followup.

Our group performed a similar analysis in 119 consecutive patients who received an ICD.[28] Forty of these patients had left ventricular EFs < .30. The 3 year overall survival rate for these 40 patients was 67%, compared to a projected survival without the ICD of 6% (p < .001). The 79 patients treated with an ICD whose left ventricular EFs were ≥ .30 had a 3 year survival of 96%, compared to a projected survival without the ICD of 46% (p < .001). Sweeney et al reported that the ICD use was associated with a lower rate of sudden death in a retrospective comparison with antiarrhythmics drugs or no drug therapy in patients awaiting a cardiac transplant; the benefit for nonsudden death was limited.[40] Finally, the recently completed MADIT trial[41] clearly showed the dramatic benefit of prophylactic ICD therapy for patients with prior myocardial infarction, low EF, nonsustained VT, and inducible non-suppressible VT/VF (as described in more detail below). Taken together, these studies strongly suggest that the ICD significantly prolonged the survival of its recipients, whether they had severe or only moderate underlying cardiac disease.

Patients with VF or hypotensive VT but with no organic heart disease also benefit from the ICD. The CEDARS investigators have shown that 24% of such patients receive an appropriate shock within the first year,[42] basically confirming the earlier findings of Meissner et al[18] and Wever et al.[33]

Argument 4: Complications of the ICD cancel out some of the benefits of the device. This argument cannot be refuted, because indeed, there is mortality associated with the use of the ICD— primarily related to perioperative death in the era of thoracotomy-requiring implantations. However, the causes of that mortality can be examined, and steps can be recommended to reduce the inherent risks of using this device.

There are several potential causes for death associated with implantation of an ICD system with epicardial leads, the most common of which are pump failure, respiratory failure, infection, and intractable ventricular tachyarrhythmias. The reported incidences of perioperative mortality 30 days after implantation of thoracotomy-requiring ICDs varies fairly widely from center to center, but usually lie in the range of 0-8%. Although Veltri et al[35] reported a perioperative mortality of 4.9% in 163 patients who received such an ICD, larger series in general tend to report perioperative mortality rates which are somewhat lower than in smaller series. Tchou et al[27] reported a mortality rate of 1.4% in 70 patients; Manolis et al[9] reported 2.6% in 77 patients; Kelly et al[43] reported 3.2% in 94 patients; Winkle et al[44] reported 1.5% in 270 patients; and our group had no perioperative deaths in 209 patients.[25] In a multicenter investigator-edited registry, the 30-day operative mortality was 3.1% in 939 recipients of thoracotomy-requiring ICDs.[45]

The incidence of perioperative mortality will depend heavily on surgical techniques, patient selection, and postoperative management.

Intraoperative techniques and procedures for implantation of ICD systems necessitating thoracotomy have been reviewed in detail,[44] and most electrophysiologists and implanting surgeons are well-versed in this area. Nonetheless, the procedures which have been adopted from center to center vary widely, from the type of incision used, to the placement of the defibrillating electrodes, to the procedures used for testing of defibrillation thresholds. While it is acceptable for each center to settle upon techniques with which they are comfortable, it is then incumbent for each center to assure that their chosen procedures yield acceptable results. A center's experience with the implantation procedure is also important, as suggested by the fact that most large series in the literature report lower incidences of perioperative mortality than most smaller series.

Patient selection as a determinant of outcome with the ICD is an issue which has been relatively neglected in the literature. Yet, patient selection is the most likely reason for the much of the disparity in reported perioperative mortalities seen among competent centers implanting epicardial-lead ICD systems. For instance, Kim et al[46] reported a perioperative mortality of 11% in 28 patients with left ventricular EFs < .30. In our series, on the other hand,[28] 40 patients with EFs < .30 received ICDs with no perioperative mortality. When considering outcomes which are this disparate, it may be helpful to examine what happened to patients who did not receive an ICD. We recently described the outcome of 38 patients who were ostensibly candidates for an ICD, but who did not receive the device.[3] These patients had survived cardiac arrests and had inducible but not suppressible ventricular arrhythmias during electrophysiologic testing. While some of these 38 refused the device, the majority did not receive an ICD because our subjective assessment was that their chances for extended survival was limited, regardless of the risk for sudden death. During a mean followup of 35 months, 8 of these 38 patients (21%) died suddenly. However, of the remaining 30 patients, 21 (70%) experienced nonsudden death. Therefore, it seems very unlikely that implantation of an ICD would have significantly improved the long-term survival of these patients. Furthermore, implanting an ICD in these sicker patients would almost certainly have substantially increased the perioperative mortality in our series. Optimal balancing of the potential risks and benefits of the ICD is obviously an important issue.

The postoperative management of patients who receive ICDs is another issue which has not received much attention in the literature. Patients who receive ICDs—primarily those requiring epicardial lead systems—can become quite unstable postoperatively. They commonly develop transient (but significant) depression of cardiac and pulmonary function. Ventricular arrhythmias which are relatively refractory to therapy are also seen after implantation of ICDs requiring thoracotomy. In fact, approximately 50% of postoperative deaths have been due to difficult-to-manage arrhythmias,[46,47] although the occurrence of such arrhythmias appears to be a less common problem with nonthoracotomy ICD implantation.[48] It is clear that postoperative management of patients receiving ICDs (particularly those requiring thoracotomy) can, potentially, be extremely difficult and challenging. Postoperative problems must be *anticipated* in any patient receiving an ICD, and any center undertaking an ICD implantation program must be prepared to offer aggressive, hands-on postoperative management.

In summary, the risk of perioperative death after ICD implantation is an inherent problem, more so with systems that require thoracotomy, a problem which does limit the potential benefit of the ICD. Every effort should be made to reduce mortality to acceptable levels. What is an "acceptable" risk for perioperative mortality with this procedure? In the author's opinion, the figure often quoted in the literature (for thoracotomy implants) of 4-5% is too high. If coronary artery bypass grafting (which involves relatively long anesthesia time and the use of cardiopulmonary bypass), can be routinely performed with a mortality of approximately 1%, a mortality rate which is 5 times higher than that seems unreasonable for the relatively simple procedure of implanting an ICD. It is essential for every center performing ICD implantation to monitor carefully their perioperative mortality figures. A perioperative mortality rate of greater than 2-3% for thoracotomy-requiring implantations (or $\geq 1\%$ for current transvenous systems) should be considered unacceptable, and should lead to a careful reassessment of patient selection criteria, operative technique and postoperative management procedures.

The current widespread use of nonthoracotomy lead systems has significantly lowered perioperative mortality. This improvement likely reflects not only a much less invasive procedure, but reduced implantation time (with less defibrillation testing) owing to concomitant use of biphasic waveforms. In one report,[19] the perioperative mortality for over 600 patients receiving Medtronic nonthoracotomy defibrillating electrodes was 0.8% (1.8% including "crossovers" to epicardial leads) vs. 4.2% (p<.001) in a similar number of epicardial implant recipients (3.6% not including crossovers, p<.05, respectively). Similarly, a perioperative mortality of 0% was reported in 151 patients receiving the CPI nonthoracotomy electrodes.[49] In a recent study of 120 nonthoracotomy ICD implants, a somewhat higher (3.3%) operative mortality was reported,[21] although device recipients in this experience were found to be older with poorer left ventricular function than observed in other series. However, one clinic compared its experience between thoracotomy and nonthoracotomy implants in a series of 146 patients.[50] While the nonthoracotomy patients had less atrial fibrillation and respiratory complications, overall survival was comparable at 2 years.

Mention should also be made of potential *long-term complications* of ICD therapy. One study reported an overall complication rate of 37 % in ICD patients.[51] These include inappropriate shocks, infection, lead-related problems, and, rarely, ICD therapy "failure" and are discussed in detail in Chaps. 9, 18, 21, 23.

Table 2. Clinical criteria for randomization to ICD vs. medical therapy in the Multicenter Automatic Defibrillator Implantation Trial (MADIT)[41]

Nonsustained VT (asymptomatic, ECG documented, 3-30 beats @ > 120 beats/min)

Prior Q-wave or enzyme positive myocardial infarction

Left ventricular EF≤ 0.35

No recent (within 3 months) indication for revascularization

Inducible sustained monomorphic VT[a] (using up to triple extrastimuli) or VF (using up to double extrastimuli) at up to 2 RV sites, *nonsuppressible* on IV procainamide or other Type IA drug[b]

---

[a] Cycle length ≤ 350 ms prior to IV procainamide, and systolic blood pressure < 80 mmHg or associated with > 50 mmHg drop in systolic blood pressure

[b] Persistently inducible sustained VT, or inducible VF (using up to double extrastimuli), after IV procainamide (15 mg/kg, followed by 4 mg/min infusion)

EP = electrophysiology; EF = ejection fraction; RV = right ventricular; MI = myocardial infarction; VF = ventricular fibrillation; VT = ventricular tachycardia

Multicenter Automatic Defibrillator Implantation Trial (MADIT)

Although adequately powered randomized clinical trials designed to assess survival with ICD vs. medical therapy in patients with documented sustained VT or VF have not yet been completed as of this writing, the results of a randomized trial investigating the role of the ICD as *prophylactic therapy* in high risk coronary artery disease patients was formally presented by Arthur Moss (Principal Investigator) at the Seventeenth Annual Scientific Sessions of the North American Society of Pacing and Electrophysiology, held in Seattle, May 1996. The Multicenter Automatic Defibrillator Implantation Trial (MADIT) focused on patients with atherosclerotic heart disease, significant left ventricular dysfunction and documented *non*sustained VT (only), who underwent electrophysiologic testing and were found to have inducible hemodynamically unstable sustained VT or VF, even after intravenous infusion of procainamide.[41] Patients with this "MADIT profile" (Table 2) were randomized to receive an ICD (initially thoracotomy-requiring and, later in the trial, transvenous systems) or "conventional" medical therapy, chosen at the discretion of the participating investigators.

The endpoint for the study was total mortality, with frequent periodic analysis of event rates in the two treatment limbs ("sequential design"). Mean left ventricular EF in both treatment arms was about 0.26. "Conventional therapy" consisted of amiodarone initially in 80% of patients so assigned. After 5 years and nearly 200 patients randomized, the trial was halted by the Data Safety and Monitoring Board because of a strikingly (>50%) lower mortality in the device-treated patients, i.e., hazard ratio of 0.47 with p=0.009. The survival benefit in patients randomized to ICD therapy was largely attributable to a reduction in arrhythmic death rate, belying the previously made argument that rescue from sustained VT or VF by the ICD would be unlikely to improve survival in patients with poor left ventricular function at high risk for cardiac death in general. The lower risk of dying in device recipients remained statistically significant even after correction for use of amiodarone, beta blockers and heart failure medication.

MADIT thus points to a whole new approach to secondary prevention, at least in a specific high risk subset of post-myocardial infarction patients. Indeed, coincident with public presentation of the MADIT findings, the U.S. Food and Drug Administration (FDA) granted the trial's sponsor, CPI/Guidant, an ICD labeling indication that covers patients with the MADIT profile. The extent to which the results of this landmark trial can be extrapolated to other high risk patient populations remains to be determined.

Quality of Life

Quality of life is an important measure of the success of ICD therapy. Most patients report an improved quality of life and would recommend the therapy to another patient.[52] In one study,[53] the proportion of patients returning to work, was 60%, similar to that following coronary artery bypass. However, a small Australian study reported only 2 of 9 working patients returned to work.

ICD patients complain of fear of being shocked in public; having pain from the shock; family role changes; and disturbance of sex life and body image.[54,55] Focus groups of *patients* also bring out concerns related to sleeping disorders, heat intolerance, fear of death, preparation for death, clothing not fitting (which should be ameliorated by the small pectoral implantable devices), and spousal overprotectiveness.[56] The primary complaints of *spouses* are fear of and preparation for death, family role changes, and being overprotective.[56] Complaints of younger patients include concerns over being able to bear children, about the device "blowing up," surgical scars, and the need for replacement surgery.[57] The most common complaints were early awakening from sleep and pain and itching along scars.[57] Financial worries, both general and specific to medical coverage, are very common.[57]

About half of all ICD patients report some degree of psychiatric morbidity[58,59] In order to separate the impact of the ICD on these problems it is helpful to compare the psychological health before and after the implant. This is done with standardized "quality of life" pyschological instruments. These include the sickness impact profile,[60] Beck depression inventory, Hamilton anxiety scale, and various subscores from the Minnesota multiphasic personality inventory.[61] The AVID trial (see below) is using, among others, the MOS 36 item health survey and the CES-D depression self report.[62]

A French study found that the ICD did not adversely affect the quality of life and that shock occurrence was not correlated with psychological well being.[61] The majority (89%) of patients in a German study (195 patients) found an unchanged or improved quality of life with an ICD but that this was negatively correlated to the shock frequency.[63] The Australian study mentioned above found that quality of life dipped at 6 months but returned to normal at 1 year. An American study used the Ferrans and Powers quality of life index which has a maximum of 30 for the overall score and sub-scores;[64] The usual complaints (listed earlier) were seen and the Psychological/Spiritual score did drop (24.8 ± 4.9 to 23.5 ± 5.9, p < .05). However, the Health/Functioning, Socioeconomic, and Family sub-scores did not drop and the overall score was not changed (23.2 ± 4.9 to 22.7 ± 5.1, NS).[65]

Driving Automobiles

A major component of quality of life in the Western World is the freedom to drive a car for work, shopping, pleasure, and worship.[66] In the U.S. only 8 states restrict driving for arrhythmia patients.[67] The vast majority (96%) of implanting physicians advise at least some ICD patients to cease driving.[68] Not surprisingly, the majority of patients ignore such advice, and 70% resumed driving (half of the ICD patients driving daily) even though most of them were not the primary household driver.[69] Other surveys report that 56-74% of ICD patients continue driving. [66,70]

Since most patients will ignore advice to cease driving, it may seem like an academic exercise to evaluate the risk of such activity. Nevertheless this has been done and with interesting results. A comparison of risk with epileptic patients has prompted one suggestion that ICD patients should be prohibited from driving for 1 or 2 years after an implant and permanently lose their license if they received tachyarrhythmia therapy during this time.[71] One sizable study covered sustained ventricular tachyarrhythmia patients (the majority of whom were on antiarrhythmic drugs; only 8% had ICDs) and counted any ICD shock delivery or a hemodynamically compromising arrhythmia as an event that could hamper the ability to control a car.[72] The event rate was 4.2% in the first month, 1.8% per month during months 2 through 7, and 0.6% per month thereafter. The suggestion was made that there be no driving during the first month and probably during the first 8 months.

The actual incidence of driving accidents with ICD patients is rather low. Based on the average reported weekly mileage of such patients and published event rates one could say that the probability of sudden death and syncopal and nonsyncopal ICD discharges are 9, 11, and 15 out of a million per kilometer driven.[70] An American survey study covering 452 physicians and 30 car accidents related to ICD shocks found that only 10.5% of ICD discharges during driving caused an accident.[73] Even though the study reported 9 fatalities the overall rate for the patients was 7.5 per 100,000 patient years which is much lower than the general population rate of 18.4 per 100,000 patient years. Similar reassuring results are seen in Europe.[74]

Given the complexities related to driving recommendations in ICD recipients, The North American Society of Pacing and Electrophysiology recently convened a symposium to address the broad issue of driving safety in patients with a variety of arrhythmias capable of impairing consciousness.[75] After weighing the available data from the literature, the writing committee recommended patients refrain from driving for 6 months following an episode of sustained ventricular tachyarrhythmia in the setting of organic heart disease—regardless of the type of antiarrhythmic treatment modality (i.e., whether or not an ICD is used).

The Future

The first decade and a half of clinical use of the ICD has shown beyond doubt that the ICD is extremely effective in doing what it was originally designed to do—preventing sudden death from cardiac tachyarrhythmias. This fact was well-established from the earliest reports on the clinical usage of the ICD, and is recognized even by the critics of the device. While there are limited completed randomized controlled studies using the ICD in patients at very high risk for sudden death, several studies using historical controls, nonrandomized contemporary control groups, and recipients of an ICD as their own controls, present strong evidence that the ICD has significantly prolonged the overall survival of appropriately selected patients.

The dramatic results of the MADIT trial would appear to vindicate the ICD supporters to date. Major ongoing prospective trials including AVID,[62,76] CIDS,[77] CASH,[78] and CABG patch[79] will hopefully continue to give further definition of the types of patients most likely to benefit from the ICD.

The AVID (Antiarrhythmics Versus Implantable Defibrillators) study aims to enroll 1200 cardiac arrest survivors and patients with serious hemodynamically compromising VT, with followup scheduled to be completed in late 1998. Enrolled patients are randomized to ICD implantation or a physician's choice of either sotalol or amiodarone. Inducibility, drug refractoriness, and ventricular function (except that class IV failure is an exclusion criterion) are irrelevant for the therapy choice and inclusion. It is possible, therefore, that the benefits of the ICD will be diluted by the inclusion of such a broad spectrum of patients who may not respond equally to ICD therapy.[80] The CIDS (Canadian Implantable Defibrillator Study) will also compare amiodarone to ICD therapy.[76,77]

The CASH (Cardiac Arrest Study Hamburg) study projects an enrollment of 400 cardiac arrest survivors. Enrolled patients were initially randomized to either amiodarone, metoprolol, propafenone, or ICD therapy. Due to a significantly higher incidence of total mortality the propafenone arm was dropped early on.[78]

It is also important to recognize that the encouraging early results with ICD therapy were achieved with relatively simple devices (nonprogrammable or minimally programmable ICDs), at centers which had a strong interest in antitachycardia devices, and with primarily thoracotomy implants. In this regard, major changes in ICD therapy have taken place.

Present tiered therapy devices offer the invitation to be configured suboptimally (e.g., to delay potentially life-saving shock in order to deliver "milder" therapies first), or inappropriately (e.g., to use pace-termination techniques which may degenerate a stable, relatively asymptomatic ventricular tachycardia into a life-threatening arrhythmia). It is thus conceivable that the outcome of patients with tiered therapy devices will not be as favorable as with the older "shock boxes."

At the same time, we are seeing the rapid expansion of ICD usage to centers which have relatively little expertise in managing complex tachyarrhythmias. It remains to be seen whether these newer, presumably less sophisticated centers can use ICDs with the kinds of results which have been reported in the literature, and which have been discussed in this chapter.

A major challenge to designers of antitachycardia devices, then, will be to develop ICDs which are flexible enough to give clinicians the features they want without making them prohibitively complex. Features such as friendly device-operator interfaces and "intelligent" programming devices (which might, for instance, suggest useful device configurations and disallow potentially dangerous ones) will be extremely important. While, on the surface, it may seem that the major engineering issues of implantable antitachycardia devices have been worked out, this remaining problem (i.e., making the devices physician-proof) may prove to be one of the most difficult yet encountered.

ACKNOWLEDGMENTS:

Figs. 1 and 2 are adapted with permission of the Journal of the American College of Cardiology.

1. Hurwitz JL, Josephson ME. Sudden cardiac death in patients with chronic coronary artery disease. Circulation 1992;95:I43-I49.
2. Furukawa T, Rozanski JJ, Nogami A, et al. Time-dependent risk of and predictors for cardiac arrest recurrence in survivors of out-of-hospital cardiac arrest with chronic coronary artery disease. Circulation 1989;80:599-608.
3. Fogoros RN, Elson JJ, Bonnet CA, et al. Long-term outcome of survivors of cardiac arrest whose therapy is guided by electrophysiologic testing. J Am Coll Cardiol 1992;19:780-788.
4. Wilber JD, Garan H, Finkelstein D, et al. Out-of-hospital cardiac arrest: Use of electrophysiologic testing in the prediction of long-term outcome. N Engl J Med 1988;318:19-24.
5. Fogoros RN, Fiedler SB, Elson JJ. The automatic implantable cardioverter-defibrillator in drug-refractory ventricular tachyarrhythmias. Ann Intern Med 1987;107:635-641.
6. Kastor JA. Michel Mirowski and the automatic implantable defibrillator. Am J Cardiol 1989;63:977-982.
7. Lown B, Axelrod P. Implanted standby defibrillators. Circulation 1972;46:637-639.
8. Mirowski M, Reid PR, Winkle RA, et al. Mortality in patients with implanted automatic defibrillators. Ann Intern Med 1983;98:585-588.
9. Manolis AS, Tan-DeGuzman W, Lee MA, et al. Clinical experience in seventy-seven patients with the automatic implantable cardioverter defibrillator. Am Heart J 1989;118:445-450.
10. Winkle RA, Mead RH, Ruder MA, et al. Long-term outcome with the automatic implantable cardioverter-defibrillator. J Am Coll Cardiol 1989;13:1353-1361.
11. Thomas AC, Moser SA, Smutka ML, et al. Implantable defibrillation: eight years clinical experience. PACE 1988;11:2053-2058.
12. Song, SL. The Billitch Report: Performance of implantable cardiac rhythm devices. PACE 1992;15:475-486.
13. Lehmann MH, Steinman RT, Schuger CD, et al. The automatic implantable cardioverter defibrillator as antiarrhythmic treatment modality of choice for survivors of cardiac arrest unrelated to acute myocardial infarction. Am J Cardiol 1988;62:803-805.
14. Akhtar M, Garan H, Lehmann MH, et al. Sudden cardiac death: management of high-risk patients. Ann Intern Med 1991;114:499-512.
15. Powell AC, Fuchs T, Finklestein DM, et al. Influence of implantable cardioverter-defibrillators on the long-term prognosis of survivors of out-of-hospital cardiac arrest. Circulation 1993;88:1083-1092.

16. Lessmeier TJ, Lehmann MH, Steinman RT, et al. Implantable cardioverter-defibrillator therapy in 300 patients with coronary artery disease presenting exclusively with ventricular fibrillation. Am Heart J 1994;128:211-218.
17. Lessmeier TJ, Lehmann MH, Steinman RT, et al. Outcome with implantable cardioverter-defibrillator therapy for survivors of ventricular fibrillation secondary to idiopathic dilated cardiomyopathy of coronary artery disease with myocardial infarction. Am J Cardiol 1993;72:911-915.
18. Meissner MD, Lehmann MH, Steinman RT, et al. Ventricular fibrillation in patients without significant structural heart disease: a multicenter experience with implantable cardioverter-defibrillator therapy. J Am Coll Cardiol 1993;21:1406-1412.
19. The PCD investigators group. Clinical outcome of patients with malignant ventricular tachyarrhythmias and a multiprogrammable implantable cardioverter-defibrillator implanted with or without thoracotomy. J Am Coll Cardiol 1994;23:1521-1530.
20. Böcker D, Block M, Isbruch F, et al. Do patients with implantable defibrillator live longer? J Am Coll Cardiol 1993;21:1638-1644.
21. Kleman JM, castle LW, Kidwell GA, et al. Nonthoracotomy versus thoracotomy implantable defibrillators. Intention-to-treat comparison of clinical outcomes. Circulation 1994;90:2833-2842.
22. Furman S. AICD benefit. PACE 1989;12:399-400.
23. Connolly SJ, Yusuf S. Evaluation of the implantable cardioverter defibrillator in survivors of cardiac arrest: the need for randomized trials. Am J Cardiol 1992;69:959-962.
24. Josephson M, Nisam S. Prospective trials of implantable cardioverter defibrillators versus drugs: are they addressing the right question? Am J Cardiol 1996;77:859-863.
25. Fogoros RN, Elson JJ, Bonnet CA. Survival of patients who have received appropriate shocks from their implantable defibrillators. PACE 1991;14:1842-1845.
26. Grimm W, Flores BT, Marchlinski FE. Shock occurrence and survival in 241 patients with implantable cardioverter-defibrillator therapy. Circulation 1993;87:1880-1888.
27. Tchou PJ, Kadri N, Anderson J, et al. Automatic implantable cardioverter defibrillators and survival of patients with left ventricular dysfunction and malignant ventricular arrhythmias. Ann Intern Med 1988;109:529-534.
28. Fogoros RN, Elson JJ, Bonnet CA, et al. Efficacy of the automatic implantable cardioverter defibrillator in prolonging survival in patients with severe underlying cardiac disease. J Am Coll Cardiol 1990;16:381-386.
29. Grimm W, Marchlinski FE. Shock occurrence and survival in 49 patients with idiopathic dilated cardiomyopathy and an implantable cardioverter-defibrillator. European Heart J 1995;16:218-222.
30. Levine JH, Waller T, Hoch D, et al. Implantable cardioverter defibrillator: use in patients with no symptoms and at high risk. Am Heart J 1996;131:59-65.
31. Hamilton RM, Dorian P, Gow RM, et al. Five-year experience with implantable defibrillators in children. Am J Cardiol 1996;77:524-526.
32. Newman D, Sauve MJ, Herre J, et al. Survival after implantation of the cardioverter defibrillator. Am J Cardiol 1992;69:899-903.
33. Wever EF, Hauer RNW, van Capelle FJL, et al. Randomized study of implantable defibrillator as first choice therapy versus conventional strategy in postinfarct sudden death survivors. Circulation 1995;91:2195:2203.
34. Myerburg RJ, Luceri RM, Thurer R, et al. Time to first shock and clinical outcome in patients receiving an automatic implantable cardioverter defibrillator. J Am Coll Cardiol 1989;14:508-514.
35. Veltri EP, Mower MM, Mirowski M, et al. Follow-up of patients with ventricular tachyarrhythmia treated with the automatic implantable cardioverter

defibrillator: Programmed electrical stimulation results do not predict clinical outcome. J Electrophysiol 1989;3:467-476.

36. Zipes DP, Roberts D, et al. Results of the international study of the implantable pacemaker cardioverter-defibrillator: a comparison of epicardial and endocardial lead systems. Circulation 1995;92:59-65.

37. Grimm W, Marchlinski FE. Shock occurrence in patients with an implantable cardioverter-defibrillator without spontaneous shocks before first generator replacement for battery depletion. Am J Cardiol 1994;73:969-970.

38. Kim SG, Maloney JD, Pinski SL, et al. Influence of left ventricular function on survival and mode of death after implantable defibrillator therapy. Am J Cardiol 1993;72:1263-1267.

39. Akhtar M, Avitall B, Jazayeri M, et al. Role of implantable cardioverter defibrillator therapy in the management of high-risk patients. Circulation 1992;85:I131-I139.

40. Sweeney MO, Ruskin JN, Garan H, et al. Influence of the implantable cardioverter/defibrillator on sudden death and total mortality in patients evaluated for cardiac transplantation. Circulation 1995;92:3273-3281.

41. MADIT Executive Committee. Multicenter automatic defibrillator implantation trial (MADIT): design and clinical protocol. PACE 1991;14:920-927.

42. Fan W, Peter CT. Survival and incidence of appropriate shocks in implantable cardioverter defibrillator recipients who have no detectable structural heart disease. 1994;74:687-690.

43. Kelly PA, Cannom DS, Garan H, et al. The automatic implantable cardioverter-defibrillator: efficacy, complications and survival in patients with malignant ventricular arrhythmias. J Am Coll Cardiol 1988;11:1278-1286.

44. Winkle RA, Stinson EB, Echt DS. Practical aspects of automatic cardioverter/defibrillator implantation. Am Heart J 1984;108:1335-1346.

45. Mosteller RD, Lehmann MH, Thomas AC, et al. Operative mortality with implantation of the automatic cardioverter-defibrillator. Am J Cardiol 1991;68:1340-1345.

46. Kim SG, Fisher JD, Choe CW, et al. Influence of left ventricular function on outcome of patients treated with implantable defibrillators. Circulation 1992;85:1304-1310.

47. Veltri EP, Mower MM, Mirowski M, et al. Follow-up of patients with ventricular tachyarrhythmia treated with the automatic implantable cardioverter defibrillator: Programmed electrical stimulation results do not predict clinical outcome. J Electrophysiol 1989;3:467-476.

48. Kim SG, Ling J, Fisher JD, et al. Comparison and frequency of ventricular arrhythmias after defibrillator implantation by thoracotomy versus nonthoracotomy approaches. Am J Cardiol 1994;74:1245-1248.

49. Ehrlich S, Endotak Investigators. Early survival and follow-up characteristics of 151 patients undergoing transvenous cardioverter defibrillator lead system implantation. J Am Coll Cardiol 1992;19:209A. (abstract)

50. Shahian DM, Williamson WA, Svensson LG, et al. Transvenous versus transthoracic cardioverter-defibrillator implantation: a comparative analysis of morbidity, mortality, and survival. J Thorac Cardiovasc Surg 1995;109:1066-1074.

51. Nunain SO, Roelke M, Trouton T, et al. Limitations and late complications of third-generation automatic cardioverter-defibrillators. Circulation 1995;91:2204-2213.

52. Luderitz B, Jung W, Deister A, et al. Patient acceptance of implantable cardioverter defibrillator devices: changing attitudes. Am Heart J 1994;127:1179-1184.

53. Kalbfleisch KR, Lehmann MH, Steinman RT, et al. Reemployment following implantation of the automatic cardioverter defibrillator. Am J Cardiol 1989;64:199-202

54. Veseth-Rogers J. A practical approach to teaching the automatic implantable cardioverter defibrillator patient. J Cardiovasc Nurs 1990;4;7-19.
55. DeBorde R, Aarons D, Biggs M. The automatic implantable cardioverter. AACN Clin Issues Crit Care Nurs 1991;2:170-177.
56. Sneed NV, Finch N. Experience of patients and significant others with automatic implantable cardioverter defibrillators after discharge from the hospital. Prog Cardiovasc Nurs 1992;7:20-24.
57. Vitale MB, Funk M. Quality of life in younger persons with an implantable cardioverter defibrillator. Dim Crit Care Nurs 1995;14:100-111.
58. Morris PL, Badger J, Chmielewski C, et al. Psychiatric morbidity following implantation of the automatic implantable cardioverter defibrillator. Psychosomatics 1991;32:58-64.
59. Fricchione GL, Olson LC, Vlay SC. Psychiatric syndromes in patients with the automatic internal cardioverter defibrillator: anxiety, psychological dependence, abuse, and withdrawal. Am Heart J 1989;117:1411-1414.
60. May CD, Smith PR, Murdock CJ, et al. The impact of the implantable cardioverter defibrillator on quality-of-life. PACE 1995;18:1411-1418.
61. Chevalier P, Verrier P, Kirkorian G, et al. Improved appraisal of the quality of life in patients with automatic implantable cardioverter defibrillator. Psychother Psychosom 1996;65:49-56.
62. AVID Investigators. Antiarrhythmics versus implantable defibrillators (AVID)—rationale, design, and methods. Am J Cardiol 1995;75:470-475.
63. Schöhl W, Trappe H-J, Lichtlen PR. Akzeptanz und lebensqualität nach implatation eines automatischen Kardioverters/Defibrillators. Z Kardiologie 1994;83:927-932.
64. Ferrans CE, Powers MJ. Psychometric assessment of the quality of life index. Res Nurs Health 1992;15:29-38.
65. Bainger EM, Fernsler JI. Perceived quality of life before and after implantation of an internal cardioverter defibrillator. Am J Crit Care1995;4:36-43.
66. Craney JM, Powers MT. Factors related to driving in persons with an implantable cardioverter defibrillator. Prog Cardiovasc Nurs 1995;10:12-17.
67. Strickberger SA, Cantillon CO, Friedman PL. When should patients with lethal ventricular arrhythmia resume driving? An analysis of state regulations and physician practices. Ann Intern Med 1991;115:560-563.
68. DiCarlo LA, Winston SA, Honoway S, et al. Driving restrictions advised by Midwestern cardiologists implanting cardioverter defibrillators: present practices, criteria utilized, and compatibility with existing state laws. PACE 1992;15:1131-1136.
69. Finch NJ, Leman RB, Kratz JM, et al. Driving safety among patients with automatic implantable cardioverter defibrillators. JAMA 1993;270:1587-1588.
70. Beauregard LA, Barnard PW, Russo AM, et al. Perceived and actual risks of driving in patients with arrhythmia control devices. Arch Intern Med 1995;155:609-613.
71. Anderson MH, Camm AJ. Legal and ethical aspects of driving and working in patients with an implantable cardioverter defibrillator. Am Heart J 1994;127:1185-1193.
72. Larsen GC, Stupey MR, Walance CG, et al. Recurrent cardiac events in survivors of ventricular fibrillation or tachycardia: implications for driving restrictions. JAMA 1994;271:1335-1339.
73. Curtis AB, Conti JB, Tucker KJ, et al. Motor vehicle accidents in patients with an implantable cardioverter-defibrillator. J Am Coll Cardiol 1995;26:180-184.
74. Jung W, Lüderitz B. European policy on driving for patients with implantable cardioverter defibrillators. PACE 1996;19:981-984.
75. Miles WM, Epstein AE, Benditt DG, et al. Personal and safety issues related to arrhythmias that may affect consciousness: implications for regulation and physician recommendations. Circulation 1996 (in press)

76. Greene HL. Antiarrhythmic drugs versus implantable defibrillators: the need for a randomized controlled study. Am Heart J 1993;127:1171-1178.

77. Connolly SJ, Jent M, Roberts RS, et al. Canadian Implantation Defibrillator Study (CIDS): study design and organization. Am J Cardiol 1993;72:103F-108F.

78. Siebels J, Kuck KH. Implantable cardioverter defibrillator compared with antiarrhythmic drug treatment in cardiac arrest survivors (the cardiac arrest study Hamburg). Am Heart J 1994;127:1139-1144.

79. Bigger JT. Future studies with the implantable cardioverter defibrillator. PACE 1991;14:883-889.

80. Fogoros RN. An AVID dissent. PACE 1994;17:1707-1711.

23

Sudden Death Despite
ICD Therapy:
Why Does It Happen?

Michael H. Lehmann, MD, Luis A. Pires, MD, Walter H. Olson, PhD, Veronica Ivan, BSEE, Russell T. Steinman, MD, John J. Baga, MD, and Claudio D. Schuger, MD.

THE PRECISE role of ICD therapy in managing patients with sustained ventricular tachyarrhythmias remains controversial and is currently an area of active investigation.[1] There is little debate, however, that ICD therapy can abort cardiac arrest due to sustained ventricular tachyarrhythmias.[1,2] Although sudden death is strikingly reduced compared to the incidence observed in historical or certain other types of control populations (Chap. 22), fatal unexpected cardiac arrest may still occur in the ICD patient.

Intuitively, one might assume (at least prior to VVI pacing via ICDs) that bradyarrhythmic events would account for the majority of sudden deaths in ICD patients, given that the implanted devices should possess the ability to cardiovert or defibrillate sustained ventricular tachyarrhythmias. In the present chapter, however, we present evidence that, during the first decade of clinical experience, mainly ventricular tachyarrhythmias were observed in association with terminal events in ICD implantees dying suddenly. Possible reasons for sudden tachyarrhythmic death in the ICD patient are discussed, and tabulated, with an eye toward reducing, perhaps further, the incidence of this uncommon but catastrophic outcome.

Terminal Events in ICD Patients Who Die Suddenly

In view of the relative paucity of data regarding the arrhythmic basis for sudden death in ICD implantees,[3-7] a multicenter study was undertaken to analyze terminal events in 51 patients who died

Table 1. Baseline clinical characteristics in 51 ICD* patients who died suddenly.

Age (mean ± SD)	58 ± 12
Male gender	94%
Atherosclerotic heart disease	84%
Left ventricular EF (mean ± SD)	.26 ± .11
New York Heart Association functional class (n = 41)	
I 15%	
II 46%	
III 37%	
IV 2%	
Presenting arrhythmia	
VF 61%	
Sustained VT with history of cardiac arrest	12%
Sustained VT without history of cardiac arrest	24%
Sustained VT with undetermined history of cardiac arrest	4%
Electrophysiologic testing	
Inducible sustained VT	84%
Inducible VF	8%
Inducible non-sustained VT or non-inducible	4%
Not done	4%

* Actually "shock only" AICD; applies to Tables 2-4 as well.

suddenly despite their having received ICDs.[8] These first generation, single zone ICD systems incorporated at least one epicardial patch defibrillation electrode and delivered committed monophasic shocks (30-32 J maximum).

Classifying deaths is an inherently imprecise undertaking that is subject to known complexities of interpretation particularly in ICD patients.[9,10] In our study,[8] we utilized a fairly conventional *definition of sudden death*, namely, death that was known or presumed to be cardiac in nature, occurring within 1 hour of symptoms in a previously medically stable patient, or death occurring during sleep or unwitnessed.

Clinical data on the 51 ICD patients who died suddenly are summarized in Table 1. Typical of the clinical profile of ICD implantees, these patients were predominantly male with underlying atherosclerotic heart disease; most had a history of cardiac arrest, and inducible sustained monomorphic ventricular tachycardia (VT) was present in the majority of cases. The mean left ventricular EF of .26 was lower, however, than the mean values of .33-.35 reported in various large ICD series,[4,11-13] suggesting that as a group the sudden death victims consisted of a subset of ICD implantees having more severely impaired myocardial function. However, the mean EF of .26 was also the mean EF in the MADIT trial. (Chap. 22)

Table 2. Implantation data and clinical course of 51 ICD recipients who died suddenly.

Concomitant bypass surgery	20%
Defibrillation threshold (DFT)	
≤ 20 J	63%
25 J 20%	
Not tested	18%
Predischarge ICD test	
Defibrillation of induced VF	19%
Conversion of induced VT	17%
Not done	65%
Antiarrhythmic drug therapy at discharge	
Amiodarone (alone or combined with IA or IB)	46%
Class IA and/or IB, only	24%
Class IC (alone or combined with IB)	4%
None	26%
History of appropriate ICD shocks up to day prior to death	78%
Months from implantation to death (median; range)	9; 0-46
Recent (3 mos.) change in clinical status	
Worsening heart failure	27%
Increased arrhythmia frequency	27%
Antiarrhythmic drug added	4%
New myocardial infarction	2%
None	40%
Preterminal symptoms (among 29 witnessed deaths)	
Palpitations	3%
Shortness of breath	7%
Chest pain	3%
None	86%
Shocks witnessed during terminal events	66%
(Among 32 patients with activated devices)	
Device in deactivated state at onset of terminal events	12%
Device Depleted* Prior to Terminal Events	19%
Autopsy Findings (n = 14)	
Acute myocardial infarction	14%
Pulmonary embolism	7%
No evidence of acute cardiopulmonary process	79%

* Unable to emit audible tones or charge the capacitor; or charge time past elective replacement time

Information pertaining to ICD implantation and subsequent clinical course is summarized in Table 2. Some of the implant practices during the study time period differed from current clinical standards,[14] reflecting an evolutionary learning curve phase in the application of ICD therapy.

For example, the defibrillation threshold (DFT) was documented to be ≤ 20 J (mean 13.4 J) in only 63% of cases, with the remainder having a DFT of 25 J or not determined. Moreover, predischarge testing of ICD function was performed in just a little over one third of the cases; in particular, such testing was undertaken in only 37% of patients in whom the intraoperative DFT was 25 J or not determined. Yet, despite less than optimal intraoperative or predischarge ICD testing, nearly 80% of patients received appropriate shocks (i.e., preceded by symptoms of near-syncope or collapse, or electrocardiographically documented sustained ventricular tachyarrhythmias) over the 9 month median time preceeding sudden death.

Consistent with the occurrence of unexpected arrhythmic death, premonitory symptoms were lacking in the great majority (86%) of witnessed cases of ICD sudden death. However, two-thirds of witnessed patients (in the setting of a device known to have been activated), experienced shocks during the terminal events, usually just prior to collapse, consistent with the occurrence of a tachyarrhythmia. Among 14 sudden death victims who underwent an autopsy, nearly 80% lacked evidence of acute cardiac or pulmonary pathology; acute myocardial infarction was implicated in only 14% of cases, a finding compatible with the absence of premonitory chest pain in most of our patient population. Although terminal acute pulmonary edema, per se, was not documented in our sudden death series, about a fourth of the patients had exhibited signs and symptoms of worsening congestive heart failure during the 3 month period prior to their demise.

Electrocardiographic monitoring was performed at some point during the terminal events in 30 (59%) of the 51 sudden deaths. A sustained ventricular tachyarrhythmia was documented in 20 (8 VT and 12 VF), comprising 66% of monitored cases; whereas asystole (in 7) or electromechanical dissociation (in 3) constituted the remainder. By analyzing the 36 cases of sudden death that were either monitored or witnessed it was possible to estimate the prevalence of a *known or presumed terminal tachyarrhythmia*, defined by the presence of terminal VT or VF, or witnessed shocks. Table 3 shows the results of this analysis. Note that no matter how the results were tabulated, whether by intention-to-treat analysis or by restriction to cases favoring optimal ICD function (activated, nondepleted devices with DFT ≤ 20 J), roughly *two thirds* of the patients succumbed to a known or presumed tachyarrhythmia. It is noteworthy that 5 (56%) of 9 patients with concomitant bradycardia pacemakers also had monitored rhythms and/or witnessed shocks compatible with tachyarrhythmic death.[8]

Table 3. Known or presumed tachyarrhythmic sudden deaths in ICD implantees

	Monitored		Witnessed*		Monitored or Witnessed*	
	n	No. with VT or VF	n	No. Shocked	n	No. with VT, VF, or shocks
All cases	30	20 (67%)	36	22 (61%)	36	29 (81%)
All cases with activated devices	26	16 (62%)	32	21 (66%)	32	25 (78%)
All cases with activated and non-depleted† devices	20	12 (60%)	25	17 (68%)	25	19 (76%)
All cases with activated/non-depleted devices *and* DFT ≤ 20 J	13	8 (62%)	16	10 (63%)	16	11 (69%)

* Includes one patient whose shocks were all "witnessed" on a Holter monitor

† Generator able to emit audible tones and charge the capacitors, with charge time less than elective replacement time

Of 19 ICD recipients who died suddenly on the basis of a known or presumed ventricular tachyarrhythmia in the setting of an activated device not known to have been depleted prior to death (third row, right-most column of Table 3), failure of the ICD to definitively convert the patient to a hemodynamically stable rhythm, despite shock delivery, was documented or suggested in 13 (68%) cases. VT/VF "storm" was documented in 2 additional patients; and non-delivery of a shock most likely contributed to sudden death in another 2 cases. (Further information regarding terminal events was not available in the remaining 2 patients.) Explanted devices were tested by the manufacturer in 14 of these 19 cases; postmortem ICD generator malfunction was identified in only 1 (7%).

The basis for known or presumed sudden tachyarrhythmic death in 27 ICD implantees, with device activation status and battery status known premortem, was investigated. As summarized in Table 4, a striking finding of this analysis was that, in 60% of the cases, 4 predisposing and potentially correctable factors could be identified in equal proportions: deactivated devices (i.e., turned "off"), depleted generators, lack of intraoperative DFT testing, or elevated DFT (25 J in the face of a maximum ICD generator output of about 30 J). Even among those patients with activated devices not known to be depleted premortem, and with intraoperative DFTs of ≤ 20 J, a variety of clinical (intrinsic or extrinsic to the patient) or hardware factors possibly contributing to sudden tachyarrhythmic death could be identified in 6 of 11 patients. Thus, from an intention-to-treat standpoint, a possible or likely explanation was lacking in only 5 (19%) of the ICD recipients who succumbed to apparent sudden tachyarrhythmic death.

Table 4. Potential factors contributing to tachyarrhythmic sudden death* in 27 implantees.

Deactivated device	4 (15%) [†]
Activated, but depleted device[#]	4 (15%)
Activated, non-depleted device, but DFT = 25J	4 (15%)[§]
Activated, non-depleted device, but DFT not tested	4 (15%)[‡]
Activated, non-depleted device, with DFT ≤ 20J	11 (41%)
Hematoma under epicardial patch	1
Pulse generator component failure	1
Drug-related DFT rise	1
Possible terminal VT below rate cut off	1
Recent worsening congestive heart failure	1
Drowning during terminal ICD shocks	1
No contributory factor identifiable	5

*   Defined by documentation of VT, VF or shocks during terminal events; 2 of 29 patients (first row, rightmost column of Table 3) were excluded owing to lack of information about battery status prior to death.

†   On autopsy, one patient had pulmonary embolism and another had acute myocardial infarction

\#   Generator unable to emit audible tones or charge the capacitors; or charge time past elective replacement time.

§   One patient had hypokalemia with adverse antitachycardia pacemaker/ICD interaction, and another had recent worsening congestive heart failure.

‡   One patient had recent worsening congestive heart failure, and 2 had signs or symptoms suggesting acute ischemia.

It should be noted that this large study of sudden death in ICD patients derives from the first generation (ICD) device experience, reflecting, in part, clinical lessons acquired during a steep learning curve in the use of ICDs. While we cannot be certain that VT and VF comprise the most common terminal arrhythmias in implantees who die suddenly with present day devices, we believe this is likely to be the case for 2 reasons. First, known or presumed tachyarrhythmias were documented during terminal events in 69% of ICD recipients under optimal conditions for successful ICD function (activated, non-depleted devices with DFT ≤ 20 J; Table 3). Second, preliminary data from the clinical investigation of a third generation ICD (Ventritex Cadence) suggests that terminal VT or VF heralded most cases of sudden death, which usually occurred *despite* eventual device-mediated conversion of the tachyarrhythmias.[15] This phenomenon may have reflected post-defibrillation electromechanical dissociation or asystole (with failed pacemaker capture) due, in part, to acute myocardial dysfunction secondary to ischemia (associated with infarction, or prolonged hypoperfusion resulting from VT/VF "storm" or delivery of initially ineffective therapy) in patients with an already severely reduced left ventricular EF.[16,17]

In a series of 17 patients dying suddenly despite having second and third generation ICDs, Pratt et al[10] using stored event data logs, found evidence of ICD discharges within 6 hours of death in 7 cases (41%)—not statistically significantly lower than that reported in the 2 larger series cited above.[8,15] Regardless, however, of the exact prevalence of terminal tachyarrhythmias in ICD patients dying suddenly, further investigation is required to distinguish (to the extent possible) primary VT/VF events from secondary tachyarrhythmias in an acutely failing heart.

Factors in ICD Therapy Success or "Failure"

Although the ultimate purpose of ICD therapy is prolongation of life, the minimum clinical expectation of an ICD system is that it convert or defibrillate sustained VT or VF, with restoration of a hemodynamically stable supraventricular (primarily sinus) rhythm in a timely fashion. Failure to achieve this minimum goal can be taken as a clinically relevant working definition of "failure" of ICD therapy. Ideally, one should differentiate between tachyarrhythmias occurring solely on the basis of chronic structural abnormalities (true failure) from those secondary to acute, reversible derangements (artifactual failure), but this is often not feasible.

The notion of ICD therapy failure is a complex one. From the high frequency of prior appropriate shocks, i.e., therapy "successes," in ICD implantees who ultimately died suddenly (Table 2), mostly with a known or presumed terminal ventricular tachyarrhythmia, it is evident that ICD efficacy can vary over time. The experience with the first generation ICD device also indicates that failure of ICD therapy cannot be presumed automatically to reflect device hardware malfunction. (Table 4)

In a broad sense, *ICD therapy must be considered a multifaceted treatment, the success of which depends on far more than simply the components of the device.* (Table 5) Both physician and patient constitute integral elements of this therapy. State-of-the-art electronic circuitry may not be sufficient to salvage a patient from sustained VT or VF if proper device function is not adequately validated at implantation, the ICD is programmed inappropriately, or generator end-of-life is not appreciated as a result of poor patient compliance with followup visits and device checks.

Table 5. Factors Contributing to Successful ICD Therapy

Device Component
- ♦ Proper electronic function of generator
- ♦ Integrity of leads and connections

Physician Component
- ♦ Proper implantation techniques (assuring appropriate lead placement and device function, avoiding infection, etc.)
- ♦ Careful post-implantation followup (periodic generator and sensing/pacing function checks; special care with device programming and with concomitant use of antiarrhythmic drugs; aggressive treatment of underlying ischemia and congestive heart failure; avoidance of potassium or magnesium depletion; patient education)

Patient Component
- ♦ Compliance regarding ICD therapy (keeping followup appointments to monitor ICD battery voltage, etc.; reporting "unusual" occurrence or increased frequency of delivered electrical therapy; awareness/monitoring for signs of possible ICD-related infection; following individualized recommendations with regard to driving, swimming, etc.; avoidance of exposure to magnetic fields or sources of electromagnetic interference [and alerting the electrophysiologist if a surgical procedure is planned, necessitating temporary ICD inactivation to avoid possible electromagnetic interference during intraoperative electrocautery])
- ♦ Compliance regarding monitoring/treatment of underlying heart disease

Diagnosis of Tachyarrhythmic Death in ICD Patients

Regardless of whether or not a patient survives a failure of ICD therapy, all efforts must be made at identifying the cause, with the aim of avoiding future recurrences. The approach to failure of ICD therapy has been mentioned in different sections of Chap. 21. In Table 6 we have attempted to bring together various facets of this problem, beginning with the basic question of whether or not the device was actually "on" at the time of therapy failure, and then proceeding systematically along the electrical pathway from ICD sensing to tachyarrhythmia detection and therapy delivery. Potentially correctable or avoidable causes of sudden tachyarrhythmic death, beyond those related solely to proper implant technique, will now be highlighted.

Deactivated ICDs

The importance of device activation for assuring optimal results with ICD therapy may seem obvious, but in the 1980's many implanting physicians routinely deactivated ICD systems in the post-operative period, so as to prevent triggering of "false positive" shocks by atrial fibrillation (a sequela of thoracotomy and epicardial patches).[18] It was disturbing to discover that some patients managed in this fashion died suddenly in the hospital.[8,11,18]

Table 6. Potential causes of sudden tachyarrhythmic death in ICD implantees.

I. Device "off"
- A. Intentionally (e.g., to avoid shocks)
- B. Accidentally (e.g., speaker magnet)
- C. Erroneously

II. Sensing or detection failure
- A. Low R-wave amplitude
  1. Intrinsic from time of implant
     - a) chronic attenuation
     - b) new local scar
  2. Dynamic
     - a) Erroneous presumption of conversion to sinus rhythm (despite persistence of VT or VF) due to pseudo-long R-R intervals resulting from signal dropout or automatic gain control related undersensing
     - b) post shock, especially in ICD system with transvenous integrated sensing/defibrillation lead
     - c) drug/electrolyte effect
- B. Sensing lead dislodgement
- C. Sensing lead fracture
- D. Loose connection of sensing lead to ICD generator
- E. Pacemaker stimulus artifact sensed during VF, and inhibiting tachyarrhythmia detection by ICD
- F. Programming-related problem
  1. Tachycardia rate cutoff zones set too high, resulting in under-("non"-) detection
  2. Lower rate tachycardia zone set too close to VT rate, periodically resetting interval counter during VT thereby preventing attainment of minimum number of intervals for satisfying tachycardia detection
  3. Fast VT with cycle length oscillating between "VF" and "VT" zones, markedly delaying declaration of tachyarrhythmia by certain algorithms*
  4. Threshold voltage for sensing set higher than actual R-wave voltage (i.e., inappropriate "sensitivity")
- G. ICD sensing circuit (i.e., electronic) malfunction

III. VT or VF rates sensed, but ICD therapy not delivered to the heart
- A. Battery depletion
  1. Expected
     - a) Early Replacement Indicator known to be attained, but generator not yet replaced
     - b) not appreciated prior to death (e.g., patient lost to followup, excessive recent utilization secondary to atrial tachyarrhythmias or VT/VF "storm", etc.)
  2. Premature (e.g., battery failure, excessive current leakage, etc.)
- B. Programming-related problem (e.g., therapy delivery held back by erroneous presumption of "supraventricular" tachyarrhythmia on the basis of "enhancement criteria" for tachycardia discrimination)

Table 6 continued.

    C.   Failure to detect true conversion to "sinus rhythm" between successive rapid VT or VF episodes which are reinitiated by recurring salvos of post-conversion nonsustained VT, with eventual automatic deactivation of VF therapy (ICD interprets independent VF episodes occurring in rapid succession as a "single event," with consecutive defibrillation "failures" leading to exhaustion of fixed allotment of (typically 4-6) shocks for such an "event")

    D.   ICD circuitry (i.e., electronic) malfunction

    E.   Loose connection between generator and antitachycardia pacing or defibrillation leads

    F.   Fracture of lead(s) for antitachycardia pacing or defibrillation

    G.   Dislodgement of antitachycardia pacing or defibrillation lead(s)

IV.   ICD therapy delivered to the heart, but patient not resuscitated

    A.   Antitachycardia pacing (ATP)

        1.   VT/VF "storm"

        2.   Incessant "pacing/shock resistant" VT (drug-related proarrhythmia)

        3.   Conversion to slower VT with reversion (in some devices) to the treatment algorithm of the "low rate zone," thereby forestalling prompt shock delivery.*

        4.   Programming-related problem (i.e., inadequate or inappropriate type of ATP specified, or inappropriately high setting for upper limit of "low" rate ("VT") zone, leading to use of ineffective therapy for very fast, poorly-tolerated VT (or VF))*

        5.   Conversion of VT to VF in a patient with marginal DFT

        6.   Failure of pacing stimuli to capture

            a)   High pacing threshold

                (1)   since implantation

                (2)   subsequent to implantation (e.g., new scar, drugs, etc.)

            b)   Inappropriate programmed pacing stimulation parameters

        7.   Inappropriate type of ATP due to circuitry (i.e., electronic) malfunction

    B.   DC shock

        1.   VT/VF "storm;" incessant VT

        2.   Elevated DFT

            a)   Since implantation

            b)   Time dependent phenomenon (related to electrode-tissue interface)

                (1)   local anatomic resistive barrier (e.g., hematoma under epicardial patch electrode)

                (2)   transient (e.g., drug-related)

                (3)   subacute or chronic (adverse) change in underlying myocardial substrate

        3.   Shock-induced conversion of VT to VF in a patient with marginal or elevated DFT*

        4.   Inappropriately low shock energy*

            a)   Programming-related

            b)   ICD circuitry malfunction

        5.   Post-shock electromechanical dissociation or asystole (possibly with failure to capture during back-up VVI pacing (due to shock itself or metabolically induced elevated pacing threshold)).

---

* Protracted time in VT or VF (due to prolonged detection time or delivery of initially ineffective therapies) may secondarily cause failure of otherwise effective electrical therapy or predispose to post-shock asystole or electromechanical dissociation, especially in patients with very poor left ventricular function.

Based on the observations of hospital-based death and a documented increased incidence of sustained ventricular tachyarrhythmias in the post-epicardial ICD system implantation period,[19,20] we[11] and others[20,21] advocated immediate device activation (perhaps with a temporarily programmed high rate cutoff) postoperatively. Although this practice cannot be proven to be safer, a shorter time to delivery of therapy would logically seem to provide the patient with the best chance of successful resuscitation. In the current era of nonthoracotomy ICD system implantations, perioperative ventricular, as well as atrial, tachyarrhythmias are not likely to pose as serious a problem as in the first decade of ICD therapy.[22]

Battery Depletion

The clinical experience with first generation ICDs emphasizes the importance of battery depletion as a potentially avoidable cause of sudden tachyarrhythmic death in ICD recipients. (Table 4) In those patients who died suddenly with depleted devices, the time to actual replacement from recognition of generator approaching end-of-life was relatively protracted (14-63 days),[8] owing largely to the historical problem of limited device availability. Nonetheless, this early experience highlights the advisability of prompt generator replacement once the need for such an intervention becomes apparent during followup, even though there is a grace period (typically ≤ 3 months, specific to each device) from appearance of an elective replacement indicator to battery end-of-life. Clinically, it may be helpful to think of ICD recipients as being, in effect, "device dependent," analogous to patients who are pacemaker-dependent.

ICD-Related Proarrhythmia

Aggravation of sustained ventricular tachyarrhythmias has been extensively described in the setting of antiarrhythmic drug administration, but is less well studied as a complication of ICD therapy. Table 7 defines the entity of ICD-related proarrhythmia. The fact that electrical therapy (either antitachycardia pacing or DC shock) may inappropriately induce a new, or worsen a preexisting, sustained ventricular tachyarrhythmia is well recognized.[4,6,23-30] Additionally, undersensing of supraventricular complexes may occur following spontaneous premature ventricular beats (which alter the amplifier automatic gain control setting), resulting in ICD-generated VVI paced beats that may, in turn, trigger VT.[31] Although in the great majority of cases, appropriate ICD function will ensure termination of such iatrogenic tachyarrhythmias, all efforts should be made to minimize the risk of ICD-related proarrhythmia—

Table 7. ICD-Related "Proarrhythmia"

VT or VF initiated by electrical therapy* delivered (mistakenly) during a supraventricular rhythm
VF or poorly-tolerated VT precipitated by electrical therapy delivered in response to a hemodynamically-stable VT

* Antitachycardia pacing, DC shock or antibradycardia pacing.[31]

especially when the problem is potentially preventable or correctable by reprogramming the ICD.[32]

Delayed Delivery of Effective Electrical Therapy

Any factor that delays the time to conversion or defibrillation of sustained VT or VF can ultimately result in failure of the ICD to resuscitate the patient. Resuscitation failure may occur on the basis of an acute time-dependent rise in DFT,[33] post-shock asystole or acute contractile dysfunction and electromechanical dissociation.[7,8,15,30] The latter phenomenon is probably more likely in patients with severe left ventricular dysfunction.[16,17] Underdetection consequent to a variety of inappropriate (not necessarily anticipatible) programming scenarios, e.g., setting of tachycardia "VT" or "VF" zone cutoff rates too high or use of detection enhancements,[34] may give rise to these problems. Newer ICDs have built-in countermeasures (e.g., "Extended High Rate [EHR]" feature in the Ventritex Contour and its predecessors and "Sustained Rate Duration [SRD]" feature in the CPI Mini and its predecessors) to safeguard against excessive delays in delivery of definitive electrical therapy. Risk-benefit trade-offs associated with programming of tachycardia detection parameters are discussed further in Chaps. 15 and 19.

Very judicious use of programmable therapy options capable of postponing shocks, such as multiple attempts at antitachycardia pacing or, utilization of a lower initial shock energy in the "VF" zone, despite the seeming benefit of a shortened charge time, may also help to prevent ICD resuscitation failure. In view of an increased risk defibrillation failure, use of submaximal shocks for VF therapy might be more appropriately reserved, if at all, for patients with at least moderately well-preserved ventricular function.

Lead Fractures and Dislodgement

Fractures of ICD leads commonly involve the sensing pathway, resulting in artifactual oversensing and inappropriate shock delivery,[30,35-41] as described in Chap. 21. If oversensing and repeated triggering of the high voltage charging circuitry occurs repeatedly, premature battery depletion may follow,[39] leaving the patient at risk for ICD "failure" during VF. Lead fractures can also contribute to tachyarrhythmic death by disruption of the electrical pathway to a defibrillation electrode predisposing to defibrillation failure[4,30,40] or, more directly, via lethal VT/VF "storm" triggered by oversensing-induced inappropriate shocks. Clearly, fracture of ICD leads often reflect certain structural limitations of the hardware, as may be seen with epicardial or subcutaneous patch electrodes,[4,37,38,40] or other lead elements.[30,39-41] On the other hand, innovations in implanting technique aimed at reducing mechanical stresses on ICD leads, especially in the region of the costoclavicular joint ("crush injury"),[42,43] merit aggressive exploration and evaluation as a means of preventing fractures. In this regard, there is already growing interest in use of the cephalic vein or a more anterolateral percutaneous approach to the subclavian vein during ICD lead placement.[44,45]

Mechanical dislodgement is another important lead-related problem that could result in failure of ICD therapy[4] or lethal mechanically-induced VT/VF "storm.[7] If recognized through X-ray or functionally (through assessment of sensing, pacing or defibrillation capability) during followup—and corrected by lead revision or replacement—potentially fatal undersensing or undertreatment of VT or VF may be averted.

Post-Shock Undersensing

Implanting physicians need to be cognizant of potential undersensing problems, described mainly in association with integrated sensing/defibrillation lead ICD systems. Undersensing following a failed defibrillation attempt, with potentially disastrous sequelae, has been reported in some patients with such nonthoracotomy ICD systems.[46-48] Although this phenomenon may be due, in part, to post-shock R-wave attenuation,[46] autogain features of the sensing amplifier are probably contributory, as evidenced by cases of persistent VF with erroneous redetection of "sinus rhythm" by a noncommitted tiered therapy ICD connected to a transvenous dedicated bipolar lead system.[49] An increased interelectrode distance between the distal (tip) electrode and the distal spring (sensing/defibrillation) electrode of the integrated transvenous system may minimize the occurrence of post-shock R-wave attenuation,[50] although it remains to be seen how favorably the sensing safety margin in such an improved lead compares with that of a dedicated bipolar transvenous sensing system.[51,52]

The correlation between identification during predischarge or followup testing of a potential underdetection problem in patients with transvenous integrated sensing/defibrillation leads and actual long-term clinical sequelae is not clear at present;[53] nor is the

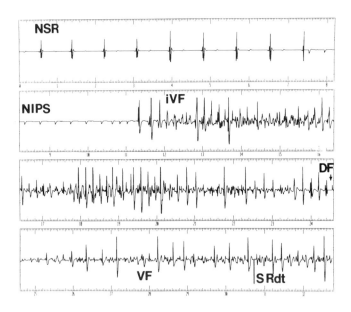

Figure 1. False redetection of sinus rhythm after a failed shock. The initial rhythm is *NSR* until a *NIPS*-induced VF (*iVF*). After the first shock delivery (*DF*), the patient remains in *VF* and the device falsely redetects a sinus rhythm at *SRdt*.

clinical utility of routine testing of this sensing lead system following subthreshold shock energy delivery during induced VF. Until these various issues are resolved, a number of prudent measures may be instituted to prevent or remedy dynamic undersensing problems in patients with integrated lead ICD systems. These measures include programming the device to maximum shock energy (or at least to a value with a "very high" safety margin) for tachyarrhythmias detected in the "high rate" zone, thereby minimizing the risk of a shock failing to defibrillate; abandonment of the noncommitted mode in select cases, so as to force shock delivery in the high rate zone, when known or suspected undersensing may lead to erroneous withholding of therapy were the ICD system to take a "second look" at the tachyarrhythmia; programming a lower tachycardia rate cutoff (i.e., longer cycle length) to render less likely transient undersensing of electrograms (erroneous registration of an R-R interval outside the tachycardia zone); and, in the case of the Ventritex Cadence device, for example, programming the "sinus" redetection algorithm to "slow" instead of "fast" (thereby requiring a greater number of long R-R intervals to be detected in order for "sinus rhythm" to be declared).

ICD-Pacemaker Interactions

Implantable ICDs can adversely affect pacemaker function and vice versa, with potentially fatal consequences. Numerous adverse effects of permanent pacemakers on ICD functions have been described[54-60] all of which may ultimately result in failure of the ICD to deliver appropriate therapy. ICD sensing of pacemaker stimulus artifacts was among the first adverse interactions noted. Such sensing may lead to normal rhythms being misinterpreted as ventricular arrhythmias or to inhibition of tachyarrhythmia detection. Double counting, caused by sensing of pacing stimulus artifacts, can lead to inappropriate ICD shocks which, in turn, may trigger ventricular tachyarrhythmias. Sensing of large stimulus artifacts in the presence of lower-amplitude VF can result in nondetection (or delays in detection) of that tachyarrhythmia.[54,55,59] Such a catastrophic adverse interaction is more likely to occur with unipolar pacemakers, since unipolar pacing stimulus artifacts are typically larger than their bipolar counterparts. It is for this reason that unipolar pacing is considered contraindicated in patients with implanted ICDs, although, in some cases, highly rigorous testing may permit its use.[61]

Strict adherence to certain implantation techniques and appropriate intraoperative and pre-discharge testing can avoid these various adverse interactions in most patients with epicardial patch-based ICD systems,[54-60] or transvenous systems.[62,64] Specifically, (1) unipolar pacemakers (and devices that revert to unipolar pacing post-shock) should be avoided; (2) in patients with transvenous ICDs, the pacemaker lead should be placed as far as possible from the defibrillating lead (usually an active-fixation lead in the right ventricular septum or outflow tract); (3) appropriate ICD sensing of VF must be demonstrated under the worst case condition of pacing (from ventricle, atrium, or both) at maximum output; (4) an adequate safety margin for pacing should be attainable at stimulation levels sufficiently low to avoid oversensing (double- or triple-counting) by the ICD; and (5) the pacemaker upper rate should be programmed below the ICD cutoff rate to prevent inappropriate ICD discharges. (See also Chaps. 14 and 17.)

Antiarrhythmic Drugs

The potential for antiarrhythmic drugs to adversely affect ICD function has been recognized for some time. The main clinical concern with the use of such agents, particularly those that have sodium channel blocking activity, is the possibility of drug-induced elevation of the DFT[65-68] and resultant defibrillation failure.[8,30] (See also Chap. 5) The ability of other antiarrhythmic agents such as sotalol to lower the DFT[68,69] may indirectly cause a problem by leading to a transiently enhanced safety margin possible false sense of security—if ICD implantation and DFT testing are performed prior to drug washout. Some antiarrhythmic agents are capable of confounding tachyarrhythmia detection. This problem can occur either as a result of tachycardia slowing on drug to a rate below the cutoff value for detection,[55] or consequent to drug-induced fluctuations in tachycardia cycle length that may fool a stability criterion into declaring the rhythm "unstable", i.e., implying "atrial fibrillation," and prompting an erroneous decision to withhold electrical therapy.[34] Clearly, the need for reassessing ICD function following addition of new antiarrhythmic drugs (and perhaps even after dosage increases) cannot be overemphasized.

Worsened Myocardial Substrate

Progression of underlying heart disease is an important factor that may adversely affect ICD function.[8] This can occur through a variety of means including ischemia, infarction, myocardial dilatation or electrolyte depletion associated with diuretic therapy, any of which may aggravate the myocardial substrate for sustained ventricular tachyarrhythmia (including precipitation of fatal VT/VF "storm")[70] or predispose to the occurrence of post-shock electromechanical dissociation. In some cases, such pathologic processes may also reduce R-wave amplitude or raise the DFT. Clinicians have the ability potentially to forestall the development of these various adverse effects on ICD function by aggressive use of appropriate medical therapy (e.g., beta blockers and angiotensin converting enzyme inhibitors) or invasive therapeutic interventions (in patients with coronary artery disease)

Finding the Cause of Actual or Aborted Sudden Death

The complex task of uncovering the cause of actual or aborted sudden cardiac death in the ICD patient requires a thorough evaluation of pre-terminal clinical events correlated with the time course and nature of ICD system responses.[8] When stored intracardiac electrograms are available, these need to be reviewed to further define the sequence of arrhythmic events associated with the cardiac arrest. In patients fortunate enough to survive through external resuscitation, ICD system function must be thoroughly reassessed, as described in Chap. 21.

Although uncommon, (Table 4)[4,8,30] the possibility of true device malfunction should be investigated. Every attempt must be made to obtain the ICD postmortem. Devices should be interrogated with a programmer and the results printed on paper or saved on floppy disk prior to explant. Care must be taken, however, to *deactivate the ICD prior to cutting the leads* so as to avoid sensing of lead noise, capable of generating artifactual terminal tachyarrhythmic events and precipitating inappropriate high voltage discharges (that could also contribute postmortem to an erroneous impression of "battery depletion"). Even though the false nature of such "events" might be recognizable (e.g., by the appearance of corresponding stored electrograms), their occurrence could still confound reconstruction of the terminal event sequence by displacing from ICD memory buffers the stored electrograms of true terminal tachyarrhythmias. Reasonable precautions should be taken to avoid mechanical or electrical damage to devices during explant and packaging. Some manufacturers provide mailer kits that ensure proper packaging for returning explanted devices. Hospital personnel, sales representatives or other field personnel should arrange for prompt shipment of returned products immediately after explant.

Detailed reasons for explanting and returning an implantable product are crucial to the analysis of returned products.[71] Minimal information is needed when devices are explanted for normal battery depletion. In contrast, when the user observes or suspects some problem or failure of the device, as in the case of sudden death, the circumstances should be described in as much detail as possible, with all supporting rhythm strips available. Clinical and followup data from the patient medical record and results of device interrogation can provide important clues for device analysis. An X-ray of the implanted system may reveal evidence of lead fracture or dislodgement, or problems with lead connections to the ICD. Any history of possible device exposure to external defibrillation, radiofrequency catheter ablation, radiation therapy, magnetic resonance imaging, hyperbaric therapy, lithotripsy, electroconvulsive shock therapy, medical diathermy, or electrosurgery also should be described--as these sources of electromagnetic interference may reset the programming of the device to default parameters (although actual damage is extremely rare).[72,73]

For all explanted devices received by manufacturers, a permanent record is created and a letter acknowledging receipt is sent to the physician. ICDs are interrogated, if possible, and all programmable parameters and stored data are recorded and analyzed.

If the ICD is still activated, it is deactivated before further processing. Devices are then sterilized and cleaned.

Routine analysis using proprietary procedures is performed on all returned ICDs. Usually this includes a *visual inspection* for physical damage such as pits, dents or large scratches, and microscopic examination when applicable including the connector module lead ports and seals, setscrews and seals. *Radiological analysis* is used to check the internal layout of components, the integrity of internal wiring, and possible foreign material. *Electrical functional tests* are conducted to determine if the device performs normally within specified tolerances. These tests involve a wide range of device parameters, including sensitivity, pacing signal characteristics, arrhythmia detection, and therapy delivery capability. The results of these tests are then compared to functional test data collected during manufacturing of the same device identified by the serial number. If the test data are within normal limits and the probable cause of the reported problem has already been identified, then the analysis is closed.

If, on the other hand, device testing reveals parameters that are not within normal limits or if special concerns or problems are identified and documented, then a plan for *specialized testing* may be undertaken. The goal of such testing is to reproduce the problem and isolate the cause using proven analysis techniques. More clinical history data may be requested, detailed manufacturing and traceability data may be collected, and specific tests may compare the device to another similar device using various analytical procedures and specialized test equipment.

Destructive analysis, if necessary, is performed only after all applicable external testing is completed and analyzed.[74,75] The metal shield halves are removed very carefully to expose internal components and circuitry. Visual inspections, electrical probing and measurements are performed to identify the specific subassembly and ultimately the specific component that caused the problem. Consultations with design engineers and manufacturing engineers are used to design specific tests that pertain to the particular problem being investigated. Sometimes the result is identification of a specific random component failure. Further tests with similar components may be performed to assure that other devices with the same type of component are not likely to develop similar failures.

When testing is completed, all of the results are summarized and reported. The physician is notified of relevant findings. If applicable, corrective action that can be taken by the physician to prevent similar failures in the future may be described. Results of device testing are then incorporated into a periodically published performance report on all returned ICDs.

Conclusions

Sudden death in the ICD patient is a particularly challenging problem at the clinical-engineering interface of ICD therapy. First generation ICD experience suggests that this unexpected event appears most commonly to be associated with the occurrence of terminal tachyarrhythmias. Failure to resuscitate the patient may result from problems at one or more levels, including hardware; device implantation, management, and followup; patient compliance; and myocardial substrate. All attempts must be made to reconstruct terminal events from clinical history, device interrogation and review of extracardiac and stored intracardiac electrograms. X-ray of the lead system and review of recent medical history and premortem ICD followup data can provide important supplementary information. The possibility of actual ICD malfunction can be investigated by device explantation with a product analysis performed by the manufacturer. Such a comprehensive approach offers the prospect of a better understanding of the uncommon problem of sudden death in ICD recipients, and, thereby, the potential for reducing its occurrence.

ACKNOWLEDGMENTS:
Thanks to Diane Szubeczak and Karen Beal for their excellent secretarial assistance. Tables 1, 2, 3, and 4 are adapted from: Lehmann MH, et al.[8] Fig. 1 is used with the permission of the Journal of the American College of Cardiology.[47]

1   Sweeney MO, Ruskin JN. Mortality benefits and the implantable cardioverter-defibrillator. Circulation 1994;89:1851-1858.
2.   Lehmann M. The results of device therapy in high-risk patients, pp 504-507. In: Akhtar M. Sudden cardiac death: management of high-risk patients. Ann Intern Med 1991;114:499-512.
3.   Luceri RM, Habal SM, Castellanos A, et al. Mechanism of death in patients with the automatic implantable cardioverter defibrillator. PACE 1988;11(II):2015-2022.
4.   Winkle RA, Mead RH, Ruder MA, et al. Long-term outcome with the automatic implantable cardioverter-defibrillator. J Am Coll Cardiol 1989;13:1353-1361.
5.   Khastgir T, Aarons D, Veltri E. Sudden bradyarrhythmic death in patients with the implantable cardioverter-defibrillator: Report of two cases. PACE 1991;14:395-398.
6.   Birgersdotter-Green U, Rosenqvist M, Lindemans FW, et al. Holter documented sudden death in a patient with an implanted defibrillator. PACE

1992;15:1008-1014.

7. Edel TB, Maloney JD, Moore SL, et al. Analysis of deaths in patients with an implantable cardioverter defibrillator. PACE 1992;15:60-70.

8. Lehmann MH, Thomas A, Nabih M, et al. Sudden death in recipients of first-generation implantable cardioverter defibrillators: analysis of terminal events. J Interven Cardiol 1994;7:487-503.

9. Epstein AE, Carlson MD, Fogoros RN, et al. Classification of death in antiarrhythmia trials. J Am Coll Cardiol 1996;27:433-442.

10. Pratt CM, Greenway PS, Schoenfeld MH, et al. Exploration of the precision of classifying sudden cardiac death: implications for the interpretation of clinical trials. Circulation 1996;93:519-524.

11. Mosteller RD, Lehmann MH, Thomas AC, et al. Operative mortality with implantation of the automatic cardioverter-defibrillator. Am J Cardiol 1991;68:1340-1345.

12. Powell AC, Fuchs T, Finkelstein DM, et al. Influence of implantable cardioverter-defibrillators on the long-term prognosis of survivors of out-of-hospital cardiac arrest. Circulation 1993;88:1083-1092.

13. Lessmeier TJ, Lehmann MH, Steinman RT, et al. Implantable cardioverter-defibrillator therapy in 300 patients with coronary artery disease presenting exclusively with ventricular fibrillation. Am Heart J 1994;128:211-218.

14. Lehmann MH, Saksena S. Implantable cardioverter defibrillators in cardiovascular practice: Report of the policy conference of the North American Society of Pacing and Electrophysiology. PACE 1991;14:969-979.

15. Pires LA, Lehmann MH, Fain ES, et al. Sudden death in patients with a third-generation implantable cardioverter-defibrillator (ICD): how and why does it happen? PACE 1995;18:942. (abstract)

16. Steinbeck G, Dorwarth U, Mattke S, et al. Hemodynamic deterioration during ICD implant: predictors of high-risk patients. Am Heart J 1994;127:1064-1067.

17. Hachenberg T, Hammel D, Mollhoff T, et al. Cardiopulmonary effects of internal cardioverter defibrillator implantation. Acta Anaesthesiol Scand 1991;35:626-630.

18. Lehmann MH, Steinman RT, Schuger CD, et al. Defibrillation threshold testing and other practices related to AICD implantation: Do all roads lead to Rome? PACE 1989;12:1530-1537.

19. Kim SG, Fisher JD, Furman S, et al. Exacerbation of ventricular arrhythmias during the postoperative period after implantation of an automatic defibrillator. J Am Coll Cardiol 1991;18:1200-1206.

20. Hii JTY, Gillis AM, Wyse DG, et al. Risks of developing supraventricular and ventricular tachyarrhythmias after implantation of a cardioverter-defibrillator, and timing the activation of arrhythmia termination therapies. Am J Cardiol 1993;71:565-568.

21. Cohen TJ, Pogo G, Goldner BG, et al. Should implantable cardioverter-defibrillators be activated immediately after implantation? Am Heart J 1994;127:480-482.

22. Kim SG, Ling J, Fisher JD, et al. Comparison and frequency of ventricular arrhythmias after defibrillator implantation by thoracotomy versus nonthoracotomy approaches. Am J Cardiol 1994;74:1245-1248.

23. Manz M, Gerckens U, Luderitz B. Erroneous discharge from an implanted automatic defibrillator during supraventricular tachyarrhythmia induced ventricular fibrillation. Am J Cardiol 1986;57:343-344.

24. Kou WH, Kirsh MM, Stirling MC, et al. Provocation of ventricular tachycardia by an automatic implantable cardioverter defibrillator. Am Heart J 1990;120:208-210.

25. Cohen TJ, Chien WW, Luire KG, et al. Implantable cardioverter defibrillator proarrhythmia: case report and review of the literature. PACE 1991;14:1326-

1329.

26. Johnson N, Marchlinski FE. Arrhythmias induced by device antitachycardia therapy due to diagnostic nonspecificity. J Am Coll Cardiol 1991;18:1418-1425.

27. Bardy GH, Poole JE, Kudenchuk PJ, et al. A prospective randomized repeat-crossover comparison of antitachycardia pacing with low-energy conversion. Circulation 1993;87:1889-1895.

28. Gillis AM, Leitch JW, Sheldon RS, et al. A prospective randomized comparison of autodecremental pacing to burst pacing in device therapy for chronic ventricular tachycardia secondary to coronary artery disease. Am J Cardiol 1993;72:1146-1151.

29. Lauer MR, Young C, Liem LB, et al. Ventricular fibrillation induced by low-energy shocks from programmable implantable cardioverter-defibrillators in patients with coronary artery disease. Am J Cardiol 1994;73:559-563.

30. Nunain SO, Roelke M, Trouton T, et al. Limitations and late complications of third-generation automatic cardioverter-defibrillators. Circulation 1995;91:2204-2213.

31. Callans DJ, Hook BG, Kleiman RB, et al. Unique sensing errors in third-generation implantable cardioverter-defibrillators. J Am Coll Cardiol 1993;22:1135-1140.

32. Pinski SL, Fahy GJ. The proarrhythmic potential of implantable cardioverter-defibrillators. Circulation 1995;92:1651-1664.

33. Echt DS, Barbey JT, Black NJ. Influence of ventricular fibrillation duration on defibrillation energy in dogs using bidirectional pulse discharges. PACE 1988;11:1315-1323.

34. Swerdlow CD, Ahern T, Chen PS, et al. Underdetection of ventricular tachycardia by algorithms to enhance specificity in a tiered-therapy cardioverter-defibrillator. J Am Coll Cardiol 1994;24:416-424.

35. Almassi GH, Olinger GN, Wetherbee JN, et al. Long-term complications of implantable cardioverter defibrillator lead systems. Ann Thorac Surg 1993;55:888-892

36. Daoud EG, Kirsh MM, Bolling SF, et al. Incidence, presentation, diagnosis, and management of malfunctioning implantable cardioverter-defibrillator rate-sensing leads. Am Heart J 1994;128:892-895.

37. Pfeiffer D, Jung W, Fehske W, et al. Complications of pacemaker-defibrillator devices: diagnosis and management. Am Heart J 1994;127:1073-1080.

38. Kleman JM, Castle LW, Kidwell GA, et al. Nonthoracotomy- versus thoracotomy-implantable defibrillators: Intention-to-treat comparison of clinical outcomes. Circulation 1994;90:2833-2842.

39. Candinas R, Hagspiel KD, MacCarter DJ, et al. Premature ICD battery depletion due to a defective lead adapter component: usefulness of extensive data logging. PACE 1993;16:2192-2195.

40. Jones GK, Bardy GH, Kudenchuk PJ, et al. Mechanical complications following implantation of multiple lead nonthoracotomy defibrillator systems: implications for management and future system design. Am Heart J 1995;10:327-333.

41. Stambler BS, Wood MA, Damiano RJ, et al. Sensing/pacing lead complications with a newer generation implantable cardioverter-defibrillator: Worldwide experience from the guardian ATP 4210 clinical trial. J Am Coll Cardiol 1994;23:123-132.

42. Jacobs DM, Fink AS, Miller RP, et al. Anatomical and morphological evaluation of pacemaker lead compression. PACE 1993;16:434-444.

43. Magney JE, Flynn DM, Parsons JA, et al. Anatomical mechanisms explaining damage to pacemaker leads, defibrillator leads, and failure of central venous catheters adjacent to the sternoclavicular joint. PACE 1993;16:445-457.

44. Byrd CL. Clinical experience with the extrathoracic introducer insertion technique. PACE 1993;16:1781-1784.

45. Magney JE, Staplin DH, Flynn DM, et al. A new approach to percutaneous subclavian venipuncture to avoid lead fracture or central venous catheter occlusion. PACE 1993;16:2133-2142.
46. Jung W, Manz M, Moosdorf R, et al. Failure of an implantable cardioverter-defibrillator to redetect ventricular fibrillation in patients with a nonthoracotomy lead system. Circulation 1992;86:1217-1222.
47. Berul CI, Callans DJ, Schwartzman D, et al. A comparison of initial detection and redetection of ventricular fibrillation in a transvenous defibrillator system with automatic gain control. J Am Coll Cardiol 1995;25:431-436.
48. Natale A, Sra J, Axtell K, et al. Undetected ventricular fibrillation in transvenous implantable cardioverter defibrillators: prospective comparison of different lead system-device combinations. Circulation 1996;93:91-98.
49. Mann DE, Kelly PA, Damle RS, et al. Undersensing during ventricular tachyarrhythmias in a third generation implantable cardioverter-defibrillator. Diagnosis using stored electrograms and correction with programming. PACE 1994;17:1525-1530.
50. Jung W, Manz M, Moosdorf R, et al. Changes in the amplitude of endocardial electrograms following defibrillator discharge: comparison of two lead systems. PACE 1995;18:2163-2172.
51. Gottlieb CD, Schwartzman DS, Callans DJ, et al. Effects of high and low shock energies on sinus electrograms recorded via integrated and true bipolar nonthoracotomy lead systems . J Cardiovasc Electrophysiol 1996;7:189-196.
52. Schwartzman D, Gottlieb CD, Callans DJ, et al. Comparative effect of shocks on the endocardial rate-sensing signals from transvenous lead systems. J Am Coll Cardiol 1995;25:15A. (abstract)
53. Ellis JR, Martin DT, Venditti FJ. Appropriate sensing of ventricular fibrillation after failed shocks in a transvenous cardioverter-defibrillator system. Circulation 1994;90:1820-1825.
54. Kim SG, Furman S, Waspe LE, et al. Unipolar pacer artifacts induced failure of an automatic implantable cardioverter/defibrillator to detect ventricular fibrillation. Am J Cardiol 1986;57:880-881.
55. Marchlinski FE, Flores BT, Buxton AE, et al. The automatic implantable cardioverter-defibrillator: efficacy, complications, and device failures. Ann Intern Med 1986;104:481-488.
56. Gottlieb C, Miller JM, Rosenthal ME, et al. Automatic implantable defibrillator discharge resulting from routine pacemaker programming. PACE 1988;11:336-338.
57. Cohen AI, Wish MH, Fletcher RD, et al. The use and interaction of permanent pacemakers and the automatic implantable cardioverter defibrillator. PACE 1988;11:704-711.
58. Epstein AE, Kay GN, Plumb VJ, et al. Combined automatic implantable cardioverter-defibrillator and pacemaker systems: implantation techniques and follow-up. J Am Coll Cardiol 1989;13:121-131.
59. Calkins H, Brinker J, Veltri EP, et al. Clinical interactions between pacemakers and automatic implantable cardioverter-defibrillators. J Am Coll Cardiol 1990;16:666-673.
60. Kim SG, Furman S, Matos JA, et al. Automatic implantable cardioverter/defibrillator: inadvertent discharges during permanent pacemaker magnet test. PACE 1987;10:579-582.
61. Haffajee C, Casavant D, Desai P, et al. Combined third generation implantable cardioverter-defibrillator with permanent unipolar pacemakers: preliminary observations. PACE 1996;19:136-142.
62. Blanck Z, Niazi I, Axtell K, et al. Feasibility of concomitant implantation of permanent transvenous pacemaker and defibrillator systems. Am J Cardiol 1994;74:1249-1253.
63. Clemo HF, Ellenbogen KA, Belz MK, et al. Safety of pacemaker implantation in

patients with transvenous (nonthoracotomy) implantable cardioverter defibrillators. PACE 1994;17:2285-2291.

64. Brooks R, Garan H, McGovern BA, et al. Implantation of transvenous nonthoracotomy cardioverter-defibrillator systems in patients with permanent endocardial pacemakers. Am Heart J 1995;129:45-53.

65. Fain ES, Dorian P, Davy JM, et al. Effects of encainide and its metabolites on energy-requirements for defibrillation. Circulation 1986;73:1334-1341.

66. Hernandez R, Mann DE, Breckinridge S, et al. Effects of flecainide on defibrillation thresholds in the anesthetized dog. J Am Coll Cardiol 1989;14:777-781.

67. Echt DS, Black JN, Barbey JT, et al. Evaluation of antiarrhythmic drugs on defibrillation energy requirements in dogs: sodium channel block and action potential prolongation. Circulation 1989;79:1106-1117.

68. Echt DS, Gremillion ST, Lee JT, et al. Effects of procainamide and lidocaine on defibrillation energy requirements in patients receiving implantable cardioverter defibrillator devices. J Cardiovasc Electrophysiol 1994;5:752-760.

69. Wang MJ, Dorian P. DL and D sotalol decrease defibrillation energy requirements. PACE 1989;12:1522-1529.

70. Tomaselli GF, Beuckelmann DJ, Calkins HG, et al. Sudden cardiac death in heart failure. The role of abnormal repolarization. Circulation 1994;90:2534-2539.

71. Mond HG. The Cardiac Pacemaker Function and Malfunction, New York Grune and Stratton, 1983.

72. Olson WH. The effects of external interference on ICD and PMs. In: Implantable Cardioverter-Defibrillators: A Comprehensive Text. Edited by PJ Wang, NAM Estes, AS Manolis. New York: Marcel Dekker, 1994, pp 139-152.

73. Nisam S, Fogoros RN. Troubleshooting Implantable Cardioverter-Defibrillator Patients. In: Implantable Cardioverter-Defibrillator. I Singer (ed). Armonk, New York: Futura Publishing Co., 1994, pp 433-455.

74. Doyle Jr, Ed, Morris, Bill, (Compiled and edited by) Microelectronics Failure Analysis Techniques, A Procedural Guide, Rome Air Development Center, Air Force Systems Command, Griffiths Air Force Base, General Electric Company, Electronics Laboratory, Syracuse, ITT Research Institute Chicago, Illinois, 1982.

75. Amerasekera EA, Campbell DS. Failure Mechanisms in Semiconductor Devices. New York, John Wiley and Sons, 1987.

24

Future Clinical Challenges

Michael H. Lehmann, MD, Mark W. Kroll, PhD

THE FUTURE for the ICD appears to highly dependent on technology progress. The major technology issues are dealt with in the preceding chapters. (Table 1) With technologic developments underway complemented by an established performance track record and clear demonstration of therapeutic efficacy, ICD therapy now poses a new series of clinical challenges.

Table 1. Areas for improvement in ICD technology — as discussed in relevant chapters.

Improvement Area	Potential Impact	Chapter
Defibrillation Waveforms	Lower DFT, implying ICD size reduction	4, 6
Leads	Increased reliability, ease of insertion, and lower DFT, implying reduced ICD size	9
Battery	Increased lifetime, decreased ICD size	10
Capacitor	Decreased ICD size	11
Sensing/Detection	Fewer inappropriate shocks	14, 15, 19

Clarification of Clinical Role of ICD Therapy

A critical question regarding ICD therapy is whether it is capable of conferring a measurable increase in the survival of patients with sustained ventricular tachyarrhythmias, individuals many of whom face a high mortality simply on the basis of the severity of their underlying cardiac disease.[1] To address this question, a number of randomized clinical trials are already underway, including the Canadian Implantable Defibrillator Study (CIDS),[2] Antiarrhythmics vs. Implantable Defibrillator (AVID),[2,3] Cardiac Arrest Study Hamburg (CASH),[4] CABG-Patch[5]. Results of these studies should become available over the next few years and, despite some methodological limitations,[6] are likely to provide some useful scientific information regarding the clinical value of ICD therapy. The preliminary results from MADIT (Multicenter Automatic Defibrillator Implantation Trial) suggest an important role for the ICD as a pro-

Table 2. Suggested actuarial-based approach for determining the role of ICD therapy.*

Patient Group	Estimated 4-yr Cumulative Incidence of Sudden Death *Without* ICD Therapy	Relative Protection from Sudden Death vs. Other Therapies
Very high risk	≥ 20%	Definitely superior.
Moderately high risk	10-20%	Generally superior, but patient subgroups most likely to benefit need to better defined.
Low risk	≤10%	Comparable to other therapies.

* For survivors of sustained VT or VF. Assumes that patients are in NYHA functional class I-III and have sufficient compliance to permit adequate ICD followup.

phylactic modality in low ejection fraction coronary patients with only nonsustained VT.[7,8]

While such studies will address the broad issue of survival in recipients of ICD therapy, more specific information will be required to aid physicians in *clinical decision making* regarding the use of the ICD as a treatment modality. Table 2 depicts the type of quantitative-actuarial framework that might serve as the basis for developing the needed management guidelines. In this schema patients are divided into 3 basic groups according to whether the results of ICD therapy are equivalent, of still undefined relationship, or superior to outcome with alternative (medical) therapy. The endpoint chosen in Table 2 is the cumulative sudden death mortality at 4 years, although other types of endpoints may be substituted for different clinical purposes. On the assumption that the ICD can be considered a "gold standard" for aborting sudden death resulting from sustained ventricular tachyarrhythmias, the strata in the Table, in effect, define 3 levels of risk. Assignment of a given patient to one of the 3 risk categories in Table 2 would be dependent upon a constellation of clinical variables, such as listed in Table 3.

A desirable future goal in the ICD therapy field would be to accumulate a sufficiently large body of data that would permit the clinician to determine risk (and, thus, treatment) category assignment in Table 2 as a function of the particular configuration of clinical variables listed in Table 3 for that patient. Sources for the needed clinical database could be derived from randomized clinical trials as well as observational studies, for both ICD and non-ICD therapies. Observational data, collected with regard to more specific patient subsets (in keeping with the clinical decision-making schema just outlined) with respect to outcome with ICD therapy have been reported for cardiac arrest survivors[9,10] and, even more specifically, survivors of ventricular fibrillation in the setting of idiopathic dilated cardiomyopathy,[11] atherosclerotic heart disease,[12] or no underlying heart disease ("primary" ventricular fibrillation).[13]

Table 3. Clinical inputs to decision-making regarding use of ICD therapy.

Age
Noncardiac co-morbidity
Underlying heart disease (if present)
    Type (coronary artery disease, dilated cardiomyopathy, other)
    Extent of treatment optimization
Left ventricular function
    Ejection fraction
    NYHA functional class
Presenting tachyarrhythmia
    Type (Sustained VT, VF, nonsustained VT, not documented [e.g., syncope])
    Maximum associated symptom severity (Table 4)
Results of electrophysiologic testing
    Inducible sustained VT or VF
    How induced [number of extrastimuli], vs. noninducible
Prior arrhythmia therapy history

VT = ventricular tachycardia, VF = ventricular fibrillation.

Table 4. Four-tier system for grading the severity of ventricular tachyarrhythmia symptoms.*

Class I	Asymptomatic or symptoms limited to palpitations or fluttering.
Class II	Lightheadedness, dizziness, chest pain, or dyspnea.
Class III	Syncope or altered mental status or other evidence of significant secondary end-organ dysfunction (including pulmonary edema, acute myocardial infarction, low-output state, or stroke).
Class IV	Cardiac arrest (absent pulse or respiration).

* It is assumed that the tachyarrhythmias are documented, ideally by ECG recordings, or at least attested to by medical or paraprofessional personnel.

Relevant data have also been reported regarding outcomes of medically or device-treated patients with sustained monomorphic ventricular tachycardia, according to the presence or absence of hemodynamic tolerance,[14-16] suggesting that, indeed, arrhythmia symptom severity (e.g., Classes III or IV vs. I or II, Table 4) represents an independent risk factor for sudden death. Continued efforts along these lines will help to define better those patient subsets most likely to benefit from ICD therapy.

Parallel developments which so far appear encouraging,[17,18] are underway to assess cost-effectiveness of ICD vs. other treatment modalities in high risk patients.

Role of the Atrial ICD

With the high incidence of stroke and embolization, atrial fibrillation is widely appreciated as an important health problem.[19,20] The limited success of antiarrhythmic drugs for atrial fibrillation has spurred work in nonpharmacological therapies. High treatment costs are also driving new therapy research.[21] The most promising nonpharmacological therapies at this time are radio frequency (RF) ablation and the atrial ICD. The RF ablation approach, still in its infancy, is focused on long linear lesions and has achieved mixed results.[22,23]

Internal atrial defibrillation is occasionally used in an acute setting in patients refractory to transthoracic cardioversion.[24] Animal (primarily sheep) studies have demonstrated the safety and efficacy of defibrillating the atrium with moderate energy shocks synchronized to the ventricular R-wave.[25]

Clinical studies using temporarily implanted leads have shown the efficacy of atrial defibrillation with endocardial leads.[26,27] Unfortunately, in one study, ventricular tachycardias were occasionally induced in spite of careful synchronization to the R-wave.[26] However, withholding the shock during R-waves with a short preceding interval may eliminate the VT induction.[27] This, unfortunately, might preclude shocking an atrial fibrillation which is conducting at a very fast rates to the ventricles. Another limitation is that patients may find shocks with energies over 1 or 2 joules to be painful.[26,27] The pain problem could be a significant factor in the clinical acceptance of the atrial ICD as the average atrial DFTs (using biphasic waveforms) are reported in the range of 8-10 joules.[26,28,29] Clinical trials of the Metrix device underway, and sponsored by InControl of Seattle, Washington should resolve many of these issues.

Optimization of Implant Techniques

With the advent of a nonthoracotomy ICD system, perioperative mortality has been significantly reduced. However, this technologic improvement should not allow implanting physicians to become complacent about the implant process. Even with nonthoracotomy lead systems, ICD-related infections and lead problems (as discussed in Chaps. 9, 18, 21) continue to be significant problems not only related to morbidity of reoperation and extended hospitalization but also because they impair quality of life and expose the patient to an increased risk of sudden death. The latter may result from lack of protection against tachyarrhythmia recurrence following ICD system explantation in the case of infection or failed defibrillation or ICD-mediated proarrhythmia in the case of lead problems.[30-32]

Greater attention will need to be focused upon pre-, intra- and post-operative phases of ICD implantation to institute measures most likely to prevent *infection* during ICD implantation or generator replacement. Consideration might also be given toward viewing device recipients, long term, as individuals deserving of prophylactic antibiotics prior to their undergoing dental or medical procedures that could predispose to bacteremia and, conceivably, intravascular, ICD lead infection. (See Chap. 18 for more detailed discussion)

Lead and connection problems are potentially catastrophic to the ICD patient. Even when they are fortunate enough to be recognized during followup, however, the corrective measure of lead revision is a potentially major undertaking, particularly if extraction of a transvenous integrated (large diameter) sensing/defibrillation lead is required. Clinical data are needed to quantify the morbidity and mortality risks associated with extraction of the latter type of lead. Also deserving of further study is the identification of certain implant techniques to reduce the risk of lead fracture, e.g., use of the cephalic vein or a more anterolateral percutaneous approach (near the lateral border of the first rib) for lead insertion into the subclavian vein.[33] Clinical guidelines also need to be developed for the followup phase to help define appropriate intervals for serial chest X-rays to aid in early identification of potential defibrillation lead/electrode problems.[34-36]

Reducing Regulatory Hurdles

Critical to progress in the ICD field will be the ability of companies to introduce innovative products to the market place in a timely fashion. Until recently, however, governmental review and approval processes related to new ICD systems have proven painfully slow, a problem with medical device approvals in general.[37] These delays have reached the point that investment capital necessary for medical product development and release is becoming increasingly scarce, with a concomitantly greater proportion of new device development and testing being conducted abroad.

Efforts to streamline the approval process clearly need to be accelerated. Recommendations to achieve this goal have been published by a broad based working group of investigators from U.S. and European Cardiological Societies.[38] The rapidity of FDA approvals of the recent crop of fourth generation ICDs as well as the "MADIT"-type indication for device therapy are encouraging signs.[39]

Legislative efforts are underway to help focus the regulatory mandate of the United States FDA and to achieve reforms in the area of medical malpractice, whose ever-present specter exerts a powerful drag on the pace of the approval process.

Rapid Access to Performance Information

Given the engineering/clinical intricacies of ICD function and the ever expanding technical sophistication and complexity of these devices, optimal management the ICD patient necessitates that physicians have up-to-the-minute, state of the art information regarding the performance of various ICDs and related lead systems. It has become increasingly clear, however, that the traditional professional medical educational vehicles, i.e., presentations at national meetings and peer reviewed published manuscripts, are inherently slow, engendering considerable delays in dissemination of evolving knowledge in the ICD field. Such a lag in availability of relevant information in a timely manner was evident recently in the controversy regarding post failed-shock sensing by a "hybrid" third generation ICD/integrated transvenous lead system;[40] and in the prolonged time to appearance of scientific information regarding the risks of tachyarrhythmia underdetection associated with use of the "stability" criterion, (Chaps. 15, 21) despite the clinical availability of this tachycardia detection "enhancement" for several years.[41,42]

It would be highly desirable, therefore, to have a common computer-based repository of ICD-related clinical/engineering information and observations *as such knowledge is generated*, available to all interested. The Internet would seem to provide a logical medium for such a rapid access information storage/retrieval system.

Such a broadened post-market release surveillance mechanism might also incorporate the activities of working groups brought together by a common desire to evaluate various aspects of ICD therapy that may not have been fully addressed during the premarket approval trials. Such areas might include performance of various hybrid ICD systems and quantitation of sensitivities and specificities of various tachyarrhythmia detection and discrimination algorithms.

ACKNOWLEDGMENTS:
Table 4 first appeared in the American Journal of Cardiology.[43]

1.   Sweeney MO, Ruskin JN. Mortality benefits and the implantable cardioverter-

defibrillator. Circulation 1994;89:1851-1858.

2. Greene HL. Antiarrhythmic drugs versus implantable defibrillators: the need for a randomized controlled study. Am Heart J 1993;127:1171-1178.

3. AVID Investigators. Antiarrhythmics versus implantable defibrillators (AVID)—rationale, design, and methods. Am J Cardiol 1995;75:470-475.

4. Siebels J, Kuck KH. Implantable cardioverter defibrillator compared with antiarrhythmic drug treatment in cardiac arrest survivors (the cardiac arrest study Hamburg). Am Heart J 1994;127:1139-1144.

5. Bigger JT. Future studies with the implantable cardioverter defibrillator. PACE 1991;14:883-889.

6. Fogoros RN, An AVID dissent. PACE 1994;17:1707-1711. (Comment in PACE 1994;17:1712-1713)

7. MADIT Executive Committee. Multicenter automatic defibrillator implantation trial (MADIT): design and clinical protocol. PACE 1991;14:920-927.

8. Moss AJ. Influence of the implantable cardioverter defibrillator on survival: retrospective studies and prospective trials. Prog Cardiovasc Dis 1993;36;85-88.

9. Powell AC, Fuchs T, Finkelstein DM, et al. Influence of implantable cardioverter-defibrillators on the long-term prognosis of survivors of out-of-hospital cardiac arrest. Circulation 1993;88:1083-1092.

10. Dolack GL for the CASCADE Investigators. Clinical predictors of implantable cardioverter-defibrillator shocks (Results of the CASCADE trial). Am J Cardiol 1994;7:27-241.

11. Lessmeier TJ, Lehmann MH, Steinman RT, et al. Outcome with implantable cardioverter-defibrillator therapy for survivors of ventricular fibrillation secondary to idiopathic dilated cardiomyopathy or coronary artery disease without myocardial infarction. Am J Cardiol 1993;72:911-915.

12. Lessmeier TJ, Lehmann MH, Steinman RT, et al. Implantable cardioverter-defibrillator therapy in 300 patients with coronary artery disease presenting exclusively with ventricular fibrillation. Am Heart J 1994;128:211-218.

13. Meissner MD, Lehmann MH, Steinman RT, et al. Ventricular fibrillation in patients without significant structural heart disease: A multicenter experience with implantable cardioverter-defibrillator therapy. J Am Coll Cardiol 1993;21:1406-1412

14. Steinman RT, Lehmann MH, Zheutlin T et al. Long term outcome of electophysiologically-guided therapy for hemodynamically-tolerated sustained ventricular tachycardias in coronary artery disease. J Am Coll Cardiol 1990;15:12A. (abstract)

15. LeClerq JF, Leenhardt A, Ruta I, et al. Esperance de vie apres une premiere crise de tachycardie ventriculaire monomorphie soutenue. Arch Mal Couer 1991;84:1789-1796.

16. Bhatt D, Kopp D, Kall J, et al. Influence of clinical presentation on survival in patients with sustained ventricular arrhythmias. PACE 1995;18:883. (abstract)

17. Kuppermann M, Luce BR, McGovern B, et al. An analysis of the cost effectiveness of the implantable defibrillator. Circulation 1990;81:91-100.

18. Wever EF, Hauer RNW, Schrijvers G, et al. Cost-effectiveness of implantable defibrillator as first-choice therapy versus electrophysiologically guided, tiered strategy in postinfarct sudden death survivors: a randomized study. Circulation 1996;93:489-496.

19. Kerr CR. Atrial fibrillation: the next frontier. PACE 1994;17:1203-1207.

20. Lüderitz B, Pfeiffer D, Tebbenjohanns, et al. Nonpharmacologic strategies for treating atrial fibrillation. Am J Cardiol 1996;77:45A-52A.

21. Roberts SA, Diaz C, Nolan PE, et al. Effectiveness and costs of digoxin treatment of atrial fibrillation and flutter. Am J Cardiol 1993;72:567-573.

22. Man KC, Daoud E, Knight B, et al. Right atrial radio frequency catheter ablation of paroxysmal atrial fibrillation. J Am Coll Cardiol 1996;27:188A.

(abstract)

23. Nakagawa H, Yamanashi WS, Pitha JV, et al. Creation of long linear transmural radiofrequency lesions in atrium using a novel spiral ribbon-saline irrigated electrode catheter. J Am Coll Cardiol 1996;27:188A. (abstract)

24. Baker BM, Botteron GW, Smith JM. Low energy internal cardioversion for atrial fibrillation resistant to external cardioversion. J Cardiovasc Electrophysiol 1995;6:44-47.

25. Levy S, Richard P. Is there any indication for an intracardiac defibrillator for the treatment of atrial fibrillation. J Cardiovasc Electrophysiol 1994;5:982-985.

26. Saksena S, Prakash A, Mangeon L, et al. Clinical efficacy and safety of atrial defibrillation using biphasic shocks and current nonthoracotomy endocardial lead configurations. Am J Cardiol 1995;76:913-921.

27. Hillsley RE, Wharton JM. Implantable atrial defibrillators. J Cardiovasc Electrophysiol 1995;6:634-648.

28. Jung W, Pfeiffer D, Wolpert C, et al. Which patients do benefit from an implantable atrial defibrillator? J Am Coll Cardiol 1996;27:301A-302A. (abstract)

29. Poole JE, Kudenchuk PJ, Dolack GL, et al. Atrial defibrillation using a unipolar, single lead right ventricular to pectoral can system. J Am Coll Cardiol 1995;25:110A. (abstract)

30. Winkle R, Mead R, Ruder M, et al. Long-term outcome with the automatic implantable cardioverter-defibrillator. J Am Coll Cardiol 1989;13:1353-1361.

31 Marchlinski FE, Flores BT, Buxton AE, et al. The automatic implantable defibrillator: efficacy, complications, and device failures. Ann Intern Med 1986;104:481-488.

32. Jones GK, Bardy GH, Kudenchuk PJ, et al. Mechanical complications following implantation of multiple lead nonthoracotomy defibrillator systems: Implications for management and future system design. Am Heart J 1995;130:327-333.

33. Magney JE, Staplin DH, Flynn DM, et al. A new approach to percutaneous subclavian venipuncture to avoid lead fracture or central venous catheter occlusion. PACE 1993;16:2133-2142.

34. Schwartzman D, Nallamothu N, Callans DJ, et al. Postoperative lead-related complications in patients with nonthoracotomy defibrillation lead systems. J Am Coll Cardiol 1995;26:776-786.

35. Drucker EA, Brooks R, Garan H, et al. Malfunction of implantable cardioverter defibrillators placed by a nonthoracotomy approach: frequency of malfunction and value of chest radiography in determining cause. Am J Roentgenol 1995;165:275-279.

36. Korte T, Jung W, Spehl S, et al. Incidence of ICD lead related complications during long-term followup: comparison of epicardial and endocardial electrode systems. PACE 1995;18:2053-2061.

37. Review & Outlook: Kessler's Devices. Wall Street J Feb. 10 1993:A12.

38. Saksena S, Epstein AE, Lazzara R. Clinical investigation of antiarrhythmic devices. Circulation 1995;91:2097-2109.

39. Leary WE. FDA gives quick approval to new uses for heart device. NY Times, May 17, 1996, p A6.

40. Lehmann MH. Hybrid nonthoracotomy ICD systems: lessons from the brouhaha. PACE 1994;17:1802-1807.

41. Swerdlow CD, Ahern T, Chen P et al. Underdetection of ventricular tachycardia by algorithms to enhance specificity in a tiered-therapy cardioverter-defibrillator. J Am Coll Cardiol 1994;24:416-424.

42. Swerdlow CD, Chen P, Kass, RM et al. Discrimination of ventricular tachycardia from sinus tachycardia and atrial fibrillation in a tiered-therapy cardioverter-defibrillator. J Am Coll Cardiol 1994;23:1342-1355.

43. Lehmann MH, Steinman RT, Meissner MD, et al. Need for a standardized approach to grading symptoms associated with ventricular tachyarrhythmias Am J Cardiol 1991;67:1421-1423.

Glossary

For unfamiliar explanatory terms used below, please consult the Index or the Glossary itself.

1CNT. Counter for lower VT zone in PRx.

1S. Single energy, single shock defibrillation threshold protocol.

2CNT. Counter for upper VT zone in PRx.

2S. Single energy, double shock defibrillation threshold protocol.

3CNT. Counter for VF zone in PRx.

3S. Single energy, triple shock defibrillation threshold protocol.

AC. Alternating current.

accordion bursts. Bursts from ATP with alternating incremental and decremental scanning.

ACNT. Counter for lower VT zone in Cadence.

action potential. The time course of the transmembrane voltage seen during electrical activation of the myocardium. Chap. 3 Fig. 1 illustrates the basic features of the cardiac action potential.

adapter. An implanted terminal block which may be required to mate replacement pulse generators to existing lead implants, mate lead/pulse generator combinations not designed by the same company nor intended to work together, or tie electrode combinations (e.g. SVC and subcutaneous patch) together as a common electrode.

adaptive burst. The rate of each ATP burst is calculated based on the rate of the VT being treated.

Aegis. Pacesetter ICD model.

AF. Atrial fibrillation.

AGC. Automatic gain control .

Ah. Ampere hour (unit of battery charge equal to 3600 coulombs).

algorithm. Decision rule (for detection in the case of the ICD) For example, rhythm onset and stability applied to the cycle length sequence.

algorithm. Decision rule.

amiodarone. A Class III agent with broad antiarrhythmic action and extremely long half life.

ampere. Unit of current equal to the flow rate of 1 coulomb per second.

amplifier. In general—a circuit that is capable of increasing the amplitude of a given signal. In the ICD it is the circuitry which senses R-wave and marks each occurrence with a digital pulse suitable for rate counting by other circuitry.

ARP. Absolute refractory period.

array electrode system. Subcutaneous electrode set consisting of two or three (e.g., three 20.5 cm long coils covering an area of about 150 cm^2).

ASIC. Application Specific Integrated Circuit—"custom" IC.

ATC. Automatic threshold control.

ATP. Antitachycardia pacing.

atrial fibrillation. A rapid (> 300 BPM) disorganized rhythm originating in the atria and conducting erratically through the AV node, yielding a very irregular ventricular response.

atrium. upper cardiac chamber (right or left).

audio transducer. See beeper

autodecremental ramp. ATP approach which produces bursts that have progressively decreasing intra-burst intervals after the first interval.

automatic gain control. Amplifier gain is increased when the signal amplitude falls.

automatic threshold control. Comparator threshold level is decreased when the electrogram signal amplitude falls—also know as ASC (automatic sensitivity control).

AV node. Conduction tissue situated at the junction between the atria and ventricles. In the absence of any disease or drug effects, transmits impulses in 1-to-1 fashion from atria to ventricles during sinus rhythm (albeit with some physiologic delay). However, may conduct only intermittently during pathologically rapid atrial rhythms (e.g., atrial fibrillation).

AV. Atrio-ventricular.

AVID. Antiarrhythmics Versus Implantable Defibrillators trial.

background current. Also known as monitoring, sensing, overhead, or idle current. This is what the ICD circuitry consumes continuously in the absence of any therapy delivery.

bandwidth. The range of frequencies over which the amplifier can accurately reproduce the signal (specifically, the difference between the high and low frequencies).

baseline voltage drift. The slow change in the average voltage impressed upon the electrogram by the electrode/electrolyte interface. Also referred to as baseline offset.

BCL. Basic (also, burst) cycle length.

BCNT. Counter for upper VT zone in Cadence.

beeper. Audio transducer in ICD for aural signaling to patient or physician.

beepograms. Phonocardiogram of ICD beeper output.

biphasic. Waveform with a distinct positive and negative portion.

BJT. Bipolar Junction Transistor: a type of electronic switch used in the amplifier and output circuit of the ICD.

blanking of amplifier input. Temporarily shorting of the inputs together to prevent disruption of the sense amplifiers during a shock.

blanking period. Time following sensed event, etc. during which sensing is not allowed. Similar to refractory period.

BPM. Beats per minute.

burping theory. An explanation for the mechanism of the biphasic defibrillation waveform which holds that the function of the second (negative) phase is to remove (i.e. "burp") the excess charge left on the cell membrane by the first (positive) phase.

burst pacing. The most common form of ATP which delivers multiple stimuli at a fixed cycle length between 50% and 100% of the tachycardia cycle length.

burst plus PES. ATP burst pacing method of adding 1 or more PES at the end of each burst, and scanning the PES coupling interval to the last pulse in the burst.

Cadence. Ventritex ICD model.

Cadet. Ventritex ICD model.

capacitance. Unit which measures capacitor charge storage ability for a given voltage.

cardioversion. Use of shock (external or via ICD) to terminate VT or atrial tachyarrhythmia; shock strength is typically lower than that for VF.

carrier frequency. Underlying radio frequency that carries the telemetered data.

CAST. Cardiac Arrhythmia Suppression Trial.

cell (electrical). A single chamber "battery;" a battery is technically only 2 or more cells.

centrifugal scanning. ATP with alternating incremental and decremental scanning bursts.

ceramic capacitor. One using a solid ceramic material for the dielectric.

charge time. The time required to bring the energy storage capacitors to a full charge in order to deliver a therapeutic shock; normally ranges from 5-18 seconds. Equal to:

$$\frac{desired\ stored\ energy + unformed\ capacitor\ losses}{(battery\ power) \bullet (inverter\ efficiency\ [\%])}$$

charging circuit. Circuitry which converts the 3-6 V typically available from the battery to the much higher voltage (usually up to 750 V) for a defibrillation shock.

charging voltage. Also called loaded voltage; represents the battery voltage during charging of the high voltage capacitors and is lower than the open circuit (or unloaded) voltage.

check characters. Uniquely matching characters generated by mathematical formulas from number theory which are used to verify the authenticity and reliability of the telemetry message to and from the ICD.

chronaxie. That duration which requires a doubling of the rheobase current in order to cause a stimulation or defibrillation.

CL. Cycle length, i.e., time between two successive depolarizations in a given cardiac chamber. (Also, statistical Confidence Limits.)

class IA agents. Sodium blocking anti-arrhythmic drugs which also slightly prolong cardiac action potential.

class IB agents. Sodium blocking anti-arrhythmic drugs which also slightly shorten or do not affect cardiac action potential.

class IC agents. Sodium blocking anti-arrhythmic drugs which primarily slow conduction without prolonging the cardiac action potential.

class III agents. Potassium blocking anti-arrhythmic drugs which primarily prolong cardiac action potential.

CLAVE. Average of the last four cycle lengths in Cadence and PRx.

clipping. Amplifier distortion in which the output attains an extremum value (minimum or maximum) and stays level at that value until the input returns to a more moderate value.

committed shock. Delivery of the shock after charging has begun, irrespective of tachyarrhythmia persistence or spontaneous termination.

comparator. A circuit element which produces a digital pulse when an input signal exceeds a preset reference voltage.

composite duration specification. Tilt followed by a fixed time extension.

composite wire. Sophisticated wires combining the conductivity of silver, or other low resistance metals with Stainless Steel (SS), MP35N (an alloy of Nickel, Cobalt, Chromium and Molybdenum), Titanium (Ti) or other high strength metal to obtain strong low resistance wire. e.g., Drawn Brazed Strand (DBS) or Drawn Filled Tube (DFT).

concertina bursts. Bursts from ATP with alternating incremental and decremental scanning.

corners of defibrillation success curve. (lower and upper) Shock amplitudes corresponding to approximately 1 and 99% defibrillation success, respectively.

coulomb. Unit of charge equal to 6×10^{18} electrons.

CPBP. Cardiopulmonary bypass pump.

critical mass hypothesis. Theory that eliminating most or all fibrillation wavefronts by stimulating excitable myocardium will cause defibrillation.

crush injury. Lead fractures caused by mechanical stresses in the region of the costoclavicular joint.

CS. Coronary sinus, especially an electrode in this cardiac venous structure.

current limiting resistor. Limits current flowing through the "truncation SCR" which rapidly discharges the energy storage capacitor in the monophasic Schuder circuit. This current limiting resistor (2-4 Ω) also helps to protect against a short on the patient leads.

current density. Current per cross sectional area. Typically expressed as amperes per cm^2.

curve width. The energy difference between the upper and lower "corners" of a defibrillation success curve.

DBS. Drawn Brazed Strand: lead conductor of high strength wire surrounding a silver core (for low resistance).

DC electrode offset voltage. Voltage generated by the electrochemical action of the electrode metal being in contact with the physiological electrolytes. Synonymous with baseline offset.

DC/DC converter. See charging circuit or inverter.

DDD. Pacing mode of dual chamber (atrial and ventricular) pacing and sensing, with inhibition of pacing in either chamber by a sensed rate above a programmed value.

decremental burst pacing. The second ATP burst cycle length is slightly faster than the first burst.

decremental ramp. ATP approach which produces bursts that have progressively decreasing intra-burst intervals after the first interval. Also called autodecremental.

decremental scanning. A form of ATP in which a programmed extrastimulus pulse is moved progressively closer to the previous systolic event.

defibrillation success curve. Plot of the probability of defibrillation vs. the shock energy.

defibrillation. Abolition of VF with the application of an electrical shock.

delivered energy. Energy delivered during a shock. Specific definition depends on the point of measurement. For example, the energy delivered from the capacitor with a biphasic shock is about 95% of the stored energy and thus essentially identical to the stored. However, the energy delivered "into" the heart (i.e., more than 1 mm past the electrodes) can be as low as 10% of the stored energy. While very popular, the usage has no physiological basis and has no consistent definition.

delta. A change in cycle length requirement which must be met before a rhythm can be declared as having a sudden onset or abrupt cycle length change.

depolarization. Electrical activation of cardiac muscle; responsible for generating intra- (and extra-)cardiac signal that can be amplified and sensed by the ICD.

detection. The processing of sensed depolarizations and noting the presence of an arrhythmia.

device based testing. Testing detection and defibrillation directly via the ICD during implantation; obviates the ECD (also called DSA or DTS).

DF-, DF+. The primary defibrillation cathode and anode connection, respectively.

DF-1. A new connector standard (also known as ISO-11318) The objective of this standard, modeled after the IS-1 pacemaker connector standard, is to ensure dimensional interchangeability of DF-1 leads and pulse generators from different manufacturers.

DFT wire. Drawn Filled Tube lead conductor of high strength wire surrounding a silver core (for low resistance).

DFT++. Defibrillation threshold confirmed by two additional shocks at the DFT energy.

DFT+. Defibrillation threshold confirmed by an additional shock at the DFT energy.

DFT. Defibrillation threshold. The "standard DFT" is measured using progressively decreasing or increasing energies during fibrillation-defibrillation testing cycles to determine the minimum energy producing defibrillation success.

dielectric constant. The measure of ability of a given insulator to store charge in a capacitor application.

dielectric strength. The maximum electrical field which an insulator or dielectric can withstand.

dielectric. Gap or insulation between the two conductors of a capacitor.

diode. Electronic component which passes current in only one direction; analogous to the aortic valve and classically (at least in England) actually referred to as "valve."

discharge curve. (for battery) The voltage as a function of time. Constantly changing chemical composition of the cathode as the cell reaction proceeds result in changes in the energetics of the reaction. This phenomenon leads to plateaus at various voltages and a general gradual decline in the voltage as discharge proceeds over time.

double counting. Sensing (counting) T-waves (or P-waves or pacemaker stimulus artifact) in addition to R-waves, resulting in an apparent rate doubling with simulation of "tachycardia."

double layer capacitor. Liquid based capacitor using electrolyte polarization to store charge.

dropout. The "disappearance" of a signal (usually a depolarization) due to physiological, lead, amplifier, or combination problems.

DSA. Defibrillation system analyzer. Synonymous with DTS and ECD.

DTS. Defibrillation test system. Synonymous with DSA and ECD.

dynamic range. Ratio of the maximum input level to the minimum input level in an amplifier.

E_1. Shock energy having only a 1% probability of defibrillating a given heart; also called the "lower corner" of the defibrillation success curve.

E_{99}. Shock energy having a 99% probability of defibrillating a given heart; also called the "upper corner" of the defibrillation success curve.

ECD. External Cardioverter Defibrillator: instrument used to determine the defibrillation threshold. Also called DSA (Defibrillation System Analyzer) or DTS (Defibrillation Test System).

ECG. Electrocardiogram. (Also abbreviated EKG.)

effective Current. The maximum rheobase current which a given pulse can satisfy.

efficacy margin. The extent to which the energy margin overestimates the safety margin.

EGM. Electrogram.

EHR. Extended High Rate (see SRD).

E_{ICD}. ICD shock energy programmed from the device.

ejection fraction. Proportion of blood volume in heart which is ejected with each contraction.

electric field. The voltage difference per distance, e.g., volts per centimeter. Also called potential gradient.

electrogram width. Width of the QRS complex which may be measured to distinguish between supraventricular tachycardias (presumably normal width) and VTs (greater width).

electrogram. Intracardiac electrical signals corresponding to cardiac activity. Internal equivalent to surface ECG.

electrolytic capacitor. One using an electrolyte solution. Employed in current ICDs.

EMD. Electromechanical dissociation: lack of correspondence between the electrical and contractile behavior of the heart.

EMI. Electromagnetic interference—includes radio frequency interference but also lower frequencies such as 60 Hz power line interference.

end of service. See EOL.

Endotak. Guidant/CPI lead model.

energy margin. Margin between device output energy and measured defibrillation threshold (E_{ICD}-DFT). Includes the (true) safety margin and an efficacy margin.

EOL. End of life voltage for a cell (battery). If this voltage is reached, the ICD may no longer be capable of functioning within specification or may be incapable of any useful function.

ERI. Elective replacement indicator. Typically a voltage measurement suggesting that the ICD battery is nearing the end of life.

ESR; equivalent series resistance. The amount of internal impedance in a voltage source (e.g. battery or capacitor) as expressed by the value of resistance which would have to placed in series with an ideal voltage source. This "ESR" reflects the decrease in output voltage from the connection of a load to the voltage source. Also called internal series resistance.

farad. Unit of capacitance—measures the ability of a capacitor to store charge as defined as the ratio of the charge (in coulombs) to the voltage.

FDI. Fibrillation detection interval. Intervals shorter than this are considered to be in the fibrillation zone.

feedthrus. Provide a conduit for electrical current from the internal circuitry to the header and leads without allowing fluid passage. Typically constructed of ceramic.

film capacitor. One made by depositing aluminum on a thin plastic film (e.g. Mylar). The aluminum forms the conductor and the plastic is the dielectric.

filtering. (Electrical) To remove (more accurately—attenuate) or accentuate various frequencies in a signal.

final voltage. Voltage (V_f) at end of pulse. Also called trailing edge voltage.

fixed burst. The rate of each ATP burst is a fixed predetermined value regardless of the rate of the VT being treated.

flyback transformer. The transformer used in an ICD charging circuit; gets its name from the fact that it delivers power through the secondary winding only during the collapse of the magnetic field—which occurs when the primary current is removed. When this happens, the secondary voltage abruptly changes polarity—or "flies back."

forming capacitor. See reforming.

FU. Followup.

FVT. Fast ventricular tachycardia. A VT which lies in the upper VT zone (between the VT and VF zone). Medtronic terminology.

gain. Amplifier output voltage divided by input voltage

Guardian. Telectronics ICD model.

H-Bridge. Biphasic waveform circuitry allowing the reversal of the direction of the voltage and current through the heart. This circuit is referred to as an "H" bridge due to the shape of the four required electronic switches and two heart connections.

half-cell potential of electrode. Voltage developed by electrode metal from being in the physiological electrolytes.

header. Block of plastic which provides the electrical and physical interface terminal blocks between the leads and the pulse generator circuitry for an ICD.

henry. Unit of inductance—measures the ability of an inductor to store energy in a magnetic field for a given electrical current.

hermetic enclosure. One that provides environmental protection (physical and fluid) to the internal electrical components. Hermeticity of the ICD is required to prevent fluid passage into the electronic assembly, which could cause corrosion of the circuitry and components as was common with epoxy potted pacemakers.

high-pass filter. Passes the high frequency and blocks the low frequency components of a signal.

holding current. The minimum current required to keep a SCR on after it has been triggered.

HV interval. His-ventricle interval.

hysteresis. A difference in system response depending on the direction of the input value changes. I.e. the system responds differently to a given input value depending upon whether or not the value was arrived at from increasing or decreasing.

ICD. Implantable cardioverter defibrillator. (Also includes, in this book, the earlier "shock-only boxes.")

idle current. See monitoring or background current.

IGBT. Insulated gate bipolar transistor, a hybrid of the BJT and the MOSFET, used in many biphasic output circuits.

impedance. The ratio of voltage across to the current through an electrical component.

incremental ramp. ATP approach which produces bursts that increase in cycle length progressively after the first interval.

inductance. The ability of an inductor to store energy in a magnetic field for a given electrical current. Also represents the ability of an inductor to inhibit high frequency signals.

input referred threshold. The comparator voltage reference divided by the amplifier gain. Gives the depolarization signal amplitude which would be required for sensing.

INR. International normalized ratio for prothrombin time (a measure of blood coagulability).

internal parallel resistance. The leakage resistance inside a battery or capacitor which continuously drains energy.

internal series resistance. The resistance inside a battery or capacitor which is in series with the output; this is what lowers the output voltage under load and is why the loaded voltage is lower than the unloaded voltage. Also called "equivalent series resistance."

intra-burst step size. The amount of change from interval to interval within an ATP incremental or decremental ramp burst.

inverter. Generates the 750 V for capacitor charging from the 3-6 V battery. Also known as DC-DC converter or charging circuit.

ischemia. Inadequate blood flow to an organ—especially to the heart where it is caused by blocked or narrowed coronary arteries.

Jewel. Medtronic ICD model.

jitter. Timing variability in sensing due to R-wave shape variability.

joule. The energy of a pulse of one volt and one ampere lasting one second. Is also about 1/4 of a calorie.

leading edge voltage. The initial voltage of a pulse (V_i). Also called peak voltage or charge voltage with present (single capacitor) waveforms since the leading edge (first) voltage is always the highest.

leakage current. Undesired (parasitic) current flows. May occur internal to the battery or capacitor. Can also occur through lead insulation.

LI. Lithium iodine. pacemaker battery chemistry.

LiSVO. Lithium Silver Vanadium Oxide: present ICD battery chemistry. Is not used in Intermedics Res-Q I.

LiVO. Lithium Vanadium Oxide: original ICD battery chemistry.

loaded voltage. The voltage of a cell (battery) while under a significant load. This is equal to the open circuit voltage less the voltage lost across the internal series resistance.

long QT syndrome. Inherited or acquired prolongation of myocardial electrical recovery; is evidenced by excessive time interval from onset of the QRS to end of T-wave. May lead to VT of torsades de pointes type.

low-pass filter. Passes low frequency and blocks high frequency components of a signal.

MADIT. Multicenter automatic defibrillator implantation trial.

Metrix. Atrial ICD being developed by InControl.

MI. Myocardial infarction.

mil. One thousandth of an inch.

Mini. Guidant/CPI ICD model.

MODE. Methoxy o-dimethyl encainide.

monitoring current. Also known as background, sensing, overhead, or idle current. This is what the ICD circuitry consumes continuously in the absence of any therapy delivery.

monitoring voltage. Also known as open circuit voltage. This is the voltage on the battery in the absence of any therapy delivery.

monomorphic. Descriptor for wide QRS tachycardia (commonly, but not exclusively, VT) in which intracardiac (or surface) electrograms exhibit a beat-to-beat uniform morphology.

monophasic. Waveform with a single polarity of the voltage.

monotonic therapy aggression. Under this tactic therapy provided by an ICD will not revert to lower energy shocks (or back to antitachycardia pacing) during a single episode of VT even if the rate is reduced (say, by conversion to a slower VT) to place it in a lower zone. Thus, a shock could be provided in such a case even though antitachycardia pacing might normally be delivered as a first line therapy for a VT of the same rate (had it begun de novo).

MOSFET. Metal Oxide Semiconductor Field Effect Transistor: electronic switch used in amplifier and some biphasic output circuits.

MP35N. A low resistance proprietary alloy of Nickel, Cobalt, Chromium and Molybdenum which is used in defibrillation lead conductors.

myocardial infarction. Death of heart tissue from deprivation of normal blood supply due to clot or chronic arterial narrowing.

NAPA. N-acetylprocainamide.

negative safety margin. Phenomenon in which a higher energy pulse is less efficacious than a lower energy pulse.

NID. Number of intervals for detection.

NIPS. Noninvasive programmed stimulation: an ICD mode which allows the device to generate pacing (or shock) pulses upon command from the programmer. NIPS is used to induce VT or VF or administer ATP.

noise floor. The intrinsic noise due to quantum mechanical and thermal effects in amplifier components — referred to as the "floor" as input signals below this level are masked by the noise and hence effectively invisible. Typical pacing or ICD amplifier has a noise floor on the order of 30 μV.

noise. Unwanted signal.

noncommitted shock. One which will not be delivered to the patient, in response to a nonsustained tachyarrhythmia, even if termination occurs after charging has begun. Also called second look shock.

notch filter. Filter which accepts (or rejects) primarily at a single frequency. E.g. a 60 Hz notch filter to reject line frequency noise on an ECG.

NSR. Normal sinus rhythm.

ODE. O-dimethyl encainide.

ODI. Onset detection interval.

ohm. Usually written Ω, is the unit of electrical resistance defined by "Ohm's law" as the ratio of the voltage to the current.

onset algorithm. Detection algorithm which attempts to prevent classification of sinus tachycardia as abnormal on the assumption that sinus tachycardia begins more gradually than VT.

open circuit voltage. The voltage of a cell (battery) while under a very small or nonexistent load. The ESR is not a factor since no current is being drawn.

overhead current. See background or monitoring current.

P-wave oversensing. Counting P-waves as ventricular depolarizations and hence deriving a falsely elevated heart rate.

P-wave. Cardiac electric waveform corresponding to atrial depolarization.

PA. Pulmonary artery.

passband. The range of frequencies accepted by an amplifier. The typical ICD amplifier accepts from 10 Hz (high-pass) to 30-100 Hz (low-pass). This range includes the majority of signal energy in the electrogram while rejecting as much interference as possible.

patch electrode. Large flat electrodes made of screen or embedded coils which are placed on the epicardium or subcutaneously.

pattern 1 defibrillation. A shock strong enough to cleanly and promptly defibrillate. Synonymous with Type A defibrillation.

pattern 2 defibrillation. A shock not strong enough to cleanly and promptly defibrillate; defibrillation ultimately occurs after a run of one or more post-shock extrasystolic activations. Synonymous with Type B defibrillation.

PCD. Medtronic ICD model.

peak detector. Creates a stored, but slowly decaying, signal which represents the peak amplitude of the previous R-wave. The information is usually stored as a voltage on a capacitor.

peak voltage. See leading edge voltage.

permittivity. Measure of dielectric constant which reflects the ability of a given insulator to store charge in a capacitor application.

PES. Programmed electrical stimulation. (Also, less commonly: programmed extrastimuli)

PG. Pulse generator.

polarization. The residual charge on the defibrillation coil from a defibrillation shock.

polymorphic. Refers to a wide QRS tachycardia (virtually always VT) in which intracardiac (or surface) electrograms exhibit a varying beat-to-beat morphology.

post-shock undersensing. Inappropriate detection of episode termination (despite tachyarrhythmia persistence) caused by delayed recovery of the post-shock electrogram amplitude or by slow response of the automatic gain control.

predischarge testing. An electrophysiologic study to reassess appropriate detection and termination of VF (and VT, when relevant) by the implanted device given before discharge from the hospital.

proarrhythmia. Worsening of an arrhythmia (becoming more frequent or more poorly tolerated) as a result of instituting putatively antiarrhythmic therapy.

probability density function. Detection algorithm which assumes that there is a loss of isoelectric time during ventricular arrhythmia and no such loss during supraventricular rhythms. These algorithms lack specificity, but have been employed with some success in certain clinical situations when the patient's normal shocking lead QRS signal is narrow.

PSA. Pacing System Analyzer.

pulse stretching. Use of a long (e.g. 100 ms) output pulse from the comparator to effect an amplifier refractory period.

PVC. Premature ventricular complex.

QRS complex. ECG manifestation of ventricular depolarization.

QT interval. Time from QRS onset to end of T-wave in ECG.

quadrifilar. Coil construction for lead conductor using four parallel filaments in a helical configuration (which creates a central lumen for stylet insertion).

R-wave. ECG manifestation of ventricular depolarization; also called QRS complex.

RA. Right atrium, especially an electrode in this location.

ramp pacing. ATP in which the cycle lengths of the pulses vary within each burst.

rate crossover. Occurs when the maximum exercise sinus rate exceeds the rate value programmed for VT detection by the ICD.

rate detection zone. The range of ventricular rhythm cycle lengths is divided into a bradyarrhythmia, a normal, and one or more (in some cases up to four) tachyarrhythmia zones. Together, these form the set of rate detection zones, for which particular ICD therapy sequences can be programmed (in tiered therapy devices). The original "shock boxes" had only two zones—normal and "VF."

rate sensing electrogram. Electrogram signal which is fed into rate sensing amplifier and thus used for rate determination and detection.

reconfirmation. After charging of the capacitors, verifying that the arrhythmia still exists.

rectification. Algebraically equivalent to an absolute value function. This function, in a sense amplifier, allows the detector to sense both positive and negative amplitude R-waves.

rectifier. Circuit element which only allows current to flow in one direction.

redetection. Process through which the ICD recognizes persistence (or appearance of new) tachyarrhythmia following therapy delivery. Algorithmic criteria typically differ somewhat from those utilized for de novo tachyarrhythmia detection.

reed switch. A thin magnetic strip (resembling a woodwind reed) and another conducting strip sealed within a slender glass cylinder. A sufficiently strong magnetic field will cause the strips to touch thus making an electrical circuit to allow external control of the ICD.

refractory period. (In a sense amplifier) Period after a detection during which the amplifier will not redetect. (In a cardiac cell) Period after depolarization during which the cell cannot be re-triggered with moderate depolarizing stimuli.

Res-Q. Intermedics ICD model.

resistance. The ratio of voltage across to the current through an electrical component. The unit of electrical resistance is the ohm which is abbreviated Ω.

RF link. Telemetry interface which is the communication means between the ICD and programmer. It is an inductive link (split transformer) and is not a "radio" link but does use low radio frequencies.

RF. Radio frequency.

rheobase. The value of the current required for an infinite duration pulse to either defibrillate or stimulate.

ring. The second most distal electrode on a pace/sense lead. Not to be confused with the distal defibrillation coil.

RR interval. Time interval between successive ventricular electrical events (depolarizations).

RV. Right ventricle, especially an electrode in this location.

RVA. Right ventricular apex, especially an electrode in this location.

safety margin. The difference between the maximum (or programmed) ICD shock energy and the minimum shock strength required for consistent defibrillation (E_{99} or E_{90}). (In common clinical parlance refers to E_{ICD} minus measured DFT, a difference termed instead, "energy margin" in this book.)

scanning step size. Amount by which each successive ATP burst pulse spacing is shortened.

Schuder circuit. Circuit using two SCRs for generating truncated monophasic shock; this was the first ICD circuit.

SCR. Silicon controlled rectifier: electronic switch used in first (monophasic) ICDs and also used for parts of some biphasic output bridges.

SDS. Step-down success defibrillation threshold protocol.

second look. Synonymous with reconfirmation and noncommitted shock.

sensing current. Monitoring or background current in the ICD.

sensing. To register the occurrence of successive cardiac depolarizations, and, thereby allow the measurement of the time interval between these cardiac depolarizations.

Sentinel. Angeion ICD model.

Sentry. Telectronics ICD model.

sequential shock. Defibrillation waveform using two closing spaced pulses of the same polarity.

setscrew. Short screw used in header to tighten and secure the terminal for the patient (defibrillation, pacing, or combined) lead.

shifting burst pacing. ATP approach in which the coupling interval between the R-wave and the first pulse in a burst is scanned.

shock on T-wave. Delivery of medium strength shock into the T-wave in order to induce fibrillation or to perform upper limit of vulnerability testing.

simultaneous shock. Programming choice with Medtronic PCD 7217 to create essentially a normal monophasic waveform as opposed to the sequential shock.

sinus redetection. Detection of normal sinus rhythm after therapy delivery.

SRD. Sustained Rate Detection protects against excessive delays in therapy delivery. Also called extended high rate (EHR). (Also may be used as abbreviation for sinus redetection.)

stability algorithm. A detection algorithm which attempts to prevent classification of atrial fibrillation with a fast ventricular response as "abnormal" (i.e., ventricular in origin) on the assumption that its cycle length variability is greater than that of a VT.

standard DFT. Energy approximating a 50-80% success probability of defibrillation; determined by inducing VF and testing progressively lower (or higher) shock energies.

stored energy. The energy stored in the ICD capacitor before the delivery of a shock. Equal to $1/2\,CV^2$.

storm (VT/VF). Repeated bouts of ventricular tachyarrhythmias occurring in rapid succession.

subcutaneous array. See array electrode system.

SubQ. Subcutaneous, especially an electrode implanted subcutaneously in mid axillary region.

summation criterion. A method of handling the zone boundary wandering problem (confounding tachycardia detection) by adding the total tachyarrhythmia interval counts in two neighboring zones.

SVC. Superior vena cava, especially an electrode in this location.

SVO. Lithium silver vanadium oxide cell (used in all current ICDs).

SVT. Supraventricular tachycardia.

synchronized shock. Used for cardioversion and delivered to coincide with a sensed ventricular event (depolarization), thereby minimizing the likelihood of inadvertently inducing VF.

syncope. Fainting.

systole. Portion of cardiac cycle during which the ventricles depolarize and contract.

T-wave oversensing. Counting T-waves as ventricular depolarizations and hence deriving a falsely elevated heart rate.

T-wave. Cardiac electric waveform corresponding to ventricular repolarization.

TACH A, TACH-0. Primary rate limit (PRL) for VT detection. Also known as TDI (tachycardia detection interval) or PCCL (primary cycle length limit).

TACH B, TACH-1. Secondary rate limit (SRL) for VT detection. Also known as FTI (fast tachycardia interval) or secondary cycle length limit (SCCL).

tachyarrhythmia sense refractory period. Each time a ventricular event is sensed, this timing period is started. If another ventricular event is sensed within this period, it is not counted. This prevents incorrect counting of device-filtered signals which typically have more waveform peaks than the original signal.

tachyarrhythmia. Rapid cardiac rhythm (VT, VF or supra ventricular tachycardia).

telemetry interface. Communication means between the ICD and programmer. It is an inductive link (split transformer) and not, as commonly believed, a "radio" link.

TENS. Transcutaneous electrical nerve stimulation.

tilt. The percentage decrease in voltage from the beginning to the end of a shock or a phase of a shock.

time constant. The amount of time for a given system (usually capacitor voltage in this book) to respond to within 37% of the final value for a new input. For a capacitor being discharged to zero volts the time constant is the time required for the voltage to decay to 37% of the initial voltage. For a automatic threshold control amplifier circuit this represent the time for the threshold to decay to 37% of an initial value.

timeout period. A period, typically 1 or 2 seconds, of no sensed depolarizations after which a tachycardia is presumed to be ongoing with signal dropout; a defibrillation shock will then be delivered asynchronously as opposed to the desired synchronous shock.

tip. The distal electrode of a pace/sense lead or of an integrated defibrillation lead.

torsade de pointes. A type of polymorphic VT occurring in the setting of prolonged duration of cardiac repolarization (increased QT interval).

trailing edge voltage. See leading edge voltage.

train pacing. Ultra rapid pacing of up to a few thousand beats per minute used to terminate reentrant tachycardias.

transformer. Electronic component which converts electrical energy into magnetic and back into electrical in order to (typically) change the voltage; uses wire coils and usually a magnetic material.

Transvene. Medtronic lead model.

trifilar. Coil construction for lead conductor using three parallel filaments in a helical configuration (which creates a central lumen for stylet insertion).

triphasic. Waveform with positive, negative, and then positive portions; alternatively negative, positive, and then negative.

triple counting. Sensing (counting) P-waves and T-waves (or pacemaker stimulus artifacts), in addition to R-waves, resulting in apparent rate tripling with simulation of "tachycardia."

truncated exponential waveform. Time course of voltage decay follows an exponential curve that is truncated upon completion of prespecified pulse width or achievement of voltage that yields a prespecified tilt. Applies to a monophasic waveform and to each phase of a biphasic waveform as seen in present ICDs.

truncation. Termination of a capacitive discharge waveform before the voltage decays excessively.

turning point morphology. (TPM) Detection algorithm which assumes that there is a loss of isoelectric time during ventricular arrhythmia and no such loss during supraventricular rhythms. Similar in philosophy to the probability density function algorithm approach.

TVL. Ventritex lead model.

twiddler's syndrome. Manipulation of the pulse generator by the patient in a manner that can dislodge the lead and possibly remove the lead from the heart entirely.

Type A defibrillation. A shock strong enough to cleanly and promptly defibrillate. Synonymous with Pattern 1 defibrillation.

Type B defibrillation. A shock not strong enough to cleanly and promptly defibrillate; defibrillation ultimately occurs after a run of one or more post-shock extrasystolic activations. Synonymous with Pattern 2 defibrillation.

Type I lead. Transvenous lead system comprising a single lead providing all defibrillation and pace/sense electrodes.

Type II lead. Transvenous lead system comprising a pair of leads, one of which has the right ventricular (RV) defibrillation electrode and the pace/sense electrode(s), the second has the superior vena cava (SVC) or right atrial (RA) defibrillation electrode.

Type III lead. Transvenous lead system comprising a pair of leads, one of which has the right ventricular (RV) defibrillation electrode and the superior vena cava (SVC) or right atrial (RA) defibrillation electrode. The second has the pace/sense electrodes,

ULV. Upper limit of vulnerability.

underdetection. Failure (or delay) of the ICD to detect a tachyarrhythmia.

underdrive pacing. Was one of the earliest ATP techniques, and relied on pacing at rates slower than the tachycardia to introduce randomly timed pacing pulses throughout diastole in an attempt to terminate the arrhythmia.

undersensing. Failing of the amplifier/lead system to mark a depolarization (or—more generally—failure to detect a local electrical variation suggestive of a fibrillation wavefront passing through).

upper limit of vulnerability hypothesis. Theory that elimination of fibrillation wavefronts by stimulating excitable myocardium (as in critical mass hypothesis) is a necessary but not sufficient condition for defibrillation.

upper limit of vulnerability. Lowest amplitude shock delivered into the T-wave which will fail to cause fibrillation.

Ventak. Guidant/CPI ICD model.

ventricle. Lower large cardiac chamber (right or left).

ventricular flutter. VT with sinusoidal morphology in the rate range of 280-300 BPM. Fatal if not terminated.

VF. Ventricular fibrillation: a very rapid (> 300 BPM) electrically disorganized rhythm originating in the ventricles. Fatal if not terminated.

VFCNT. Counter for VF zone in Medtronic Jewel and Ventritex Cadence.

volt. Unit of voltage which is electrical pressure analog and represents the force driving the current through its path.

voltage delay. Phenomenon in which the SVO cell voltage at the start of a capacitor charging cycle is lower than at the end. This is due to a resistance-increasing coating growing on the cell cathode from insufficient use of the cell.

volume resistivity. The ratio of the electric field to the current density. Also the resistance between facing sides of a 1 cm cube of a given material. The unit is the $\Omega \cdot cm$

VOO. Pacing mode of continuous ventricular pacing.

VT. Ventricular tachycardia: rapid rhythm (< 280 BPM) originating in one of the ventricles. Typically more organized (monomorphic) than VF. Clinical manifestations may vary widely (from asymptomatic to fatal), depending on extent and duration of associated hemodynamic compromise.

VTCNT. Counter for VT zone in Medtronic Jewel. There are one each for VT and FVT.

VVI. Pacing mode of ventricular sensing and ventricular pacing with inhibition of pacing by sensed rate above a programmed value.

Wolff-Parkinson-White syndrome. (WPW). Presence of an accessory conducting pathway from the atria to the ventricles ("bypassing" the AV node). Potentially dangerous as it could allow rapid transmission of impulses to the ventricles during atrial fibrillation; the pathway could itself support a reentrant tachycardia.

X out of Y. Basic detection algorithm which requires X out of Y intervals to be in a certain zone; e.g., 9 out of 12 intervals must be in the VT zone for VT to be detected.

Y adapter. Connector block with two female ports and one male plug to allow the use of both an SVC lead and a SubQ patch since some ICDs have only two high-voltage connections.

zone boundary wandering. Consecutive VT intervals straying above and below the preset VT detection interval; can readily lead to delays in VT therapy.

Index

—E—

a.   As the various models of each manufacturer share more similarities than differences,
it is advised to scan the index for all models of a
given manufacturer if a desired model and feature
does not appear where expected.

—N—

—O—

—P—

—T—

—X—